Anatomy
for
Dental Students

Anatomy
for
Dental Students

Dr R K Zargar

MS
Peoples' Medical College
Bhopal (MP)
Ex. Professor & Head
Departement of Anatomy
Armed Forces Medical College
Pune-411040

Lt Col SUSHIL KUMAR

MBBS, MS (Anatomy)
Reader
Departement of Anatomy
Armed Forces Medical College
Pune-411040

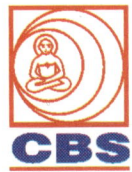

CBS

CBS PUBLISHERS & DISTRIBUTORS
NEW DELHI • BANGALORE (INDIA)

DEDICATION

The all pervading presence of Almighty
Benevolence of our revered Gurus
Blessings of our respected teachers
Care of our loving Parents
Affections of our understanding family members
Best wishes of our inspiring friends
&
Impetus of our adorable students
have made it possible to present this
humble offering

ISBN : 81-239-1334-6

First Edition : 2006

Copyright © **Author & Publisher**

Publishing Director : Vinod K. Jain

Published by :
Satish Kumar Jain for CBS Publishers & Distributors,
4596/1-A, 11 Darya Ganj, New Delhi - 110 002 (India)
E-mail: cbspubs@vsnl.com • Website: www.cbspd.com

Branch Office :
2975, 17th Cross, K.R. Road, Bansankari 2nd Stage, Bangalore-70
Fax : 080-26771680 • E-mail : cbsbng@vsnl.net

Composed by :
LineArt Graphics, Delhi-110091

Printed at :
Asia Printograph, Delhi

Preface

Medical education is growing in multifold. This is to keep pace with the requirement of health care system in the country. The aspirations of younger generations despite newer avenues, lead them to join a health care institute.

The Dental Council of India has a structured detailed syllabus. By and large the books of Anatomy for students cover more than the laid down the curriculum required for the dental students.

At times referring to these books is time consuming and more than adequate with the result a dental student finds it convenient and not student friendly for learning anatomy in the first year.

In view of these constrains faced by the students this books has been conceived and written to make learning of anatomy more purposeful. The students and the faculty will surely find it different from other books as individual topics are presented as per the syllabus. The deficiency of schematic diagrams strongly felt but it is desirable that the students should evolve their own schematic diagrams after they have gone through the description, which builds up the anatomical concepts and understanding.

The hardwork gone in the preparation of this book is ditigently contributed by ex colleague Lt Col Sushil Kumar of Armed Forces Medical College, Pune-40. His drive and perseverance have been instrumental in meeting the deadline set by publisher.

I wish to extend my sincere thanks to Mr. B.R. Sharma of CBS Publisher & Distributors for having belief and confidence in me. He has been full of energy and is blessed with great capacity to stoke the academic pursuits. His sincerely is commendable. I wish to acknowledge Mr. S.K. Jain, Managing Director of CBS Publisher & Distributor for his efforts in publishing this book.

Jan 2006   Dr R K Zargar

v

Contents

Preface .... *v*

Chapter 1. **Introduction** 3-15

Chapter 2. **Skin and Fasciae** 16-21

Chapter 3. **Muscles** 22-28

Chapter 4. **Bone** 29-34

Chapter 5. **Cartilage/Gristle** 35-37

Chapter 6. **Joints** 38-47

Chapter 7. **Nervous System** 48-52

Chapter 8. **Autonomic Nervous System** 53-56

Chapter 9. **Cranial Nerves** 57-60

Chapter 10. **Cardiovascular System** 61-65

Chapter 11. **Lamphatic System** 66-69

Chapter 12. **The Skull** 73-74

Chapter 13. **Norma Verticalis** 75-76

Chapter 14. **Norma Frontalis** 77-79

Chapter 15. **Norma Occipitalis** 80-81

Chapter 16. **Norma Lateralis** 82-85

Chapter 17. **Vault of Skull** 86-87

Chapter 18. **Cranial Fossae** 88-95

Chapter 19. **Norma Basalis** 96-100

Chapter 20. **Mandible** 101-104

Chapter 21. **Maxilla** 105-108

Chapter 22. **Sphenoid Bone** 109-113

Chapter 23. **Parietal Bone** 114-115

Chapter 24. **Frontal Bone** 116-118

Chapter 25. **Temporal Bone** 119-121

Chapter 26. **Ethmoid Bone** 122-123

Chapter 27. **Palatine Bone** 124-126

Chapter 28. **Zygomatic Bone** 127-128

Chapter 29. **Vomer** 129

Chapter 30. **Hyoid Bone** 130-131

Chapter 31. **Lacrimal Bone** 132

Chapter 32. **Inferior Nasal Concha** 133-134

Chapter 33. **Nasal Bone** 135-136

Chapter 34. **Foetal Skull** 137-140

Chapter 35. **Cervical Vertebrae** 141-145

Chapter 36. **Scalp and Temple** 149-153

Chapter 37. **Cervical Fascia** 154-156

Chapter 38. **Face** 157-169

Chapter 39. **Posterior Triangle of Neck** 170-175

Chapter 40. **Back** 176-180

Chapter 41. **Anterior Triangle of Neck** 181-192

Chapter 42. **Deep Dissection of Neck** 193-217

Chapter 43. **Parotid Region** 218-221

Chapter 44. **Temporal and Interatemporal Fossae** 222-236

Chapter 45. **Submandibular Region** 237-240

Chapter 46. **Mouth and Pharynx** 241-251

Chapter 47. **Nasal Cavity** 252-258

Chapter 48. **Tongue** 259-264

Chapter 49. **Larynx** 265-272

Chapter 50. **Orbit** 273-284

Chapter 51. **Ear** 285-291

Chapter 52. **Eye** 292-295

Chapter 53. **Meanings and Blood Vessels** 299-312

Chapter 54. **Medula Oblongata** 313-315

Chapter 55. **Pons** 316-318

Chapter 56. **Cerebellum** 319-322

Chapter 57. **Midbrain** 323-324

Chapter 58. **Cerebrum** 325-332

Chapter 59. **Thalamus and Hypothalamus** 333-335

Chapter 60. **Limbic System** 336-337

Chapter 61. **Spinal Cord** 338-345

Chapter 62. **Autonomic Nervous System** 346-350

Chapter 63. **Epithelium** 353-359

Chapter 64. **Connective Tissue** 360-364

Chapter 65. **Cartilage** 365-366

Chapter 66. **Bone** 367-368

Chapter 67. **Muscle** 369-370

Chapter 68. **Blood Vessels** 371-373

Chapter 69. **Nervous Tissue** 374-377

Chapter 70. **Salivary Glands** 378-381

Chapter 71. **Lymphoid Tissue** 382-386

Chapter 72. **Integumentary System** 387-389

Chapter 73. **Lip, Tooth and Tongue** 390-392

Chapter 74. **Gastrointestinal Tract** 393-395

Chapter 75. **Respiratory System** 396-398

Chapter 76. **Endocrine Glands** 399-404

Chapter 77. **General Aspects** 407-415

Chapter 78. **Gametogenesis : Conversion of Germ Cells into Male and**

　　　　　　 Female Gametes 416-432

Chapter 79. **Developments of Systems** 433-464

Chapter 80. **Glossary : Germ Layer Derivatives** 465-466

Chapter 81. **Critical Periods of Human Development** 467-473

Chapter 82. **Correlated Human Development** 474-487

Chapter 83. **Head and Neck** 491-502

Chapter 84. **Conventional Radiology** 503-506

Chapter 85. **Special Radiological Investigations** 507-512

　　　　　　 Index 513-518

Section-I
General Anatomy

CONTENTS

1. Introduction   3-15

2. Skin and Fasciae   16-21

3. Muscles   22-28

4. Bone   29-34

5. Cartilage/Gristle   35-37

6. Joints   38-47

7. Nervous System   48-52

8. Autonomic Nervous System   53-56

9. Cranial Nerves   57-60

10. Cardiovascular System   61-65

11. Lamphatic System   66-69

Introduction

Anatomy is the study of the structures of the body and the relationship of its constituent parts to each other. The term, "Anatomy", is derived from a Greek word (**ana = up, tome = cutting**). The term, "dissection (**dis = a sunder, secare = to cut**)" is a Latin equivalent of the Greek anatome. But it should be noted that anatomy and dissection are not synonymous. Dissection is a technique while anatomy is a wide and vast subject. All descriptions of human body are described on the assumption that the body is in "**anatomical position**".

SUBDIVISIONS

Gross anatomy

It is also known as **macroscopic anatomy**. The various body parts and their relationship to each other are studied with the naked eye.

There are two approaches for study of gross anatomy

Systemic anatomy

The body is studied under various systems e.g.:
- Study of nervous system (**Neurology**)
- Study of vascular system (**Angiology**)
- Study of skeletal system (**Osteology**)
- Study of respiratory, digestive, endocrine and urogenital system (**Splanchnology**)

Regional anatomy

The body is studied under various regions/parts as:
- Upper limb and lower limb
- Thorax
- Abdomen and pelvis
- Head and neck
- Brain

Microscopic anatomy

This is also known as **histology**. It is the study of various body structures with the help of a microscope using various stains.

Developmental anatomy

Also known as **embryology**, but the use of this term should be restricted. This branch deals with prenatal and postnatal developmental changes in an individual. Two terms should be noted:
- **Ontogeny** - developmental history
- **Phylogeny** - evolutionary history

Surface anatomy

This is also known as **topographic anatomy**. In this, various deeper parts of the body are projected on to the surface of body

Radiological anatomy

It is the study of various deep organs e.g., soft and hard parts by plain and contrast radiography.

Living anatomy

It is studied on living human beings either by clinical methods e.g., inspection, palpation, percussion and auscultation or by using some investigating means e.g., bronchoscopy, endoscopy, radiography, electromyography.

Applied anatomy (Clinical anatomy)

Anatomy considered with special reference to its medical and surgical bearing is known as **applied anatomy**.

Comparative anatomy

This branch deals to explain the change in form and morphology of different animals including man.

Physical anthropology

This branch deals chiefly with the external features i.e. measurements of various features of different races and groups of people.

Racial anatomy

It is a sub branch of physical anthropology.

Statistical anatomy

Study of data on variations encountered is termed statistical anatomy.

Experimental anatomy

It deals with study of various facts influencing and determining the form, structure and functions of different parts of the body.

ANATOMICAL NOMENCLATURE

In 1895, German Anatomical Society met in Basle and approved a list of about 5000 terms known as **Basle Nomina Anatomica** (B.N.A.). Following six rules were set by the commission:

- Each part shall have *one name*
- Each term shall be *in Latin*
- Each term shall be as *short and simple* as possible

- The terms shall be merely *memory signs*
- *Related terms* shall, as far as possible, be similar e.g., femoral artery, femoral vein, femoral nerve
- *Adjectives* in general shall be arranged as opposite e.g., major and minor, superior and inferior.

In **1950** at Oxford (5th) International Congress of Anatomists, a new body - **Internal Anatomical Nomenclature Committee** was instituted. The Anatomical nomenclature was grouped into:

- Nomina Anatomica
- Nomina Histologica
- Nomina Embryologica

BODY POSITIONS

Anatomical position

Person is standing erect, with the arms by the sides and the face and palms of the hands directed forwards. The lower limbs are parallel with the toes pointing forwards. The eyes look straight to the front. All the body structures and their relationship to each other are described in relation to body being in anatomical position.

Supine position

The body is in recumbent position e.g., lying down with the face directed upwards.

Prone position

The body is in recumbent position e.g., lying down with the face directed downwards.

Lithotomy position

The body is in supine position with buttocks at the edge of the examination table. The hips and knees are flexed and the thighs are wide apart. This position is used in perineal surgeries and normal vaginal deliveries.

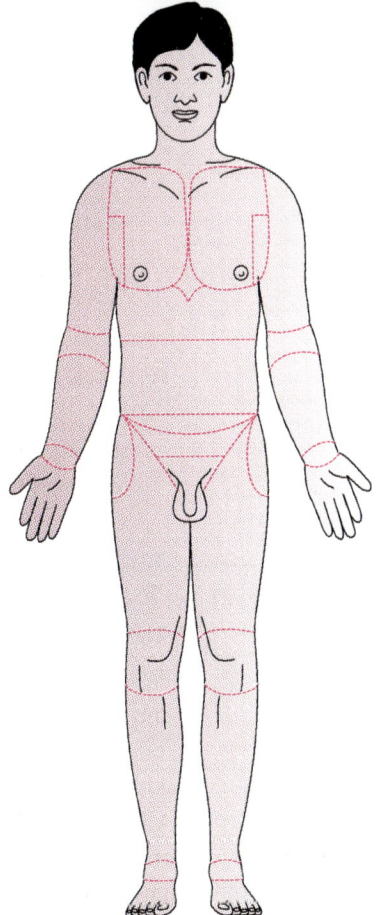

Fig. 1.1 : Anatomical Position

PLANES OF REFERENCE

Median plane

This is an imaginary vertical plane that passes longitudinally through the body and divides it into right and left halves. The median plane intersects the surface of the front and the back of the body into anterior and posterior median lines.

Sagittal plane (L = Sagitta → arrow)

Any vertical plane through the body, that is parallel with the median plane. The sagittal planes are named after the sagittal suture of the skull, to which they are parallel. This should be noted that the term "parasagittal" is redundant. Anything parallel with sagittal plane is still sagittal.

Coronal plane

This is also known as **frontal plane**. Any vertical plane that intersects the median plane at right angle and separates the body into front and back parts is termed as coronal / frontal plane.

Horizontal plane

A plane at right angle to both the median and coronal planes, separating the body into upper and lower parts is termed as horizontal plane.

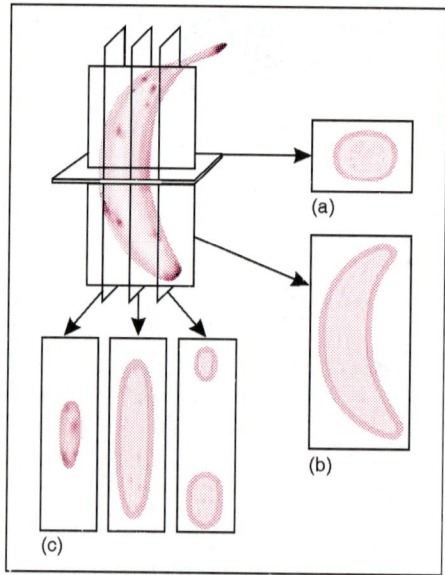

Planes of reference, a) Transverse Plane, b) Sagittal Plane, c) Coronal Plane

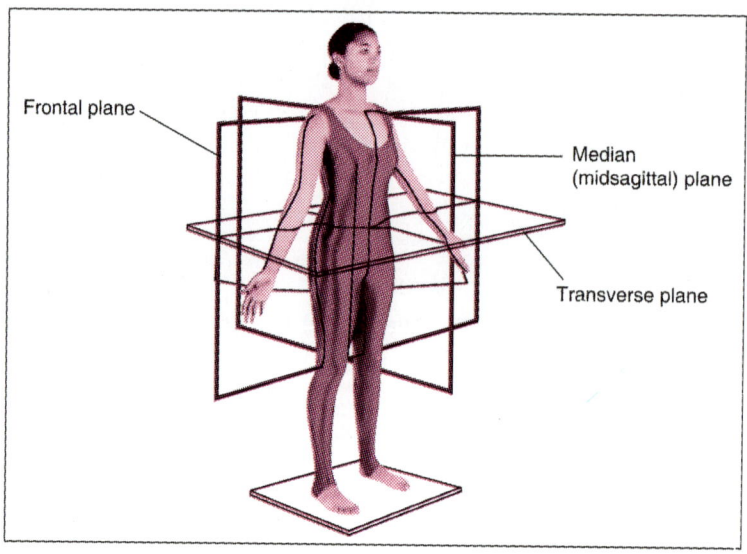

Fig. 1.2 : Planes of reference

Transverse plane

The transverse plane passes at right angle to the longitudinal axis of a structure. Thus, a transverse section through an artery is not necessarily horizontal. A transverse section through the hand is horizontal, whereas a transverse section through the foot is coronal.

TERMS OF REFERENCE

Superior: Near the head end i.e. cranial.

Inferior: Near the tail end i.e. caudal.

Anterior or ventral: Nearer the front of the body.

Posterior or dorsal: Nearer the back.

Middle: Used for a structure lying between two others those are anterior and posterior or superior and inferior.

Median: Used for a structure lying or situated at median plane.

Medial: Nearer to the median plane.

Lateral: Farther from the median plane.

Intermediate: Lying between two structures, one is medial and the other lateral.

Ipsilateral: Of the same side, right or left.

Contralateral: Of the opposite side.

Cranial or cephalic: Nearer the upper end of the body may be used in place of superior.

Caudal: Nearer the lower end used sometimes in place of inferior.

Proximal and distal: Used in limbs. Indicate nearer to and farther from a fixed point.

- **Proximal:** Nearer to the fixed point
- **Distal:** Farther from the fixed point

Superficial: Towards the surface.

Deep: Away and inner to the surface.

- These terms (superficial and deep) denotes the relative distances of structure from the surface of the organ.

Internal: Nearer to the center of an organ or a cavity.

External: Farther from the center of an organ or a cavity.

- The terms internal and external are used to describe the relative distance of a structure from the center of an organ or cavity.

Invagination: Inward protrusion.

Evagination: Outward protrusion.

TERMS USED FOR LIMBS

Radial or Pre-axial border: Outer border of upper limb.

Ulnar or Post-axial border: Inner border of upper limb.

Tibial or Pre-axial border: Inner border of lower limb.

Fibular or Post-axial border: Outer border of lower limb.

Palmar: Pertaining to the palm of hand.

Plantar: Pertaining to the sole of foot.

MOVEMENTS

Flexion

- To flex is to bend or to make an angle.
- Approximation of flexor surfaces whereby the angle of the joint is reduced.
- Takes place in a sagittal plane
- Usually an anterior movement, but is occasionally posterior e.g., flexion at knee joint.

Extension

- To extend is to stretch out or to straighten.
- Opposite of flexion
- Angle at the joint is increased
- Usually takes place in a posterior direction

Lateral flexion

- Movement of the trunk in a coronal plane
- This may be right or left lateral flexion

Adduction (Latin **Ad = to duco = I**)

- Movement towards the median plane or central axis

Abduction (Latin **Ab = from duco = I**)

- Movement away from the median plane or central axis

Circumduction (Latin **Circum = around**)

- Movements of flexion, abduction, extension and adduction taking place in a sequence, thereby describing a cone.

Rotation

- Term applied to the movement of a part of the body around its long axis.

Medial rotation

- Movement that results in the anterior surface of the part facing medially (**inward rotation**)

Lateral rotation

- Movement that results in the anterior surface of the part facing laterally (**outward rotation**)

Supination

- Lateral rotation of the forearm from the pronated position, so that the palm of the hand comes to face anteriorly (**A beggar supinates**)

Pronation

- Medial rotation of the forearm in such a manner that the palm of the hand faces posteriorly (**A king pronates**).

Inversion

- Movement of the foot in such a manner so that medial border is raised and the sole faces medially or inwards.

Eversion

- Opposite to inversion, in which lateral border of foot is raised and the sole faces laterally or outwards

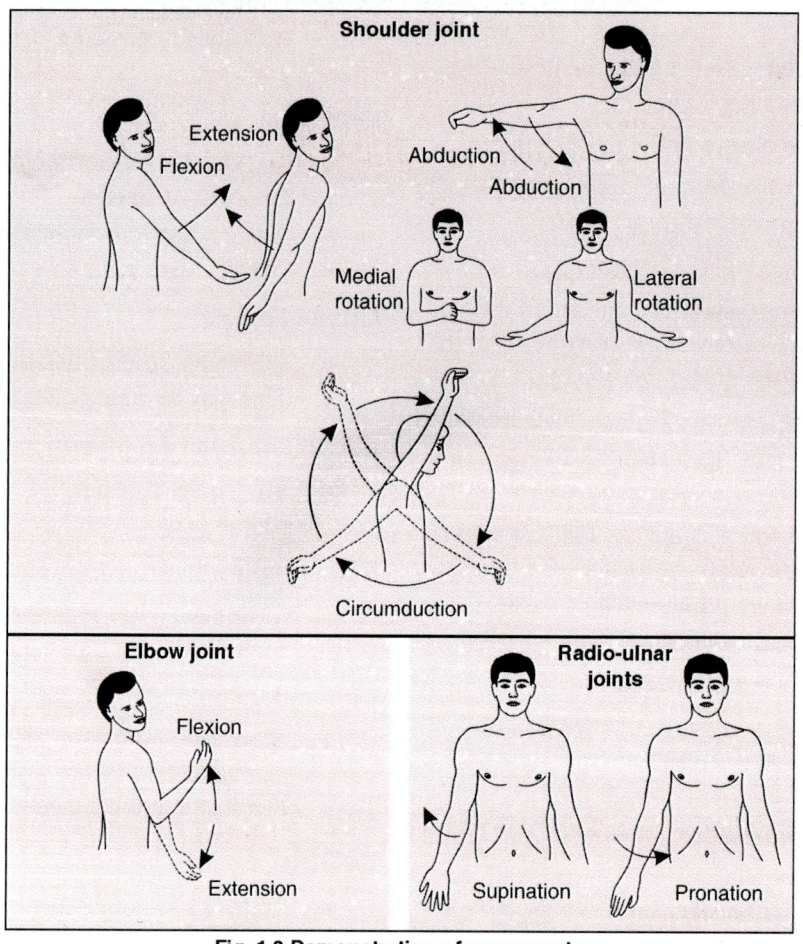

Fig. 1.3 Demonstration of movements

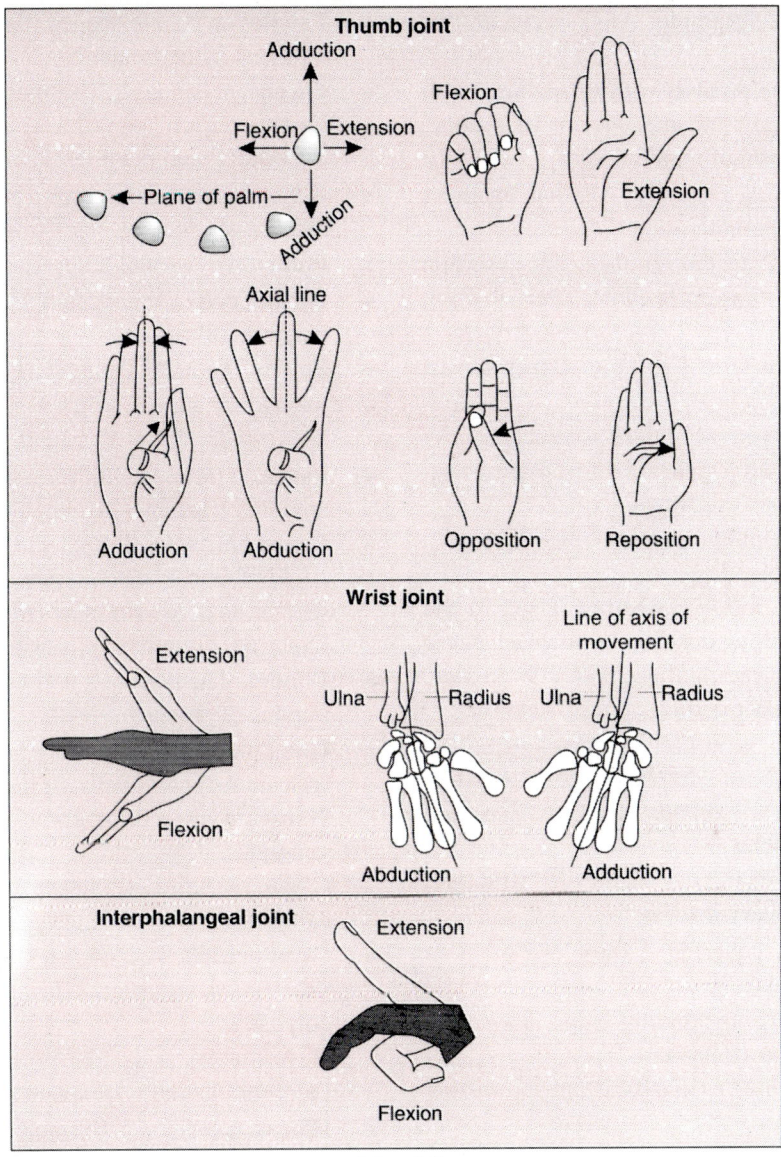

Fig. 1.4

GENERAL ANATOMICAL TERMS

- **Acinus**. The smallest unit of a compound gland; more commonly called an **alveolus**. <u>Example</u>: Lung alveoli.

- **Aditus**. The entrance into a cavity. <u>Example</u>: Aditus to mastoid antrum.

- **Afferent**. Used to indicate that a structure leads towards the organ it supplies. In the ner-vous system corresponds to sensory nerves.

- **Ala**. A wing like projection. <u>Example</u>: Ala of vomer bone.

- **Alveolus**. The smallest air spaces of the lungs; synonymous with acinus.

- **Ampulla.** A flask. Hence the dilated portion of a tube. <u>Example</u>: Ampullary part of fallopian tube.

- **Ansa.** A loop. Example: Ansa cervicalis of cervical nerves.
- **Antrum**. A cave. A cavity with air and lined with mucous membrane in the interior of a bone. Example: Antrum of maxilla bone.
- **Annulus.** A ring. Example: Annular ligament of superior radio-ulnar joint.
- **Aponeurosis**. A tendinous sheet like insertion of a muscle. Example: External oblique aponeurosis.
- **Brachium.** An arm. Example: Brachium of upper limb.
- **Bursa.** A collapsed sac of fluid present generally where a tendon or skin slides over bone. Example: Sub deltoid bursa.
- **Canaliculus.** Diminutive of a canal. Example: Tympanic canaliculus.
- **Commissure.** Joining together. Used in the nervous system to indicate bundles of nerve fibres crossing the midline from side to side. Example: Anterior commissure of cerebrum.
- **Condyle.** A. knuckle. Smooth rounded eminence of a bone which is articular in nature and covered with articular cartilage. Example: Condyles of femur.
- **Corona.** A crown. Thus encircling structure. Example: coronary arteries.
- **Cortex.** Outer covering. Example: Cortex of supra renal gland.
- **Crista.** A sharp upstanding ridge. Example: Crista terminalis of heart.
- **Crus.** A leg or used as to indicate any projecting process.
- **Cystic.** Generally pertaining to a bladder (cyst).
- **Dens.** A tooth. Example: Odontoid process of axis vertebra.
- **Efferent.** The opposite of afferent. In the nervous system corresponds to motor nerves.
- **Epicondyle.** The prominence placed above a smooth articular eminence which is always extra capsular in nature. Example: Epicondyles of femur.

- **Falciform.** Sickle-shaped. Example: Falciform ligament of peritoneum.
- **Fascia.** A bandage. The membrane of fibrous tissue which sheaths tissues. Example: Superficial and deep fascia.
- **Filum.** A thread. Example: Filum terminale of spinal cord.
- **Folliculus.** A small bag.
- **Foramen.** A hole or opening. Example: Foramen magnum of skull.
- **Fornix.** An arch. Example: Fornix of vagina.
- **Fossa.** A shallow depression. Example: Subscapular fossa of scapula.
- **Fovea.** A pit or small depression which may be articular. Example: Fovea on the head of femur.
- **Frenulum.** A small ligament. Usually used for a fold of skin or mucous membrane limiting the separation of the structures to which it attached. Example: Frenulum of tongue.
- **Fundus.** The base of a hollow organ. Example: Fundus of stomach.
- **Ganglion.** A swelling. In the nervous system any collection of nerve cells outside the central nerve system is termed ganglion. Example: Ciliary ganglion.
- **Genu.** A bend. Example: Genu of corpus callosum.
- **Glomerulus.** A tight meshwork usually of vessels. Example: Glomerulus of renal corpuscle.
- **Hamulus**. A hook like projection. Example: Pterygoid hamulus of sphenoid bone.
- **Hiatus.** A slit or gap. Example: Hiatus for greater petrosal nerve.
- **Hilum.** A depression where blood vessels and nerves enter an organ. Example: Hilum of spleen.
- **Incisura.** A notch. Example: Incisura angularis.
- **Infundibulum.** A funnel. Example: Infundibulum of right ventricle.
- **Isthmus.** A narrow strip joining two larger pieces; narrowing of a canal. Example: Isthmus of fallopian tube.

- **Labium or Lip.** The raised margin of an orifice. <u>Example</u>: Labium majus of vagina.
- **Labrum.** A brim. <u>Example</u>: Acetabular labrum of hip bone.
- **Labyrinth.** A maze of communicating spaces or canals. <u>Example</u>: Bony labyrinth of internal ear.
- **Lacuna.** A pit or hole.
- **Lamina or Lamella.** A thin plate or sheet. Example: Lamina terminalis.
- **Ligament.** A band joining two structures generally used for fibrous band but may be composed of any tissue. <u>Example</u>: Ilio-femoral ligament of hip joint and gastro-splenic ligament (double layered fold of peritoneum)
- **Limbus.** A border or margin. <u>Example</u>: Limbus fossa ovalis of right atrium.
- **Lingula.** A tongue-shaped projection. <u>Example</u>: Lingula of mandible.
- **Macula.** A spot or stain. <u>Example</u>: Macula of the eye.
- **Meatus.** A passage or a short canal. <u>Example</u>: Middle meatus of nose.
- **Medulla.** The central portion of any organ where its structure is different from the outer layer or cortex. <u>Example</u>: Medulla of supra renal gland.
- **Mesentery.** Double layered fold of peritoneum which suspends the small intestine from the posterior abdominal wall.
- **Node.** A knot or a small swelling having a spherical aggregation of cells. <u>Example</u>: SA node of conducting of heart.
- **Nucleus.** The internal body of a cell. In the central nervous system it is referred to a collection of nerve cells.
- **Ostium.** An entrance; the opening into a tube. <u>Example</u>: Osteum of fallopian tube.
- **Papilla.** The nipple. Nipple-shaped elevation <u>Example</u>: Major duodenal papilla.
- **Parenchyma.** The proper tissue of an organ distinct from accessory structures such as its fibrous capsule. <u>Example</u>: Parenchyma of mammary gland.
- **Pedicle.** Stalk or a tube joining two structures.
- **Pelvis.** A basin. <u>Example</u>: Bony pelvis.
- **Plexus.** A plaited structure of vessels or nerves. <u>Example</u>: Brachial plexus.
- **Plica.** A fold. <u>Example</u>: Plica triangularis of palatine tonsil.
- **Ramus.** A horn like projection. <u>Example</u>: Ramus of mandible.
- **Raphe.** A seam. The interlocking aponeurosis of two muscles. <u>Example</u>: Mylohyoid raphe.
- **Rete.** A net. Communicating channels. <u>Example</u>: Rete testis.
- **Retinaculum.** A tie. A band of connective tissue (ligament) which holds tendons in place <u>Example</u>: Flexor retinaculum at wrist.
- **Rima.** A cleft. <u>Example</u>: Rima glottidis of larynx (slit between vocal cords)
- **Scaphoid.** Boat shaped. <u>Example</u>: Scaphoid bone.
- **Septum.** A thin partition. <u>Example</u>: Septum pellucidum.
- **Sinus.** A hollow or creek. Air-filled cavities of the cranial bones (**maxillary sinus**) or large venous spaces within the skull (**superior sagittal sinus**) or dilatations of blood vessels (**coronary sinus**)
- **Spine.** A sharp-pointed projection. <u>Example</u>: Spine of sphenoid.
- **Somatic.** Pertaining to the body wall. <u>Example</u>: Somatic nerves.
- **Splanchnic.** Pertaining to the GIT. <u>Example</u>: Splanchnic nerves.
- **Squamous.** Scaly. <u>Example</u>: Squamous plate of frontal bone.
- **Stria.** A stripe or line. <u>Example</u>: Stria terminalis.
- **Styloid.** Like stake. <u>Example</u>: Styloid process of radius.
- **Sulcus.** A furrow. <u>Example</u>: Sulcus for superior sagittal sinus.

- **Synovia.** Fluid present in joint cavities, bursae and tendon sheaths.
- **Taenia.** A band or ribbon. Example: Taenia coli of large intestine.
- **Tegmen.** A cover. Example: Tegmen tympani of temporal bone.
- **Tela.** A web or thin mesh. Example: Tela choroidea of lateral ventricle.
- **Torus.** A swelling. Example: Torus palatinus (swelling on the posterior part of hard palate).
- **Trabecula.** A small beam. Generally used for the pieces which make up the lattice of cancellous bone.
- **Trochlea.** A pulley-shaped surface. Example: Trochlea of ulna.
- **Tuber. Tubercle. Tuberosity**. A swelling. For any kind of rounded swelling these three terms are used without much distinction. Example: Greater tubercle of humerus, tuberosity of ulna.
- **Vagina.** A sheath.
- **Velum.** A curtain. Example: Tensor veli palatine.
- **Vesica.** A bladder especially the urinary bladder. Example: Ectopia vesicae.
- **Villus.** Shaggy hair. Fine processes projecting from a surface. Example: Chorionic villi of placenta.
- **Visceral.** Pertaining to organs. Example: Referred visceral pain.
- **Zona.** A belt. A circular or ring-like structure. Example: Zona orbicularis of capsule of hip joint.

TERMS USED IN CLINICAL PRACTICE

Symptom is a subjective indication of a disease as perceived by the patient. **Primary symptoms** are symptoms that are intrinsically associated with the disease process. **Secondary symptoms** are a consequence of the disease process.

Sign is an objective finding as perceived by an examiner, such as fever or a rash.

Diagnosis is the identification of a disease by scientific evaluation of physical signs, symptoms, clinical history and laboratory tests. The diagnosis may be **clinical diagnosis, differential diagnosis** and **laboratory diagnosis.**

Prognosis is the prediction of the probable outcome of a disease. It is based on the condition of the person and the usual course of the disease.

Fever is an abnormal elevation of the temperature of the body above 37° C (98.6° F) because of disease. Fever results from an imbalance between the elimination and the production of heat. Temperature of healthy people may be increased by exercise, anxiety and dehydration. Various Infections, neurological diseases, malignancies and many drugs may cause the development of fever.

Inflammation is the protective response of the body to injury. Inflammation may be acute or chronic. It is characterized by **redness, heat, swelling, pain** and **loss of function**.

Oedema (**swelling**) is the abnormal accumulation of fluid in interstitial spaces of tissues. Edema may be caused by **increased capillary fluid pressure, venous obstruction** and **inflammatory reactions**. Edema may also occur because of loss of serum protein due to various causes.

Thrombosis is an abnormal vascular condition in which a thrombus develops within a blood vessel leading to intravenous coagulation of blood.

Embolism is an abnormal circulatory condition in which an embolus (detached and circulatory thrombus) travels through the bloodstream and becomes lodged in a blood vessel leading to its complete or partial obstruction. Types of embolism include **air embolism** and **fat embolism.**

Ulcer is a circumscribed, craterlike lesion of the skin or mucous membrane. This result from necrosis accompanies some inflammatory, infectious, or malignant processes.

Sinus is a cavity or channel - cavity within a bone, a dilated channel for venous blood or a blind tract lined by epithelium which opens at one end permitting the escape of purulent material.

Fistula is an abnormal passage from an internal organ to the body surface or between two internal organs- **pulmono-peritoneal fistula.** The fistula may be caused by a congenital defect, injury or infection

Necrosis is the localized tissue death that occurs in response to disease or injury. **Coagulation necrosis** - blood clots block the flow of blood and causes tissue ischemia distal to the clot, **Gangrenous necrosis** - ischaemia combined with bacterial action causes putrefaction leading to necrosis.

Degeneration is the gradual deterioration of normal cells.

Gangrene means necrosis or death of tissue which is due to ischemia (loss of blood supply), bacterial infection and putrefaction. **Dry gangrene** - late complication of diabetes mellitus with arteriosclerosis in which the affected extremity becomes cold, dry and eventually turns black. **Moist gangrene** may be seen after a crushing injury or an obstruction of blood flow by an embolism or tight bandages.

Infarction is the development and formation of an infarct causing obstruction of the blood vessel leading to tissue necrosis. Types of infarction include **myocardial infarction** and **pulmonary infarction.**

Atrophy is the wasting or diminution of size of a part of the body because of disease or other causes.

Hypertrophy is an increase in the size of an organ caused by an increase in the size of the cells rather than the number of cells. Types of hypertrophy include **adaptive hypertrophy, compensatory hypertrophy, and physiologic hypertrophy.**

Hyperplasia is an increase in the number of cells of a body part.

Hypoplasia is the underdeveloped organ or tissue. This results from a decrease in the number of cells

Aplasia is the developmental failure resulting in the absence of an organ or tissue.

Syndrome Also called **symptom complex.** It is a complex of signs and symptoms to present a clinical picture of a disease or congenital abnormality.

Paralysis is the loss of muscle function or the loss of sensation, or both. It may be due to trauma, disease and poisoning. Paralyses may **flaccid paralysis** or **spastic paralysis.**

Hemiplegia is the paralysis of one side of the body. It may be **cerebral hemiplegia, facial hemiplegia** or **spastic hemiplegia.**

Paraplegia is the paralysis in the lower limbs and trunk which is characterized by motor or sensory loss.

Quadriplegia is the paralysis of the arms, legs and trunk of the body below the level of an associated injury to the spinal cord. This is usually caused by injury to the spinal cord commonly in the area of the fifth to the seventh vertebrae

Anaesthssia is the absence of normal sensation as induced by an anesthetic agent. Anesthesia induced for medical or surgical purposes may be **topical, local, regional** or general.

Hyperesthesia is an exaggerated sensitivity such as pain or touch.

Paraesthesia is the subjective sensation, experienced as numbness, tingling or a 'pins and needles' feeling. It may be termed as **acroparesthesia.**

Coma is the deep unconsciousness. Coma is characterized by the absence of spontaneous eye openings, response to painful stimuli and verbal command. The person cannot be aroused. Coma may result from trauma, space-occupying lesions of brain, toxic metabolic conditions, and encephalitis or brain ischaemia.

Tumour is also called **neoplasm.** It is a new growth of tissue characterized by progressive and uncontrolled proliferation of cells. The tumour may be benign or malignant.

Benign means mild (illness or growth) and thus not an immediate threat though treatment eventually may be required for health.

Malignant means severe (illness or growth). A malignant tumour is invasive and metastatic in nature.

Carcinoma is the malignant epithelial growth which invades surrounding tissue and metastasizes to distant regions of the body. The tumour is firm, irregular, and nodular with a well-defined border.

Sarcoma is the malignant growth of the soft tissues (**mesodermal in origin**) arising in fibrous, fatty, muscular, synovial, vascular, or neural tissue. This generally presents as a painless swelling.

Metastasis the process by which tumour cells spread to distant parts of the body.

Convalescence is the period of recovery after an illness, injury or surgery.

Therapy is the treatment of any disease.

GLOSSARY OF PREFIX AND SUFFIX

Prefix	Meaning	Examples
• a -	Without	Aphasia
• ab-	Away	Abduction
• ad-	Toward	Adduction
• ante-	Before	Ante-cubital
• anti-	Against	Antibiotics
• bi-	Two	Bicondylar
• circum-	Around	Circumflex
• contra-	Opposed	Contralateral
• di-	Two	Diencephalon
• dia-	Between	Diaphragm
• dis-	Apart	Disarticulation
• dys-	Difficult	Dyskinesia
• ec-	Out of	Ectopic
• ecto-	Outer	Ectoderm
• endo-	Within	Endoderm
• epi-	Over	Epidermis
• hemi-	Half	Hemiplegia
• hyper-	Excessive	Hyperactive
• hypo-	Under	Hypothyroidism
• infra-	Below	Infraorbital
• inter-	Between	Intercostal
• intra-	Within	Intra pleural
• mes-	Middle	Mesencephalon
• meta-	Beyond	Metaphysis
• neo-	New	Neonatal
• pan-	Entire	Panophthalmitis
• para-	Beyond	Paracentesis
• peri-	Around	Periosteum
• poly-	Many	Polycystic
• post-	After	Postoperative
• pre-	Before	Prenatal
• pseudo-	False	Pseudo stratified
• re-	Again	Regurgitation
• retro-	Behind	Retrosternal
• semi-	Half	Semiconscious
• sub-	Under	Subcutaneous
• supra-	Above	Suprarenal
• sym-	Together	Symphysis
• trans-	Across	Transection
• ultra-	Beyond	Ultrasound
• -algia	Pain	Neuralgia
• -cele	Protrusion (hernia)	Cystocele
• -centesis	Surgical puncture to remove fluid	Paracentesis
• -ectomy	Cutting out	Cholecystectomy
• -emesis	Vomit	Hematemesis
• -emia	Blood condition	Leukemia
• -genesis	Origin	Pathogenesis
• -graphy	Recording	Echocardiography
• -itis	Inflammation	Rhinitis
• -logy	Science	Osteology
• -oma	Tumour	Carcinoma
• -penia	Deficiency	Leucopenia

- **-plexy** — Fixation — Orchidoplexy
- **-phagia** — Eating — Polyphagia
- **-phobia** — Abnormal fear — Hydrophpbia
- **-plasty** — Surgical repair — Rhinoplasty
- **-pnoea** — Breathing — Dyspnoea
- **-ptosis** — Prolapse — Proctoptosis
- **-rrhage** — Excessive flow — Haemorrhage
- **-rrhaphy** — Suturing in place — Herniorrhaphy

- **-rrhea** — Flow or discharge — Rhinorrhea
- **-rrhexis** — Rupture — Enterorrhexis
- **-scope** — Instrument for examination — Bronchoscope
- **-scopy** — Examination — Bronchoscopy
- **-stomy** — Surgical opening — Colostomy
- **-tome** — Instrument for Cutting — Cystotome
- **-tomy** — Cutting — Cystotomy

2

Skin and Fasciae

SKIN

- It is the largest organ of the body.
- It is the outer or external covering of the body.
- It is continuous with mucous membranes of the body at orifices.
- It accounts for seven percent of body weight.

Consists of three major regions

Epidermis – Outermost superficial region

Dermis – Middle region

Hypodermis – Deepest region

Epidermis

- Outer portion of the skin which is exposed to the external environment and its main function is protection.
- Composed of keratinized stratified squamous epithelium consisting of four distinct cell types and four or five layers.
- Cell types include **keratinocytes**, **melanocytes**, **Merkel cells**, and **Langerhans'** cells.

Cells of epidermis

- **Keratinocytes** – Produce **keratin**.
- **Melanocytes** – Produce **melanin**.

- **Langerhans' cells** – Epidermal macrophages help in activation of the immune system.
- **Merkel cells** – Function as touch receptors in association with sensory nerve endings

Dermis

- It is true skin. Also called corium.
- Second major skin region which contains connective tissue.
- Cell types include fibroblasts, macrophages, and occasionally mast cells and white blood cells.
- Composed of two layers – Papillary and Reticular.

Papillary layer

- Composed of areolar connective tissue with collagen and elastic fibres.
- Its superior surface contains peg like projections - **dermal papillae**.
- Dermal papillae contain capillary loops, Meisner's corpuscles and free nerve endings.

Reticular layer

- This accounts for approximately 80% of the skin thickness.

- Collagen fibres in this layer add strength and resiliency to the skin.
- Elastin fibers provide stretch-recoil properties.

Three pigments contribute to skin color

Melanin – Yellow to reddish-brown to black pigment which is responsible for dark skin colors.

Carotene – Yellow to orange pigment in the palms and soles.

Hemoglobin – Reddish pigment responsible for the pinkish hue of the skin.

APPENDAGES OF THE SKIN

Hair

- Helps maintain warmth, alerts the body to presence of insects on the skin
- Guards the scalp against physical trauma, heat loss and sunlight
- Made up of the shaft projecting from the skin and the root embedded in the skin
- Consists of **medulla**, **cortex** and outermost **cuticle**

Types of hair

Vellus are pale fine body hair found in children and adult females.

Terminal hairs are coarse long hair of eyebrows, scalp, axilla and pubic region.

NAILS are scale-like modification of epidermis. It is made of hard keratin.

Parts of the nail:

- Free edge
- Body
- Root
- Nail folds
- Eponychium – cuticle

SEBACEOUS GLANDS

- Occur over entire body **except** in palms and soles.
- Secrete sebum - an oily secretion
- Simple alveolar glands of **holocrine type**
- Entire cell breaks up to form secretion
- Most are associated with a hair follicle

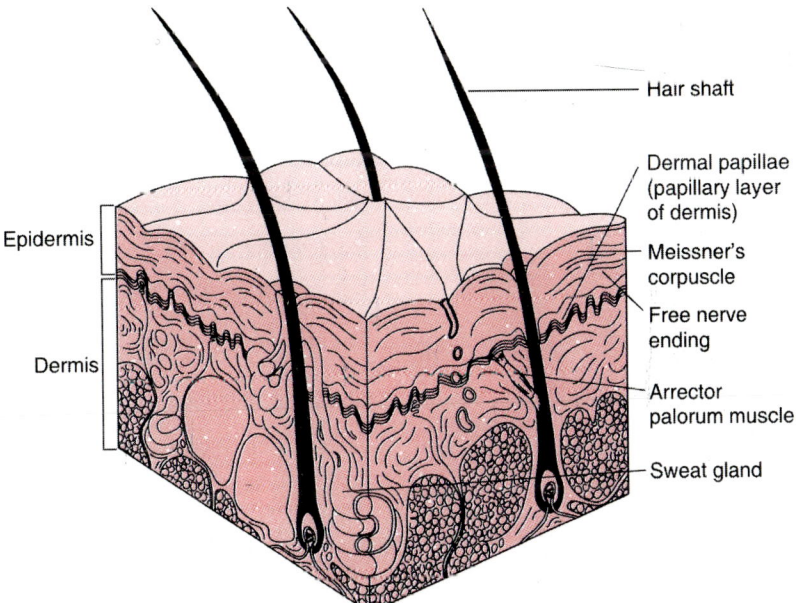

Fig. 2.1: General structure of Skin

Functions of sebum

Collects dirt; softens and lubricates hair and skin.

SWEAT GLANDS

Different types: Prevent overheating of the body; Secret cerumen and milk

Eccrine sweat glands – Found in palms, soles of the feet, and forehead

Apocrine sweat glands – Found in axillary and anogenital areas

Ceruminous glands – Modified apocrine glands in the external ear canal which secrete cerumen

Mammary glands – Specialized sweat glands that secret milk

FUNCTIONS OF INTEGUMENTARY SYSTEM

1. **Protection** – Chemical, physical, and mechanical barrier
2. **Body temperature**
   - Regulated by dilation (cooling) and constriction (warming) of dermal vessels
   - Sweat glands increase secretions to cool the body
3. **Cutaneous sensation** – Exoreceptors for touch and pain
4. **Metabolic functions** – Synthesis of vitamin D in dermal blood vessels
5. **Blood reservoir** – Skin blood vessels store up to 5% of the body's blood volume
6. **Excretion** – Limited amounts of nitrogenous wastes are eliminated from the body in sweat

CLINICAL CONSIDERATIONS

Burns

First-degree – Only the epidermis is damaged

- Symptoms include localized redness, swelling, and pain

Second-degree – Epidermis and upper regions of dermis is damaged

- Symptoms mimic first degree burns, but blisters also appear

Third-degree – Involve entire thickness of the skin

- Burned area appears gray-white, cherry red, or black, and there is no initial edema nor pain (since nerve endings are destroyed)

Estimation of the severity of burns

Burns considered critical if:
- Over 25% of the body has second-degree burns
- Over 10% of the body has third-degree burns
- There are third-degree burns on face, hands, or feet

RULE OF NINE

The area of skin involved in burns can be determined by this.

Upper limb: 9 percent X 2 = 18

Lower limb: 18 percent X 2 = 36

Front of trunk: 18 percent

Back of trunk: 18 percent

Head and neck: 9 percent

Perineum: 1 percent

Du Bois formula

This is used to calculate the surface area of a person.

A = W x H x 71.84

A: Surface area in square cm

W: Weight in kilogram

H: Height in cm

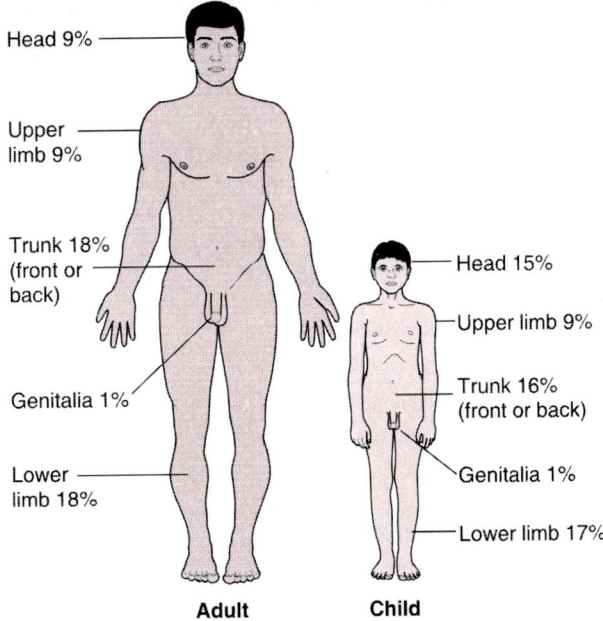

Fig. 2.2: Rule of nine in estimation of burns

Adult labels:
Head 9%
Upper limb 9%
Trunk 18% (front or back)
Genitalia 1%
Lower limb 18%

Child labels:
Head 15%
Upper limb 9%
Trunk 16% (front or back)
Genitalia 1%
Lower limb 17%

Adult   Child

FASCIA

It is a sheet of fibro-fatty tissue, placed deep to skin, and invests muscles and other deep structures. It varies widely in structure and thickness according to the functional requirement.

The fascia is a packing material (**connective tissue**) that remains between areas of more specialized tissue, such as muscle.

Most fascial layers are sparingly supplied by free nerve endings and simple, small, encapsulated endings.

When fasciae lie over non-expansile parts (e.g., muscles of pelvic wall, prevertebral muscles) they are:

- Well developed demonstrable membranes
- Can be sutured after incision

When, fasciae lie over expansile parts (e.g., cheek, and pharynx) they:

- Do not exist as demonstrable membranes
- Indefinite and thin collections of loose areolar tissue

Classification

Fascia is classified into

- Superficial fascia
- Deep fascia

SUPERFICIAL FASCIA

Hypodermis / subcutaneous tissue / tela subcutanea

- It is the fibrous mesh filled with fat which connects skin to the underlying deep fascia. It is the general coating of the body beneath the skin. It comprises of:

Fat and areolar tissue

Cutaneous vessels, nerves and lymphatics

- Thickness of superficial fascia varies with the amount of fat present. Fat is abundant in gluteal & lumbar regions, front of thigh and anterior abdominal wall below umbilicus, etc.

- Distribution of fat in superficial fascia varies with sex. The smoother outline of a female's figure is due to greater amount of fat (subcutaneous) - a secondary sexual character.

- Fat is absent from the eyelids, external ear, penis, scrotum, etc.
- The subcutaneous layer of fat is known as **Penniculus adiposus (PA)**. This acts as a barrier to the heat loss from the body (fat is a poor conductor of heat). The P.A. contains flat sheet of muscles called PENNICULUS CARNOSUS (PC). One end of each muscle fibre is attached to the skin and the other end to the deep fascia or bone.
- In humans, the remnants of **Penniculus Carnosus** are well developed and highly differentiated at some places e.g. muscles of scalp and face, platysma, palmaris brevis, corrugator cutis ani, dartos muscle, muscles of nipple.

Modifications of superficial fascia

- Mammary gland
- Platysma
- Dartos
- Palmaris brevis
- Corrugator cutis ani

Contents of superficial fascia

In addition to fibro-fatty tissue, the superficial fascia also contains

1. Small blood vessels, lymphatics, lymph nodes, etc.
2. Various modifications in the form of:
   - Mammary gland
   - Subcutaneous muscles of fascia (Dartos, Platysma)
3. Deeply situated sweat glands

Functions of superficial fascia:

1. Conserves body heat
2. Facilitates movements of skin
3. Serves as a soft medium for the passage of blood vessels and nerves to the skin

DEEP FASCIA

It is the dense inelastic membrane which separates superficial fascia from the underlying deeper structures. It invests the body beneath superficial fascia.

Features

- It is continuous with fibers of superficial fascia
- Sends partitions (septae) between muscles from its deep surface, forming intermuscular septa, thus dividing limbs into various compartments
- Sends prolongations in the form of fibroareolar sheaths for the muscles, vessels and nerves
- It is devoid of fat and is very sensitive
- It never crosses a subcutaneous bone, but blends with its periosteum. Thus it is continuous with periosteum (no deep fascia covering bones)

Distribution of deep fascia

It varies widely in thickness. In the ilio-tibial tract of fascia lata it is very well developed. Over rectus sheath it is quite thin and barely demonstrable. It is entirely absent in face and ischiorectal fossa.

It is well defined in the limbs and forms tight and tough sleeve. In the neck forms a collar

Modifications of deep fascia

1. *In relation to muscles*

   It forms intermuscular septa which form separate compartments for functionally different groups of muscles. It covers each muscle. These septae arise from intermuscular septum known as *EPIMYSIUM* which in turn sends septae to cover each muscle fasciculus. These septae are known as *PERIMYSIUM*. From the perimysium septae are known as *ENDOMYSIUM*. Blood vessels, nerves and lymphatics travel to each muscle fiber through these septae.

2. In relation to blood vessels

It forms sheaths (**perivascular sheaths**) around large arteries and veins e.g., carotid sheath, axillary sheath and femoral sheath. The fascial covering is dense around the arteries and loose around the veins allowing distention of veins.

3. In relation to nerves

The deep fascia sends prolongation or extensions to cover nerves. The deep fascia covering the nerve is *EPINEURIUM* and that covering each nerve fascicle is called *PERINEURIUM*. The fascial covering of each nerve fiber is known as *ENDONEURIUM*.

Functional aspect:

- Carries capillaries and lymphatics.

4. In relation to

The deep fascia modifies to form

- Synovial membrane
- Capsule
- Bursae

At places, where tendons cross over a joint, the fascia thickens to form **retinaculum**. This acts as a pulley and also keeps tendons in position. Also forms tendons sheath and bursae. These devices prevent wear and tear of the tendons and minimize friction.

5. In relation to palm and sole

Deep fascia thickens to form aponeurosis which protects the underlying structures e.g., nerves, blood vessels and delicate tendons.

6. In relation to bones

Deep fascia becomes continuous with periosteum. The fascia between two adjacent bones sometimes condenses to form **interosseous membrane** (e.g., of forearm and leg) which keeps the bones at optimal distance, increases the surface area for attachments of muscles and in upper limb, helps in weight transmission.

Functions of deep fascia

1. Keeps underlying structures in position
2. Preserves characteristic surface contour of the limbs
3. Provides extra surface for muscle attachments
4. Helps in venous and lymphatic return
5. Assists muscles in their action by tension and pressure exerted by it on to muscles (their surfaces)
6. Retinacula acts as pulleys and serve to prevent loss of power. Friction is also minimized by keeping tendons in position
7. Ligaments give strength and stability to the joints

CLINICAL CONSIDERATIONS

- The course taken by the deeply accumulated pus is determined by the fascial planes and neurovascular bundles.
- Damage to deep fascia of leg can affect the venous return leading to accumulation of blood and fluid in the leg termed as oedema.

Muscles

(Latin – Mus = Mouse) (Gk = Mys)

They are so named because many resemble a mouse along with their tapering ends (tendons) representing tail

It is a contractile tissue which brings about a movement

Truly they are regarded as motors of body

TYPES

Three types

1. Skeletal muscle
2. Smooth muscle
3. Cardiac muscle

SKELETAL MUSCLE

Striped / striated / somatic / voluntary

Examples: Muscles of limbs and body wall

Features

- Most abundant
- Attached to skeleton
- Supplied by somatic (cerebrospinal) nerves and hence under voluntary control
- Responds quickly to stimuli
- Capable of rapid contraction and hence easily fatigued

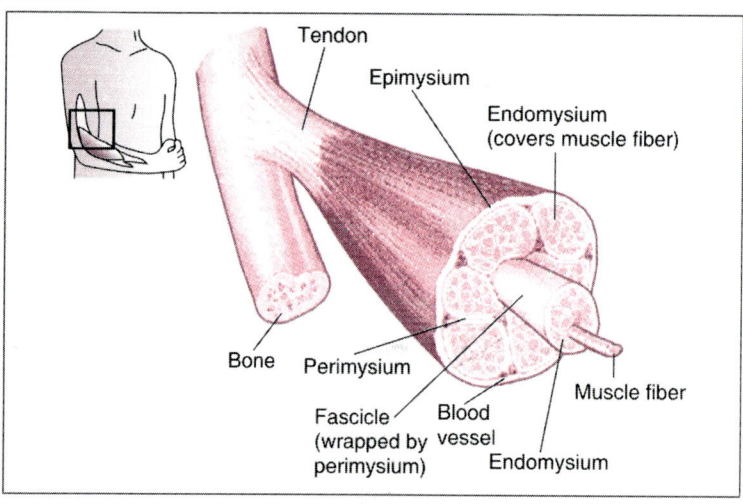

Fig. 3.1: Skelelatal Muscle

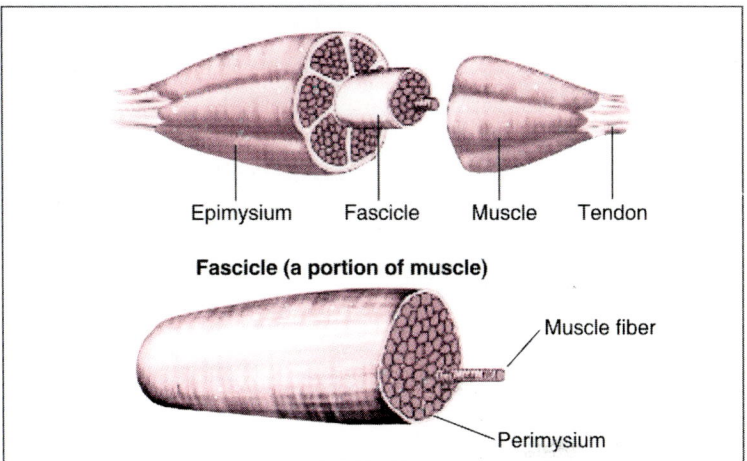

Epimysium   Fascicle   Muscle   Tendon

Fascicle (a portion of muscle)

Muscle fiber

Perimysium

Fig. 3.2: Skelelatal Muscle

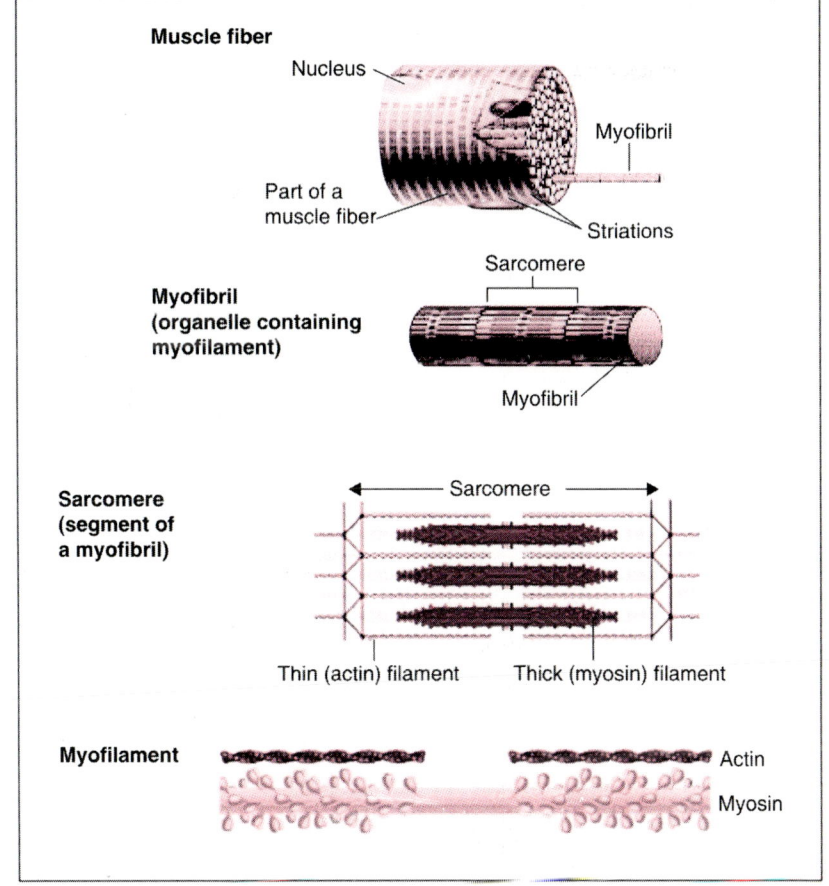

Muscle fiber

Nucleus

Myofibril

Part of a
muscle fiber

Striations

Sarcomere

**Myofibril
(organelle containing
myofilament)**

Myofibril

**Sarcomere
(segment of
a myofibril)**

Sarcomere

Thin (actin) filament   Thick (myosin) filament

Myofilament

Actin

Myosin

Fig. 3.3: Structure and organization of skeletal muscle

- Help the individual in adjusting to external environment
- They are under highest nervous control of cerebral cortex

Microscopically

- Exhibit cross striations
- Each muscle fiber is a multinucleated cylindrical cell, containing groups of myofibrils separated by **Cohnheim's areas**

SMOOTH MUSCLE

Plain / unstriped / non-striated / visceral / involuntary

Examples:

- Muscles of digestive and urogenital systems
- Muscles of blood vessels
- Arrector pili muscles of the skin

Features

- Surround or encircle the viscera.
- Supplied by autonomic nerves and hence not under voluntary control
- Respond slowly to stimuli
- Capable of sustained contraction and hence do not fatigue

- Provide motive power for regulating internal environment, related to digestion, circulation, excretion, etc.
- Less dependent on nervous control, being capable of contracting automatically, spontaneously and rhythmically

Microscopically

- Do not exhibit cross striations
- Each muscle fiber is an elongated and spindle shaped cell with a single centrally placed round nucleus
- Myofibrils show longitudinal striations

CARDIAC MUSCLE

Features

- Forms myocardium of heart
- Intermediate e.g., striated but involuntary
- Meant for automatic and rhythmic contractions

Microscopically

- Each muscle fiber, having a single centrally placed nucleus, branches and anastomosis with neighboring fibers at intercalated discs (**apposed cell membranes**)
- Cross striations are less prominent

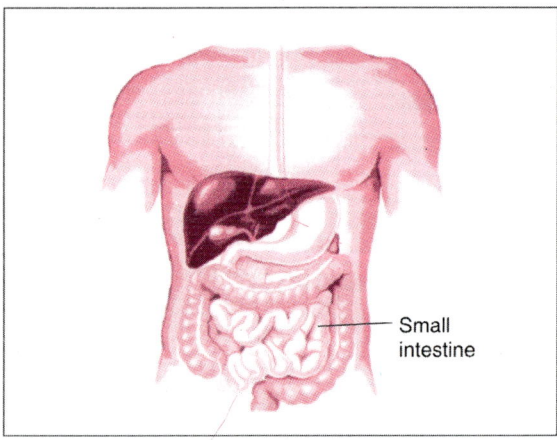

Small intestine

Fig. 3.4: Skelelatal Muscle

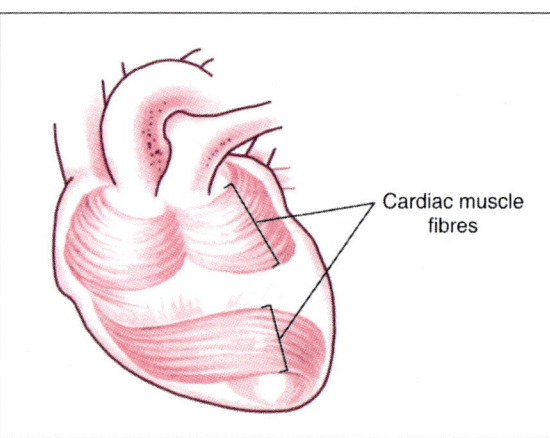

Cardiac muscle fibres

Fig. 3.5: Cardiac Muscle

SKELETAL MUSCLE

Consists of

Two ends

Origin – End of muscle which is relatively fixed during contractions.

Insertion – End of muscle which moves during contraction.

In limbs, origin is usually proximal to insertion.

Parts

Fleshy: Contractile, called **belly**

Fibrous: Non contractile which may be

- *Tendon*: cord like
- *Aponeurosis*: Flattened sheet

Nomenclature

The muscles have been named according to:

1. **Shape:** Trapezius, Rhomboideus, Deltoid
2. **Number of heads:** Biceps, Triceps, Quadriceps
3. **Structure:** Semimembranosus, Semitendinosus
4. **Location:** Temporalis, Supraspinatus
5. **Attachments:** Stylohyoid, Cricothyroid
6. **Function:** Adductor longus, Flexor carpi ulnaris, Abductor pollicis longus
7. **Direction of fibers:** Rectus abdominis, Transversus abdominis

Nerve supply

Nerve supplying a muscle is called **motor nerve**

Motor point

Site where motor nerve enters muscle

May be one or more

Electrical stimulation at this point is more effective

MOTOR UNIT

It is the single alpha motor neuron together with muscle fibers supplied by it.

Size depends upon precision of muscle contraction.

Small motor units (5-10 muscle fibers) are seen in extra ocular muscles.

Large motor units (100-200 muscle fibers) seen in muscles of limbs.

NEUROMUSCULAR JUNCTION

- Cholinergic in nature.
- On approaching muscle the axons of motor nerve lose their myelin sheath and break up into no of branches to supply individual muscle fibers.
- This specialized motor nerve ending (rich in Ach) is of **two types:**

En plaque terminals: (Plaque = plate)

- Are plates like
- Known as motor end plate
- Found in most of skeletal muscles of body

En grappe' terminalis (Grappe = grape)

- Resembles a bunch of grapes.
- Found in extra-ocular muscles, trail endings of muscle spindles.
- At neuromuscular junction, muscle fiber is also specialized into a SOLE PLATE which is a localized collection of granular sarcoplasm containing many nuclei and mitochondria. This also presents "**synaptic gutters**" for the end plates.
- Motor end plate and sole plate are separated by an ultramicroscopic gap.
- Sarcolemma folds (**sub-neural clefts**) in synaptic gutters are rich in acetyl cholinesterase which destroys the liberated acetylcholine after each neuromuscular transmission of impulse.

BLOOD SUPPLY OF MUSCLES

- Blood supply is derived from muscular branches of from neighbouring arteries.
- Arteries, veins and motor nerve pierce the

muscle at **neurovascular hilum** that is fairly constant point.

- Subsidiary arteries may enter muscle near the ends
- Arteries divide repeatedly to form arterioles in the perimysium and capillaries in the endomysium for "nutritive circulation".
- Arteriovenous anastomoses are abundant in epimysium and perimysium for "non nutritive circulation" during muscular contraction.

Lymphatics

- These accompany the vessels and drain into neighboring nodes.

ACTIONS OF MUSCLES

- Generally during muscle contraction, its belly length shortens by 1/3 (**30%**) and thus brings about a movement.
- The range of movement depends upon:
- Length of fleshy fibers
- Power or force of movement on number of fibres
- During contraction, length may decrease or remain unchanged or increases. It depends upon functional demand of body
- Each movement at a joint is brought about by a coordinated activity of different groups of muscles.

Muscles are classified as under

1. *Prime mover*

- It is a muscle or group of muscles that directly bring about a desired movement.
- Gravity may also act as a prime mover e.g.:Brachialis as flexor at elbow joint

2. *Antagonist (Opponents)*

- This is a muscle or group of muscles that directly oppose the movement under consideration (Triceps brachii that is extensor of forearm when acting as a prime mover is the antagonist to flexor of forearm). Depending upon rate and force of movement, antagonists may be relaxed, or by lengthening while contracting, they may control movement and make it smooth, free from jerkiness and precise. These muscles cooperate rather than oppose.
- Gravity may act as an antagonist

3. *Fixators / Fixation muscles*

- They stabilize points or parts and thereby maintain posture or position while the prime movers act.
- They stabilize proximal joints so that desired movement at the distal joint may occur smoothly **e.g.:** muscles holding scapula steady are acting as fixator while deltoid moves humerus.

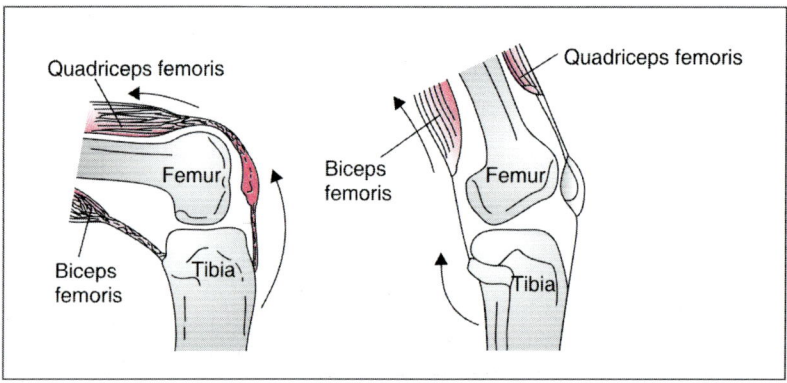

Fig. 3.6: Primemover and Antagonist

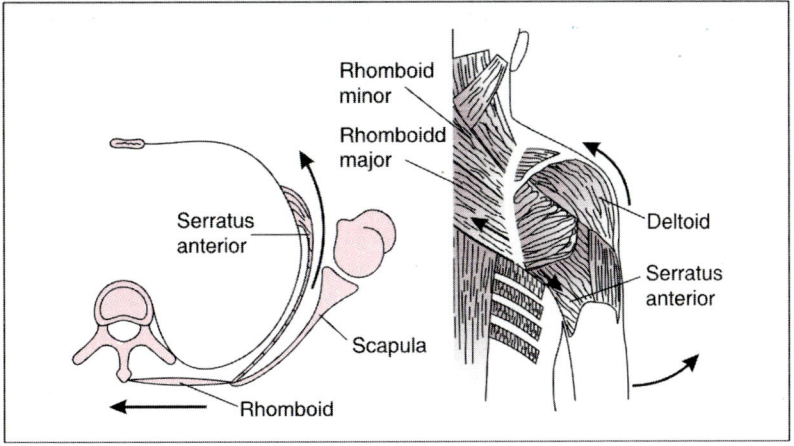

Fig. 3.7: Prime mover and Antagonist

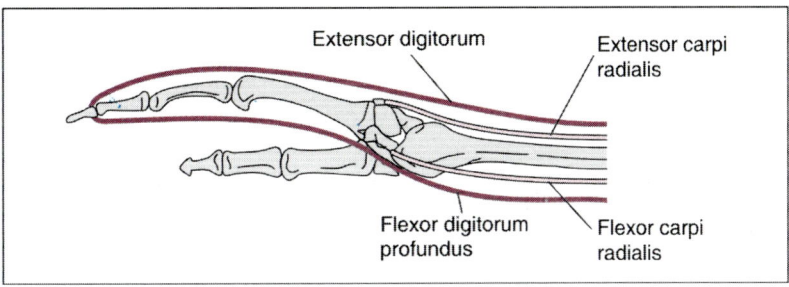

Fig. 3.8: Synergist

4. *Synergists*

- Special class of fixation muscles.
- Partial antagonist to prime mover.
- When a prime mover crosses two or more joints, synergists prevent undesired actions at intermediate joints. **e.g.:** long flexor that flexes fingers would at the same time flex the wrist if the wrist were not stabilized by extensors of wrist – synergists in this movement.

LEVER SYSTEM

- **Bones** – Act as levers
- **Joints** – Act as fulcrums
- **Muscle contraction** – Provides effort

First class – The fulcrum is between the load and the effort.

Second class – The load is between the fulcrum and the effort.

Third class – The effort is applied between the fulcrum and the load. Most of the muscles are placed in this group.

CLINICAL CONSIDERATIONS

Paralysis

Loss of motor power (power of movement)

Muscles are unable to contract:

There is damage to motor neural pathways leading to Upper motor neuron (**UMN**) or Lower motor neuron (**LMN**) paralysis.

UMN **Paralysis:** Spastic paralysis that exaggerated tendon jerks

LMN paralysis: Flaccid paralysis that is loss or decrease tendon jerks

Muscular spasm

It May be

Localized – commonly caused by a "muscle pull"

Generalized – seen in tetanus and epilepsy

- These are quite painful
- To relieve its pain muscle should be relaxed by appropriate treatment

Disuse atrophy

Muscles not used for long time, become thin and weak.

Reduction in size (**muscular wasting**) is a feature of

- UMN paralysis
- Generalized debility

Hypertrophy

Excessive use of a particular muscle may result in better development or even hypertrophy.

Regeneration

Muscle is capable of limited regeneration.

If large regions are damaged regeneration does not occur and damaged part is replaced by connective tissue.

Myopathy

This is characterized by muscle weakness, wasting and microscopic changes within muscle tissue. Myopathy is distinct from a muscle disorder caused by nerve dysfunction. The specific diagnosis of any myopathy is made by **electromyographic studies** and **muscle biopsy**.

TENDON

It is the fibrous and non contractile part of a muscle.

- The attachment of muscle to bone is usually by a long cord like or cylindrical structure, known as **tendon**.
- Composed of more or less parallel bundles of collagenous fibers. Its length varies.
- Surrounded by *EPITENDINEUM* - thin, fibro elastic sheath of loose connective tissue which extends between the bundles
- Supplied by sensory nerve fibers, reaching them from muscle nerves. Also receive sensory fibers from overlying superficial fascia or from nearby deep nerves.
- Usually supplied by arteries that anastomose within by veins and lymphatic vessels. The vascular needs are very small.
- Certain tendons can be used for tendon transfer and transplantation.
- They are destroyed very slowly by inflammatory processes and infected tendons heal very slowly.

APONEUROSIS

- The attachment of a muscle to bone by means of a thin, broad sheet is known as aponeurosis.
- Like tendon, aponeurosis is also composed of move or less parallel bundles of collagenous fibers.
  e.g.: Exterior oblique aponeurosis.

RAPHE

- It is a fibrous band which is formed by **interdigitating fibers** of an aponeurosis.
- It is stretchable.
  e.g.: Mylohyoid raphe

Bone

Latin word = Os, Greek = Osteon

DEFINITION

Connective tissue and along with cartilage constitute skeleton. Together they form the main supporting framework of the body.

Features

1. A bone of a living person is it self a living thing.
2. It has blood vessels, lymph vessels and nerves.
3. It grows.
4. It is subject to disease.
5. It heals itself when damaged.
6. It can mould it self according to change in stress and strain.

Structure and components

- Bone is also known as osseous tissue.
- Rigid form of connective tissue.
- Consists of cells and specialized connective tissue coat known as periosteum.

CELLS

Three cell types
1. Osteoblasts

These are associated with bone formation and are found in relation to bone surface where osseous matrix is being deposited.

2. Osteocytes

These are bone cells. These are **osteoblasts** which have been imprisoned within bone matrix

3. Osteoclasts

They are multinucleated giant cells of varying size. They are involved in bone resorption, although mechanism involved in this is unclear.

BONE MATRIX

Comprises following components:

Organic portion

- Forms 35% of weight of bone
- Composed chiefly of **osteo-collagenous fibres** which are difficult to see in ordinary preparation
- Makes bone tough and resilient (flexible that can afford resistance to tensile force)

Inorganic portion

- Forms 65% of weight of bone
- Composed of minerals principally as crystals of calcium phosphate and partly calcium carbonate and other salts
- Makes bone hard and rigid that can afford resistance to compressive forces

Bone matrix is arranged characteristically in layers / lamellae. The Lamellae result from concentrically deposited matrix. Fibers in any lamella are parallel to each other and take a spiral loop.

Periosteum

It is the fibrous sheath that envelops bone except articular surfaces. It is consists of two layers, although not sharply defined

Outer layer – composed of dense fibrous tissue, containing network of blood vessels.

Inner layer – contains numerous spindle shaped connective tissue cells (**osteoprogenitor cells**) which on stimulation become activated as in fracture.

Endosteum

Delicate layer lining marrow cavities and extends as lining into canal system of compact bone.

Consists of condensed reticular tissue that has both osteogenic and hemopoietic potencies.

CLASSIFICATION OF BONES

A. REGIONAL CLASSIFICATION

A. Axial bones
- **Skull**
  Cranium - 8
  Face - 14
  Auditory ossicles - 6
- Vertbral column - 26

B. Thorax
Sternum - 1
Ribi - 24

Appendicular bones

Upper limb: Girdle and Free bones - 64
Lower limb: Girdle and Free bones - 62

This number is not exact but varies. There may be fusion of lunate and triquetral or of two vertebrae. A bone may be suppressed or congenitally absent

Example: Absent phalanx or vertebra.

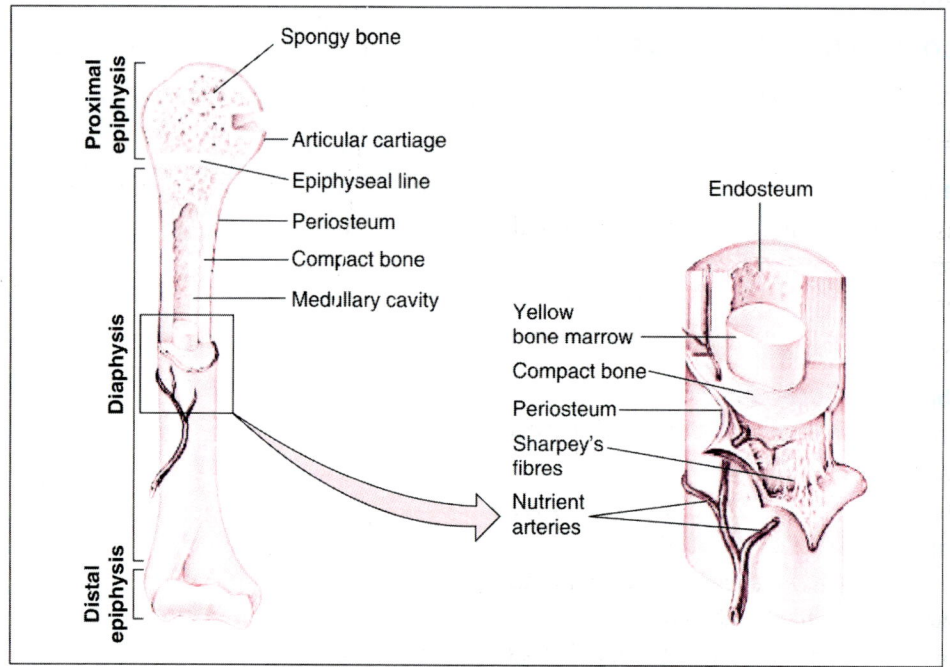

Fig. 4.1: Parts of a bone and its structure

B. STRUCTURAL CLASSIFICATION

Macroscopically the bone may be

1. Compact bone
2. Cancellous bone

Features of Compact bone

- Dense in texture
- Extremely porous
- Best developed in cortex of long bones

Features of Cancellous bone

- Open in texture
- Made up of meshwork of trabeculae, between that are marrow containing spaces present
- Adaptation to compressive forces

Microscopically the bone may be

- Lamellar
- Fibrous
- Dentine
- Cement

C. DEVELOPMENTAL CLASSIFICATION

Membrane (dermal) bone

Cartilaginous bone

Membrane bone

- Ossify in membrane (mesenchymal ossification)
- Derived from mesenchymal condensation
  e.g.: Bones of skull vault and facial bones

Intramembranous ossification

- Formation of most of the flat bones of the skull and the clavicles
- Fibrous connective tissue membranes are formed by mesenchymal cells
- An ossification center appears in the fibrous connective tissue membrane
- Bone matrix is secreted within the fibrous membrane
- Woven bone and periosteum form
- Bone collar of compact bone forms, and red marrow appears

Cartilaginous bone

- Ossify from cartilage (endochondral ossification)
- Derived from pre formed cartilage models.
  e.g.: Bones of limbs and vertebral column.

Endochondral ossification

- Begins in the second month of development.
- Uses hyaline cartilage "bones" as models for bone construction.
- Requires breakdown of hyaline cartilage prior to ossification.
- Formation of bone collar.
- Cavitations of the hyaline cartilage.
- Invasion of internal cavities by the periosteal bud, and spongy bone formation.
- Formation of the medullary cavity; appearance of secondary ossification centers in the epiphyses.
- Ossification of the epiphyses, with hyaline cartilage remaining only in the epiphyseal plates.

D. MORPHOLOGICAL CLASSIFICATION

According to shape/morphology

1. **Long** – peculiar to limbs
2. **Short** - peculiar to limbs
3. **Flat** – peculiar to skull vault
4. **Irregular** – peculiar to axial skeleton and girdles
5. **Pneumatic** – peculiar to skull
6. **Sesamoid** – develops in certain tendons

Long Bones

Features

- Serve as levers for muscles
- Develops from one primary centre of ossification in cartilage

- Ends develop from one or more secondary center of ossification

Long bone may be

1. **Typical** long bone e.g. Humerus
2. **Miniature** long bone – one epiphysis e.g., Metatarsals
3. **Modified** long bone – no medullary cavity e.g., Clavicle

Exceptions

- Clavicle and ribs do not possess medullary cavity
- Vertebrae are classified as irregular but their bodies possess most of the features of long bone

Short Bones

Features

- Modified cubes and are confined to carpus and tarsus
- They have generally six surfaces; out of that four (or less) are articular, leaving two (or more) for attachments of ligaments and for blood vessels to ends
- Develop in cartilage
- Begin to ossify after birth
  e.g.: Carpals and tarsals

Flat Bones

Features

- Consists of two layers of compact bone and marrow spread between them
- Most flat bones help to form walls of rounded cavities and therefore are curved
  e.g.: Bones of skull vault, Scapula

Irregular Bones

Features

- Are irregular or mixed shaped

- Composed of spongy bone and marrow that in compact covering bone
  e.g.: Vertebrae, Hip bone

Pneumatic Bone

Features

- Bones containing air spaces lined with mucous membrane
- Typically seen in skull bones
- They impart resonance to voice
  e.g.: Maxilla, Ethmoid

Sesamoid Bone (Arabic seed like)

- Develops in tendon
- No periosteum present, hence no regeneration
- Free surface is covered with articular cartilage
- Appear after birth

Functionally

- Minimize friction
- Alter direction of pull of muscle
- Resist pressure
- Maintain local circulation

Accessory Bones/Supernumerary Bones

- Not always present
- May occur as ununited epiphysis
- Developed from extra centre of ossification
  e.g.: Sutural bones, Os trigonum

Importance: May be mistaken for fracture

FUNCTIONS

1. Forms rigid supporting framework of body, giving shape to it
2. Serves as levers for muscles
3. Afford protection to certain viscera. e.g., brain, spinal cord, heart and lungs
4. Store house of calcium and phosphorus

5. Contain marrow - factory for blood cells
6. Provide surface for attachments of muscles, tendons, ligaments, etc.
7. Contain reticulo-endothelial cells which are phagocytic in nature
8. Para nasal sinuses (PNS) impart resonance to voice

BLOOD SUPPLY

1. Nutrient artery

- It is the main artery of the shaft. Also known as **medullary artery**.
- It enters bone through nutrient foramen and runs obliquely through cortex.
- After entering, it divides into ascending and descending branches in medullary cavity.
- Each branch further subdivides into a number of small parallel channels that terminate in adult metaphysis.
- It supplies medullary cavity, inner two third of cortex and metaphysis.
- The blood flow through cortex runs in centrifugal directions

2. Periosteal twigs

- These enter shaft at many points.
- These run in small longitudinal (**Haversian**) canals and supply outer 1/3rd of the cortex.

3. Twigs from articular arteries

These are derived from epiphyseal arteries and metaphyseal arteries:

- **Epiphyseal arteries are** derived from peri-articular vascular arcade (**circulus vasculosus**).
- **Metaphyseal arteries** are derived from neighboring arteries which pass directly to metaphysis and reinforce metaphyseal branches of nutrient artery.

In general, articular arteries (twigs) that anastomose around the joint, usually between bone and synovial membrane supply epiphysis and metaphyseal region.

RESPONSE TO MECHANICAL STRESS

Wolff's law states that a bone grows or remodels in response to the forces or demands place upon it.

Observations supporting Wolff's law:

1. Long bones are thickest midway along the shaft where bending stress is greatest
2. Curved bones are thickest where they are most likely to buckle
3. Trabeculae form along lines of stress
4. Large bony projections occur where heavy active muscles attach

MEDICO LEGAL CONSIDERATIONS

1. Estimation of age from bones

Age of an individual can be determined with fair accuracy by doing radiological examination of certain bones (ends of long bones and carpals). The age by which various epiphyses fuse with rest of the bone is fairly constant. The fusion takes place about two to three years earlier in females than males.

2. Estimation of sex

Pelvis and skull are important bones to establish the sexing. The sexual differences are well marked in these bones more so in pelvis. It has been worked out that other bones can be used in the absence of pelvis and skull in sex determination e.g. sternum and limb bones.

3. Estimation of height

The height of an individual can be determined from certain bones by using formulae. The important bones are long bones of limbs.

CLINICAL CONSIDERATIONS

Defective membranous ossification

- May be seen in "**cleidocranial dysostosis**" with
- Clavicle aplasia.
- Increase in transverse diameter of cranium.
- Retardation of fontanalle – defective ossification.

Paget's disease

- Characterized by excessive bone formation and breakdown.
- Pagetic bone with an excessively high ratio of woven to compact bone is formed.
- Pagetic bone, along with reduced mineralization, causes spotty weakening of bone.
- Osteoclasts activity wanes, but osteoblast activity continues to work.
- Usually localized in the spine, pelvis, femur and skull.
- Cause is not known (possibly viral).

Osteoporosis

- Characterized by low bone mass.
- Bone resorption outpaces bone deposition.
- Occurs mostly in women after menopause.

Rickets

- This condition is caused by the deficiency of vitamin D in infancy and childhood.
- This is characterized by abnormal bone formation.
- Features include soft pliable bones causing bone deformities - **bowlegs** and **knock-knees**, enlarged skull, chest deformities, spinal curvature, enlargement of the liver and spleen with general tenderness of the body.

Osteomalacia

- Occurs in adults.
- Abnormal condition of the lamellar bone characterized by a loss of calcification of the matrix resulting in softening of the bone.
- This is accompanied by weakness, fracture and pain.
- The condition is the result of an inadequate amount of phosphorus and calcium available in the blood for mineralization of the bones.
- This deficiency may be caused by a diet lacking these minerals or vitamin D or by a lack of exposure to sunlight thus person is unable to synthesize vitamin D.

Osteosarcoma

- Malignant bone cancer

5

Cartilage/Gristle

Greek word = Chondros

DEFINITION

It is a connective tissue in which a solid ground substance that is more resilient than bone forms the matrix. It is composed of cells (**chondrocytes**) and fibers (**collagen** or **yellow elastic**) that are embedded in a firm gel like matrix that is rich in mucopolysaccharide.

Features

1. Have no blood vessels or lymphatics
2. Nutrition diffuses through matrix
3. Have no nerves thus insensitive to pain
4. Surrounded by perichondrium which is similar to periosteum
5. When calcified, chondrocytes die and cartilage is replaced by bone

TYPES

Hyaline Cartilage (Greek: **hyalos** - a transparent stone)

- White and resilient.
- Potential bone.
- All bones (except clavicle and certain skull bones) performed in hyaline cartilage. Thyroid, cricoid and 1st costal cartilages begin to calcify at about 40th year.

- Persists in adult at:
  - Articular ends of bones as articular cartilage - no perichondrium.
  - At sternal ends of ribs as costal cartilage.
  - Cartilages of nose, trachea, bronchi and larynx

Fibro-Cartilage

- Has same structure as fibrous tissue with addition of cartilage ground substance (bears same resemblance to fibrous tissue as a starched collar bears to a soft collar).
- Whenever fibrous tissue is subjected to great pressure, it is replaced by fibro cartilage that is tough, strong and resilient.
- Appears white and opaque due to abundance of dense collagen fibers.

e.g.: Intervertebral discs, articular discs (e.g., menisci of knee joint).

It lines certain bony grooves in which tendons are placed.

Elastic Cartilage

- In this type, cartilage cells are numerous and the solid ground work is pervaded by yellow elastic fibers, making it more pliable.
  Found only in:
  - External ear

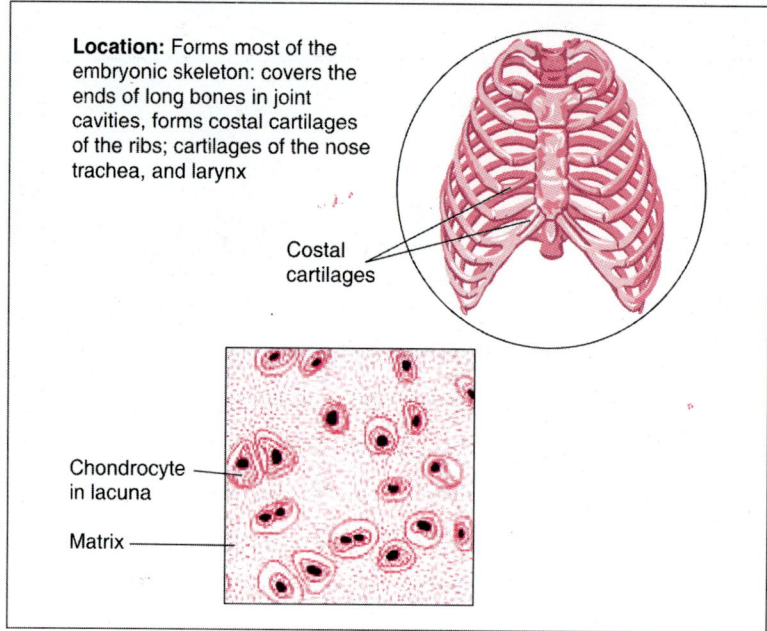

Location: Forms most of the embryonic skeleton: covers the ends of long bones in joint cavities, forms costal cartilages of the ribs; cartilages of the nose trachea, and larynx

Costal cartilages

Chondrocyte in lacuna

Matrix

Fig. 5.1: Hyaline cartilage

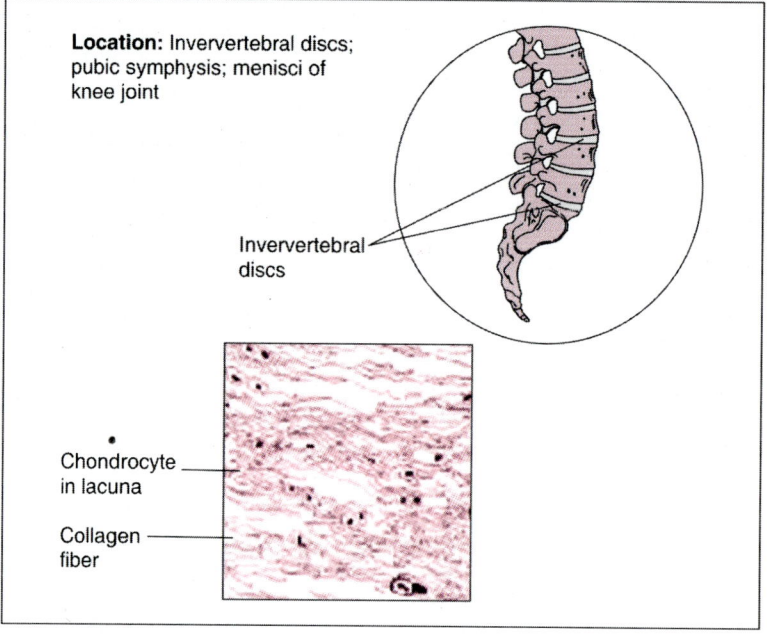

Location: Inververtebral discs; pubic symphysis; menisci of knee joint

Inververtebral discs

Chondrocyte in lacuna

Collagen fiber

Fig. 5.2: Fibro-cartilage

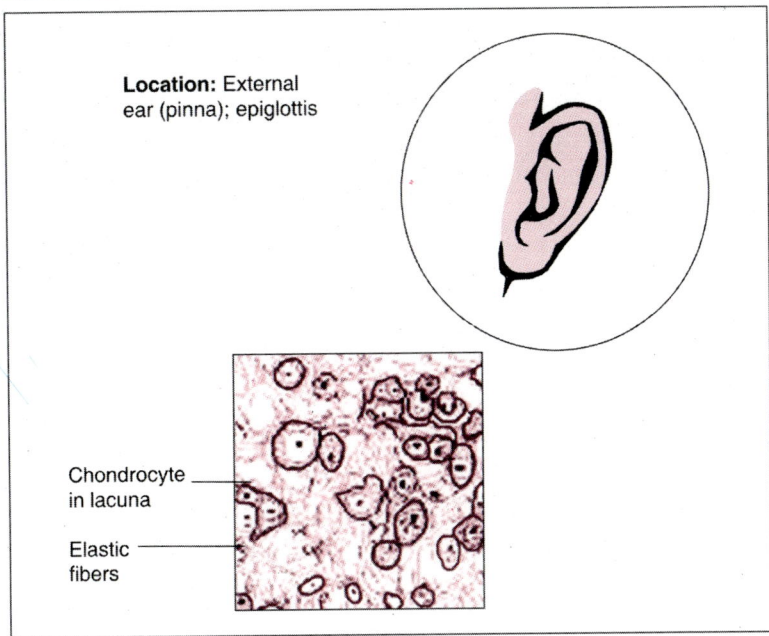

Location: External ear (pinna); epiglottis

Chondrocyte in lacuna

Elastic fibers

Fig. 5.3: Elastic cartilage

- Pharyngo-tympanic tube
- Small cartilages guarding entrance of larynx.

Functionally: Maintains the shape of the structure while allowing great flexibility.

CLINICAL CONSIDERATIONS

Achondroplasia

It is a disorder of cartilage growth in the epiphyses of the long bones and skull resulting in premature ossification, permanent limitation of skeletal development and dwarfism. This is characterized by protruding forehead with short arms and legs. The trunk is normal. Onset starts in foetal life. Familial achondroplasia is inherited as an autosomal dominant disorder. This can be diagnosed antenatally.

Chondrodystrophy

It is a group of disorders in which there is abnormal conversion of cartilage to bone particularly in the epiphyses of the long bones. Patients are dwarfed, with normal trunks and shortened extremities.

6

Joints

Greek = Arthron – Arthrology, Arthritis
Latin = Articulatio (A joint)
Latin = Junctura (A joint)

DEFINITION

A joint (or articulation) said to exist whenever two or more bones or cartilages meet. Thus a joint is a junction between bones or cartilages. It is a device to permit movements. The immovable joints are meant for growth and permit moulding during childbirth.

CLASSIFICATION

A. **STRUCTURAL :** On the basis of intervening tissue
  1. **Fibrous**
  2. **Cartilaginous**
  3. **Synovial**

B. **FUNCTIONAL :** On the basis of movements permitted
  1. **Synarthroses** (immovable) e.g., fibrous joints
  2. **Amphiarthroses** (slightly movable) e.g., cartilaginous joints
  3. **Diarthroses** (Freely movable) e.g., synovial joints

C. **REGIONAL :** On the basis of location
  1. **Skull type** – Immovable
  2. **Vertebral type** – Slightly movable
  3. **Limb type** – Freely movable

CLASSIFICATION OF JOINTS

Fibrous	**Cartilaginous**	**Synovial**
Fixed (*Synarthroses*)	Slightly movable (*Amphiarthroses*)	Freely movable (*Diarthroses*)
Types	**Types**	**Types**
1. Sutures	1. Pri.cart. joints	1. **Plane**
• Plane	(*Synchondroses*)	2. **Hinge** (*Ginglymi*)
• Squamous		3. **Pivot** (*Trochoid*)
• Limbous	2. Sec.cart. joints	4. **Bicondylar**
• Serrate	(*Syndesmoses*)	5. **Ellipsoid**
• Dentate		6. **Saddle** (*Sellar*)
2. Gomphosis		7. **Ball & socket**
3. Syndesmosis		
4. Schindylesis		

STRUCTURAL JOINTS

Fibrous Joints/Fixed Joints/Synarthrosis

They are generally limited to skull.

They are of following varieties

A. Sutures

- Skull bones are lined outside by a membrane called pericranium and on inside by another membrane called endocranium (**outer layer of dura mater**).
- These membranes pass across from one bone to other, uniting them.
- Some fibrous tissue intervenes that passes from one side to the other and is continuous with pericranium termed as **sutural ligament**.
- Provide necessary rigidity and geometry in the upper neurocranium, nasofacial and palatine skeleton.
- Sutures start disappearing (by **bone fusion**) around 30 years of age. Fusion starts on inner surface and gradually extends to outer surface.

Types

1. **Plane suture :** In this type there is simple apposition of contiguous surfaces which are usually rough and reciprocally irregular.

   e.g.: Intermaxillary

   Inter palatine   **cruciform suture**

   Palatomaxillary

2. **Squamous suture :** Adjacent bone surfaces are reciprocally bevelled.

   e.g.: Anterior Squamous, Temporal and parietal sutures.

3. **Limbus suture :** Adjacent bone surfaces are reciprocally bevelled and mutually ridged or serrated.

   e.g.: Posterior Squamous, Temporal and parietal sutures.

4. **Serrate suture :** Edges are like serrations of a saw.

   e.g.: Sagittal and corona sutures.

5. **Dentate suture :** Edges have small tooth projections. These often widen towards their ends to provide even more effective interlocking.

   e.g.: Lambdoid suture

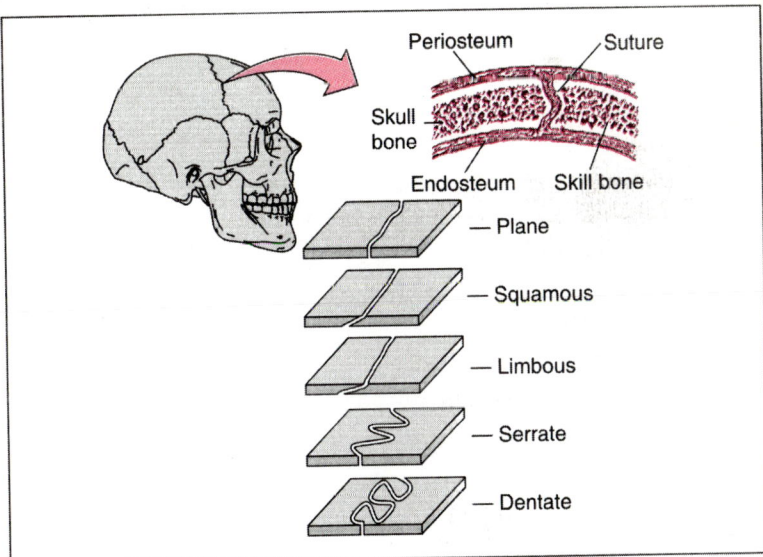

Fig. 6.1: Sutures

B. Schindylesis

Wedge and groove
e.g.: Rostrum of sphenoid and ala of vomer.

C. Gomphosis (Articulatio dentoalveolaris)

Also called "peg and socket joint"

The cavity in jaw and root of teeth, connected by some fibrous tissue (collagen of periodontium connects dental cement that is alveolar bone)

e.g.: Joint between tooth and jaw (Alveolar socket)

D. Syndesmosis

It is a fibrous articulation in which bony surfaces are bound together by an interosseous ligament, a slender fibrous cord or an aponeurotic membrane.

Examples include:

- Inferior Tibiofibular joint
- Middle radio ulnar joint

Following joints are also included in syndesmosis

- Pterygospinous
- Stylohyoid
- Interspinous
- Inter-transverse

- Ligamentum flava
- Ligamentum nuchae

CARTILAGINOUS / SLIGHTLY MOVABLE / AMPHIARTHROSES

Primary Cartilaginous Joint/Synchondrosis/ Hyaline Cartilage Joint

Features

1. Bones are united by a plate of hyaline cartilage (two ossifying ends are closely bonded by a specialized hyaline growth cartilage).
2. Joint is immovable but strong.
3. Temporary in nature because cartilage plate is replaced by bone later, process known as **synostosis**.

Functionally: Synchondrosis is primarily a growth mechanism although they also contribute to slightly more flexible skeleton in youth (resist – forces, compression, tension shear or torsion).

Examples include:

- Joints between diaphysis and epiphysis
- Neurocentral synchondrosis
- 1st costochondral joint

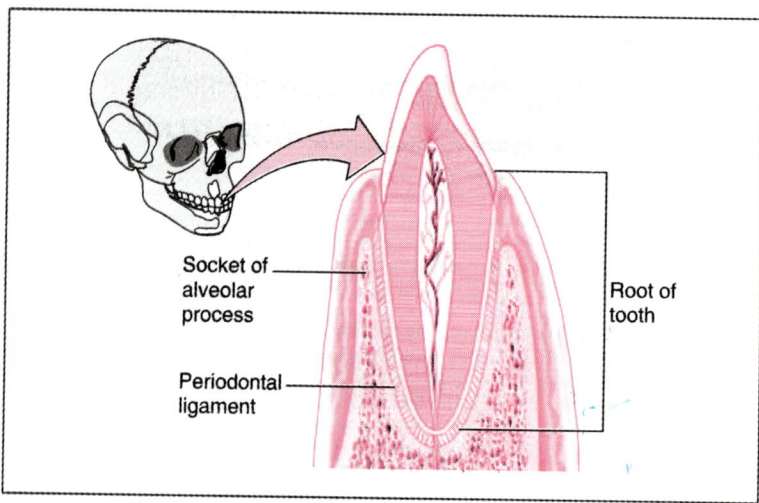

Socket of alveolar process

Root of tooth

Periodontal ligament

Fig. 6.2: Gomphosis

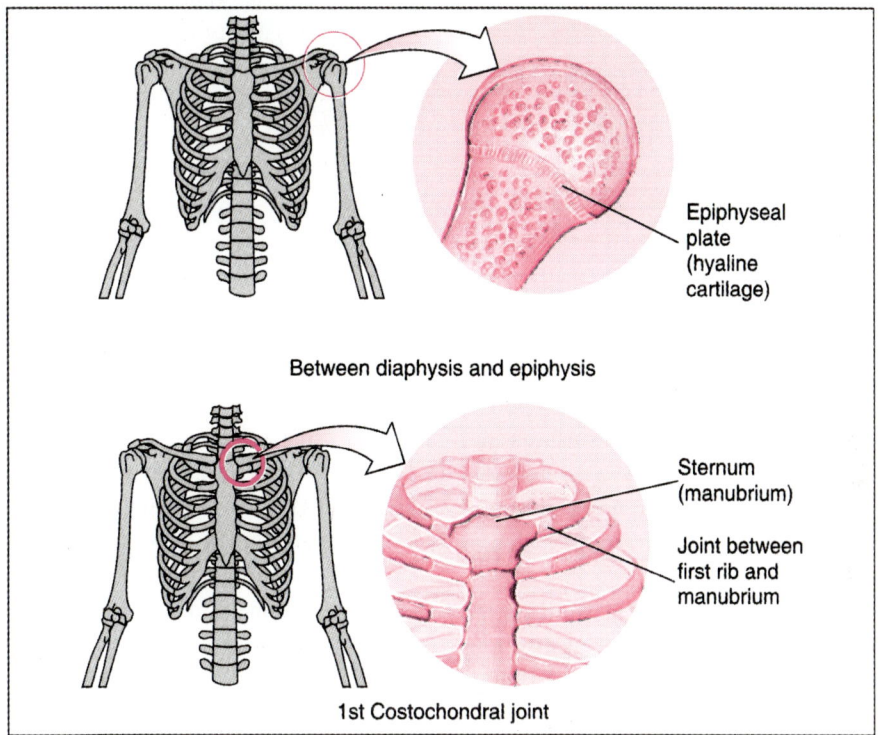

Between diaphysis and epiphysis

Epiphyseal plate (hyaline cartilage)

Sternum (manubrium)

Joint between first rib and manubrium

1st Costochondral joint

Fig. 6.3: Primary cartilaginous joint

Secondary Cartilage Joint/Symphysis/Fibro-Cartilaginous Joint

Features

1. Bone ends forming such joints are covered with a thin layer of hyaline cartilage united by an intervening layer of fibro cartilage.
2. Bones are bound together by intervening disc of fibro-cartilage.
3. Ligaments join the bones but fail to form the capsule.
4. They are permanent and persist through out life.
5. Typically seen in midline and permit limited movements due to compressible pad of fibro-cartilage.
6. Thickness of fibro-cartilage is directly proportional to range of movement.
7. These joints represent an intermediate stage in the evolution of synovial joints

Examples include:

Joints between bodies of vertebrae
Pubic symphysis

SYNOVIAL / FREELY MOVABLE / DIARTHROSES

Features

1. Most evolved and most mobile joints in the body
2. Large majority of joints come in this category
3. Bony ends are not directly connected by any tissue
4. Have smooth articular surfaces covered with hyaline or articular cartilages
5. Bones are held together by a capsule made up of fibrous tissue called fibrous or articular capsule

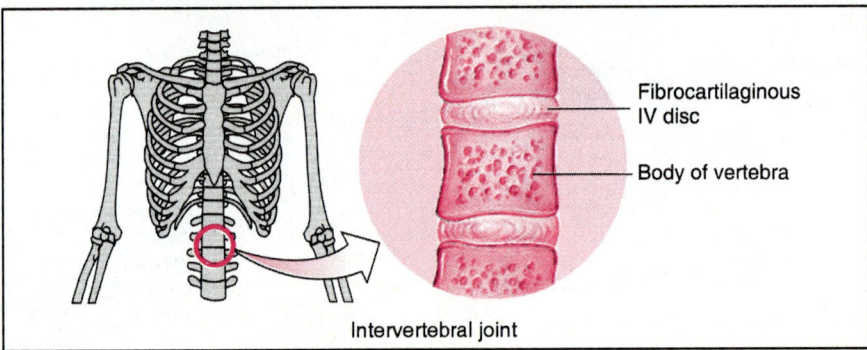

Fibrocartilaginous
IV disc

Body of vertebra

Intervertebral joint

Fig. 6.4: Secondary cartilaginous joint

6. Capsule encloses the articular surfaces in a joint cavity
7. Inside of capsule is lined by a synovial membrane which is absent over articular surfaces
8. Joint cavity is filled with a fluid called synovial fluid, serving lubricating and nutritive functions. The viscosity of fluid is due to hyaluronic acid, secreted by **A-cells** of the synovial membrane
9. Fibrous capsule is richly innervated and thus is sensitive to stretches imposed by movements
10. Fibrous capsule is reinforced by true ligaments or accessory ligaments.

True ligaments represents thickening of fibrous capsule. These may be intracapsular or extra capsule.

Accessory ligaments are placed away from the capsule.

FIBROUS CAPSULE

- Consists of parallel and interlacing bundles of white collagen fibers (connective tissue fibers) on the periphery of articular surfaces
- Perforated by articular vessels and nerves. May present one or more perforations through the synovial membrane, protrudes to form a pouch or sac (**bursae**)
- Fibrous capsule shows two or more thickenings in the constituent fiber bundles

that are generally parallel to one another. These thickenings are called capsular (intrinsic) ligaments of the joint and they are named according to their position or attachment

- In some joints, fibrous capsule is reinforced by tendons or expansions from tendons of neighboring muscles
- Due to its rich innervation, capsule is pain sensitive to stretches imposed by movements. This sets up appropriate reflexes to protect the joint from any sprain. This is known as "**watch dog action**" of capsule
- Capsule is reinforced by true and accessory ligaments

SYNOVIAL MEMBRANE

- Derived from embryonic mesoderm. Lines the interior of synovial joint:
  Capsule
  Non articular parts
  But not articular surface
- Also lines synovial bursae (pouch) and synovial tendon sheaths.
- Apposed surfaces are lubricated by a fluid (like egg albumin) that is secreted and absorbed by synovial membrane (**A cells**).
- It is pink, shiny and smooth through out.

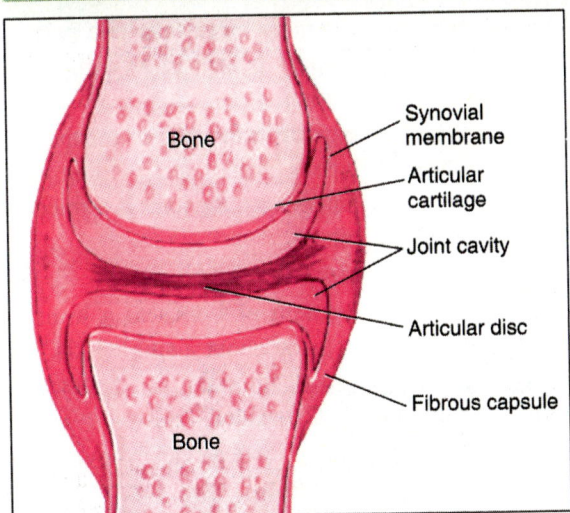

Fig. 6.5: Section of typical synovial joint

- Inner surface bears occasional small finger like projections called synovial villi which increase in size and number with age.
- This membrane is thrown into folds that projects into joint cavity (some are constant and named:
  - Alar folds
  - Ligamentum mucosum of Knee joint
- It is absent from intra-articular discs or menisci and ceases at the margins of articular cartilages peripheral few mm of which are a structural transitional zone between synovial membrane and articular cartilage.

SYNOVIAL FLUID

- It is a clear or pale yellow viscous fluid.
- It has slightly alkaline pH.
- It consists of small mixed population of cells and some amorphous metachromatic particles.
- In man, its volume is quite low. Usually less than 0.5 ml can be aspirated from a large joint

- It is present in the cavities of
  Synovial joints
  Synovial bursae
  Tendon sheaths

Functions
1. **Nutritive source** for
   - Articular cartilage
   - Disc, menisci
   - Synovial membrane
2. **Lubrication**
   - Increases efficiency.
   - Decreases friction.
   - Decreases erosion of surfaces (wear and tear).
3. **Provides** liquid environment

ARTICULAR PAD OF FAT

- Accumulation of adipose tissue occurs in the synovial membrane in many joints. Such pads are flexible, elastic and displaceable cushions occupying potential spaces and irregularities in joints that are not wholly filled with synovial fluid. During movement they accommodate to the changing shape and volume of irregularities.
- Villi and other folds increase the surface area and they promote an adequate distribution of lubricant synovial fluid over the articular surfaces.
- Villi are fewer in number in normal joints. They are more numerous where membrane rests on areolar tissue near articular marking and surfaces of folds and fringes. They increase in number as age advances and become very prominent in certain pathological conditions.

Structurally: essentially consists of
- Cellular intima, resting upon
- Vascular (fibro-vascular) sub-intimal lamina (sub synovial tissue)

Two types **A and B cells** have been recognized in synovial membrane:

Type A – predominate.

Type B – various cytoplasmic structures are poorly developed but contain glycogen deposit.

Function

Both cell types are concerned with secretion and absorption of synovial fluid and removal of other substances.

STABILITY OF SYNOVIAL JOINT

Various factors are important. It is multifactorial mechanism. These factors are

1. **Muscles**
    - Most important and indispensable factor
    - Tone of different groups of muscles acting on the joint

2. **Ligaments**
    - Important not only in stability but also in preventing any over movement
    - They also guard against sudden excessive accidental movement
    - They are not helpful against constant stress because once they are stretched; they tend to remain in elongated position

3. **Bones**
    - Important especially in firm type/secure type of joint **e.g.:** Hip joint
    - In other, they have very little to negligible role to play **e.g.:** Shoulder joint

4. **Gravity**
    - May play a role in stability of joint

CLASSIFICATION OF SYNOVIAL JOINTS

1. **Complexity of organization/form**
    - Many synovial joints possess only two articular surfaces and are termed as simple joints **e.g.:** Shoulder joint

- A joint possessing more than one pair of articular surfaces is termed as compound **e.g.:** Elbow joint
- When an intra-articular disc or menisci of fibro-cartilage is present and dividing joint into two components, the joint is termed as complex joint.

2. **Degree of freedom of joints**
    - When movement of bones at a joint is limited to rotation about a **single axis** the joint is termed as "**uniaxial**" and it possesses "one degree of freedom"
    - When completely independent movements can occur around **two axes**, joint is termed as "**biaxial**" and it possesses "two degrees of freedom".
    - When independent movements can occur around **three axes**, joint is termed as "**polyaxial**" and it possesses "three degree of freedom"

3. **Translation**
    - One articular surface slides across its partner and there may be slight element of rotation or angulation **e.g.:** Plane joint
    - Translation is also a feature of many joints in association with large angulation changes **e.g.:** Shoulder joint

GROSS MORPHOLOGICAL CLASSIFICATION OF SYNOVIAL JOINTS

A. **Plane/Gliding joints**
B. **Uniaxial**
    1. Hinge
    2. Pivot
C. **Biaxial**
    1. Condylar
    2. Ellipsoid
    3. Saddle or Seller
D. **Polyaxial / Multiaxial**
    1. Ball and socket

PLANE/GLIDING JOINTS

- Formed by fairly flat articular surfaces.
- Permit gliding movements (translation) in various directions.
- No axis in these joints.
  e.g.: Intercarpal joints, joints between articular processes of vertebrae

HINGE /GINGLYMUS JOINTS

- Uniaxial (transverse axis).
- Articular surfaces are so moulded as to largely restrict to and fro movements in one plane and generally they are pulley shaped.
- Sides of joints are typically provided with strong collateral ligaments
- Movements are around a transverse axis.
  e.g.: Elbow joint (humero-ulnar component), Interphalangeal joints.

In their profiles they are not arcs by varyingly spiral therefore the main to and fro swing includes some conjunct rotation.

Rotation is of two types

Conjunct - an integral and inevitable accompaniment of the main movement.

Adjunct - can occur independently and may or may not accompany the principal movement.

PIVOT / TROCHOID JOINTS

- Uniaxial (longitudinal axis).
- Comprises a central bony pivot surrounded by an osteoligamentous ring.
- Movement is restricted to rotation around a longitudinal axis, passing through centre of pivot.
- Pivot may rotate with in the ring e.g., Radio-ulnar joints.
- Ring may rotate around the pivot e.g., Middle atlanto-axial joint.

CONDYLAR JOINT

- Articular surfaces include condyle shaped articular surface (male surfaces) fitting into reciprocally concave female surface some times called condyles.
- Generally uniaxial in nature, having principal movements occurring largely in one plane, but in addition, limited amount of rotation is possible about a second axis - orthogonal (set at 90^0) to the first or principal axis.
- Movements mainly around a transverse axis, but rotation can occur around the vertical axis.
  e.g.: Knee joint -condyles almost parallel within a common fibrous capsule.
  Temporo-mandibular joint - condyles well apart in separate capsules.

ELLIPSOID JOINT

- Biaxial in nature.
- Formed by the reception of an oval convex male surface into an elliptical female concavity.
- Primary movements are possible in two axes set at right angle. (Flexion/Extension and Adduction/Abduction).
- Combination produces circumduction
  e.g.: Wrist joint (Radio-carpal joint)
  Atlanto-occipital joint

SADDLE / SELLAR JOINT

- Biaxial in nature, but for all practical purposes, considered as polyaxial joint.
- Opposing articular surfaces are concavo-convex.
- In articulated joint, convexity of larger (male) surface is opposed to concavity of smaller (female) surface and vice versa.

- Primary movements occur in two planes set at right angles but because of their articular geometry, these are accompanied by rotation. Such "**conjunct rotation**" can not occur independently but they must not be regarded as simply a by product of imperfect mechanics. It is functionally important in habitual positioning and limitation of movement. **e.g.:**
  – 1st carpo-metacarpal joint (Thumb joint)
  – Calcaneo-cuboid joint

BALL AND SOCKET / SPHEROIDAL JOINT

- Multiaxial in nature, having three degree of freedom.
- Formed by the reception of globular head (male surface) in to a cup shaped socket (female surface).
- Movements occur around a number of axes independently, that have a common center e.g. all axes passing through a common center.
- Flexion / extension, adduction / abduction, medial / lateral rotations and circumduction occur quite freely.
- Their surfaces, though resembling parts of spheres are not strictly spherical but slightly avoid. Consequently in most positions congruence is not perfect but occurs only in one position at the end of the commonest movement.
  Examples include:
  – Shoulder joint and hip joint

BLOOD SUPPLY

- From a peri-articular arterial plexus formed by articular and epiphyseal branches.
- Numerous branches from this plexus perforate the fibrous capsule and form a rich vascular plexus in deeper parts of synovial membrane.

- Blood vessels of synovial membrane terminate around articular margins in looped anastomoses known as circulus articularis vasculosus (**circularis vasculosus**).
- This plexus supplies capsule, synovial membrane and epiphyses.
- Articular cartilage is avascular.
- After epiphyseal fusion communication between circulus vasculosus and end arteries of metaphysis is established. Thus chances of osteomyelitis in metaphysis are minimized.

NERVE SUPPLY

- Capsule and ligaments have rich nerve supply thus sensitive to pain.
- Synovial membrane has poor nerve supply.
- Articular cartilage is non nervous and insensitive to pain.
- Articular nerves contain sensory and autonomic fibers.
- Some sensory fibers are proprioceptive in nature and these are sensitive to position and movement. They are concerned with reflex control of posture and locomotion.
- Other sensory fibers are sensitive to pain.
- Autonomic fibers are vasomotor or vasosensory.

HILTON'S LAW

It states that a motor nerve to the muscle acting on joint tends to give a branch to that joint and another branch to the skin covering the joint. This concept was further elucidated by Gardner (1948) and accordingly each nerve innervates a specific region of the capsule and that the part of the capsule that is rendered taut by a given muscle is innervated by the nerve supplying its antagonists. Thus, the pattern of innervation is concerned with the maintenance of an efficient stability at the joint.

CLINICAL CONSIDERATIONS

Dislocation

Articular surfaces are abnormally displaced, so that one surface loses its contact completely from the other. If partial contact is still retained it is termed as subluxation, caused by trauma. Commonly seen features are:

- Pain and swelling
- Deformity
- Loss of function

Sprain

In this condition there is severe pain in the joint caused by ligamentous tear without any dislocation or fracture. Tear leads to effusion into the joint, causing severe pain. Movements at the joint are restricted.

Neuropathic joint

Due to complete dennervation so that all reflexes are eliminated.

Joint is left unprotected and liable to mechanical damage.

The affected joint shows:

- Painless swelling
- Excessive mobility
- Destruction

This is caused by:

- Leprosy
- Tabes dorsalis
- Syringomyelia

Bursitis

An inflammation of a bursa, usually caused by a blow or friction

Symptoms are pain and swelling

Treated with anti-inflammatory drugs; excessive fluid may be aspirated

Tendonitis

Inflammation of tendon sheaths typically caused by overuse

Symptoms and treatment are similar to bursitis

Arthritis

Inflammation of a joint is termed as arthritis.

Common causes include:

- Rheumatic
- Rheumatoid
- Osteo-arthritis
- Tuberculous

Involved joint is

- Swollen
- Movement are restricted and painful

7

Nervous System

It is a system which:
- Controls and co-ordinates whole body
- Controls all voluntary and involuntary activities of body
- Adjusts the body to the surrounding

To meet these requirements, the nervous system should have specialized tissue with properties of:
- Sensitivity
- Conductivity
- Responsivity

Nervous system is divided into:

A. CENTRAL NERVOUS SYSTEM
- Consists of **Brain** which lies within the skull and **Spinal cord** lies within vertebral canal
- Surrounded by 3 layers /meninges – Pia, Arachnoid and Dura mater (from inside out)

B. PERIPHERAL NERVOUS SYSTEM

Divided into:
1. **Cerebrospinal nervous system** with:
   - Cranial nerves (12 pairs)
   - Spinal nerves (31 pairs)
2. **Autonomic nervous system with sympathetic and parasympathetic components**
   - Includes splanchnic nerves innervating viscera, glands, blood vessels and smooth muscles

- These nerves are connected to CNS by somatic nerves.

CELLS OF NERVOUS SYSTEM

Two types
- Excitable cells
- Non excitable cells

NEURON

These are excitable cells and consists of cell body and processes
- **Afferent**: Dendrites
- **Efferent**: Axon

Structural classification

1. **Multipolar**
   - Possess more than two processes
   - Numerous dendrites and one axon
2. **Bipolar**
   - Possess two processes
   - Rare neurons – found in some special sensory organs
3. **Unipolar (pseudounipolar)**
   - Possess one short, single process
   - Start as bipolar neurons during development

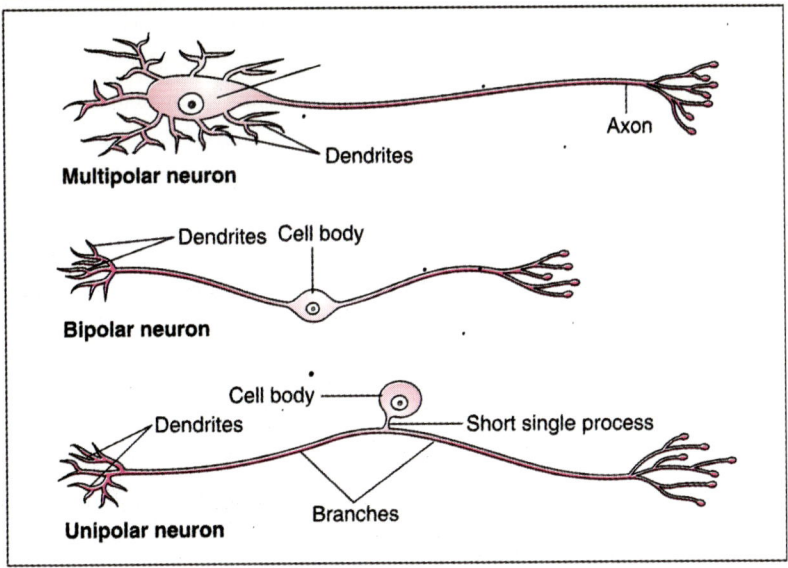

Fig. 7.1: Structural classification of neurons

According to the direction the nerve impulse travels

1. **Sensory (afferent) neurons:** Transmit impulses toward the CNS
   - Virtually all are **unipolar** neurons
   - Cell bodies are located in the ganglia outside the CNS
   - Short, single process divides into:

   Central process – runs centrally into the CNS

   Peripheral process – extends peripherally to the receptors

2. **Motor (efferent) neurons**
   - Carry impulses away from the CNS to effector organs.
   - Most motor neurons are multipolar.
   - Cell bodies are situated within the CNS.
   - Form junctions with effector cells.
   - Interneurons (**association neurons**) – most are multipolar which lie between motor and sensory neurons.
   - Confined to central nervous system.

   According to the length of axon

   Golgi type 1 - have long axon

   Golgi type 2 - have short axon

Non excitable cells: Supporting cells

Six types of supporting cells

Four in the CNS

Two in the PNS
   - Provide supportive functions for neurons
   - Cover non synaptic regions of the neurons

Types of neuroglial cells

1. **ASTROCYTES**
   - Most abundant glial cell type
   - Take up and release ions to control the environment around neurons
   - Recapture and recycle neurotransmitters

2. **MICROGLIA**
   - Smallest and least abundant
   - Phagocytes – the macrophages of the CNS
   - Engulf invading microorganisms and dead neurons
   - Derived from blood cells called monocytes

3. **EPENDYMAL CELLS**
   - Line the central cavity of the spinal cord and brain

- Bear cilia which to help circulate the cerebrospinal fluid

4. OLIGODENDROCYTES
- Have few branches
- Wrap their cell processes around axons in CNS.
- Produce myelin sheaths

5. SATELLITE CELLS
- Surround neuron cell bodies within ganglia

6. SCHWANN CELLS (Neurolemmocytes)
- Surround axons in the PNS.
- Form myelin sheath around axons of the PNS

Myelin sheath

It is a whitish, fatty segmented sheath around most long axons; surrounds thicker axons.

Functions:
1. Form an insulating layer.
2. Prevent leakage of electrical current.
3. Increase the speed of impulse conduction.

Myelin sheath in PNS
- Formed by Schwann cells.
- Develop during fetal period and in the first year of postnatal life.
- Schwann cells wrap in concentric layers around the axon and cover the axon in a tightly packed coil of membranes.
- **Neurilemma** – material external to myelin layers.

Functions of Supporting Cells
1. Mechanical support to neurons
2. Acts as insulator between neurons
3. Phagocytic function
4. Repair function by gliosis – proliferation
5. Myelination by oligodendrocytes
6. Maintains metabolic and ionic environment
7. Exchanges of material between brain and CSF by ependymal cells

REFLEX ARC

It is the basic functional unit of neuron by which an integrated neural activity can be performed.

It has five basic components:
1. **Receptor** – Site where stimulus acts
2. **Sensory neuron** – Transmits afferent impulses to the CNS
3. **Integration center** – Consists of one or more synapses in the CNS
4. **Motor neuron** – Conducts efferent impulses from integration center to an effector
5. **Effector** – muscle or gland cell which responds to efferent impulses by contracting or secreting

Types of Reflexes
1. **Monosynaptic reflex** – simplest of all reflexes
   - Just one synapse

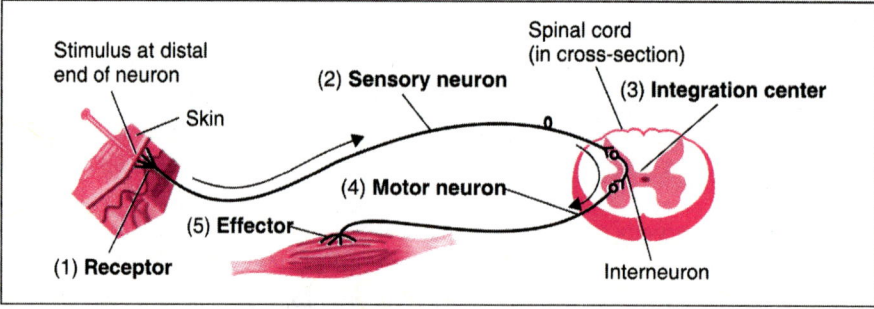

Fig. 7.2: Components of Reflex Arc

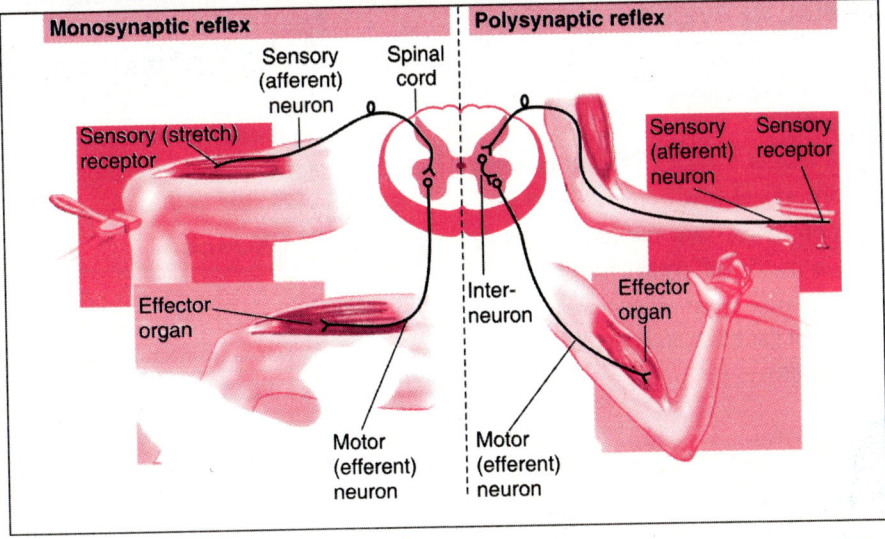

Fig. 7.3: Types of reflexes

- The fastest of all reflexes
  Example – knee-jerk reflex
2. **Polysynaptic reflex** – more common type of reflex
   - Most have a single interneuron between the sensory and motor neuron
     Example – withdrawal reflexes

SPINAL CORD

- Extension of the medulla oblongata of the brain.
- Long and nearly cylindrical.
- Placed in the vertebral canal.
- Extends from the foramen magnum at the base of the skull to the lower border of L-2 vertebra. Until the third month of foetal life, the cord occupies the entire length of the vertebral canal. Thereafter, the canal growth exceeds that of the cord. By the sixth month of foetal month, the caudal end of the cord reaches the upper margin of sacrum. At birth it is at the level of the L-3 vertebra.
- Adult cord is approximately 1 cm in diameter with an average length of 45 cm.
- Conducts sensory and motor impulses to and from the brain and controls many reflexes.
- Thirty-one spinal nerves originate from the cord: **8 Cervical, 12 Thoracic, 5 Lumbar, 5 Sacral** and **1 Coccygeal**.
- Enclosed by three protective membranes called meninges: **Dura mater, Arachnoid** and **Pia mater**.
- Develops from the ectoderm - caudal portion of the embryonic neural plate.
- **Cut section** shows internal **Grey matter** – 'H' shaped having dorsal horn and ventral horn – contains cell bodies of neurons. **White matter** – surrounds grey matter and contains processes of neurons.

Conus medullaris – Terminal portion of the spinal cord

Filum terminale – Fibrous extension of the pia mater which anchors the spinal cord to the coccyx

Denticulate ligaments – Delicate sleeves of pia mater which attach the spinal cord to the vertebrae

Cauda equina – Collection of nerve roots at the inferior end of the vertebral canal

ROOTS OF SPINAL NERVES

- Each spinal nerve connects to the spinal cord via two roots
- Each root forms a series of rootlets that attach to the spinal cord
- Ventral roots arise from the anterior horn and contain motor (**efferent**) fibres
- Dorsal roots arise from sensory neurons in the dorsal root ganglion and contain sensory (**afferent**) fibres

Dorsal root:

- Attached dorsal at on each side
- Contains sensory fibers
- Presence of ganglion – cell bodies of sensory neurons

Ventral root:

- **Sympathetic system**
- **Parasympathetic system**
- Contains motor fibers
- No ganglion, cell bodies of motor neurons in ventral horn.

At the intervertebral foramen, dorsal and ventral roots unite to form a mixed spinal nerve, which then gets distributed to various body structures.

SPINAL NERVES

Thirty-one pairs of mixed nerves arise from the spinal cord and supply all parts of the body except the head.

They are named according to their point of issue

8 cervical (C-1 to C-8)
12 thoracic (T-1 to T-12)
5 Lumbar (L-1 to L-5)
5 Sacral (S-1 to S-5)
1 Coccygeal (Co)

Rami of spinal nerves

The short spinal nerves branch into three or four mixed rami:

- Small dorsal ramus
- Larger ventral ramus
- Small meningeal branch
- Rami **communicantes** at the base of the ventral rami in the thoracic region

NERVE PLEXUSES

- All ventral rami **except T-2 to T-12** form interlacing nerve networks called *plexuses*
- Plexuses are found in the **Cervical**, **Brachial**, **Lumbar** and **Sacral** regions.
- Each resulting branch of a plexus contains fibers from several spinal nerves.
- Fibers travel to the periphery via several different routes.
- Each muscle receives a nerve supply from more than one spinal nerve.
- Therefore damage to one spinal segment cannot completely paralyze a muscle.

DERMATOMES

Dermatome is the area of skin innervated by the cutaneous branches of a single spinal nerve
All spinal nerves except C-1 participate in dermatomes

STRETCH REFLEX

- Stretching the muscle activates the muscle spindle.
- Excited γ motor neurons of the spindle cause the stretched muscle to contract.
- Afferent impulses from the spindle result in inhibition of the antagonist.
  Example: patellar reflex
- Tapping the patellar tendon stretches the quadriceps and starts the reflex action
- The quadriceps contract and the antagonistic hamstrings relax

8

Autonomic Nervous System

- Motor part of ANS is concerned with innervations of cardiac and smooth muscles and glands. It differs from somatic system in that the pathway from nerve cells in the CNS to the target organ is interrupted in a ganglion. The pre-ganglionic cell bodies are always within the CNS.

- In sympathetic system they are in lateral horn cells of all thoracic and upper two lumber spinal segments (thoraco-lumber outflow). The post ganglionic cell bodies are situated in the ganglia in PNS.

- In parasympathetic system the ganglia are either in sympathetic trunk or within the walls of the viscera. In the case of certain system in head and neck structures, four ganglia are situated a little away from the structures innervated. This system controls involuntary activities of the body – gut motility. It consists of

- Pre-ganglionic fibers
- Ganglia for relay
- Post-ganglionic fibers

AUTONOMIC SYSTEM IS DIVIDED INTO

Sympathetic component

Parasympathetic component

These systems present ganglia – sites of synapses of neurons. These are preganglionic fibers and postganglionic fibers. Cell bodies of postganglionic fibers lie in the ganglion.

SYMPATHETIC NERVOUS SYSTEM

The **Sympathetic trunk** extends from base of skull to coccyx. Theoretically there is one ganglion for each spinal nerve but fusion occurs, thus:

Division	Origin of Fibers	Length of Fibers	Location of Ganglia
Sympathetic	Thoracolumbar region of the spinal Cord	Short preganglionic and long postganglionic	Close to the spinal cord
Parasympathetic	Brain and spinal cord	Long preganglionic and short postganglionic	In the visceral effect or organs

53

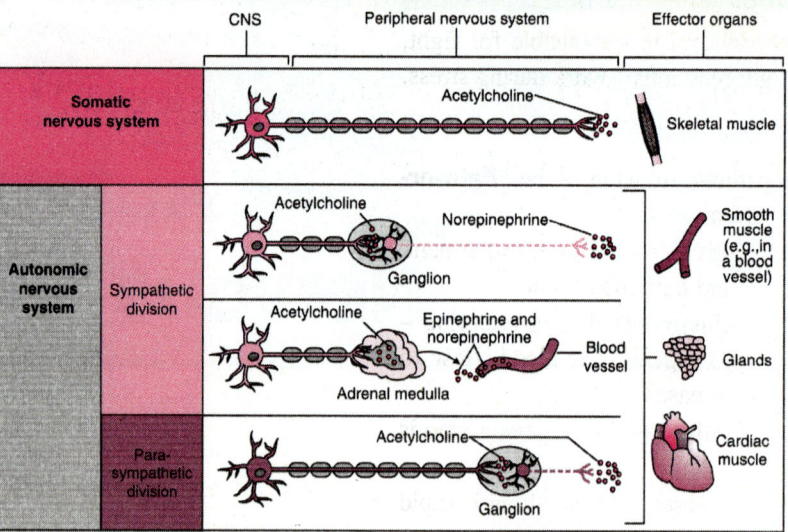

Fig. 8.1: Nervous system and its divisions

Cervical region:

- Superior cervical ganglion (Fusion of C-1 to C-4)
- Middle cervical ganglion (Fusion of C-5 and C-6)
- Inferior cervical ganglion (fusion of C-7 to T-1)

Thoracic region – 11

Lumbar region – 4

Sacral region – 4

- Each sympathetic trunk ganglia has a visceral branch called splanchnic nerve in thoracic lumbar and sacral region and cardiac branch in cervical region. Cardiac branches descend to the cardiac plexus which is supplemented by fibers from upper thoracic ganglia.
- From lower thoracic ganglia splanchnic nerves pierce diaphragm to reach the coeliac plexus.
- Upper lumber splanchnic nerves reach superior hypogastric plexus and this divides to enter the right and left inferior hypogastric plexuses. They are joined by sacral splanchnicus. These plexuses are joined by parasympathetic nerves.

- Preganglionic fibers – cell – bodies in lateral horn (intermediate column) of spinal cord from T-1to L-2 or L-3 to form **Thoraco lumbar outflow.**
- Ganglia from two chains - one on either side of vertebral column called sympathetic chain / trunk.
- Preganglionic fibers are short while post ganglionic fibers are long
- Post ganglionic fibers pass through spinal nerves.
- Supply blood vessels, sweat glands and arrector pilorum muscle of skin. Some preganglionic fibers form **splanchnic nerves** which synapse on distant ganglia called collateral ganglia or terminal ganglia and supply the viscera.
- Sympathetic fibers use adrenaline and noradrenaline as their neurotransmitters (**adrenergic**) except postganglionic fibers supplying sweat glands and blood vessels of skeletal muscle (**cholinergic**)

- Symptoms system is responsible for fight, flight, fright reactions – work during stress.

Role of sympathetic activity

1. The sympathetic division is the "**fight-or-flight**" system
2. Involves **E** activities – exercise, excitement, emergency, and embarrassment
3. Promotes adjustments during exercise – blood flow to organs is reduced, flow to muscles is increased
4. Its activity is illustrated by a person who is threatened
5. Heart rate increases, and breathing is rapid and deep
6. The skin is cold and sweaty, and the pupils dilate

PARASYMPATHETIC NERVOUS SYSTEM

- Preganglionic fibers – cell bodies in cranial nerve nuclei or in lateral horn of spinal cord from S-2, 3, 4 segments to form **cranio-sacral out flow.**
- Nuclei of IIIrd, VIIth, IXth and Xth cranial nerves are associated with parasympathetic ganglia. These are **Ciliary**, **Pterygo-palatine**, **Otic** and **Submandibular** ganglia.
- The pre-ganglionic fibers of cranial origin of these ganglia have their cell bodies in:
  Edinger Westphal nucleus (**III CN**)
  Superior slivatory nucleus (**VII CN**)
  Lacrimatory nucleus (**VII CN**)
  Inferior slivatory nucleus (**IX CN**)
  Dorsal nucleus of Vagus (**X CN**)
- Postganglionic cells lie in:
  Ciliary ganglion
  Pterygopalatine ganglion
  Otic ganglion
  Submandibular ganglion

- The pre-ganglionic fibers of sacral origin arise from **S-2, 3, 4** and constitute **pelvic splanchnic nerves**. These join the inferior hypogastric plexuses. From here they supply the pelvic viscera and hindgut.
- These parasympathetic ganglia lie nearer to the viscera or gland they supply.
- Preganglionic fibers are long and postganglionic fibers are short.
- Parasympathetic fibers use acetylcholine as their neurotransmitter (**cholinergic**)
- "All the smooth muscles in the body except those of blood vessels and all the glands except sweat glands are supplied by parasympathetic nervous system."
- Parasympathetic system is responsible for anabolic (building up) activities – digestion, absorption, conservation of energy, and facilitates acts of micturition, defecation and sexual function.

Role of Parasympathetic activity

1. Concerned with keeping body energy use low
2. Involves the **D** activities – digestion, defecation, and diuresis

Its activity is illustrated in a person who relaxes after a meal

- Blood pressure, heart rate, and respiratory rates are low
- Gastrointestinal tract activity is high
- The skin is warm and the pupils are constricted

VISCERAL REFLEXES

- These reflexes have the same elements as somatic reflexes
- They are always polysynaptic pathways
- Afferent fibers are found in spinal and autonomic nerves

Cranial outflow	Cranial Nerve	Ganglion	Effector Organ(s)
	Oculomotor (III)	Ciliary	Eye
	Facial (VII)	Pterygopalatine Submandibular	Salivary, nasal, and lacrimal glands
	Glossopharyngeal (IX)	Otic	Parotidsalivary glands
	Vagus (X)	Located within the walls of target organs	Heart, lungs, and most visceral organs
Sacral outflow	S_2-S_4	Located within the walls of the target	Large intestine, urinary bladder, ureters, and reproductive organs

REFERRED PAIN

- Pain arising from the viscera but is perceived as somatic in origin
- This may be due to the fact that visceral pain afferents travel along the same pathways as somatic pain fibres

AUTONOMIC NERVOUS SYSTEM CONTROL

- The hypothalamus is the main integration center of ANS activity
- Subconscious cerebral input via limbic lobe connections influences hypothalamic function
- Other controls come from the cerebral cortex, the reticular formation, and the spinal cord

9

Cranial Nerves

- Twelve pairs of cranial nerves arise from the brain.
- They have sensory, motor or both sensory and motor functions.
- Each nerve is identified by a number (I through XII) and a name.
- Four cranial nerves carry parasympathetic fibers that supply muscles and glands in the head and neck region.

CRANIAL NERVES

Arise from ventral aspect of brain except **4th—Trochlear** which arises from dorsal aspect of the brain.

A functional aspect of cranial nerves is as under:

1st **Olfactory** – Sense of smell.

2nd **Optic** – Sense of vision.

3rd **Oculomotor** – Extra ocular muscles of eye ball.

4th **Trochlear** – Extra-ocular muscle of eye ball.

5th **Trigeminal** – Muscles of mastication and sensory to face and scalp.

6th **Abducent** – Extra-ocular muscle of eye ball.

7th **Facial** – Muscles of facial expression.

8th **Vestibulocochlear** – sense of hearing and balance and equilibrium.

9th **Glossopharyngeal** – Sensations from oral cavity, face, Larynx

10th **Vagus** – Movements of pharynx and larynx

11th **Accessory** – Parasympathetic control of CVS, respiratory system and gut

12th **Hypoglossal** – Muscles of tongue

OLFACTORY NERVE

- Arises from the olfactory epithelium.
- Passes through the cribriform plate of the ethmoid bone.
- Fibers run through the olfactory bulb and terminate in the primary olfactory cortex.
- Functions solely by carrying **afferent impulses for the sense of smell**.

OPTIC NERVE

- Arises from the retina of the eye.
- Optic nerves pass through the optic canals and converge at the optic chiasm.
- They continue to the thalamus where they synapse.
- From there, the optic radiation fibers run to the visual cortex.
- Functions solely by carrying **afferent impulses for vision**.

OCULOMOTOR NERVE

- Fibers extend from the ventral midbrain, pass through the superior orbital fissure, and supply **extrinsic muscles of eye ball**.
- **Functions** in raising the eyelid, directing the eyeball, constricting the iris and controlling lens shape.

TROCHLEAR NERVE

- Fibers emerge from the dorsal midbrain and enter the orbits via the superior orbital fissures.
- Innervate the superior oblique muscle.
- Primarily a motor nerve that directs the eyeball.

TRIGEMINAL NERVE

- Composed of three divisions: **Ophthalmic** (V-1), **Maxillary** (V-2) and **Mandibular** nerve (V-3).
- Fibers run from the face to the pons via the superior orbital fissure (V-1), the foramen rotundum (V-2) and the foramen ovale (V-3).
- Conveys sensory impulses from various areas of the face (V-1) and (V-2) and supplies motor fibers (V-3) for mastication.

ABDUCENT NERVE

- Fibers after leaving the inferior pons enter the orbit via the superior orbital fissure.
- Primarily a **motor nerve** innervating the **Lateral Rectus** muscle.

FACIAL NERVE

- Fibers leave the pons and travel through the internal acoustic meatus.
- Emerges through the stylomastoid foramen.
- **Mixed nerve** with five major branches.
- **Motor functions** include facial expression, and the transmittal of autonomic impulses to lacrimal and salivary glands
- **Sensory function** is to carry taste sensations from the anterior two-thirds of the tongue.

VESTIBULO-COCHLEAR NERVE

- Fibers arise from the hearing and equilibrium apparatus of the inner ear and pass through the internal acoustic meatus.
- Enter the brainstem at the junction of pons and medulla.
- **Two divisions** : Cochlear (hearing) and Vestibular (balance)
- **Functions** are solely sensory for the sense of **equilibrium** and of **hearing**.

GLOSSOPHARYNGEAL NERVE

- Fibers emerge from the medulla and leave the skull via the jugular foramen.
- Distributed in the neck.
- Nerve IX is a mixed nerve with **motor and sensory functions**.
- **Motor**: innervates part of the tongue and pharynx, and provides secreto-motor fibers to the parotid salivary gland.
- **Sensory**: carries taste and general sensory impulses from the tongue and pharynx.

VAGUS NERVE

- The only cranial nerve that extends beyond the head and neck.
- Fibers emerge from the medulla and leave via the jugular foramen.
- The vagus is a mixed nerve.
- Most **motor fibers are parasympathetic** fibers to the heart, lungs, and visceral organs

- **Sensory function** is to carry taste sensations from posterior most part of the tongue.

ACCESSORY NERVE

- Formed from two roots: **Cranial root** emerging from the medulla and a **Spinal root** arising from the upper cervical segments of the spinal cord.
- Spinal root passes upward into the cranium via the foramen magnum.
- Accessory nerve leaves the cranium via the jugular foramen.
- Primarily a **motor nerve** supplying:
  - Larynx, pharynx and soft palate
  - Innervates the **Trapezius** and **Sternocleidomastoid**

HYPOGLOSSAL NERVE

- Fibers arise from the medulla and exit the skull via the hypoglossal canal
- Innervates both **extrinsic and intrinsic muscles of the tongue**

TERMS USED IN CLINICAL NEUROANATOMY

- **Adiadochokinesia.** Inability to perform rapidly alternating movements.
- **Agnosia.** Lack of ability to recognize the significance of sensory stimuli which may be auditory, visual, tactile, etc.
- **Agraphia.** Inability to express thoughts in writing due to a central lesion.
- **Alexia.** Loss of power to grasp the meaning of written or printed words and sentences.
- **Anopsia.** A defect of vision.
- **Aphasia.** A defect of the power of expression by speech or of comprehending spoken or written language.
- **Apraxia.** Inability to carry out purposeful movements in the absence of paralysis.
- **Astereognosis.** Loss of ability to recognize objects or to appreciate their form by touching or feeling them.
- **Asynergy.** Disturbance of the proper association in the contraction of muscles that ensures that the different components of an act follow in proper sequence, at the proper moment, and or the proper degree, so that the act is executed accurately.
- **Ataxia.** A loss of power of muscle coordination, with irregularity of muscle action.
- **Athetosis.** Degenerative changes in the corpus striatum and cerebral cortex which is characterized by bizarre, writhing movements of the fingers and toes.
- **Bradykinesis.** Abnormal slowness of movements.
- **Brain stem.** Denotes the medulla, pons and midbrain.
- **Cauda equina.** The lumbar and sacral spinal nerve roots in the lower part of the spinal canal.
- **Cerebellum.** A large part of the brain with motor functions, situated in the posterior cranial fossa.
- **Cerebrum.** The principal portion of the brain. including the diencepabalon and the cerebral hemispheres.
- **Chordotomy.** Division of the spinothalamic tract for intractable pain (tractotomy).
- **Chorea.** A disorder characterized by irregular, spasmodic, involuntary movements of the limbs or facial muscles. This is due to degenerative changes in the neo-striatum.
- **Cortex.** Outer layer of gray matter of the cerebral hemispheres and cerebellum
- **Diencephalon.** Consist of the thalamus, epithalamus, sub thalamus and hypothalamus.
- **Diplopia.** Double vision.

- **Dyskinesia.** Abnormality of the motor function, characterized by involuntary and purposeless movements.
- **Dysmetria.** Disturbance of the power to control the range of movement in muscular action.
- **Engram.** Used in psychology to mean the lasting trace left in the psyche by previous experience(a latent memory picture)
- **Ganglion.** A swelling composed of nerve cells. Also used for certain regions of gray matter in the brain e.g. basal ganglia of the cerebral hemisphere.
- **Hemiballismus.** A violent form of motor restlessness involving one side of the body, caused by destructive lesion involving the sub thalamic nuclei.
- **Hemiplegia.** Paralysis of one side of the body.
- **Homeostasis.** A tendency toward stability in the internal environment of the body.
- **Hydrocephalus.** Excessive accumulation of cerebrospinal fluid.
- **Hyperacusis.** Abnormal loudness of perceived sounds.
- **Interoceptor.** One of the many sensory end organs within viscera.
- **Kinesthesia.** The sense of perception of movement.
- **Macrosmatic.** Acutely developed sense of smell.
- **Microsmatic.** Having a sense of smell, but of relatively poor development
- **Mimetic.** The muscles of facial expression. Supplied by the facial nerve. Sometimes referred to as mimetic muscles.
- **Neurobiotaxis.** Pertaining to memory.
- **Neuroglia.** Accessory or interstitial cells of the central nervous system; includes astrocytes, oligodendrocytes, microglial cells and ependymal cells.

- **Neuron.** The morphological unit of the nervous system, consisting of the nerve cell body and its processes (dendrites and axon).
- **Nociceptive.** Responsive to injuries stimuli.
- **Nystagmus.** An involuntary oscillatory movement of the eye.
- **Paralysis.** Loss of voluntary action.
- **Paraplegia.** Paralysis of both legs and lower part of trunk.
- **Paresis.** Partial paralysis.
- **Pneumoencephalography.** The cerebrospinal fluid is replaced by air, followed by X-ray visualization of the ventricles and subarachnoid space. This technique has been replaced by CT scan.
- **Proprioceptor.** One of the sensory endings in muscles, tendons, and joints; provides information concerning movement and position of body parts (proprioception).
- **Ptosis.** Drooping of the upper eyelid.
- **Quadriplegia.** Paralysis affecting all four limbs.
- **Somatic.** Used denote the body, exclusive of the viscera.
- **Somesthetic.** The consciousness of having a body. Somesthetic sensations are the general senses of pain, temperature, touch, pressure, position, movement and vibration.
- **Strabismus.** A constant lack of parallelism of the visual axes of the eyes (Squint)
- **Synapse.** The site of contact between neurons, at which site one neuron is excited or inhibited by another neuron.
- **Syringomyelia.** A condition characterized by central cavitation of the spinal cord and gliosis around the cavity.
- **Tetraplegia.** Paralysis affecting the four limbs. Also called quadriplegia.
- **Tomography.** Sectional roentgenography. Computerlsed tomography (CT scan) is a valuable diagnostic technique.

10

Cardiovascular System

Cardiovascular system is a transport system of body supplying nutrients to all tissues and carrying metabolites to excretory organs through a liquid medium called blood.

Features

- Closed system of tubes
- Lined from inside by endothelium

COMPONENTS

HEART

- Muscular organ which pumps blood into arteries
- Four chambered organ consisting of two receiving chambers (**atria**) and two pumping chambers (**ventricles**)
- Left side carries oxygenated blood
- Right side carries deoxygenated blood

ARTERIES

- Distributing channels
- Carry blood away from heart
- Carry oxygenated blood (**except pulmonary artery**)
- Show branching like a tree

- Have 3 coats: from inside out these are
  - Tunica intima - Endothelium
  - Tunica media - Muscle coat
  - Tunica externa - Fibrous coat

Muscular arteries –deliver blood to body organs – distributing vessels.

- Diameters range from 1 cm to 0.3 mm.
- Includes most of the named arteries.
- Thick tunica media with more smooth muscle and less elastic tissue
- Active in vasoconstriction
- Unique features include: internal and external elastic laminae

ARTERIOLES

- Smallest arteries just visible to naked eye
- Muscle coat is thick
- Break up to form capillaries
- Larger arterioles possess all three tunics
- Diameters range from 0.3 mm to 10 μm
- Diameter of arterioles is controlled by:
  - Local factors in the tissues
  - Sympathetic nervous system
  Lead to capillary beds
  - Control flow into capillary beds via vasodilatation and constriction

CAPILLARIES

- Capillaries are the smallest blood vessels.
  - Diameter from 8–10 μm
  - Walls consisting of a thin tunica interna, one cell thick
  - Allow only a single RBC to pass at a time (single file)
  - Pericytes on the outer surface stabilize their walls
- Connect arteries to veins through venules.
- Form anatomosing network.
- Allow exchanges (metabolites, tissue fluid etc.)
- Site-specific functions of capillaries

In the lungs – Oxygen enters blood, carbon dioxide leaves

In the small intestines – Receive digested nutrients

In endocrine glands – Pick up hormones

In the kidneys – Removal of nitrogenous wastes

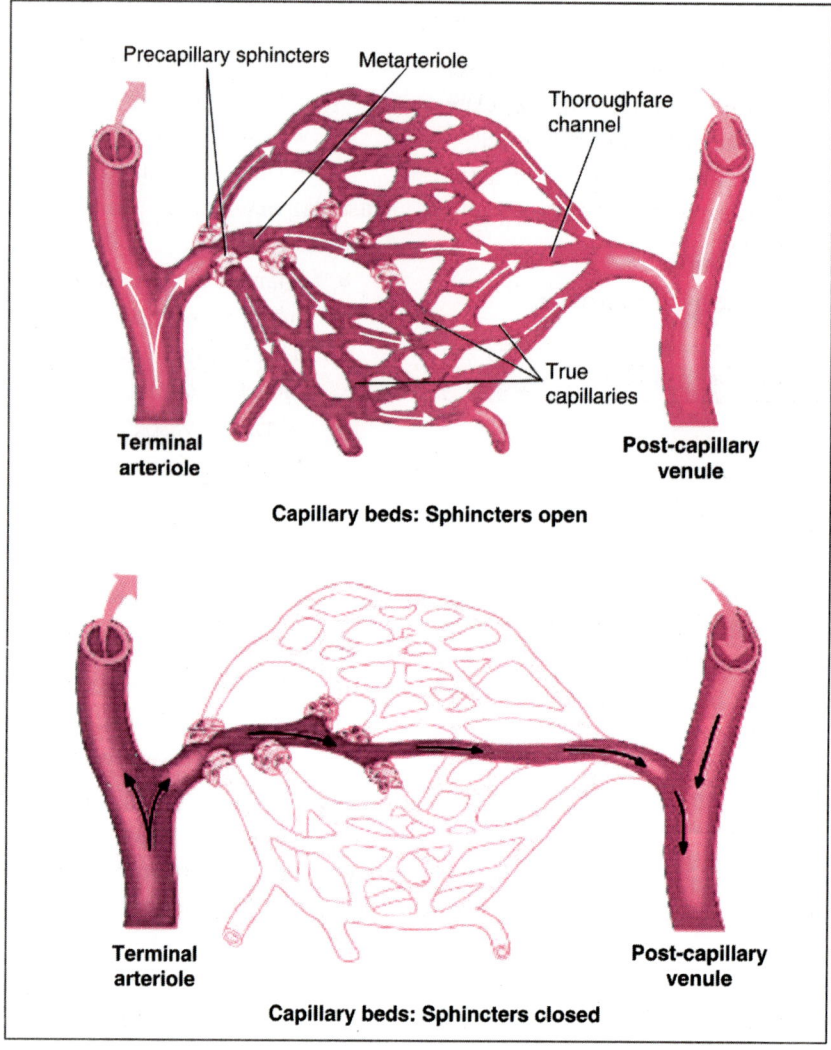

Precapillary sphincters   Metarteriole
Thoroughfare channel
True capillaries
Terminal arteriole
Post-capillary venule
Capillary beds: Sphincters open

Terminal arteriole
Post-capillary venule
Capillary beds: Sphincters closed

Fig. 10.1:

CAPILLARY BEDS

A microcirculation of interwoven networks of capillaries, consisting of:

Vascular shunts – metarteriole are thoroughfare channel connecting an arteriole directly with a post capillary venule.

True capillaries – 10 to 100 per capillary bed, capillaries branch off the metarteriole and return to the thoroughfare channel at the distal end of the bed.

BLOOD FLOW THROUGH CAPILLARY BEDS

Precapillary sphincter forms cuff of smooth muscle that surrounds each true capillary. This regulates blood flow into the capillary and to the tissues.

Blood flow is regulated by vasomotor nerves and local chemical conditions, so it can either bypass or flood the capillary bed

THREE TYPES OF CAPILLARY

Continuous – most common
Fenestrated – have pores
Sinusoids

1. **CONTINUOUS CAPILLARIES**

   Continuous capillaries are abundant in the skin and muscles and have:
   - **Endothelial cells** that provide an uninterrupted lining.
   - **Adjacent cells** that are held together with tight junctions.
   - **Intercellular clefts** of unjoined membranes that allow the passage of fluids.

   Continuous capillaries of the brain:
   - Constitute the blood-brain barrier.
   - Endothelial cells held together by complete tight junctions and desmosomes all around.
   - No intercellular clefts are present.
   - Vital molecules pass through by a highly selective transport mechanisms.
   - Not a barrier against oxygen, carbon dioxide and some anesthetics.

2. **FENESTRATED CAPILLARIES**
   - Found wherever active capillary absorption or filtrate formation occurs (e.g., small intestines, endocrine glands and kidneys).
   - **Characterized by**:
   - An endothelium riddled with pores (**fenestrations**).
   - Greater permeability to solutes and fluids than other capillaries.

3. **SINUSOIDS**

   Are wide, leaky capillaries found in some organs with following features:
   - Usually fenestrated
   - Intercellular clefts are wide open
   - Highly modified
   - Large lumens
   - Have a large diameter and twisted course
   - Found in the liver, spleen, bone marrow, lymphoid tissue and in some endocrine organs.
   - Allow large molecules (proteins and blood cells) to pass between the blood and surrounding tissues.
   - Blood flows sluggishly which allows for modification in various ways

VENULES

- Smallest veins are called venules with diameters from 8–100 μm.
- Smallest venules are called post capillary venules
- Are formed when capillary beds unite
- Conduct blood from capillaries toward the heart
- Allow fluids and white blood cells to pass from the bloodstream to tissues
- Venules join to form veins.

- Tunica externa is the thickest tunic in veins.
- Post capillary venules are the smallest venules, composed of endothelium and a few pericytes.
- Large venules have one or two layers of smooth muscle (tunica media).
- Blood pressure is much lower than in arteries.

VEINS

- Formed when venules converge.
- Composed of three tunics, with a thin tunica media and a thick tunica externa consisting of collagen fibers and elastic networks.
- Capacitance vessels (blood reservoirs) that contain 65% of the blood supply.
- Accompany arteries but without branching, having tributaries.
- Carry blood towards the heart.
- Carry deoxygenated blood (**except pulmonary vein**).
- Have valves within them to prevent backflow (especially in leg)
- Veins have much lower blood pressure and thinner walls than arteries
- To return blood to the heart, veins have special adaptations:

Large diameter of lumen which offer little resistance to flow

Valves which prevent backflow of blood

Venous sinuses are specialized, flattened veins with extremely thin walls (e.g., coronary sinus of the heart and dural sinuses of the brain).

ANASTOMOSIS

- Communication between neighboring vessels in addition to communication through capillaries which may be **pre capillary** or **post capillary**

- The circulation through them is called **collateral circulation**
- If blood vessel gets occluded compensation of blood supply to some extent possible

TYPES OF ANASTOMOSIS

1. **Arterial**: To maintain blood supply of a joint during movement e.g., **palmar arch** and plantar arch
2. **Venous**: To serve as alternative routes for drainage of an organ. e.g., **dorsal venous arch**
3. **Arteriovenous**: For adjustment of blood supply according to the need. e.g., skin of nose, lips, external ear, uterus, etc.

END ARTERIES

Anatomical: Arteries which do not anastomose with their neighbors e.g., central artery of retina.

Physiological: Arteries which anastomose with neighboring vessels but anastomoses are very poor. Inefficient in acute/sudden blockage of an artery but in long term ischemia, collateral circulation can open up to supply the need e.g., arteries of heart and other organs: e.g., kidneys, liver and spleen.

TYPES OF CIRCULATION

Systemic

Blood is pumped by left ventricle to the body parts and returns to the right atrium.

Pulmonary

Blood is pumped by right ventricle through the lungs to the left atrium and returns to the left atrium after oxygenation.

Portal

It is a part of systemic circulation in which the blood passes two sets of capillaries before draining into a systemic vein.

CLINICAL CONSIDERATIONS

Thrombophlebitis

It is the inflammation of a vein generally accompanied by formation of blood clot. It occurs most commonly after trauma to the vessel, postoperative venous stasis, immobilization or a long period of intravenous catheterization. It is suspected when the vessel feels hard and cordlike and is extremely sensitive to pressure. The entire limb may be pale and swollen. Deep vein thrombophlebitis (**DVT**) is characterized by cramping pain especially in the calf.

Blood pressure (BP)

It is the pressure exerted by the circulating blood on the walls of the arteries, veins and the chambers of the heart. The pressure in the aorta and the large arteries of a young adult is approximately **120 mm Hg during systole** and **80 mm Hg in diastole**. The **pulse pressure** is approximately **50 mm Hg**

The blood pressure is measured by auscultation using sphygmomanometer and stethoscope. The cuff is placed around the upper arm and inflated to a pressure greater than the systolic pressure to occlude the brachial artery. The diaphragm of the stethoscope is placed over the **brachial artery in the cubital fossa** medial to the tendon of biceps brachii. The pressure in the cuff is slowly released. No sound is heard until the cuff pressure falls to the systolic pressure in the artery. At that point a pulse is heard. As the cuff pressure continues to fall slowly, the pulse continues. These **sounds of Korotkoff** are produced by turbulence of the blood flowing through a vessel that is partially occluded. When the cuff pressure reaches the diastolic pressure pulse disappears. Thus the cuff pressure at which the first sound is heard is the **systolic blood pressure** and the cuff pressure at which the sounds stop is the **diastolic blood pressure**.

Haemangiomas

These are benign tumour consisting of a mass of blood vessels.

Types

1. Capillary haemangioma
2. Cavernous haemangioma
3. Nevus flammeus

Aneurysm

It is the localized dilatation of the vessel wall. This is usually caused by **atherosclerosis** and associated hypertension. This may be seen after **trauma** or **infection. Congenital weakness** of the vessel wall may results in aneurysm. Aneurysms are common in the aorta but can occur in peripheral vessels. Arterial aneurysm results in a pulsating swelling. An aneurysm may rupture causing fatal hemorrhage.

Types

1. Aortic aneurysm
2. Berry's aneurysm
3. Dissecting aneurysm
4. Varicose aneurysm
5. Ventricular aneurysm

Angiography

It is the radiological visualization of the blood vessels and interior of the heart after the intravascular introduction of radio-opaque contrast medium. The procedure is used in the diagnosis of

1. Myocardial infarction
2. Vascular occlusion with atherosclerotic changes
3. Cerebro-vascular accident
4. Renal artery stenosis
5. Pulmonary emboli

The contrast medium is injected into an artery or vein or introduced into a catheter inserted in a peripheral artery.

11

Lamphatic System

FEATURES

- Drainage system accessory to venous system (absent in central nervous system).
- The fluid exuded through capillaries gets absorbed back by the veins but some (10-20%) of it becomes tissues fluid and is absorbed through lymphatics.
- Superficial lymphatics follow veins **except** in tongue.
- Deep lymphatics follow arteries.

Consists of two semi-independent parts
1. A network of lymphatic vessels
2. Lymphoid tissues and organs scattered throughout the body.

Returns interstitial fluid and leaked plasma proteins back to the blood.

LYMPH

- Interstitial fluid once it has entered lymphatic vessels.
- Clear fluid similar to blood plasma.
- After passage through lymph nodes may contain lymphocytes.

Flow of lymph:

Tissue fluid – network of lymph capillaries regional

lymph nodes – larger lymphatics – thoracic duct or right lymphatic duct – Great veins near the heart.

Lymph vessels

- A one-way system in which lymph flows toward the heart.
- Lymph vessels **include**:
- Microscopic, permeable blind-ended capillaries.
- Lymphatic collecting vessels.
- Trunks and ducts.

LYMPHATIC CAPILLARIES

These are similar to blood capillaries with modifications:

- Remarkably permeable
- Loosely joined endothelial mini valves
- Withstand interstitial pressure and remain open

The mini valves function as one-way gates that:

- Allow interstitial fluid to enter lymph capillaries
- Do not allow lymph to escape from the capillaries

During inflammation, lymph capillaries can absorb:

- Cell debris
- Pathogens

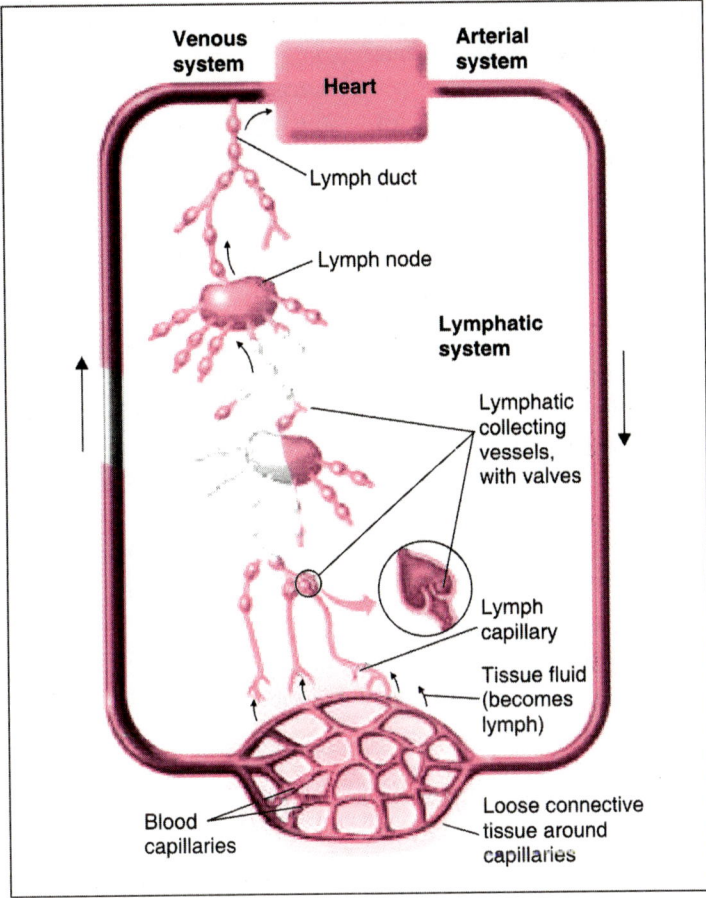

Fig. 11.1: Lymphatic system

- Cancer cells

Cells in the lymph nodes:

- Cleanse and "examine" this debris

Lacteals are specialized lymph capillaries present in intestinal mucosa

- Absorb digested fat and deliver chyle to the blood

LYMPHATIC TRUNKS

Lymphatic trunks are formed by the union of the largest collecting ducts.

Major trunks include:

- Paired lumbar, bronchomediastinal, subclavian and jugular trunks.

- A single intestinal trunk.

Lymph is delivered into one of two large trunks:

Right lymphatic duct – Drains the right upper arm and the right side of the head and thorax.

Thoracic duct – Arises from the cisterna chyli and drains the rest of the body.

LYMPHATIC TISSUE

Diffuse lymphatic tissues are scattered reticular tissue elements in every body organ

- Larger collections appear in the lamina propria of mucous membranes and lymphoid organs

Lymphatic follicles (nodules) are solid, spherical bodies consisting of tightly packed reticular elements and cells.

- Have a germinal center composed of **dendritic** and **B cells**.
- Found in isolation and as part of larger lymphoid organs.

LYMPHATIC ORGANS

Lymphoid organs are discrete, encapsulated collections of diffuse lymphoid tissue and follicles.

Examples include the Lymph nodes, Spleen, and Thymus.

LYMPH NODES

- Nodes are imbedded in connective tissue and clustered along lymphatic vessels.
- Aggregations of these nodes occur near the body surface in inguinal, axillary and cervical regions of the body.
- Present along lymph vessels/lymphatics.
- Size pinhead to olive size. Flattened shaped.
- Act as filters for lymph.

Their basic functions are:

1. **Filtration** of plasma - Macrophages destroy microorganisms and debris
2. **Immune system activation** – Concentration and monitor for antigens and mount an attack against them (**immune response**)
3. Lymphatics and lymphoid tissue are important in **rejection of grafts**

Structure

Nodes are bean shaped and surrounded by a fibrous capsule Trabeculae extended inward from the capsule and divide the node into compartments. Nodes have two histologically distinct regions:

- – **Cortex**
- – **Medulla**

SPLEEN

Largest lymphoid organ, located on the left side of the abdominal cavity beneath the diaphragm

It extends to curl around the anterior aspect of the stomach

It is served by the splenic artery and vein which enter and exit at the hilus

Functions

1. Site of lymphocyte proliferation
2. Immune surveillance and response
3. Cleanses the blood
4. Stores breakdown products of red blood cells
5. Spleen macrophages salvage and store iron for later use by bone marrow
6. Site of foetal erythrocyte production which normally ceases after birth
7. Stores blood platelets

Structure

- Surrounded by a fibrous capsule. It has trabeculae that extend inward and contains lymphocytes, macrophages and large numbers of erythrocytes.
- Two distinct areas of the spleen are:
- **White pulp** is the area containing mostly lymphocytes suspended on reticular fibers and involved in immune functions.
- **Red pulp** is the remaining splenic tissue concerned with disposing of worn-out red blood cells and blood borne pathogens.

THYMUS

- It is a bilobed organ which secrets **thymosin** and **thymopoietin hormones** that causes T lymphocytes to become immunocompetent.
- The size of the thymus varies with age:
- In infants, it is found in the lower part of neck and extends into superior mediastinum.

- It increases in size and is most active during childhood.
- It stops growing during adolescence and then gradually atrophies.

Structure

- Thymus has an outer cortex and inner medulla.
- The cortex contains densely packed lymphocytes and scattered macrophages.
- The medulla contains fewer lymphocytes and thymic (**Hassall's**) corpuscles.

CLINICAL CONSIDERATIONS

Lymphangitis

It is the inflammation of one or more lymphatic vessels usually resulting from an acute infection of one of the limbs. It is characterized by fine red streaks seen extending from the infected area to the axilla or groin. The infection may spread to the bloodstream.

Lymphadenitis

It is the inflammation of the lymph nodes. This usually results from neoplastic disease, bacterial infection or other inflammatory condition. The nodes may be enlarged, hard, smooth or irregular. The location of the affected node is indicative of the site or origin of the disease.

Filariasis

This disease is caused by the presence of microfilaria in the tissues of the body. They infest the lymph glands and channels after the mosquito bite or other insect. The infection is characterized by occlusion of the lymphatic vessels, with swelling and pain of the limb distal to the blockage. In a long standing case the limb may become greatly swollen.

Elephantiasis

It is the end-stage of filariasis. This is characterized by massive swelling usually of the legs. The overlying skin becomes thick and coarse. Elephantiasis results from long standing filariasis.

Lymph nodes enlargement

When there is an infection in the area of drainage of lymph nodes they tend to enlarge.

Graft rejection

The lymphatics and lymphoid tissue are important in graft rejection.

Section-II
Osteology

CONTENTS

12. **The Skull**   73-74

13. **Norma Verticalis**   75-76

14. **Norma Frontalis**   77-79

15. **Norma Occipitalis**   80-81

16. **Norma Lateralis**   82-85

17. **Vault of Skull**   86-87

18. **Cranial Fossae**   88-95

19. **Norma Basalis**   96-100

20. **Mandible**   101-104

21. **Maxilla**   105-108

22. **Sphenoid Bone**   109-113

23. **Parietal Bone**   114-115

24. **Frontal Bone**   116-118

25. **Temporal Bone**   119-121

26. **Ethmoid Bone**   122-123

27. **Palatine Bone**   124-126

28. **Zygomatic Bone**   127-128

29. **Vomer**   129

30. **Hyoid Bone**   130-131

31. **Lacrimal Bone**   132

32. **Inferior Nasal Concha**   133-134

33. **Nasal Bone**   135-136

34. **Foetal Skull**   137-140

35. **Cervical Vertebrae**   141-145

12

The Skull

INTRODUCTION

The skeleton of the head is formed by the skull. Excluding the mandible rest of the skull forms the cranium. The upper part of the cranium encloses the brain and is called calvaria. The remainder of the skull constitutes the facial skeleton including the mandible. The lower part of facial skeleton is freely movable - temporomandibular joints. Rest of the skull is made up of large number of bones (flat, irregular and pneumatic) which are joined by sutures – immovable joints. With advancing age some of the sutures may get obliterated.

ANATOMICAL POSITION

Frankfort's plane

A horizontal plane passing anteriorly along inferior margin of bony orbit to the upper margin of external acoustic meatus posteriorly

Reid's base line

Another methodology for holding the skull in anatomical position is following the Reid's base line which is also kept in horizontal plane. It passes anteriorly along the lower margin of bony orbit and posteriorly through the middle of external acoustic meatus.

METHODS OF STUDY OF SKULL

Skull as a whole can be studied in the following manners

OUTER ASPECTS

NORMAS:

- Norma frontalis – from in front
- Norma verticalis – from above
- Norma lateralis – from the side
- Norma occipitalis – from behind
- Norma basalis – from below

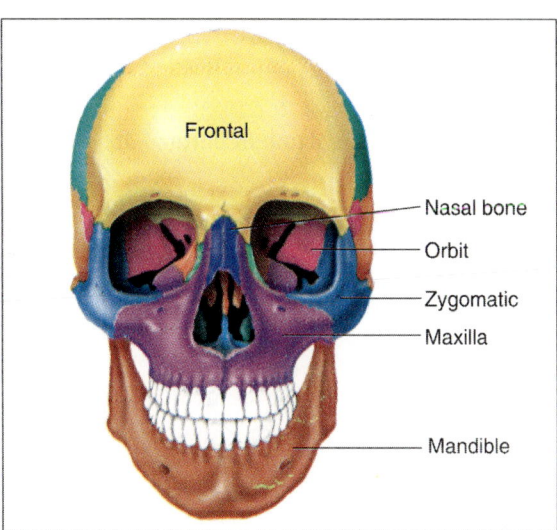

Fig. 12.1: The Skull

INNER ASPECT

The roof of calvaria is called skull cap. On removing the skull cap, the interior can be seen – floor of calvaria (base of the skull). It shows three natural subdivisions. From before backward they are

- Anterior cranial fossa
- Middle cranial fossa
- Posterior cranial fossa

INDIVIDUAL BONES

Can be studied in the intact skull or as a disarticulated bone

Cranial points

The different points on the skull from which the commoner measurements are taken are listed below:

In the Middle Line

- **Gnathion** – The point of the chin.
- **Prosthion** – The lowest point on the upper jaw between the central incisors.
- **Akanthion** – The anterior nasal spine
- **Nasion** – Junction of nasal and frontal bones.
- **Glabella** – Mid point at level of superciliary arches.
- **Bregma** – Junction of coronal and sagittal sutures.
- **Lambda** – Junction of sagittal and lambdoid sutures.
- **Opsthocranion** – The most posteriorly projecting point on the occipital bone.
- **Inion** – The external occipital protuberance.
- **Opisthion** – The central point of the posterior edge of the foramen magnum.

- **Basion** – The central point of the anterior edge of the foramen magnum

At the side of the Skull

- **Dacryon** – Junction of lacrimo- maxillary and fronto -maxillary sutures
- **Gonion** – The outer side of the angle of the mandible.
- **Pterion** – Region where frontal, parietal, greater wing of sphenoid and squamous part of temporal meet.
- **Porion** – a point on the posterior root of the zygomatic arch above the middle of the upper border of the external auditory meatus.
- **Asterion** – Region where occipital, parietal, and temporal meet.

Frankfurt plane is a horizontal plane passing through both poria and the lowest point on the left inferior orbital margin. When comparisons are being made between different skulls it is useful to have a standard place of orientation and the Frankfurt plane is the one most commonly used.

CLINICAL CONSIDERATION

Sexing of the Skull

Medico legal importance for medico legal practice determination of the sex of the diseased from the bone/bones is essential. Certain features of the skull help in determining the use of an individual. Besides the usual indicators such as one all size and muscular markings, the following features are taken into consideration

- Superciliary arches
- Frontal eminence
- Mastoid process

13

Norma Verticalis

INTRODUCTION

When seen from above the outline of skull is more or less oval but it is variable in different races.

Bones taking part

From before backwards, the bones are

- Frontal
- Parietal (right and left)
- Occipital

SUTURES

There are **three sutures** joining these bones

- **Coronal suture** - Between frontal and right and left parietal
- **Sagittal suture** - Between two parietal bones in the median plane
- **Lambdoid suture** -Between posterior border of two parietals and occipital bone

FEATURES

Vertex

The highest point on Norma verticalis is termed as vertex

Bregma

The point where coronal and sagittal sutures meet is termed as bregma. In foetal skull, anterior fontanalle is placed as a membrane filled gap at the site of bregma. It is diamond shaped.

Lambda

It is situated at the junction of sagittal and lambdoid sutures. In foetal skull this site is represented by posterior fontanalle which is a membrane filled smaller gap. It is triangular in shape.

Parietal foramen

About 3.5 cm in front of the lambda, parietal bone presents foramen near the sagittal suture on either side. This foramen may be absent in one or both the sides. A small emissary vein passes through it connecting superior sagittal sinus with the veins of the scalp.

Parietal eminence

The maximum convexity of parietal bone appears as parietal eminence.

Temporal lines

On the lateral part of normal verticalis, running across from frontal onto parietal bones are temporal lines (superior and inferior).

CLINICAL CONSIDERATIONS

Fontanellae

The bones of the vault of foetal skull are held together by flexible fibrous joints. The bones are soft at this stage. Hence during child birth they can slide over each other. This process is called moulding. It helps in the passage of foetal skull smoothing through the birth canal during delivery. The change in the shape of vault of skull is not permanent.

Nature of bones and the presence of fontanalle permit the skull to undergo remodeling keeping pace with the growth of the brain during infancy and childhood. The cranial capacity increases until 16 years as thereafter the bones thicken.

Parietal Emissary Foramen

Parietal foramen transmits an emissary vein connecting the veins in the scalp to the superior sagittal sinus. The emissary vein lacks valves and the blood can flow in either direction. Thus this is possibility of spread of infection from the scalp to the cranium.

14

Norma Frontalis

INTRODUCTION

Skull viewed from front is termed as Norma frontalis. Main features are:
- **Bony orbits** - for eye balls
- **Anterior nasal aperture**
- **Oral aperture** between maxillae and mandible

BONES TAKING PART

From above downwards
- Frontal
- Nasal
- Maxilla
- Lacrimal
- Sphenoid (greater and lesser wings)
- Zygomatic
- Mandible

SUTURES

The vertical growth of facial skeleton is due to growth along the suture sites (fronto maxillary suture), appearance of dentition and appearance of paranasal air sinuses.

Metopic suture – The frontal bone develops in two halves. Normally they fuse with each other to form a single frontal bone. However, in 7 to 8% cases (figure is variable) the two halves are joined by a well marked midline suture which does not get obliterated, known as metopic suture.

FEATURES

Superciliary arch – seen above medial part of each orbit as smooth and arched elevation.

Glabella – A median elevation where two superciliary arches meet.

Nasion – Below the glabella the nasal bones meet the frontal bone by front nasal suture. The two nasal bones are joined with each other by internasal suture. Nasion is the point where the internasal and frontonasal sutures meet.

Frontal eminences – Above the superciliary arches on each side, slight rounded elevation in the middle of the forehead are seen. They are well marked in females.

LOWER PART OF FACE

Nasal notch – The anterior bony aperture of nose is seen as a notch in each maxilla.

Anterior nasal spine – Marked as a sharp prominent projection where nasal notch meet in the midline.

Infraorbital foramen – About 1 cm below the infraorbital margin, the maxilla presents infra orbital foramen – transmits terminal parts of infra orbital vessels and nerve.

Prominence of cheek – Below and lateral to the orbit, zygomatic bone forms a prominence.

Maxilla – Contribute a larger share in the formation of facial skeleton. It is joined with each other below the anterior nasal aperture, on the sides with zygomatic bone, above and medially with nasal bones and superiorly with frontal bone and posteromedially with lacrimal and behind with ethmoid bone.

Frontal process – Joins medially with nasal bone, superiorly with frontal bone and posterolaterally with lacrimal bone.

Zygomatic process –It is a stout process from the superolateral part of the bone. Zygomatico-maxillary suture articulates the bones along this process.

Alveolar process – Provides sockets for upper teeth. The stout root of canine causes an elevation – canine eminence. It separates the canine fossa on its lateral side from the incisive fossa on its medial side.

Zygomatic bone – The prominence of the cheeks is attributed to the zygomatic bones which are placed inferolateral to the orbit. Each bone has two processes and three surfaces.

PROCESSES

Frontal - Projects upwards to articulate with frontal bone

Temporal - Extents horizontally backwards to articulate with temporal one forming the zygomatic arch.

Surfaces

Orbital, temporal and lateral.

Orbital opening

Appears as quadrangular in shape formed by

Supraorbital margin

It is formed entirely by frontal bone. Supraorbital notch / foramen is seen on its superomedial part.

Lateral margin

It is formed by frontal process of zygomatic bone and corresponding process of frontal bone. The suture appears as a slight depression which can be readily palpated.

Infraorbital margin

 It is formed by zygomatic bone laterally and the maxilla medially. This margin can also be felt easily through the skin.

Medial orbital margin

It is not as distinct as other margins. It is formed from above downwards by

- Frontal bone
- Lacrimal crest of frontal process of maxilla.

The lacrimal crest is sharp and distinct in lower portion only.

ORBITAL CAVITY

The eyeballs with their muscles, vessels and nerves are packed in orbit. The fat in the orbit also lodges lacrimal apparatus. The orbital opening on the face forms the base of pyramidal shaped orbital cavity. Since the long axis of the orbit is directed backwards and medially, the lateral walls are convergent. The medial walls are parallel to each other. That besides the orbit presents the roof, floor and an apex.

CONTENTS

- Eye ball and its vessels and nerves
- Extra ocular muscles
- Orbital fascia

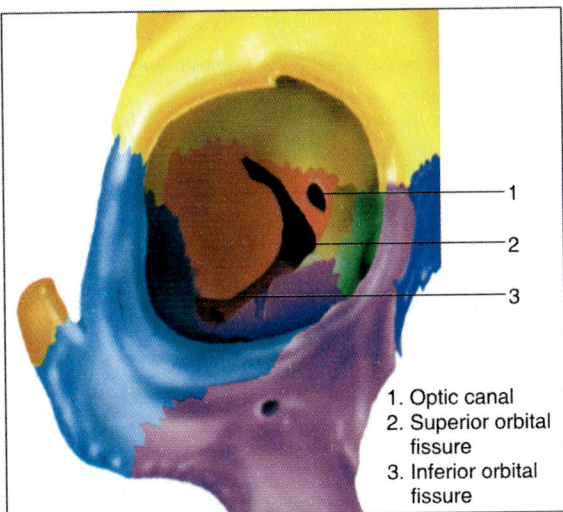

1. Optic canal
2. Superior orbital fissure
3. Inferior orbital fissure

Fig. 14.1: Bony orbit

- Orbital fat
- Greater part of lacrimal apparatus

BOUNDARIES

Roof of orbit

It is formed by orbital plate of frontal bone and lesser wing of sphenoid. It is a thin plate of frontal bone (orbital plate) separates the orbit from the part of the brain in the anterior cranial fossa. Anteromedial part of the roof is related to the frontal air sinus. In the anterolateral part lacrimal fossa is situated – for lacrimal gland. At the posterior end the roof joins the medial wall – **optic canal**, for the passage of optic nerve and ophthalmic artery. Along the superior, medial and lower margins of the optic canal, a tendinous ring (of **Zinn**) is attached. It provides attachment to extra ocular muscles of eye ball.

Floor of orbit

Formed by orbital surface of maxilla and its anterolateral part is formed by zygomatic bone. A triangular area posteriorly – orbital process of palatine bone – forms a part of floor where it meets medial wall. Between the floor and lateral wall, inferior orbital fissure is seen. Along the floor, the infra orbital groove runs between inferior orbital fissure posteriorly and infra orbital foramen anteriorly. This groove is seen as a canal in its anterior part. The groove, canal and foramen transmit infraorbital nerve and vessels.

Medial wall of orbit

It is formed anteroposterior by

- Frontal process of maxilla having lacrimal crest
- Lacrimal bone
- Orbital plate of ethmoid (largest contribution) and
- Part of frontal bone joining maxilla.

This is thin all over except its posterior part. It slopes downward and laterally to merge with the floor. From anterior to posterior it presents:

Lacrimal groove – for lacrimal sac

Below the groove **nasolacrimal canal** is seen which connects the lacrimal sac with nasal cavity through nasolacrimal duct.

Ethmoidal air sinuses intervene between the orbital cavity and nasal cavity.

Lateral wall of orbit

It is formed by zygomatic bone anteriorly and greater wing of sphenoid posteriorly. Posteriorly the lateral wall is separated from the roof by superior orbital fissure. This gap is bounded by

Above - Lesser wing of sphenoid

Below - Greater wing of sphenoid

Medially - Body of sphenoid

The lateral part of tendinous ring divides superior orbital fissure into three portions which transmit cranial nerves for the orbit (motor and sensory) along with ophthalmic veins.

Apex of orbit

It is at the medial end of superior orbital fissure.

15

Norma Occipitalis

INTRODUCTION

The skull appears like an arc when it is seen from behind

BONES TAKING PART

- Occipital bone
- Posterior part of parietal bones
- Mastoid process of temporal bones

SUTURES

- The lambdoid suture can be seen in its entire extent

- Occipitomastoid suture is placed inferiorly as part of lambdoid suture

- Parietomastoid suture is not a part of lambdoid. It is seen at posteroinferior angle of parietal bone

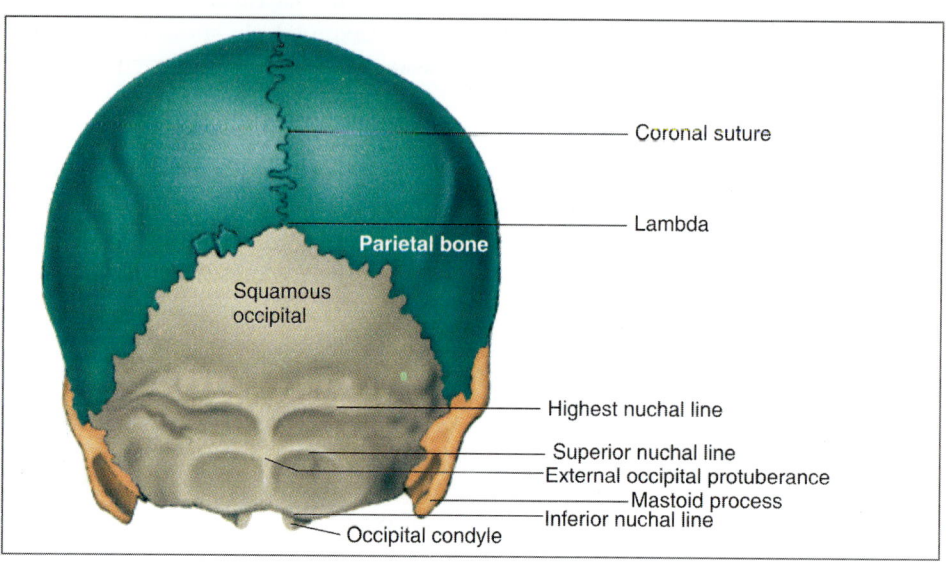

Fig. 15.1: Norma Occipitalis

FEATURES

External occipital protuberance

It is the most prominent bony landmark on the occi-pital bone in the mid line. Inion is the most prominent point on the external occipital protuberance.

Highest nuchal lines

These are curved bony ridges commencing at the superior part of the protuberance. They appear as highly arched ridges.

Superior nuchal lines

They pass laterally from the protuberance as bone ridges. They demarcate the scalp and the back of the neck.

External occipital crest

It is a raised ridge extending from the external occipital protuberance to the posterior margin of foramen magnum.

Inferior nuchal lines

Arched ridges on either side commencing from external occipital crest midway between superior nuchal lines and posterior margin of foramen magnum

Mastoid process

Inferolateral part of Norma occipitalis. Shows well marked mastoid process as part of temporal bone.

16

Norma Lateralis

INTRODUCTION

When the skull is examined without the mandible from the side **Norma lateralis** is seen. It also includes adjoining parts of norma frontalis, verticalis and occipitalis. Thus only its central part having important features is described.

BONES TAKING PART

Bones in view are greater wing of sphenoid and temporal bone
The other bones are

- Maxilla
- Zygomatic
- Frontal
- Parietal and
- Occipital are contributing in adjacent parts of Norma frontalis, verticalis and Norma occipitalis.

SUTURES

An arched suture runs antero posteriorly joining squamous part of temporal with greater wing of sphenoid (squamo-sphenoid suture)
Parietal bone (squamo-parietal suture)

Posteriorly, the mastoid part of temporal bone joins posteroinferior angle of parietal (parietomastoid suture)
Occipital bone (inferior part of lambdoid suture)

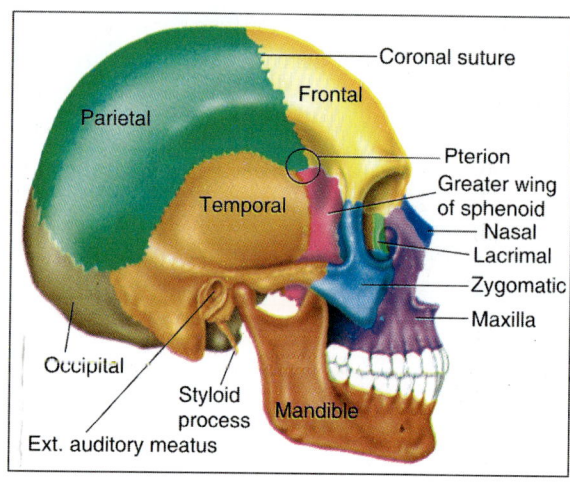

Fig. 16.1: Norma Lateralis

FEATURES

Temporal lines

From the zygomatic process of temporal bone, the two temporal lines arch upwards and backwards across the coronal suture onto the parietal bone. Posteriorly upper temporal line disappears and the lower one extends downwards and forwards on the squamous part of temporal bone until the mastoid part. The line continues as supramastoid crest which becomes continuous with posterior root of zygomatic process. It bounds suprameatal triangle superiorly. The upper temporal line provides attachment to strong temporal fascia. The area between two temporal lines and lower temporal line are for temporalis muscle.

Zygomatic arch

It can be felt in front of the ear where the cheek and temple meet. It is formed by temporal process of zygomatic bone and zygomatic process of temporal bone. Its lower border and deep surface give attachment to masseter muscle. The zygomatic process of temporal bone posteriorly widens as anterior and posterior roots. The anterior root is in front of articular fossa, placed medially, for the head of the mandible. Here the anterior root presents smooth articular eminence which is in front of articular fossa. This eminence is termed as tubercle of *root of zygoma*. The posterior root passes backward and is continuous with the supramastoid crest. These structures can be seen distinctly when the skull is viewed from below.

External acoustic meatus

It is placed below the posterior root of zygoma. The cartilaginous part of the auditory tube is attached to the anterior and inferior margins of external acoustic meatus. The tympanic plate is formed by anterior, inferior and the posterior margins. Squamo-tympanic fissure is distinctly seen anterosuperior to the opening along the inferior aspect. Behind and above the meatus, the suprameatal spine is seen as a small depression with a bony spicule. It lies in the suprameatal (**McEvan's**) triangle – bounded by:

- Supramastoid crest – above
- Posterior superior margin of meatus – in front
- Vertical tangent on postero superior margin. The triangle leads to mastoid air cells.

Mastoid part of temporal bone

It is placed behind the external acoustic meatus.

Asterion

Also known as lateral fontanalle. It is the meeting point of three bones namely:

- Posteroinferior angle of parietal
- Mastoid part of temporal
- Squamous part of occipital

Mastoid process

It is strong finger tip like projection. It is below the external acoustic meatus. It is felt behind the auricle. The prominence of mastoid process is due to pull of sternomastoid muscle – traction epiphysis. Other muscles attached to the mastoid process are splenius capitis and longissimus capitis. The groove medial to mastoid process gives attachment to posterior belly of digastric. Mastoid foramen is seen near the upper part of occipito- mastoid suture to transmit an emissary vein that connects sigmoid sinus.

Styloid process

It is a slender spinous projection of variable length. It is a part of mastoid portion of temporal bone. It is placed medial to mastoid process. Its base is embedded in the tympanic plate while the tip is directed downwards, forwards and medially. Being placed deeper, the ramus of the mandible conceals part of styloid process. The styloid apparatus consists:

- Stylohyoid muscle
- Styloglossus muscle
- Stylopharyngeus muscle
- Stylohyoid ligament
- Stylomandibular ligament

TEMPORAL FOSSA

It is placed between the zygomatic arch, frontal process of zygomatic bone and the temporal lines.

BOUNDARIES

Superiorly – Temporal lines

Anteriorly – Formed by zygomatic bone, greater wing of sphenoid and frontal bone

Inferiorly – It communicates freely with infratemporal fossa.

PTERION

In the anterior part of the fossa, an irregular H shaped suture – Pterion is seen. Here the following bones meet: frontal, sphenoid, squamo-temporal and parietal. It is 3.5 cm behind the fronto zygomatic suture and about 3.5 cm above the zygomatic arch.

CONTENTS OF TEMPORAL FOSSA

- Temporal fascia and temporalis
- Middle temporal vessels
- Zygomatico temporal nerve
- Temporal branch of mandibular nerve

Fossa communicates with

- **Infra temporal fossa**
- **Pterygo-palatine fossa** through pterygo-maxillary fissure

INFRATEMPORAL FOSSA

This space is placed below the level of zygomatic arch

BOUNDARIES

Anterior all – Posterior surface of body of maxilla

Medial wall – Lateral pterygoid plate

Posteriorly – Styloid apparatus

Roof – Infratemporal crest and infratemporal surface of greater wing of sphenoid

Laterally – Ramus of the mandible

Pterygomaxillary fissure is a gap between anterior and medial walls. It leads into pterygo-palatine fossa. The upper end of pterygomaxillary fissure is continuous with posterior limit of inferior orbital fissure.

CONTENTS

Muscles

- Temporalis
- Lateral pterygoid
- Medial pterygoid
- Masseter

Artery

- **Maxillary artery** and its branches from its first and second parts

Vein

- Pterygoid venous plexus

Nerves

- Mandibular nerve and its branches
- Chorda tympani
- Posterior superior alveolar

Ligament

- Sphenomandibular ligament

Ganglion

- Otic ganglion

COMMUNICATIONS

Superiorly – with temporal fossa

Anteriorly–with pterygopalatine fossa through pterygomaxillary fissure

Through pterygomaxillary fissure, the infratemporal fossa is connected to the orbit along the posterior end of inferior orbital fissure.

PTERYGOPALATINE FOSSA

This small space is placed below the apex of the orbit. It is better seen in a sagittally cut skull.

BOUNDARIES

Roof - Body of sphenoid and palatine bone

Posteriorly of pterygoid process

Medially - Perpendicular plate of palatine bone

Anteriorly - Upper part of posterior surface of maxilla

Laterally - Through pterygomaxillary fissure, communicates with Infra temporal fossa

Floor - Meeting of anterior and posterior walls

CONTENTS

Maxillary nerve

Sphenopalatine (*Pterygopalatine*) **ganglion** and its branches

Third part of maxillary artery and its branches

COMMUNICATIONS

With the orbit – Inferior orbital fissure

With infratemporal fossa – Pterygo-maxillary fissure

With middle cranial fossa
- Foramen rotundum
- Pterygoid canal

With posterior nasal aperture
- Palatovaginal canal
- Sphenopalatine foramen
- Greater and lesser palatine foramina

CLINICAL CONSIDERATIONS

Pterion

This land mark is clinically important because

- Anterior division of middle meningeal vessels lies between the layers of dura mater on the internal aspects. Hence the vessels are vulnerable to damage due to fracture at this site.
- The rupture of vessels leads to extradural hematoma which compresses the cerebral cortex. To decompress and to ligate the bleeding vessels, burr hole is made near the pterion.

Trigeminal Neuralgia - Injection Routes

Pain over the distribution area of one or more divisions of trigeminal nerve is termed trigeminal neuralgia.

Alcohol injection

90% alcohol is injected (1 ml) into the Gassarian (trigeminal) ganglion. The needle is inserted from definite land marks which lead it to the foramen ovale. The local infiltration gives immediate relief which lasts from 6 months to 2 years. Repeated injections may cause fibrosis. This would necessitate undertaking surgical intervention.

The **surgical treatment** involves
- Ablation of the central root / affected division of the nerve
- Medullary tractotomy – to cut the descending fibres of trigeminal nerve

17

Vault of Skull

INTRODUCTION

Brain along with meninges is placed in the cranial cavity. The bones coming in contact with the brain are frontal, parietal, sphenoid, temporal and occipital. These bones are lined on the inside by endocranium (endosteal layer of dura mater) and on the outer surface by pericranium. The sutural ligaments anchor these layers.

BONES TAKING PART

- Frontal
- Parietal on either side
- Occipital

SUTURES

- Coronal
- Sagittal
- Lambdoid

The sutures start obliterating from inner aspect. This process starts after forty years and completed by sixty years on the external aspect.

FEATURES

Frontal crest

Projecting backwards in the midline, this raised bony crest attaches falx cerebri. It presents a groove – sagittal sulcus which lodges commencement of superior sagittal sinus.

Granular fovealae / pits

On tracing the sagittal sulcus backwards, granular pits are seen as irregular depressions on each side. They are caused by arachnoid granulations. These are tuft like projections of arachnoid mater into the superior sagittal sinus. Through these the cerebrospinal fluid (**CSF**) is discharged into superior sagittal sinus. To start with they are minute finger like projections. As the age advances their number increases and appears as granulations which cast well marked impressions in aged skull.

Vascular impressions

The inner aspect of cranium is characterized by well marked vascular impressions. These are caused by the meningeal vessels. One cm behind the lateral limit of coronal suture, the endocranium shows the impression of anterior branch of middle meningeal artery.

Parietal foramen

About 3.5 cm in front of lambdoid suture near the sagittal groove parietal foramen is seen on either side. An emissary vein passes through this foramen to connect superior sagittal sinus with veins of the scalp.

CLINICAL CONSIDERATIONS

Fractures of the Skull

Direct hard blow to the skull causes skull fracture. The fracture lines are seen radiating away from the point of impact. They are seen running in different directions. When the skull shows fracture opposite to the site of blow is termed counter coup/counter blow fracture.

Age Estimation by Suture Fusion on Calvaria

With advancing age sutures of the skull vault start obliterating. It begins first on the inner surface between 30 to 40 years. On the outer surface the obliteration is about 10 years later. This shows variations.

Obliteration generally follows a sequence whereby lower part of coronal suture is first to show obliteration followed by posterior part of sagittal suture. Lambdoid suture is lost to obliterate.

In X-ray skull the diploic canals containing the diploic veins may be mistaken for fracture of the cranium.

The calvarium is vulnerable to fracture where it is thin. The diploic canals containing the diploic veins appear in a radiograph as discontinuity of the bone especially in the parietal area.

18

Cranial Fossae

INTRODUCTION

The inner aspect of base of skull shows three subdivisions arranged at higher to lower level as one examines the skull from anterior to posterior. These are called cranial fossae – anterior, middle and posterior. These fossae present undulations that are due to cerebral gyri. The dura mater – endosteal layer is firmly adherent to the cranial fossae. The endocranium (endosteal dura) is continuous with the pericranium through the foramina and fissures seen in the cranial fossae.

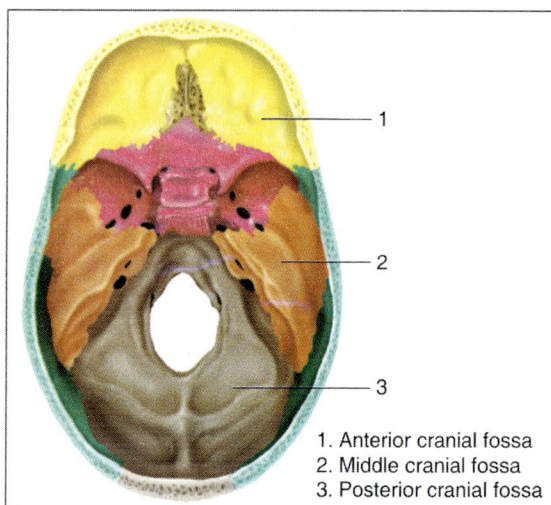

1. Anterior cranial fossa
2. Middle cranial fossa
3. Posterior cranial fossa

Fig. 18.1: Cranial Fossae

ANTERIOR CRANIAL FOSSA

BOUNDARIES

Anteriorly and by the sides - By frontal bone

    Floor - Orbital plate of frontal with cribriform plate of ethmoid in between lesser wing and anterior part of body of sphenoid form the posterior part of the floor demarcating it from posterior cranial fossa.

FEATURES

Cribriform plate of ethmoid

It lies between two orbital plates of frontal bone. It forms roof of nasal cavity. Thus it separates anterior cranial fossa from nasal cavity. The sieve like openings receives 15 to 20 olfactory nerve rootlets from upper nasal mucosa. These synapse in the olfactory bulb that rests over the cribriform plate. The suture between the cribriform plate of ethmoid and orbital plate of frontal bone presents anterior and posterior ethmoidal foramina. These transmit corresponding nerves and vessels.

Crista galli

It is a median crest (tooth like projection) giving attachment to double fold of dura mater – falx cerebri. This sickle shaped fold of dura mater separates the adjoining medial surfaces of two cerebral hemispheres. Its convex attached margin encloses superior sagittal sinus while inferior sagittal sinus is along its concave inferior free border in its posterior two third.

Foramen caecum

In front of base of crista galli, a blind foramen – foramen caecum is present. At times, when it is patent, an emissary vein connects superior sagittal sinus with nasal mucosal vein.

Orbital plate of frontal

It forms major part of floor of anterior cranial fossa. Frontal air sinus at times can be seen on the anteromedial aspect of the frontal bone between two laminae.

Sphenoid bone

The posterior part of floor behind the orbital and cribriform plates presents the following features of the sphenoid bone.

- **Jugum sphenoidale** – Formed by anterior part of upper surface of body of sphenoid. Underneath this lies the sphenoidal air sinus.
- **Sulcus chiasmaticus/optic groove** – It is a transverse wall marked groove over the body of sphenoid immediately behind jugum sphenoidale. It lodges optic chiasma which on tracing laterally leads into optic foramen – seen in middle cranial fossa.
- **Lesser wing** – Forms posterior part of floor of anterior cranial fossa. Its posterior margin is curved, free and overhangs anterior part of middle cranial fossa. When traced medially, the margin ends in anterior clenoid process. The free margin of tentorium cerebelli is attached to it. The free margin of lesser wing of sphenoid laterally reaches the suture between the frontal bone

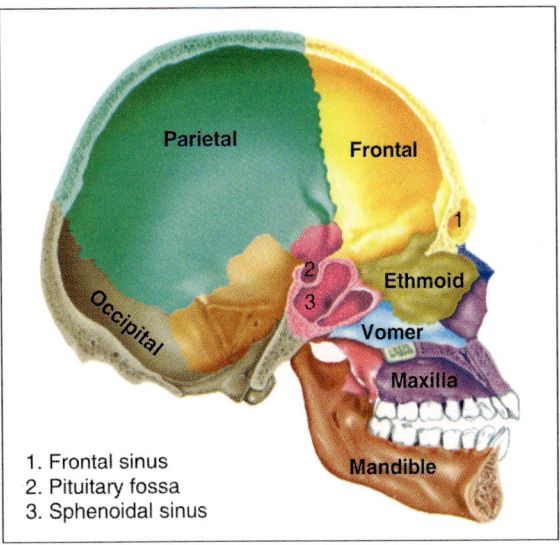

1. Frontal sinus
2. Pituitary fossa
3. Sphenoidal sinus

Fig. 18.2: Cranial Fossae: Lateral Profile

and greater wing of sphenoid. It also bounds superior orbital fissure.

MIDDLE CRANIAL FOSSA

BOUNDARIES

Anteriorly

Posterior free border of lesser wing, anterior clenoid processes and anterior margin of sulcus chiasmaticus

Posteriorly

Superior border of petrous part of temporal bone and dorsum sallae of sphenoid (plate of bone projects upwards and forward posterior to hypophyseal fossa)

On each side

Squamous temporal, anteroinferior angle of parietal bone and greater wing of sphenoid

Floor

Body of sphenoid, cerebral surface of greater wing of sphenoid, cerebral surface of squamous temporal and anterior surface of petrous temporal bone

FEATURES MEDIAN PART

Sulcus chiasmaticus

The optic chiasma and the meningeal coverings of the optic nerve are related to it. Since the optic chiasma lies above and behind the sulcus chiasmaticus it is to be noted that the sulcus does not lodge the optic chiasma.

Optic canal

It is directed forward, laterally and slightly downwards.

It **transmits:**

- **Optic nerve** with all three meningeal coverings
- **Ophthalmic artery**

To see this foramen, one has to view it from the front of orbit or from posterior side by tilting the skull down anteriorly.

Sella turcica

Shaped like a saddle. It is a part of body of sphenoid

Hypophyseal fossa

The upper surface of body of sphenoid is hollowed out to lodge the hypophysis cerebri (pituitary gland) – hypophyseal fossa

Dorsum sallae

Behind the hypophyseal fossa, the body of sphenoid presents a plate of bone projecting upwards and forwards – dorsum sallae.

Posterior clenoid process

At the superolateral angle, the dorsum sallae is expanded to form posterior clenoid process. Attached margin of tentorium cerebelli is anchored here.

Carotid sulcus

It is present on the lateral side of sella turcica starting from foramen lacerum.

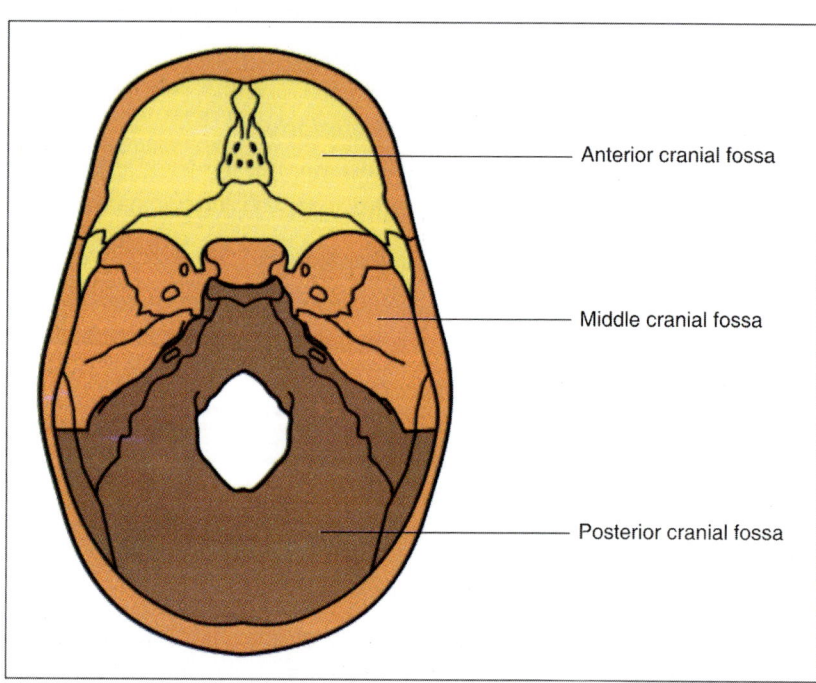

Fig. 18.3: Cranial Fossae

- Anterior cranial fossa
- Middle cranial fossa
- Posterior cranial fossa

LATERAL PART

It lodges temporal lobes of cerebrum. It presents following features.

Superior orbital fissure

This obliquely placed fissure (long axis is directed upwards, laterally and forwards) is wider at its medial end. It is bounded by lesser wing, body and greater wing of sphenoid. It transmits structures which enter or leave the orbit namely –

Nerves

- Terminal branches of V1 (ophthalmic division of trigeminal nerve)
- III, IV & VI cranial nerves

Vessels

- Superior and inferior ophthalmic veins

CAVERNOUS SINUS

On either side of sloping part of body of sphenoid lies the cavernous sinus. It is formed by separation of meningeal layer of dura mater from endosteal dura mater. The floor and lower part of medial wall is formed by endosteal dura while roof and lateral wall is formed by meningeal dura At its anterior end, this sinus receives superior and inferior ophthalmic veins and sphenoparietal sinus. At its posterior end it issues superior petrosal sinus which is a two way channel connecting it with transverse sinus. The inferior petrosal sinus connects the cavernous sinus to sigmoid sinus. At its superior aspect it receives superficial middle cerebral vein. It is also connected to superior sagittal sinus by a two way channel along its superior aspect. Inferiorly a set of emissary vein connect this sinus to pterygoid venous plexus. The two cavernous sinuses are interconnected medially by anterior and posterior inter-cavernous sinuses – circular sinus. The cavernous sinus like other dural venous sinuses drains into the veins outside the cranium. Thus its various connections are clinically significant.

GREATER WING OF SPHENOID

Presents the following features:

Foramen rotundum

It is the anterior most round foramen in greater wing of sphenoid. It is below and behind the medial end of superior orbital fissure. The maxillary nerve (V-2) leaves middle cranial fossa through this foramen to enter pterygopalatine fossa.

Foramen ovale

Placed posterolateral to foramen rotundum, this oval foramen is anterolateral to foramen lacerum – which is a gap between apex of petrous temporal and posterior part of body of sphenoid. Through foramen ovale, following structures pass to and fro to middle cranial fossa and infratemporal fossa:

- Mandibular nerve
- Lesser petrosal nerve
- Accessory meningeal artery
- Emissary vein

Foramen spinosum

It is immediate posterolateral to foramen ovale. It is named so as it is seen close to spine of sphenoid (spine is appreciated in normal basalis). This small foramen transmits following structures:

- **Middle meningeal artery** and its accompanied vein
- **Nervous spinosum** – sensory nerve from trunk of mandibular nerve and carries sensory impulses from dura mater in the base of middle cranial fossa. The middle meningeal vessels produce well marked grooves in the floor and lateral wall of middle cranial fossa.

Foramen lacerum

It is an interosseous space with haggard margins. This foramen is bounded by the bulk of apex of petrous temporal, by the body and part of greater wing of sphenoid. At its anterior pole it communicates with pterygoid canal. Its posterior pole receives internal carotid artery which enters middle cranial fossa through the upper opening of foramen lacerum. The inferior opening of foramen lacerum (Norma basalis view) is closed by a plate of cartilage. Thus no important structure passes through the lower opening except an emissary vein and meningeal branch of ascending pharyngeal artery.

Emissary sphenoidal foramen

Infrequently present small foramen near the root of greater wing of sphenoid in between the foramen rotundum and ovale – foramen of Vaselius. It transmits an emissary vein connecting cavernous sinus to pterygoid venous plexus.

Canaliculus innominatus

It is an accessory foramen at times seen between foramen ovale and spinosum. It transmits lesser petrosal nerve from middle cranial fossa to otic ganglion in the upper part of infratemporal fossa.

FEATURES OF SUPERIOR SURFACE OF PETROUS TEMPORAL BONE

Trigeminal impression

A shallow depression is seen on the anterior surface near the apex of petrous temporal. It is immediately behind and lateral to foramen lacerum. It occupies a space of dura mater – cavum trigerminale. It lodges trigeminal ganglion in cavum trigerminale.

Hiatus and groove for greater petrosal nerve (*Fallopian hiatus*)

It is a minute opening lateral to trigeminal impression. It leads into a narrow groove that runs towards the foramen lacerum. The greater superficial petrosal nerve comes out through this hiatus to run in the groove to reach pterygoid canal at the anterior pole of foramen lacerum.

Hiatus and groove for lesser petrosal nerve

Anterolateral to fallopian hiatus and groove for lesser petrosal nerve, there is an opening in tegmen tympani and a groove running towards foramen ovale. It transmits and lodges lesser petrosal nerve.

Arcuate eminence

Posterolateral to trigeminal impression is the arcuate eminence which is seen as rounded transversely placed elevation. It is caused by underlying superior semicircular canal of internal ear.

Tegmen tympani

A thin sheet of bone forms the roof of tympanic cavity – tegmen tympani. This is seen anterolateral to arcuate eminence. The sheet of bone extends anteromedially above the pharyngotympanic tube. The roof of tympanic antrum is formed by posterior part of tegmen tympani lateral to arcuate eminence.

Superior border of petrous part of temporal bone

It separates middle cranial fossa from posterior cranial fossa. It is grooved by superior petrosal sinus along its entire course.

Cavum trigeminale

In front of starting part of groove for superior petrosal sinus there is a shallow smooth notch (trigeminal notch) is seen. This notch leads into trigeminal impression. The roots of trigeminal nerve are seen between superior petrosal sinus above and the endosteal dura covering the bone below. The trigeminal notch extends forwards and medially as a bony projection. It gives attachment to petroclenoid ligament which extends up to posterior clenoid process. The VI th cranial nerve (Abducent) presents second sharp bend across the upper border of temporal bone in front of bony spicule. Thus the nerve lies under petroclenoid ligament and by the side of dorsum sallae. (**Dorollo's canal**). It is joined by internal carotid artery to run in the floor of cavernous sinus.

POSTERIOR CRANIAL FOSSA

INTRODUCTION

This is deepest and most extensive of all the three cranial fossae.

BOUNDARIES

Anteriorly

- Dorsum sallae
- Clivus
- Basisphenoid
- Basiocciput

Posteriorly

- Lower part of squamous part of occipital bone

Each side

- Petromastoid part
- Condylar part of occipital bone

Posterosuperiorly

- Postero inferior angle of parietal bone

CONTENTS OF POSTERIOR CRANIAL FOSSA

Contains the hind brain
- Pons and medulla (in front)
- Cerebellum (behind)

FEATURES

IN CENTRAL OR MEDIAN PART

Clivus

The anterior wall is related to network of basilar sinuses which is connected to
- inferior petrosal sinus
- internal vertebral venous plexus

The sloping surface of clivus is related to anterior parts of pons and medulla together with the meninges. The petro occipital fissure separates the clivus from the petrous temporal bone. The fissure leads into jugular foramen behind. The inferior petrosal sinus runs along the fissure.

Foramen magnum

It is the largest foramen in the floor of the fossa. It is surrounded by components of occipital bone
- Basilar part of occipital in front
- Condylar part on each side
- Squamous part behind

Its narrow anterior part is above the dens of axis while wider posterior part has the passage of medulla that becomes continuous with the spinal cord in the vertebral canal. The medial aspect of occipital condyles encroach the anterior part of foramen magnum making it narrower.

Internal occipital crest & protuberance

Behind the foramen magnum in the median plane is placed the internal occipital crest. Superiorly it is traced as an irregular elevation – internal occipital protuberance. Wide shallow grooves produced by transverse sinuses are seen lateral to the internal occipital protuberance. Usually the right groove is deeper. The lateral part of these grooves becomes continuous with the groove for sigmoid sinuses. Below these grooves the squamous part of occipital bone lodges cerebellar hemispheres in the well marked hollowed fossae. To internal occipital crest the falx cerebelli is attached containing occipital sinus while the internal occipital protuberance is marked by the meeting of sinuses – **confluence of sinuses.**

The tentorium cerebelli is a tent like double fold of meningeal layer of dura mater having an attached margin which encloses the transverse sinus between its two layers. The free margin surrounds the mid brain. The anterior ends of free margin are attached to anterior clenoid process. The posterior clenoid process and superior border of petrous temporal give attachment to two layers of tentorium cerebelli with the superior petrosal sinus in between. In the posterior part of cranial fossa above the attached margin of tentorium cerebelli are fossae for the occipital lobe of cerebrum. Thus the attached margin of tentorium cerebelli extends from posterior clenoid process onto superior border of petrous temporal, along the groove for transverse sinus until the internal occipital protuberance.

IN LATERAL AREA

Jugular tubercle

The condylar part of occipital bone shows a rounded elevation – jugular tubercle – which lies medial to lower border of jugular foramen. Below and behind the jugular tubercle, the inner end of anterior condylar canal is seen.

Hypoglossal canal (*Anterior condylar canal*)

It transmits hypoglossal (XII CN) nerve and meningeal branch of ascending pharyngeal artery.

Posterior condylar canal (if present)

It opens in the posterior cranial fossa behind and lateral to the opening of hypoglossal canal. An emissary vein runs in it to connect sigmoid sinus with sub occipital venous plexus.

PART FORMED BY POSTERIOR SURFACE OF PETROUS PART OF TEMPORAL BONE

Jugular foramen

On tracing the petro occipital fissure, the jugular foramen is seen at its posterior end. It is an irregular gap between upper and lower borders. The lower border is smooth while upper border is irregular and sharp. It presents a notch for the Glossopharyngeal nerve. The foramen is divided into three parts – anterior most part transmits superior petrosal sinus, the middle part provides passage for IX, X & XI cranial nerves (from anterior to posterior) while the posterior wide part transmits

sigmoid sinus and inferior petrosal sinus. The sigmoid sinus beyond jugular foramen continues as internal jugular vein receiving inferior petrosal sinus as its first tributary.

Internal acoustic meatus

On the anterolateral wall of posterior cranial fossa above the jugular foramen – internal acoustic (auditory) meatus is present. It is a slit like opening transmitting motor and sensory root (nervous intermedius) of facial nerve along with Vestibulocochlear nerve. The sensory root of facial nerve is placed over the VIII cranial nerve and under motor root of facial nerve. Hence it is called as nervous intermedius.

MASTOID PART OF TEMPORAL BONE

Sigmoid sulcus

Tracing the anterolateral wall of posterior cranial fossa posteriorly a gentle **S shaped wide groove** is seen from the lateral limit of the groove for the transverse sinus to the posterior limit of jugular foramen. It occupies the sigmoid sinus. At times mastoid foramen is seen near its posterior margin (mastoid foramen) connecting emissary vein from the sigmoid sinus. The right sigmoid sulcus is deeper.

CLINICAL CONSIDERATIONS OF ANTERIOR CRANIAL FOSSA

Fracture of Orbital Plate of Frontal Bone

This causes trickling of blood under the conjunctiva – subconjunctival haemorrhage. The other fractures in the anterior cranial fossa may present a complex clinical picture due to involvement of frontal, ethmoidal and sphenoidal air sinuses. There may be bleeding into the nose or mouth. Tearing of meninges would cause leakage of CSF from the nose. Meningitis may appear due to communication with the exterior through the nasal cavity.

Foramen Caecum

When it is patent it transmits a vein from the nasal mucosa to the superior sagittal sinus. Thus it is a potential site for transmission of infection from the nasal cavity to the cranium.

CLINICAL CONSIDERATIONS OF MIDDLE CRANIAL FOSSA

Radiographic Studies of Sella Turcica and Hypophyseal Fossa

Aneurysm of internal carotid artery, tumours of pituitary and raised intracranial pressure demand radiographic/imaging investigation. Decalcification is observed in dorsum sellae.

Fracture of Middle Cranial Fossa

It is characterized by multiple features of bleeding through ear, CSF leakage from the ear, bleeding into the mouth and involvement of abducent (medial squint and diplopia). Facial and auditory nerves may be involved.

CLINICAL CONSIDERATION OF POSTERIOR CRANIAL FOSSA

Fractures

These can cause extravasations of blood in the sub occipital region. A swelling appears at the back of the upper part of the neck due to this bleeding. Ninth, tenth and eleventh cranial nerves may get injured in the jugular foramen.

19

Norma Basalis

INTRODUCTION

The inferior surface of skull is termed as normal basalis. It presents many foramina. It presents very irregular surface and has no distinct subdivisions.

BOUNDARIES

In front: Incisor teeth of maxilla
Behind: Superior nuchal lines
On each side
- By other teeth
- Zygomatic arch and is posterior root
- Mastoid process

SUBDIVISIONS

Anterior Part

It is formed by complete alveolar arch and hard palate

Middle Part

It is placed between posterior margins of hard palate anteriorly to a transverse line posteriorly passing through the anterior margin of foramen magnum.

Posterior Part

Behind the transverse line passing through anterior margin of foramen magnum

ANTERIOR PART OF NORMA BASALIS

FEATURES

Alveolar arch of maxilla

It presents (in adult) 16 sockets for the roots of the teeth. Each half has 2,1,2,3 sockets respectively for incisors, canine, premolars and molars. The size and depth of all sockets is not uniform.

Hard palate

Formation – By the palatine processes of maxillae and the horizontal plates of palatine bone.

Sutures – The palatine processes and palatine bone are joined by cruciform suture (inter maxillary, interpalatine and palatomaxillary sutures)

Incisive fossa – Behind the incisors, a deep inverted funnel shaped fossa – incisive fossa lies in the median plane. This leads into incisive canals (right and left). The incisive fossa transmits (a) Long nasopalatine nerve from floor of nasal cavity to the palate (b) Terminal branches of greater palatine vessels ascending of the nasal cavity.

Greater palatine foramen – It is seen behind the palatomaxillary suture medial to last molar tooth. It transmits vessels and nerve of the same name

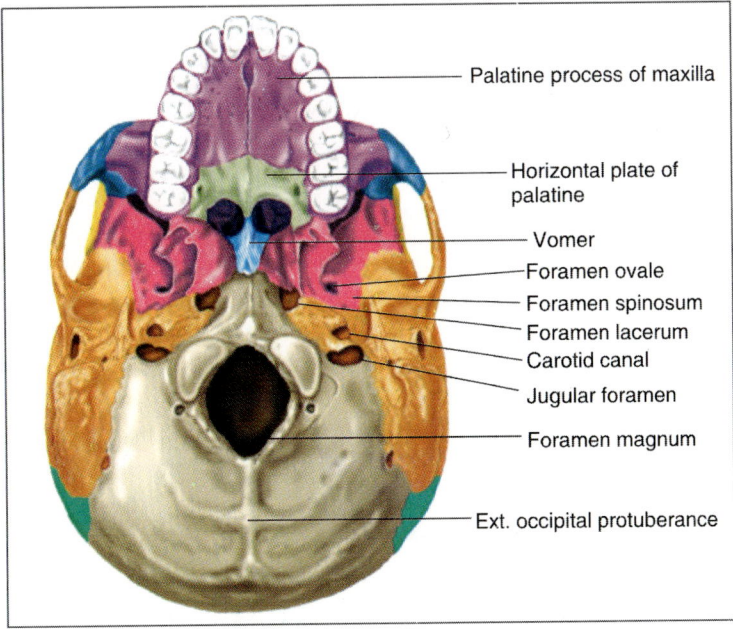

Fig. 19.1: Norma Basalis

Lesser palatine foramina- They are situated behind the greater palatine foramen, transmitting vessels and nerve of the same name.

Posterior nasal spine – The posterior border of hard palate is free. Its median projection is termed as posterior nasal spine. The palatine aponeurosis is attached to the free margin of hard palate.

Palatine crest – It is a raised ridge situated behind the greater palatine foramen.

MIDDLE PART OF NORMA BASALIS

On tracing anteriorly lateral to midline it leads into posterior nasal apertures with posterior border of vomer is in between.

FEATURES OF MEDIAN AREA

Union of basi-occiput and basi-sphenoid – In front of anterior margin of foramen magnum in an adult, the basilar part of occipital bone and body of sphenoid are joined by synostosis. Its anterior part in the midline presents pharyngeal tubercle. Highest fibers of superior constrictor of pharynx are attached here.

FEATURES OF LATERAL AREA

Pterygoid process

Between the greater wing and body of sphenoid two vertical laminae of bone are seen separated posteriorly from each other by pterygoid fossa. Anteriorly the two pterygoid plates are fused to each other. On the lateral side the fused laminae are separated from the maxilla by pterygomaxillary fissure.

Medial pterygoid plate

It projects directly posteriorly. The medial surface bounds posterior nasal aperture. This plate presents following features.

Scaphoid fossa

The upper end of posterior border of the plate encloses shallow boat shaped fossa – scaphoid fossa.

Pterygoid hamulus

In the lower part the posterior border projects as a hook like projection – pterygoid hamulus. Its root is grooved laterally by the tendon of tensor veli palati.

Lateral pterygoid plate

It projects posterolaterally. Its lateral surface bounds the infratemporal fossa while superiorly it is continuous with the greater wing of sphenoid.

FEATURES OF GREATER WING OF SPHENOID

Infratemporal surface & infratemporal crest

It forms anterior part of roof of infratemporal fossa. The infratemporal crest is placed at anterolateral part of greater wing. It marks the upper limit of infratemporal fossa. Articulations of greater wing (a) **laterally** - with squamous temporal (b) **posteromedially** - with petrous temporal. This wing bears important foramina and a spine.

Spine of sphenoid

It appears at the posterolateral arch of external surface of greater wing. Medial surface of the spine is flat. The spine is related to following nerves.
- **Medially – Chorda tympani**
- **Laterally – Auriculotemporal nerve**

The spine provides **attachment to**
- Sphenomandibular ligament
- Anterior ligament of maleus

Foramen ovale

It is placed posterolateral to upper end of posterior margin of lateral pterygoid plate.

Foramen spinosum

It is posterolateral to foramen ovale medial to the spine of sphenoid.

Emissary sphenoidal foramen

When present it is in between foramen ovale and scaphoid fossa.

Canaliculus innominatus

It is occasionally seen. It is situated between foramen ovale and spinosum.

Sulcus tubae

An anterolateral groove is seen bounded by posterior border of greater wing and petrous temporal bone. The cartilaginous part of pharyngo-tympanic tube is placed in this groove. When traced posterolaterally the groove leads to the canal for the tube which runs in the petrous part of temporal bone.

FEATURES OF INFERIOR SURFACE OF PETROUS TEMPORAL

Foramen lacerum

Medial to the groove for auditory tube, it is the gap between the apex of petrous temporal, greater wing of sphenoid and basilar part of occipital bone. The gap forms one cm long canal. Its posterior wall receives the anterior end of carotid canal.

Carotid canal

Posterolateral to foramen lacerum is the opening of carotid canal. The internal carotid artery along with sympathetic plexus enters the carotid canal. Within the petrous temporal the canal turns forwards and medially to reach the posterior wall of foramen lacerum. The internal carotid artery presents two bends at each end of carotid canal.

Squamo-tympanic fissure

It runs posterolaterally between the tympanic plate and the articular fossa of squamous temporal bone. It is lateral to the base of spine of sphenoid. The lower border of tegmen tympani enters the squamo-tympanic fissure to **divide** it into
- Petro-tympanic fissure (posteriorly)
- Petro-squamous fissure (anteriorly)

The chorda tympani nerve comes out through petrotympanic fissure and lies medial to. spine of sphenoid. It also transmits anterior tympanic artery.

Mandibular fossa

It has two parts anterior articular and posterior nonarticular. The head of the mandible with the articular disc of TM Joint occupies the articular part of mandibular fossa. The fossa is restricted in front by a transverse rounded elevation – articular tubercle. This is continuous laterally with anterior root of zygoma.

Tubercle of root of zygoma

When viewed from lateral aspect the commencement of anterior root is seen as a tubercle – tubercle of root of zygoma. It gives attachment to lateral ligament of TM joint.

FEATURES OF TYMPANIC PART OF TEMPORAL BONE

Behind the squamotympanic fissure external acoustic meatus is seen. The tympanic part of temporal bone separates the articular fossa from the external auditory meatus. The tympanic part is triangular in shape, its apex being close to root of spine of sphenoid. Its free lower border surrounds anterolateral margin of carotid canal. The tympanic part extends backwards and laterally until the root of styloid process to form sheath of styloid process. The tympanic part is fused with mastoid part of temporal bone posteroinferiorly.

POSTERIOR PART OF NORMAL BASALIS

Foramen magnum

It occupies anteromedian part of posterior portion of Norma basalis. The foramen is oval due to greater anteroposterior diameter. To anterior margin of foramen magnum anterior atlanto occipital membrane is attached while to the posterior margin posterior atlanto occipital membrane along with alar ligament is attached. It communicates posterior cranial fossa with vertebral canal. For descriptive purposes it can be divided into two parts:

Anterior part is for
- Apical ligament of dens
- Membrana tectoria

Wider posterior part is for
- Lower end of medulla with meninges in subarachnoid space
- Vertebral arteries
- Spinal accessory nerve
- Posterior spinal arteries
- Anterior spinal artery
- Lower portions of tonsils of cerebellum (at times)

Occipital condyles

Placed anterolateral to the margin of foramen magnum, overlapping it are the occipital condyles. Each condyle is oval in shape and is to form atlanto occipital joint for" Yes" movement. They articulate with superior articular facets on the lateral mass of atlas.

Anterior condylar canal (*Hypoglossal canal*)

Running anterolaterally above the anterior part of occipital condyle the anterior condylar canal is seen. It transmits hypoglossal nerve.

Posterior condylar fossa

Behind the occipital condyle is the condylar fossa. It may be pierced by posterior condylar canal for the passage of emissary vein from the sigmoid sinus.

Jugular process

Lateral to the condyle an irregular part of occipital bone (jugular process) articulates with petrous temporal.

Jugular foramen

The anterior border of jugular process bounds the jugular foramen posteriorly. The large foramen is situated at the posterior end of petro occipital suture. Anteriorly a raised ridge separates it from the carotid canal. Laterally it is close to the sheath of styloid process. Medially a thin plate of bone separates it from anterior condylar canal. The axis of the foramen is directed anteromedially. The foramen is larger on the right side usually.

Jugular fossa

A depression of variable depth is seen in petrous temporal. It is seen posterolateral to the jugular foramen. The floor of the fossa lodges superior bulb of internal jugular vein separating it from the tympanic cavity

Cochlear canaliculus & Notch

The inferior ganglion of Glossopharyngeal nerve is occupied in a triangular depression seen on the upper boundary of jugular foramen medially. The opening of cochlear canaliculus lies at the apex of the notch. The edges of the notch may divide the jugular foramen into three parts. The cochlear canaliculus communicates the perilymph with the cerebrospinal fluid.

Tympanic canaliculus

The bony bridge between carotid canal and jugular fossa presents a small opening – tympanic canaliculus. Tympanic branch of Glossopharyngeal nerve (**Jacobson's nerve**) enters the middle ear cavity.

Styloid process

A slender projection of variable length extends downwards, forwards and medially placed medial to the tympanic plate. Its proximal part (tympanohyal) is covered anterolaterally by the bony sheath of tympanic plate. Its distal part (stylohyal) gives attachment to structures constituting styloid apparatus. They are **muscles** – Stylohyoid, stylopharyngeus and styloglossus and **ligaments** – stylohyoid and stylomandibular.

Stylomastoid foramen

It is seen between mastoid process and styloid process. It is the lower opening of facial canal for the exit of motor root of facial nerve.

Mastoid process & notch

Behind and lateral to stylomastoid foramen, the mastoid process projects downwards and forwards. It forms the lateral wall of an oblique groove – mastoid notch. The posterior belly of digastric arises from this notch. Medial to the notch, the bone may be grooved by the occipital artery.

External occipital crest

Behind the foramen magnum in the median plane a linear ridge – external occipital crest is present. It extends posteriorly until the external occipital protuberance. The ligamentum nuchae is attached to this crest. From the middle of the crest, curved lines diverge backwards and laterally running parallel to superior nuchal lines.

External occipital protuberance

This bony projection is most prominent land mark limiting the Norma basalis posteriorly. This landmark is used in craniometry.

CLINICAL CONSIDERATIONS

Fracture of Spine of Sphenoid

The spina of sphenoid is related to two nerves auriculotemporal nerve and chorda tympani. Damage to auriculotemporal nerve would result in dry mouth (postganglionic parasympathetic pathway to the parotid gland will be disrupted).

Involvement of chorda tympanis causes loss of taste sensations from the anterior two third of the tongue (gustatory to the tongue).

Arnold Chiari Syndrome

This is the most common congenital anomaly involving cerebellum. The vermis of cerebellum herniates into the vertebral canal through foramen magnum. This anomaly results in communicating type of hydrocephalus. The interference of absorption of cerebrospinal fluid results in dilatation of the entire ventricular system of brain. This anomaly is frequently associated with spina bifida with meningomyelocele.

20

Mandible

INTRODUCTION

It is a bone of face having a curved more or less horizontal body that is continuous with two broad rami from the posterior end of the body. They project upwards and participate in temporomandibular joints. Mandible is required for mastication. Hence it is very strong.

BODY OF MANDIBLE

Shaped like a horse shoe having two borders (upper border and lower) and two surfaces (internal and external)

OUTER SURFACE

Rough and shows the following features:

Symphysis menti

It represents midline fusion of the two halves. It is a misnomer since it is not a secondary cartilaginous joint.

Mental protuberance

The ridge of the symphysis menti encloses a triangular area close to the lower border. It is raised on each side as mental tubercles.

Mental foramen

On the anterolateral aspect of the body on each side below the second premolar is the mental foramen. Mental nerve and vessels emerge through this foramen.

Mental fossa

Between the mental tubercles the midline triangular depression is termed as mental fossa.

Oblique line

A faint line runs upwards and backwards from the mental tubercle to become continuous with the anterior margin of the ramus of mandible. This line is well marked in its posterior part.

UPPER BORDER

It is formed by the hollow of the sockets for the roots of the teeth. Hence it is termed as alveolar border. In an adult mandible each half presents eight sockets for **Incisors (2) Canine (1) Premolars (2) and Molars (3)**

LOWER BORDER

It is also termed as the base of the mandible. It is thick and rounded. It extends backwards and laterally from the symphysis menti to continue as lower border of the ramus beyond last molar tooth.

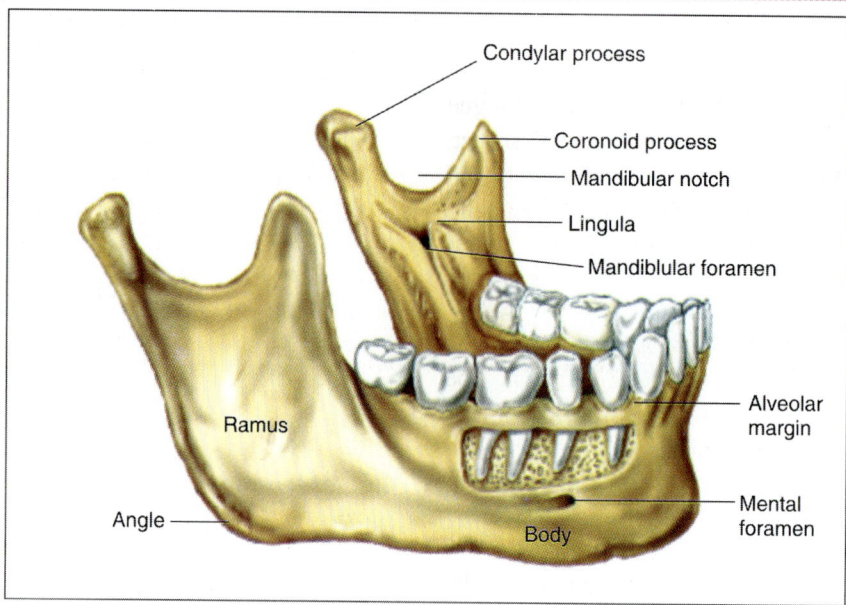

Fig. 20.1: Mandible

INNER SURFACE

It shows following features:

Mylohyoid line

An oblique ridge – mylohyoid line divides the inner surface into upper and lower parts. It is well marked posteriorly below the molar teeth, starting from behind and below the third molar tooth. It runs forwards and downwards to reach the interval between the digastric fossae below the genial tubercle.

Sublingual fossa

It is a triangular shallow area situated above the anterior part of mylohyoid line which lodges the sublingual salivary gland.

Submandibular fossa

Below the mylohyoid line in its posterior half the surface shows a hollow – submandibular fossa which lodges submandibular salivary gland.

Genial tubercles

In midline above the anterior ends of mylohyoid lines, genial tubercles are present – two on each side and called upper and lower tubercles.

Digastric fossa

It provides attachment of anterior belly of digastric muscle.

Mylohyoid groove

Below the posterior end of mylohyoid line, mylohyoid groove is seen which is well marked as it is traced upwards and backwards on the inner surface of the body of mandible.

RAMUS OF MANDIBLE

Quadrilateral part that is continuous with the body of the mandible anteriorly

Outer surface

This flat surface bears oblique ridges in the lower part – Masseter is attached here.

Inner surface

Mandibular foramen

An irregular opening guarded by a thin small tongue like projection is seen on its anteromedial aspect. It transmits inferior alveolar (dental) nerve and vessels. These run in the mandibular canal situated within the ramus and body of mandible.

Lingula

The mandible develops from Meckel's cartilage and the mesenchymal membrane covering it. The lingula represents part of remnant of Meckels cartilage. Sphenomandibular ligament is attached to the lingula.

Area below & behind mandibular foramen

This roughened area is for medial pterygoid muscle.

BORDERS OF RAMUS

Inferior

It is continuous anteriorly with the base of mandible in line with the third molar tooth. Behind it is continuous with posterior border at the angle of the mandible. In males the angle is everted.

Posterior

It is a round and thick border which bears a gentle concavity in the middle with convexity in its upper and lower parts. It extends from the angle of mandible upwards to the back of condyloid process (head of the mandible)

Superior

It is relatively thin and bounds mandibular notch. It ends anteriorly at the coronoid process.

Anterior

From the anterior border of coronoid process it begins as a thin curved border that becomes thick as it continues as the oblique line on the body of mandible.

PROCESSES OF MANDILE

Condyloid process

The postero superior part arising from quadrilateral ramus of mandible is termed the condyloid process. Its expanded upper part is head of mandible. It is convex in all directions and is greater in transverse diameter than antero posterior diameter. It articulates with mandibular fossa of temporal bone. The articular disc intervenes the two articular surfaces. The head of mandible can be palpated in front of tragus during movements of TM joint. A constricted part below the head is neck of the mandible. The neck in its anterior part bears a concavity – pterygoid fovea for lateral pterygoid muscle.

Coronoid process

Tracing the upper border anteriorly a flattened triangular projection is seen directed upwards and forwards. To its margins and medial surface the medial pterygoid muscle is attached.

Mandibular canal

This can be viewed only on resecting the bone downwards and forwards from the mandibular foramen. It extends from the ramus to the body. It contains inferior dental nerve and vessels. These issue branches for the roots of the teeth. Mental and incisive canals arise from the mandibular canal in line with the root of second premolar tooth.

OSSIFICATION

It ossifies from the mesenchymal membrane covering the outer surface of **Meckel's cartilage**. The part of the bone which ossifies from the Meckel's cartilage is as under:

Parts ossifying in cartilage
- Lingula and Sphenomandibular ligament
- Genial tubercles

Parts ossifying in membrane
- Rest of the bone ossifies in the membrane.

GROWTH OF MANDIBLE

Height of the mandible is gained with growth of the ramus and downward and forward growth of the body.

Height is further gained by the appearance of alveolar processes and teeth together.

Circumferential growth of the body and ramus is carried out by the well regulated processes of accretion and deposition i.e. new bone is deposited on the outer surface while along the inner surface accretion takes place.

AGE CHANGES IN MANDIBLE

In medico-legal practice, the mandible is a definite clue to the age of the individual. Sex of the individual can also be ascertained in conjunction with features of other bones.

CLINICAL CONSIDERATIONS

Fractures of Mandible

Usually the fractures of mandible occur on the opposite side of the blow. Commonly affected sites are (a) coronoid process (b) neck of mandible (c) angle of mandible (d) body of mandible in front of mental foramen. Frequently these fractures are bilateral.

Patterns of Fracture of Mandible

- Neck of condyle - most common followed by

- Angle o' .andible through the last tooth
- Region .w the canine tooth (butterfly fractur'

Dislocation

The head of the mandible may dislocate into the infratemporal fossa. It may be unilateral or bilateral. This forward dislocation is possible when the mouth is wide open (Yawning) or a blow). The reduction is done by pressing the mandible down with the thumbs on the last molar teeth (to bring the head of the mandible down). Upward pressure is applied at the chin (closure of mouth) which guides the head of the mandible into the mandibular fossa.

Mandibular Nerve Block

The extra oral approach for the mandibular nerve block is injecting the local anaesthetic agent in the mandibular nerve as it emerges from the foramen ovale. The needle is passed through the mandibular notch into the infratemporal fossa.

Inferior Alveolar/Lingual Nerve Block

To anaesthetize the lower teeth, floor of the mouth and anterior two third of the tongue adequately for small operations (tooth extraction, root canal treatment), the inferior alveolar / lingual nerve is anaesthetized. About half inch above the crown of last molar tooth and just medial to the ramus of the mandible, the needle is passed backwards and slightly outwards. This will infiltrate the posterior division of mandibular nerve just above it enters the mandibular canal.

21

Maxilla

It is the largest facial bone except the mandible. It forms

- Upper jaw
- Buccal roof
- Floor and lateral wall of nasal cavity
- Floor of orbit
- Part of infratemporal fossa
- Pterygopalatine fossa
- Inferior orbital fissure
- Pterygomaxillary fissure

IT CONSISTS OF BODY

Four processes

- Zygomatic
- Frontal
- Alveolar
- Palatine

BODY

It is roughly pyramidal and presents four surfaces

- Anterior
- Infratemporal (posterior)
- Orbital
- Nasal

These surfaces enclose the maxillary sinus

Anterior surface

It faces anterolaterally and shows inferior elevations which overlie the roots of teeth.

Incisive fossa is seen above incisors in depressor septi is attached. To the alveolar border a slip of orbicularis oris is attached, and superolateral to nasalis is attached.

Canine fossa (lateral to incisive fossa) is separated from incisive fossa by the canine eminence. In the canine fossa levator anguli oris is attached.

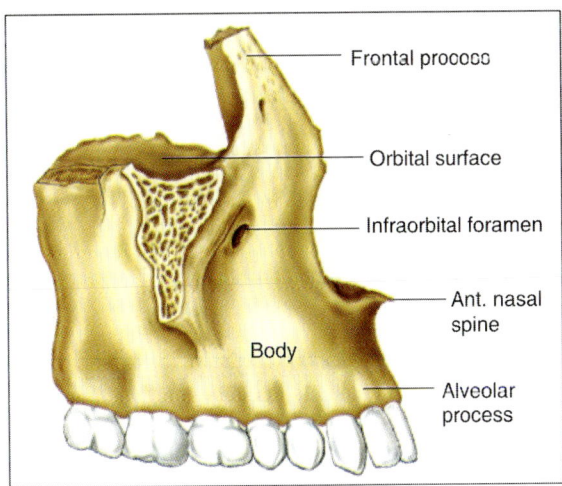

Frontal process

Orbital surface

Infraorbital foramen

Ant. nasal spine

Body

Alveolar process

Fig. 21.1: Maxilla

Infraorbital foramen is seen above the canine fossa. It transmits infraorbital vessels and nerve.

Medially the anterior surface ends at nasal notch and ends in a pointed process which, with opposite side forms the **anterior nasal spine**. To the anterior surface near the notch, nasalis and depressor septi are attached.

Infratemporal surface

It faces posterolaterally and forms the anterior wall of the infratemporal fossa. It is separated from the anterior surface by zygomatic process of maxilla. Near its centre there are openings of two or three alveolar canals which contain posterior superior alveolar vessels and nerves. Maxillary tuberosity is see posteroinferiorly. It is rough superomedially where it joins the pyramidal process of palatine bone. Few fibres of medial pterygoid are attached to it. Above this anterior boundary of the pterygopalatine fossa is there which is grooved by the maxillary nerve as it passes laterally and slightly upwards into the infraorbital groove on the orbital surface.

Orbital surface

This smooth and triangular surface forms most of the floor of orbit. Anteriorly its medial border has a lacrimal notch, behind which it joins with the lacrimal bone and the orbital plate of ethmoid while posteriorly with the orbital process of palatine bone. Its posterior border forms most of the anterior edge of the inferior orbital fissure and in the central infraorbital groove is seen.

Its anterior border forms part of the orbital margin and continuous medially with the lacrimal crest of the frontal process of maxilla. The infraorbital groove transmits infraorbital vessels and nerve. It begins midway on the posterior border and continuous with a groove on the posterior surface. It passes forwards into the infraorbital canal, which opens on the anterior surface below the infraorbital margin.

Near its midpoint the canal has a small lateral branch (**canalis sinuosus**) for the anterior superior alveolar nerve and vessels. It descends in the orbital floor lateral to the infraorbital canal and curves medially in the anterior wall of the maxillary sinus. It passes below the infraorbital foramen to the margin of the anterior nasal aperture in front of the anterior end of the inferior concha. Then it follows the lower margin of aperture to open near the nasal septum in front of the incisive canal.

Nasal surface

It shows large, irregular maxillary hiatus posterosuperiorly which leads into the maxillary sinus. At the upper border of hiatus parts of air sinuses are completed by the ethmoid and lacrimal bones. Below the hiatus it forms part of the inferior meatus. Behind it a rough surface meets the perpendicular plate of palatine. This surface is traversed by a groove which descends forwards from the midpoint of posterior border. It is converted into greater palatine canal by the perpendicular plate of palatine bone.

Anterior to the hiatus a deep groove is continuous above with the lacrimal groove and forms about two-thirds of the circumference of the nasolacrimal canal. This canal leads the nasolacrimal duct to the inferior meatus. More anterior oblique conchal crest is seen for the inferior nasal concha.

MAXILLARY SINUS

This is a large pyramidal cavity. Its thin walls correspond to orbital, alveolar, facial and infratemporal aspects of the maxilla. Its apex is directed laterally which extends into the zygomatic process. Its base is placed medially and forms the lateral wall of the nasal cavity and shows the maxillary hiatus.

The hiatus is reduced in living persons by

- **Above** - Uncinate process of ethmoid and descending part of the lacrimal

- **Below** - Maxillary process of the inferior nasal concha
- **Behind** - Perpendicular plate of palatine

The maxillary sinus is connected with the middle meatus, usually by two small openings, one of which is usually closed by mucous membrane.

Its posterior wall contains alveolar canals which transmit posterior superior alveolar vessels and nerves to molar teeth. Its floor is formed by the alveolar process and its lowest part is about 1.25 cm below the nasal floor. The infraorbital canal usually ridges the sinus from roof to anterior wall.

PROCESSES

ZYGOMATIC PROCESS

Into this pyramidal projection anterior, infratemporal and orbital surfaces converge. In front it merges into the facial surface of the body of maxilla. Behind it is concave and continuous with the infratemporal surface. Above it is serrated for the articulation with the zygomatic bone. Below an arched border separates facial (anterior) and infratemporal surfaces.

FRONTAL PROCESS

It projects posterosuperiorly between the nasal and lacrimal bones.

Lateral surface is divided by a vertical anterior lacrimal crest for the attachment of the medial palpebral ligament and is continuous below with the infraorbital margin. At the junction of the crest and orbital surface a small palpable tubercle is seen - guide to the **lacrimal sac**. The smooth area anterior to the lacrimal crest merges below with the anterior surface of body and part of **orbicularis oculi** and **levator labii superioris alaeque nasi** are attached here. Behind the crest a vertical groove joins the lacrimal bone to complete the lacrimal fossa.

Medial surface forms part of the lateral wall of nose. A rough subapical area joins with the ethmoid and closes anterior ethmoidal air cells. Below this ethmoidal crest articulates posteriorly with the middle nasal concha.

The frontal process joins above with the nasal part of frontal bone, anterior border with the nasal bone and its posterior border joins with the lacrimal bone.

ALVEOLAR PROCESS

It is thick and arched and contains sockets for roots of teeth. There are eight sockets on each side which vary according to contained teeth (for canine –deepest, for molars - widest and subdivided into three by septa, for incisors and second premolar - single, for the first premolar sometimes double).

Buccinator is attached to the outer alveolar aspect up to the first molar. In articulated maxillae the processes form the **alveolar arch**.

PALATINE PROCESS

It is thick, strong and placed horizontally. It projects medially from the lowest part of the medial maxillary aspect. It forms a large part of the floor of nose and palate.

Inferior surface is concave and with the opposite side it forms anterior three-fourth of the hard palate. It has numerous vascular foramina and depressions for palatine glands. Posterolaterally it contains two grooves which contain greater palatine vessels and nerves.

Between the maxillae behind the incisor teeth a median places intermaxillary palatal suture is seen.

In the incisive fossa there are openings of two lateral incisive canals. Each canal ascends into its half of the nasal cavity and transmits terminations of the greater palatine artery and nasopalatine nerve.

Occasionally two additional median openings are present - anterior and posterior incisive foramina which transmit the nasopalatine nerves.

Superior surface is concave transversely and forms most of the floor of nasal cavity.

Lateral border is continuous with the body of maxilla.

Medial border is raised into a nasal crest which with the opposite side forms a groove for the vomer. The front of nasal crest rises higher as incisor crest which is prolonged forwards into a sharp process. Two processes forms anterior nasal spine.

Posterior border is serrated for the horizontal plate of palatine bone.

OSSIFICATION

It ossifies in mesenchyme from three centres.

One centre for the main maxillary mass - Appears above the canine fossa during 6th week of intrauterine life.

Two centres for the premaxillary region (**os incisivum**) which corresponds in position with a true premaxilla.

Out of these two premaxillary centres, the principal centre appears above the incisor tooth germs during 7th week of intrauterine life. The second centre (**paraseptal** or **prevomerine**) begins in the medial wall of a paraseptal cartilage which fuses soon with the palatine process of maxilla.

The bone formed by the principal premaxillary centre is overgrown by bone developed from the main maxillary mass which fuses along its anterior limit with alveolar process of maxilla (**interalveolar suture of Farmer**).

The maxillary sinus appears as a shallow groove on the nasal aspect during 4th month of intrauterine life.

AGE CHANGES

At birth
- Transverse and sagittal dimensions are greater than vertical dimensions
- Frontal process is prominent
- Body of maxilla is just little more than an alveolar process and its alveoli reach almost to the orbital floor
- Maxillary sinus is just a furrow on the lateral wall of nose

In adults
- Vertical dimension is greatest due to the development of the alveolar process and enlargement of the maxillary sinus

When all teeth are lost
- Bone reverts to the infantile shape
- Its height diminishes
- Alveolar process is absorbed
- Lower parts of the bone is contracted and reduced in thickness

Differences in the mode of alveolar absorption in maxilla and mandible are of practical importance in fitting dentures.

CLINICAL CONSIDERATION

The walls of the sinus are very thin. Thus a tumour may push upwards into the orbital floor and displace the eyeball – exophthalmos. It may project into the nasal cavity, protrude onto the cheek or spread backwards into the infratemporal fossa or downwards into the mouth.

Extraction of molar teeth may damage the floor, and the impact may fracture its walls.

22

Sphenoid Bone

This bat shaped bone is wedged between the frontal, temporal and occipital bones. It consists of a body, greater and lesser wings and pterygoid processes which descent from the junctions of the body and greater wings.

BODY

Cuboidal shaped body contains two large air sinuses, separated by a bony septum. Superior (cerebral) surface articulates in front with the cribriform plates of ethmoid.

FEATURES

Jugum sphenoidale

It is related to gyri recti and olfactory tracts. It is bounded behind by the anterior border of the sulcus chiasmaticus which leads laterally to the optic canals. **Tuberculum sellae**

It is behind jugum sphenoidale

Sella turcica

It is behind tuberculum sallae which contains the hypophysis cerebri in the hypophyseal fossa. Its anterior edge is completed laterally by two middle clinoid processes, posteriorly by dorsum sellae. The superior angles of dorsum sallae have posterior clinoid processes – attachment of the tentorium cerebelli.

Posterior to dorsum sellae the body slopes into basioccipit together they form the clivus.

Lateral surfaces - united both with the greater wings and the medial pterygoid plates.

Above the root of each wing a broad carotid sulcus lodges ICA and cavernous sinus with closely related nerves. It is deepest posteriorly, overhung medially by the petrosal process and has a sharp lateral margin, the lingula, which continues back over the posterior opening of the pterygoid canal.

Anterior surface – a median triangular sphenoidal crest is seen which forms a small part of the nasal septum.

Anterior border joins the perpendicular plate of ethmoid

Sphenoidal sinuses are two large, irregular cavities within the body which are separated by an asymmetrical septum. They varying in form and size and each sinus is partially divided by bony laminae.

CLASSIFICATION OF SPHENOIDAL SINUSES

- **Conchal** - small sinus separated from the sella turcica by about 10 mm of trabecular bone

- **Presellar** - sinus not extended posteriorly to the tuberculum sellae
- **Sellar** - sinus extended at variable distances beyond the tuberculum

Each half anterior surface of the body is consists of:

- A superolateral depressed area joined to the labyrinth of ethmoid which completes the posterior ethmoidal sinuses
- Its lateral margin articulates with the orbital plate of ethmoid above and orbital process of palatine below
- An inferomedial triangular area forms the posterior nasal roof and near its superior angle is the opening of sphenoidal sinus is present

Inferior surface – has a median triangular sphenoidal rostrum. Posterior ends of the sphenoidal conchae flank the rostrum which articulates with alae of vomer. On each side of the posterior part of the rostrum, behind the apex of sphenoidal concha, a thin vaginal process projects medially from the base of the medial pterygoid plate.

GREATER WINGS

These curve superolaterally from the body. Posteriorly it fits the angle between petrous and squamous parts of the temporal bone at a sphenosquamosal suture.

Cerebral surface – anterior part of the middle cranial fossa.

Foramen rotundum is anteromedian which transmits maxillary nerve.

Foramen ovale is placed posterolateral to foramen rotundum.

It transmits

- Mandibular nerve
- Accessory meningeal artery
- Lesser petrosal nerve
- Emissary vein from the cavernous sinus

Foramen spinosum is placed anteromedial to the spine of sphenoid.

It transmits

- Middle meningeal artery
- Meningeal branch of the mandibular nerve

Lateral surface is divided by a transverse infratemporal crest into

- Temporal surface
- Infratemporal surface

Infratemporal surface presents the foramen ovale and foramen spinosum.

Spine of the sphenoid - its medial side shows a faint anteroinferior groove for the chorda tympani. Sphenomandibular ligament is attached to its tip.

Orbital surface faces anteromedially (posterior part of the lateral orbital wall). Its serrated upper edge articulates with the orbital plate of frontal while its serrated lateral margin articulates with the zygomatic bone.

Smooth inferior border is the posterolateral edge of the inferior orbital fissure. **Medial margin** forms the inferolateral edge of the superior orbital fissure. Here, a small tubercle gives partial attachment of the common tendinous ring of Zinn. Below the medial end of superior orbital fissure a grooved area forms the posterior wall of the pterygopalatine fossa which is pierced by the foramen rotundum.

The margin of the greater wing (from the body to the spine) in its medial half forms anterior limit of the foramen lacerum and displays the posterior aperture of the pterygoid canal. Its lateral half articulates with the petrous temporal bone at a sphenopetrosal synchrondrosis.

Sulcus tubae contains the cartilaginous part of auditory tube.

Anterior to the spine of sphenoid the concave margin is serrated for articulation with the squamous part of temporal bone. The tip of the greater wing articulates with the sphenoidal angle of parietal bone at pterion.

Medial to this, a triangular rough area articulates with the frontal bone and its medial angle is continuous with the inferior boundary of the superior orbital fissure.

LESSER WINGS

These are triangular, pointed plates which project laterally from the anterosuperior regions of the body.

Superior surface of each is smooth and related to the cerebral frontal lobe.

Inferior surface is a posterior part of the roof of orbit and upper boundary of the superior orbital fissure. It overhangs the middle cranial fossa.

Posterior border projects into the lateral cerebral fissure; its medial end is the anterior clinoid process, for attachment of the anterior end of the free tentorial border.

Anterior and middle clinoid processes are sometimes united to form a **caroticoclinoid foramen**.

The lesser wing is connected to the body by an anterior root (thin and flat) and posterior root (thick and triangular). Between them the optic canal is placed which contains the optic nerve and ophthalmic artery

SUPERIOR ORBITAL FISSURE

This triangular opening connects the cranial cavity and orbit.

It is bounded
- **Medially** by body of sphenoid
- **Above** by lesser wing
- **Below** by medial margin of orbital surface of greater wing
- Completed laterally by frontal bone

PTERYGOID PROCESSES

The pterygoid processes descend perpendicularly from the junctions of the greater wings and body, consists of medial and lateral plates. The upper parts of the plates fused anteriorly while they are separated below by the angular pterygoid fissure - margins articulate with the pyramidal process of palatine bone. The plates diverge behind and the pterygoid fossa between them contains the medial pterygoid and tensor veli palatini muscles.

Above a small, oval, shallow scaphoid fossa is seen which is formed by division of the upper posterior border of the medial plate - tensor veli palatini is attached.

The anterior surface of the root of the pterygoid process is broad and triangular and forms the posterior wall of pterygopalatine fossa which is pierced by the anterior opening of the pterygoid canal.

Lateral pterygoid plate

The lateral pterygoid plate is broad, thin and everted.

Lateral surface forms part of the medial wall of the infratemporal fossa - attachment of the lower head of the lateral pterygoid.

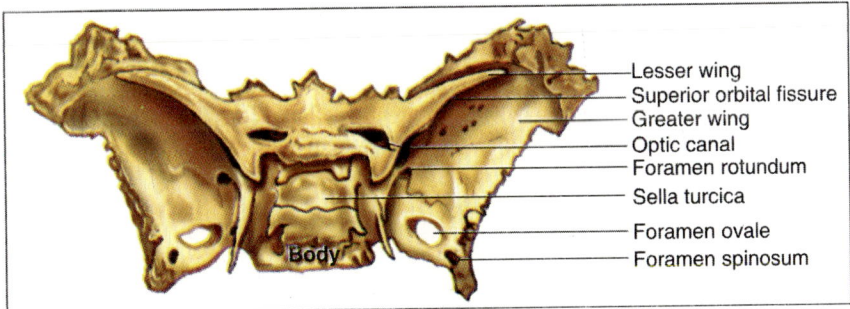

Fig. 22.1: Sphenoid: Superior Aspect

Medial surface forms the lateral wall of the pterygoid fossa – attachment of medial pterygoid.

Upper part of its anterior border forms the posterior boundary of the pterygomaxillary fissure. Its lower part articulates with the palatine bone and the posterior border is free.

Medial pterygoid plate

It is narrower and longer than the lateral plate. Its lower end curves into pterygoid hamulus around which the tendon of the tensor veli palatini winds and the pterygomandibular raphe is attached to it.

Lateral surface forms the medial wall of the pterygoid fossa.

Medial surface forms the lateral boundary of the posterior nasal aperture.

The medial plate is prolonged above on the inferior aspect of the body of sphenoid as the thin vaginal process which articulates anteriorly with the sphenoidal process of palatine and medially with the ala of vomer. Inferiorly it has a furrow which is converted into a canal anteriorly by the sphenoidal process of palatine – palatovaginal canal.

Palatovaginal canal transmits
- Pharyngeal branches of the maxillary artery
- Pterygopalatine ganglion

To the posterior margin of medial pterygoid plate the pharyngobasilar fascia is attached while to its lower end the superior pharyngeal constrictor is attached.

At its upper end a small pterygoid tubercle is seen just below the posterior opening of pterygoid canal.

In the lower part anterior margin of the plate articulates with the posterior border of the perpendicular plate of palatine bone.

SPHENOIDAL CONCHAE

These are two thin, curved plates which are attached anteroinferiorly to the body of sphenoid.

Superior concave surface of each concha is the anterior wall and part of the floor of a sphenoidal sinus. Each has anterior (vertical, quadrilateral) and posterior (horizontal, triangular) parts.

Anterior part consists of

- A superolateral depressed area, completing the posterior ethmoidal sinuses and joining below with the orbital process of a palatine bone
- An inferomedial area, smooth and triangular and part of the nasal roof, perforated above by the round opening connecting the sphenoidal sinus and sphenoethmoidal recess.

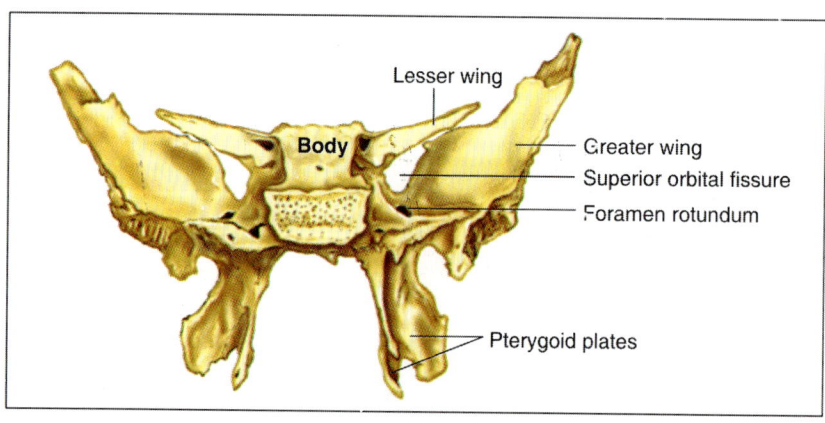

Fig. 22.2: Sphenoid: Posterior view

Anterior parts of the two bones meet in the midline - sphenoidal crest.

Posterior part

It appears in the nasal roof and completes the sphenopalatine foramen. Its medial edge articulates with the rostrum of sphenoid and ala of vomer while its apex is directed posteriorly, is superomedial to the vaginal process of the medial pterygoid plate and joins the posterior part of the ala.

OSSIFICATION

Most of the bone is preformed in cartilage.

Till 7th month of intrauterine life the body of sphenoid consists of

- **Presphenoidal part** - anterior to the tuberculum sellae with which the lesser wings are continuous
- **Postsphenoidal part** - comprise the sella turcica and dorsum sellae and with which the greater wings and pterygoid processes are continuous

There are six ossification centres for the presphenoidal part

There are eight ossification centres for postsphenoidal part

Pre-sphenoidal part

During the 9th week of intrauterine life a centre appears in each lesser wing. Thereafter two bilateral centres appear in the presphenoidal part of body.

Each sphenoidal concha has a centre which appears during 5th month of intrauterine life. This enlarges and it partly surrounds a posterosuperior expansion of the nasal cavity, which becomes the sphenoidal sinus.

During 4th year the concha fuses with the labyrinth of ethmoid bone and before puberty with the sphenoid and palatine bones. Its anterior deficiency persists as an opening for the sphenoidal sinus.

Post-sphenoidal part

One centre appears bilaterally in the greater wing during 8th week of intrauterine life. This centre forms only the root of the wing and the rest of greater wing ossifies in the mesenchyme. During 4th month of intrauterine life two centres appear which flank the sella turcica and soon fuse.

The medial pterygoid plates are also ossify in membrane. For each plate a centre appear during 9th week of intrauterine life.

Medial and lateral pterygoid plates join during 6th month of foetal life. During 4th month a centre appears for each lingula which soon joins the body.

23

Parietal Bone

INTRODUCTION

It bounds the skull on the sides and the roof. Four borders and angles make it somewhat quadrilateral in shape. It has external convex surface and internal concave surface. The medial upper border forms sagittal suture. The anterior border forms coronal suture. The anterior border leads to anteroinferior angle wherein on the inner aspect groove for anterior division of middle meningeal vessel is seen. The posterior border participates in the lambdoid suture. The inferior border articulates anterior to posterior with (a) greater wing of sphenoid (b) squamous temporal and mastoid part of temporal bone. The bone on the inner aspect shows groove for sigmoid sinus.

ANATOMICAL POSITION

- Outer surface is convex
- Concave border inferiorly
- Groove for sigmoid sinus at postero inferior angle.

The bone is held in anatomical position by securing the anteroinferior angle with thumb and index finger of the side it belongs.

FEATURS

External Surface

Parietal eminence/ tuber

Near the centre a slight elevation is seen on the convex smooth external surface. Foetal growth is monitored by measuring biparietal diameter (between two parietal eminences) by ultrasound.

Temporal lines

Superior and inferior temporal lines appear as curved lines extending as arches upwards and backwards in the middle of superior and inferior borders. Temporal fascia is attached to superior temporal line while the temporalis is attached to the area between the two temporal lines.

Parietal foramen

These are situated close to the sagittal (superior) border at the posterior part. It is not always present. It transmits emissary vein connecting superior sagittal sinus.

Internal Surface

It presents impressions of gyri on superolateral surface of cerebrum. The surface is marked by grooves for middle meningeal vessels seen running from the anteroinferior angle towards the upper border. Along the upper border a longitudinal groove for lodging the superior sagittal sinus is seen as a shallow impression. This sagittal sulcus has a number of granular pits which lodge arachnoid granulations better seen in old people. The postero inferior angle bears the groove for sigmoid sinus.

ANGLES

Antero-superior (FRONTAL)
- Forms Bregma (anterior fontanalle till 1 ½ years) with the meeting of coronal and sagittal sutures.

Antero-inferior (SPHENOIDAL)
- Forms pterion (antero-lateral fontanalle till 6 months)

Postero-superior (OCCIPITAL)
- Forms lambda (posterior fontanalle till 1 year) with the meeting of sagittal and lambdoid sutures

Postero-inferior (MASTOID)
- Forms Asterion (postero-lateral fontanalle)

OSSIFICATION

It ossifies in membrane from two centres. These appear at the parietal eminence. The ossification extends gradually in a radial manner towards the periphery of the bone. The angles get ossified later than rest of the bone. Hence fontanalle are formed around four angles.

CLINICAL CONSIDERATIONS

Commonly involve the maximum convexity of the bone – parietal tubers/eminence. This may be due to direct blow or in vehicular accidents.

This foramen (one in each parietal bone close to sagittal suture) transmits emissary veins connecting superior sagittal sinus with the vein of scalp. These channels are valve less. The blood can flow in either direction. Thus an infection of the scalp may pass through emissary veins to superior sagittal sinus resulting in thrombosis of the sinus or meningitis.

24

Frontal Bone

INTRODUCTION

It forms the forehead and looks like a cockle-shell. It also forms roof of the orbital cavity

PARTS

SQUAMOUS – Expanded part that forms major part of the bone.

ORBITAL PLATES - Each orbital plate extends backwards as a shelf like projection to form the roof of the orbital cavity.

NASAL – From the lower aspect in the midline the projecting nasal spine is seen.

ANATOMICAL POSITION

This is an impaired bone.

- Convex external surface (squamous part) to face forwards
- Orbital plates project horizontally backwards.

FEATURES

SQUAMOUS PART

External surface

Shows following features

Frontal eminence

On each side about 3 cm above the supra orbital margin rounded elevations are seen.

Superciliary arches

Below the frontal eminence shallow grooves separate superciliary arches from the frontal eminence.

Glabella

A smooth elevation is seen in the midline where the two superciliary arches meet.

Supraorbital margin

Under the superciliary arches, the upper border of orbital opening is formed by a sharp supraorbital

116

margin. The medial one third of supra orbital margin is rounded and bears supraorbital notch/foramen at the junction of medial one third and lateral two third. It transmits supra orbital vessels and nerve.

Zygomatic process

The supraorbital margin on tracing laterally continues in zygomatic process. This prominent and strong process articulates with zygomatic bone.

Superior and inferior temporal lines

Are seen arising from zygomatic process.

Internal surface

This concave surface is related to the frontal lobe. Hence it is named cerebral surface. This is marked by impressions of frontal lobe gyri.

Sagittal sulcus

It is a vertical groove in the upper part of the median plane. The margins of this sulcus when traced below form the frontal crest. The falx cerebri is attached to frontal crest and the margins of sagittal sulcus. The sulcus lodges anterior part of superior sagittal sinus.

Foramen caecum

The frontal crest leads into a small notch which is completed into foramen caecum with the articulation of ethmoid bone.

Granular foveolae

These are seen on the floor of the sagittal sulcus for arachnoid villi /granulations.

Notch for ethmoid bone

The orbital plates are thin triangular shelf like parts that are separated from each other by a wide gap-ethmoid notch (for ethmoid bone)

Temporal surface

The temporal lines separate the frontal surface and the temporal surface. This area below and behind the temporal lines forms the anterior part of temporal fossa.

ORBITAL PART

Orbital surface of orbital part

When viewed from below the orbital plates appear smooth, concave and have a fossa in its anterolateral part for the lacrimal gland. Anterior to the articulation with the ethmoid bone the lacrimal bone articulates with frontal bone by fronto lacrimal suture. Midway between the suture and supraorbital notch is a small depression for fibro cartilaginous pulley of superior oblique muscle.

Ethmoidal notch

It intervenes between two orbital plates. The ethmoid articulates in the ethmoid notch.

Frontal sinus

On either side of midline two irregular cavities extend backwards, upwards and laterally between the two tables of the bones. On surface these can be marked at the medial part of superciliary arches.

Posterior border

The thin and serrated border articulates with lesser wing of sphenoid.

NASAL PART

This part of bone projects downwards between the supra orbital margins. It is marked by nasal notch for articulation with nasal bone (medially), frontal processes of maxilla and lacrimal bone (laterally) from medial to lateral and anterior to posterior. From the centre of the nasal notch posteriorly a sharp nasal spine extends downwards and forwards. It articulates in front with the nasal bone and behind with the nasal septum and the perpendicular plate of ethmoid bone.

OSSIFICATION

Like other bones of the vault of skull, frontal bone also ossifies in membrane except the orbital plates.

The ossification begins from two centres placed at the frontal eminence. Thus two halves are separated by frontal/metopic suture. This suture usually gets obliterated by eighth year. However, in 7-9% cases it may persist.

CLINICAL CONSIDERATIONS

Metopic suture

The inferior part of metopic suture may persist in about 5% of individuals. In a radiograph of skull (AP view) it may be mistaken for a fracture.

Compression of supraorbital nerve

The supraorbital nerve emerges from supraorbital foramen/notch. Compression of nerve here causes considerable pain. This fact is used by anaesthetist to determine the depth of anaesthesia/consciousness.

Fracture of frontal bone

In an adult localized injury to the bone causes a depressed comminuted fracture. The severity of the impact causes bleeding in the subaponeurotic space of the scalp. This results in indirect black eye.

25

Temporal Bone

INTRODUCTION

Contributes in Norma basalis and lateralis. Morphologically it has four parts which get fused.

PARTS

Squamous

- Mastoid
- Petrous
- Tympanic
- Styloid process

The squamous is thin and expanded. Mastoid part forms posterior part of the bone. Petrous part is hard and triangular. Tympanic part is placed below the squamous part and in front of the mastoid process as a curved plate. Styloid process projects downwards and forwards from the under surface of the bone as a slender pointed and elongated projection.

FEATURES

Squamous part

Outer surface — Temporal surface

Smooth and slightly convex. The middle temporal artery runs in a vertical groove seen above and in line with external acoustic meatus. Supramastoid crest above and behind external acoustic meatus - curved line the running backwards and upwards. Temporal fascia and temporalis muscle are attached.

Suprameatal triangle

A depression posterosuperior to external acoustic meatus and below the anterior part of supramastoid crest. Tympanic antrum lies in the depth of the triangle.

Zygomatic process

It projects anteriorly from the lower portion of the temporal surface. Its anterior end is free and articulates with zygomatic bone to complete zygomatic arch. Its posterior part is triangular in shape with superior and inferior surfaces. The superior surface forms a part of temporal fossa. Inferior surface is bounded by two roots. The tubercle of root of zygoma is placed where the two roots meet. The anterior root bears semi cylindrical body. The superior border of zygomatic process attaches temporal fascia. Masseter arises from the deep surface and lower border of the zygomatic arch.

The mandibular fossa/articular fossa is divided into anterior articular and posterior non articular parts by squamo-tympanic fissure. The articular eminence forms the anterior boundary of mandibular fossa.

MASTOID PART

Forms posterior part of temporal bone

FEATURES

Mastoid process
Lower projection that gives attachment to the muscles. Before backward these are (a) **Sternocleidomastoid** (b) **Semispinalis** (c) **Splenius capitis**

Mastoid notch
The deep groove on the medial surface of the bone is for posterior belly of digastric muscle.

Occipital groove
Medial to mastoid notch, this shallow groove occupies the occipital artery.

Mastoid foramen
Present near the posterior border of mastoid process for the passage of emissary vein connecting sigmoid sinus and a small artery from the occipital artery for the dura mater.

Mastoid air cells
The composition of bone includes small spaces collectively termed as mastoid air cells which communicate with the middle ear cavity through its posterior wall by aditus.

TYMPANIC PART

It is placed externally between squamous and mastoid parts. In the depth it is fused with the petrous part and is seen in the angle between the petrous part and squamous part. Posteriorly it fuses with squamous part and mastoid part. The anterior surface forms the posterior wall of mandibular fossa. An enlarged parotid gland finds it way between this surface and temporomandibular joint making opening of mouth difficult and painful. The lower border is sharp and encloses the root of styloid process termed sheath of styloid process.

External acoustic meatus – This 16 mm long bony canal is directed anteromedially as well as downwards. The tympanic part of temporal bone forms its anterior wall, floor and lower part of posterior wall. The roof and upper part of posterior wall are formed by squamous temporal. Its medial end has the tympanic membrane while the lateral/outer end is bounded above by posterior root of zygomatic process.

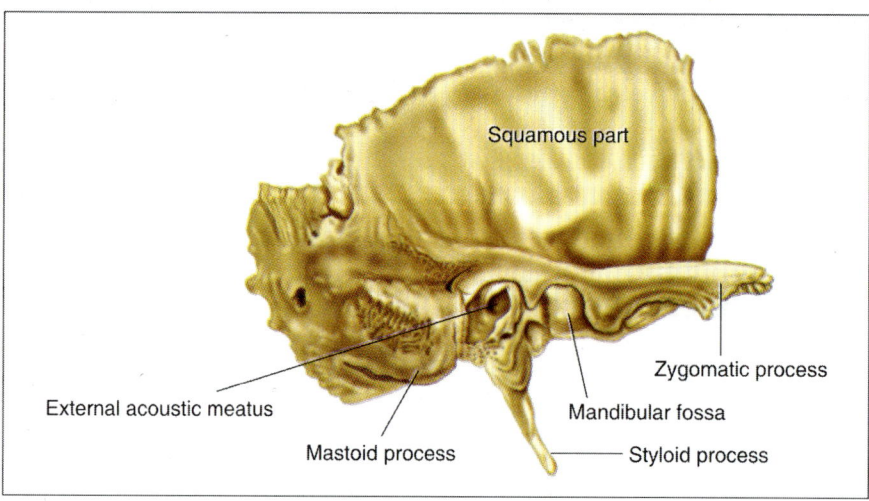

Fig. 25.1: Temporal Bone

PETROUS PART

In the base of skull petrous part of temporal bone is seen wedged between sphenoid and occipital bones. It has a base, an apex, three surfaces and three borders. It contains middle ear and internal ear. Base is directed backwards and apex is placed anteromedially. Anterior surface forms floor of middle cranial fossa. Posterior surface has in its middle the internal auditory meatus. Inferior surface forms part of external surface of base of skull and has following features:

- Groove for pharyngotympanic tube
- Carotid canal
- Jugular fossa
- Tympanic canaliculus
- Stylomastoid foramen

The superior border is grooved by superior petrosal sinus. The tentorium cerebelli is attached here. Posterior border has following features from medial to lateral (a) groove for inferior petrosal sinus (b) Jugular fossa (c) notch for IX cranial nerve. The anterior border is articular- laterally with squamous temporal and medially with greater wing of sphenoid.

Trigeminal impression

Behind the apex is a slight depression for trigeminal ganglion which is lodged in the cavum trigeminale.

Arcuate eminence

It is placed posterolateral to trigeminal impression. This elevation is caused by underlying superior semicircular canal of internal ear.

Tegmen tympani

Lateral to the arcuate eminence a thin plate of bone forms roof of the tympanic antrum – tegmen tympani.

Groove for greater petrosal nerve

On the tegmen tympani a groove runs to reach the foramen lacerum. This medially placed groove is for greater superficial petrosal nerve.

Groove for lesser petrosal nerve

Lateral to the groove for greater superficial petrosal nerve, another groove occupying the lower petrosal nerve extends towards foramen ovale.

Internal acoustic meatus

It transmits VII and VIII cranial nerves along with labyrinthine vessels.

STYLOID PROCESS

From the undersurface of temporal bone slender and pointed bony projection extending downwards and forwards is styloid process. It has a proximal part (tympanohyal) which is ensheathed by part of tympanic plate. Its distal part (stylohyal) gives attachment to muscles and ligaments together termed styloid apparatus.

CLINICAL CONSIDERATIONS

Injury to Facial Nerve

The mastoid process (traction epiphysis) grows with the age. When the child starts holding his neck it implies that the sternocleidomastoids are adequately strong to prevent falling of the head in any direction. This milestone is reached by sixth month. Prior to this, the facial nerve as it comes out through stylomastoid foramen is relatively unprotected. Exposure to cold causes oedema of facial nerve at this site. It leads to infranuclear facial nerve palsy (Bell's palsy).

McEvan's Triangle

Suprameatal triangle is an important landmark. It demarcates the tympanic antrum which lies medial to it. It is about half inch deep to the triangle. Thus to drain the pus from the tympanic antrum an opening is made in the suprameatal triangle. In children a thin layer of bone covers the tympanic antrum at the suprameatal triangle.

26

Ethmoid Bone

This cuboidal shaped fragile bone is placed anteriorly at the base of cranium.

It forms
- Medial walls of bony orbit
- Nasal septum
- Roof and lateral walls of the nasal cavity

It comprises
- Cribriform plate
- Median perpendicular plate
- Two labyrinths

CRIBRIFORM PLATE

This fills the frontal ethmoidal notch and forms part of the roof of nasal cavity. **Crista galli** projects upwards from this and to its posterior border falx cerebri is attached.

Anterior border joins the frontal bone by two small alae which complete the foramen caecum.

Its sides are bulged by air cells. On both sides of the crista galli the cribriform plate is narrow, depressed and related to the gyrus rectus and olfactory bulb.

Its numerous foramina transmit olfactory nerves. Anteriorly on each side of the crista is a small slit occupied by dura mater. A foramen is seen anterolateral to the slit through which anterior ethmoidal nerve and vessels pass to the nasal cavity.

A groove runs forwards to it from the anterior ethmoidal canal.

PERPENDICULAR PLATE

This thin, flat, quadrilateral median plate descends from the cribriform plate which forms the upper part of the nasal septum.

Its anterior border meets nasal spine of frontal and crest of the nasal bones. Its posterior border

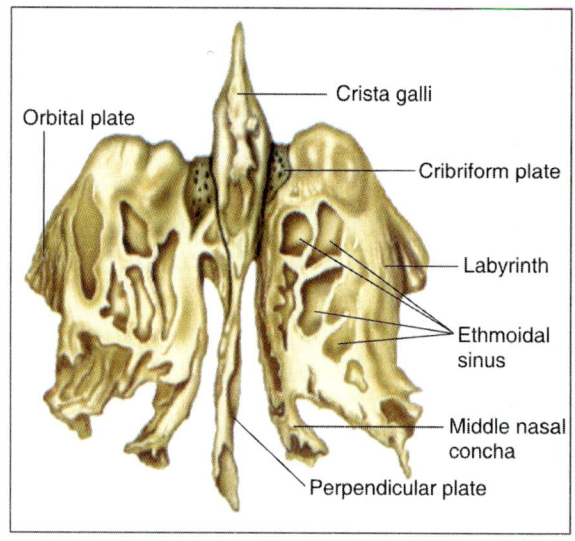

Fig. 26.1: Ethmoid Bone

joins sphenoidal crest above and vomer below. The inferior border is attached to the nasal septal cartilage.

ETHMOIDAL LABYRINTHS

These consist of thin-walled ethmoidal air cells. The ethmoidal air cells are as

- Anterior group
- Middle group
- Posterior groups

Superior surface shows open air cells, completed by edges of the frontal ethmoidal notch. It is crossed by two grooves which complete anterior and posterior ethmoidal canals with the frontal bone.

On the posterior surface large air cells are completed by sphenoidal conchae and the orbital process of palatine bone.

Lateral surface – orbital plate (forms part of the medial wall of orbit) which covers the middle and posterior ethmoidal air cells. It articulates

- **Superiorly** with the orbital plate of frontal bone
- **Inferiorly** with the maxilla and orbital process of palatine
- **Anteriorly** with the lacrimal
- **Posteriorly** with the sphenoid bone

Few air cells which are placed anterior to the orbital plate, their walls are completed by the lacrimal bone and frontal process of the maxilla.

Uncinate process projects posteroinferiorly from the labyrinth which appears in the medial wall of the maxillary sinus as it crosses maxillary hiatus to join the ethmoidal process of inferior nasal concha.

Medial surface of the labyrinth forms part of the lateral wall of nasal cavity. A thin lamella descends from the inferior surface of the cribriform plate to end as middle nasal concha. Posteriorly it is divided by superior meatus and bounded above by the superior nasal concha. Posterior ethmoidal air cells open into this meatus.

Middle ethmoidal air cells produce bulla ethmoidale on the lateral wall of the middle meatus. On the bulla middle ethmoidal cells open into the middle meatus. An infundibulum extends upwards and forwards from the middle meatus which communicates with anterior ethmoidal sinuses. It continues upwards as the frontonasal duct.

OSSIFICATION

Ossifies in cartilage from three centres

- One in the perpendicular plate
- One in each labyrinth

The centres in labyrinth appear in the orbital plates between 4th and 5th months of intrauterine life.

At birth only the labyrinths are partially ossified and the rest of the bone is cartilaginous.

During the first year the perpendicular plate and crista galli begin to ossify from the median centre and fuses with the labyrinths during second year.

The cribriform plate ossifies partly from the perpendicular plate and partly from the labyrinths.

The ethmoidal air cells begin to develop during foetal life. In the newborn these can be appreciated as narrow pouches.

QUESTIONS: ETHMOID

- Name the bones which articulate with ethmoid bone - start from crista galli and proceed in a clockwise direction.
- Which nasal conchae are formed by the ethmoid bone?
- Which part forms the medial wall of the orbit?

27

Palatine Bone

It is placed posteriorly in the nasal cavity between the maxillae and pterygoid processes of sphenoid.

It forms

- Floor and lateral wall of nose
- Hard palate
- Floor of orbit
- Pterygopalatine and pterygoid fossae
- Inferior orbital fissure

It resembles a letter L.

It consists of horizontal and perpendicular plates, with three processes:

- Pyramidal
- Orbital
- Sphenoidal

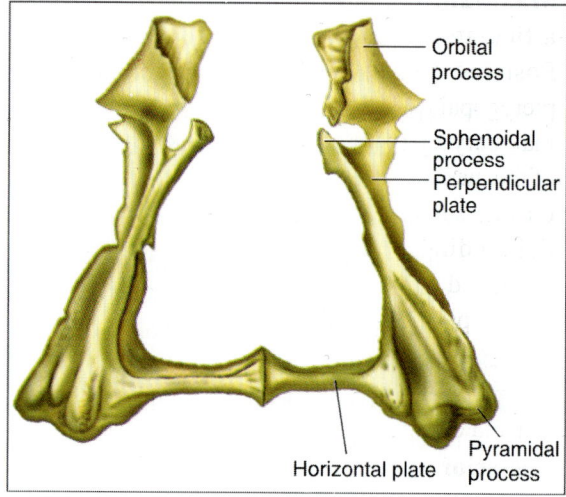

Fig. 27.1: Palatine Bone

It is quadrilateral in shape.

It consists of

- Two surfaces
- Four borders.

Nasal surface forms the posterior floor of nose

Palatine surface with its fellow forms a posterior one fourth of the hard palate.

Posterior border is thin and concave which behind the palatine crest provide attachment of the expanded tendon of tensor veli palatini. Medially the posterior border with its fellow forms median posterior nasal spine - attachment of the musculus uvulae.

Anterior border is serrated which articulates with the palatine process of maxilla

Lateral border is continuous with the perpendicular plate

Medial border is thick and serrated. It articulates with its fellow in the midline and forms the posterior part of the nasal crest. This crest articulates with the posterior part of the lower edge of vomer.

PERPENDICULAR PLATE

The perpendicular plate is thin and oblong.
It has -

- Two surfaces
- Four borders

Nasal surface shows a depression inferiorly - part of the inferior meatus. Above this the horizontal conchal crest articulates with the inferior concha and above this again a shallow depression forms part of the middle meatus. This depression is limited above by ethmoidal crest for the middle concha.

Maxillary surface is rough and irregular. It articulates with the nasal surface of maxilla. Posterosuperiorly it forms medial wall of the pterygopalatine fossa. Its anterior area overlaps the maxillary hiatus from behind to form posterior part of the medial wall of the maxillary sinus. Posteriorly on this surface there is a deep, obliquely placed descending greater palatine groove which is converted into a canal by the maxilla. It transmits greater palatine vessels and nerve.

Anterior border is thin and irregular and behind the maxillary process of the inferior concha articulates with it.

Posterior border presents a serrated suture to articulate with the medial pterygoid plate. It is continuous above with the sphenoidal process of palatine and expanded below into pyramidal process of palatine bone.

Superior border - orbital and sphenoidal processes project from here which are separated by the sphenopalatine notch. The notch is converted into a foramen by the body of sphenoid. This foramen connects the pterygopalatine fossa to the posterior part of the superior meatus and transmits sphenopalatine vessels and the posterior superior nasal nerves.

Inferior border is continuous with the lateral border of the horizontal plate.

PROCESSES

Pyramidal process

It slopes down posterolaterally from the junction of the horizontal and perpendicular plates of palatine into the angle between the pterygoid plates. On its **posterior surface** a smooth triangular area is seen which is limited on each side by rough articular furrows articulating with the pterygoid plates. This completes the lower part of the pterygoid fossa. Anteriorly the **lateral surface** articulates with the maxillary tuberosity. The **inferior surface** near its junction with the horizontal plate shows the lesser palatine foramina for the corresponding nerves and arteries.

It is directed superolaterally from in front of the perpendicular plate.

It presents
- Three articular surfaces
- Two non-articular surfaces

- **Anterior (maxillary) surface** faces downwards and anterolaterally which articulates with the maxilla
- **Posterior (sphenoidal) surface** directed upwards and posteromedially. It communicates with the sphenoidal sinus which is completed by sphenoidal concha.
- **Medial (ethmoidal) surface** faces anteromedially. It articulates with the labyrinth of ethmoid.

- **Superior (orbital) surface** is directed superolaterally to the posterior part of the orbital floor
- **Lateral surface** is oblong which faces the pterygopalatine fossa. It is separated from the orbital surface by a rounded border. This

surface may present a groove (directed superolaterally) for the maxillary nerve. It is continuous with the groove on the posterior surface of maxilla.

Sphenoidal process

It is a thin plate which is directed superomedially.

Superior surface articulates with the sphenoidal concha and, above it, with the root of the medial pterygoid plate.

Inferomedial surface is part of the roof and lateral wall of nose.

Lateral surface articulates posteriorly with the medial pterygoid plate. Its anterior region forms part of the medial wall of the pterygopalatine fossa.

Posterior border articulates with the vaginal process of the medial pterygoid plate.

Anterior border is the posterior edge of the sphenopalatine notch.

Medial border articulates with the ala of vomer.

Sphenopalatine notch (between the two processes) is converted into a foramen by articulation with the body of sphenoid.

OSSIFICATION

Ossifies in mesenchyme from one centre which appears during 8th week of intrauterine life in the perpendicular plate

Ossification spreads into all parts.

At birth the height of the perpendicular plate is equal to the width of the horizontal part but in adults it is almost twice the size.

28

Zygomatic Bone

It forms the prominence of cheek.

It contributes to

- Lateral wall and floor of orbit
- Walls of temporal and infratemporal fossae
- Complete the zygomatic arch

It is roughly quadrangular with anteromedial and frontal processes.

It presents

- Three surfaces
- Five borders
- Two processes

Lateral surface is convex and pierced near its orbital border by the zygomaticofacial foramen (often double) for the zygomaticofacial nerve and vessels. Below the foramen zygomaticus minor and, posteriorly, zygomaticus major are attached. The foramen may be absent.

Posteromedial (temporal) surface has a rough anterior area which articulates with the maxilla and a smooth posterior area seen extending upwards posteriorly on its frontal process as the anterior aspect of the temporal fossa. It also extends back on the medial aspect of the temporal process as an incomplete lateral wall for the infratemporal fossa. Zygomaticotemporal foramen pierces this surface near the base of the frontal process.

Orbital surface is smooth and concave. It forms the anterolateral part of the orbital floor and adjoining lateral wall. It presents zygomatico-orbital foramina -openings of canals leading to zygomatico-facial and temporal foramina.

Anterosuperior (orbital) border forms the inferolateral circum-ference of the orbital opening which separates the orbital and lateral surfaces.

Anteroinferior (maxillary) border articulates with the maxilla. Its medial end tapers to a point above the infraorbital foramen.

Posterosuperior (temporal) border is sinuous and continuous with the posterior border of the frontal process and upper border of the zygomatic arch. The temporal fascia is attached to it.

Posteroinferior border is roughened by attachment of masseter.

Posteromedial (serrated) border articulates with the greater wing of sphenoid above, and orbital surface of the maxilla below.

Frontal process is thick and serrated. It articulates above with the zygomatic process of frontal and behind with greater wing of sphenoid. On its orbital aspect (within the orbital opening) about one cm below the frontozygomatic suture, a tubercle is present for the attachment of

- Lateral palpebrae ligament
- Suspensory ligament

- Aponeurosis of levator palpebrae superioris (LPS)

Temporal process is directed backwards which has an oblique, serrated end. It articulates with the zygomatic process of temporal to complete the zygomatic arch.

OSSIFICATION

Ossifies from one centre which appears during 8th week of intrauterine life. The bone may be divided by a horizontal suture into larger (upper) and smaller (lower) divisions.

QUESTIONS: ZYGOMATIC BONE

- What are zygomatic bones commonly known as?
- What parts of the orbit are formed by the zygomatic bones?
- What complications can occur with fracture of the infraorbital plate?

Vomer

It is a thin and flat unpaired bone which forms the postero-inferior part of the nasal septum. It presents

- Two lateral surfaces
- Four borders

Lateral surfaces are marked by grooves for nerves and vessels. One groove is obliquely antero-inferior for the nasopalatine nerve and vessels.

Superior border is thickest having a deep furrow between projecting alae which articulate with the rostrum of sphenoid.

Alae articulate with

- Sphenoidal conchae
- Sphenoidal processes of palatine bones
- Vaginal processes of medial pterygoid plates

Each ala is placed between the body of sphenoid and vaginal process; its inferior surface forms the vomerovaginal canal.

Inferior border articulates with the median maxillary and palatine nasal crests. **Anterior border** is longest and it articulates in its upper half with the perpendicular plate of ethmoid; its lower half is cleft to receive the inferior margin of the septal cartilage of nose.

Posterior border is concave which separates the posterior nasal apertures. It is thick and bifid above and thin below. Its anterior end articulates with the posterior margin of the incisor crest of maxilla and descends between the incisive canals.

OSSIFICATION

Ossifies from two centres; appear during 8th week of intrauterine life which unites during 12th week.

Hyoid Bone

It is a U-shaped bone which is suspended from the tips of the styloid processes by the stylohyoid ligaments.

It consists of a body, two greater and two lesser cornua.

BODY

It is irregular, elongated and quadrilateral.

Anterior surface is convex which faces anterosuperiorly. It is crossed by a transverse ridge with a slight downward convexity.

Posterior surface is smooth, concave and faces posteroinferiorly. It is separated from the epiglottis by the thyrohyoid membrane.

GREATER CORNUA

These project backward from the lateral ends of the body. They taper posteriorly and each ends in a tubercle.

These are connected to the body in early life by cartilage, but after middle age they are united by bone.

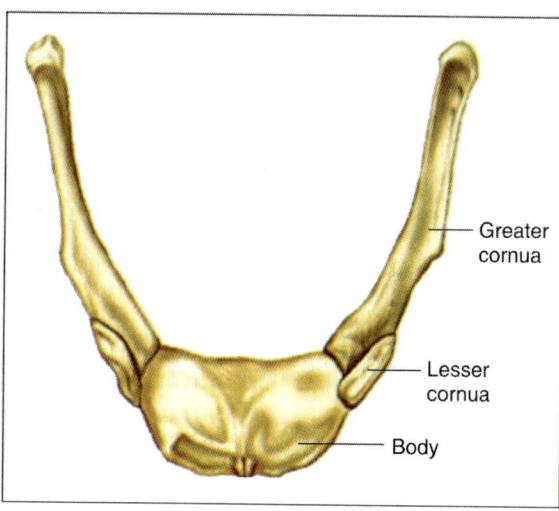

Fig. 30.1: Hyoid Bone

The greater cornua can be identified and the bone can be moved from side to side when the throat is griped between finger and thumb.

LESSER CORNUA

These are two small, conical projections placed at the junctions of the body and greater cornua. These are connected at their base to the body by fibrous tissue and occasionally to the greater cornua by synovial joints.

ATTACHMENTS

Anterior surface of body - Geniohyoid

Lower anterior surface - Mylohyoid, above the sternohyoid (medially) and omohyoid (laterally)

Superior border - Lowest fibres of the genioglossus, hyoepiglottic ligament and thyrohyoid membrane

Inferior border - Sternohyoid (medially) and omohyoid (laterally)

Upper surface of each greater cornu - Middle constrictor of pharynx and hyoglossus (laterally)

Near the junction of cornu with body – Stylohyoid, lateral to hyoglossus and little posterior is the fibrous loop of digastric tendon

Medial border - Thyrohyoid membrane

Lateral border - Thyrohyoid

Posterior and lateral aspects of the lesser cornua - Middle constrictors of pharynx

Apices of lesser cornua - Stylohyoid ligaments

OSSIFICATION

Develops from the cartilages of the second and third branchial arches

- **Lesser cornua** develops from the second arch
- **Greater cornua** develops from the third arch
- **Body** develops from the fused ventral ends of both arches

Ossifies from six centres - two for the body, two for each cornu.

Commencement

- **In greater cornua** at the end of 9th month of intrauterine life
- **In the body** just before or after birth
- **In lesser cornua** about puberty

Apex of greater cornua remains cartilaginous till third decade of life, later they fuse with the body.

Synovial joints between the greater and lesser cornua are replaced by ossification in later life.

31

Lacrimal Bone

It is the smallest and most fragile cranial bone which is placed anteriorly in the medial wall of orbit.

It has

- Two surfaces
- Four borders

Lateral (orbital) **surface** is divided by a vertical posterior lacrimal crest anterior to which is a vertical groove. Its anterior edge meets the posterior border of the frontal process of the maxilla to complete the fossa for the lacrimal sac. The medial wall of groove is prolonged by a descending process which helps to form the nasolacrimal canal by joining the lips of the maxillary nasolacrimal groove and lacrimal process of the inferior nasal concha. Behind the crest is part of the medial wall of orbit. To this surface and crest the lacrimal part of orbicularis oculi is attached. The surface ends below in the lacrimal hamulus which, with the maxilla, completes the upper opening of the nasolacrimal canal.

Anteroinferior part of medial (nasal) **surface** forms part of the middle meatus **Posterosuperior part** joins with ethmoid to complete anterior ethmoidal air cells.

Anterior (lacrimal) **border** articulates with the frontal process of the maxilla

Posterior border articulates with the orbital plate of ethmoid

Superior border articulates with the frontal bone

Inferior border articulates with the orbital surface of maxilla

It develops in mesenchyme. It ossifies from one centre which appears during 12th week of intrauterine life around the nasal capsule.

32

Inferior Nasal Concha

It is a curved horizontally placed bone placed in the lateral wall of nose.

It has

- Two surfaces
- Two borders
- Two ends

Medial surface is convex and much perforated.

Lateral surface is concave and forms part of the inferior meatus.

Superior border is thin and irregular. It is divided into three regions.

Anterior - articulates with the conchal crest of maxilla

Posterior - articulates with the conchal crest of palatine

Middle - articulates with three processes

- **Lacrimal process** placed at the junction of the anterior with the posterior three-fourths of the border which articulates with a descending lacrimal process and with the edges of the nasolacrimal groove on the maxillary surface of maxilla - completes the nasolacrimal canal.

- **Ethmoidal process** ascends to the uncinate process of ethmoid.

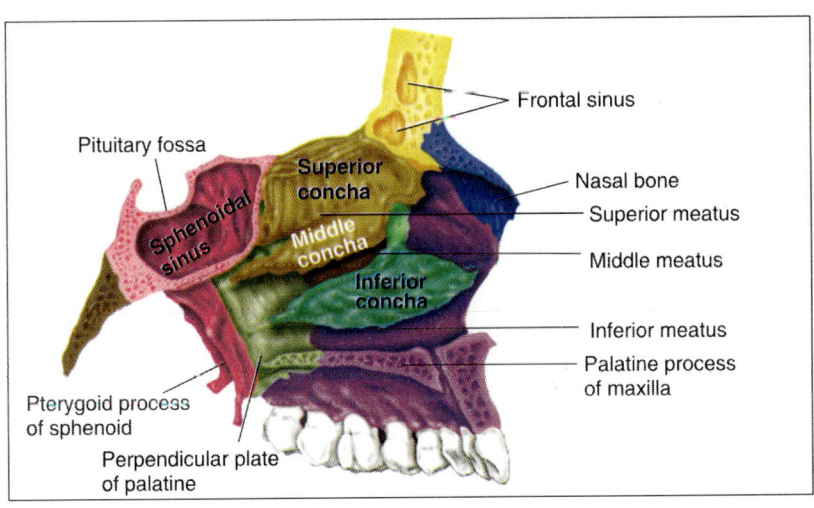

Fig. 32.1: Lateral wall of nose

133

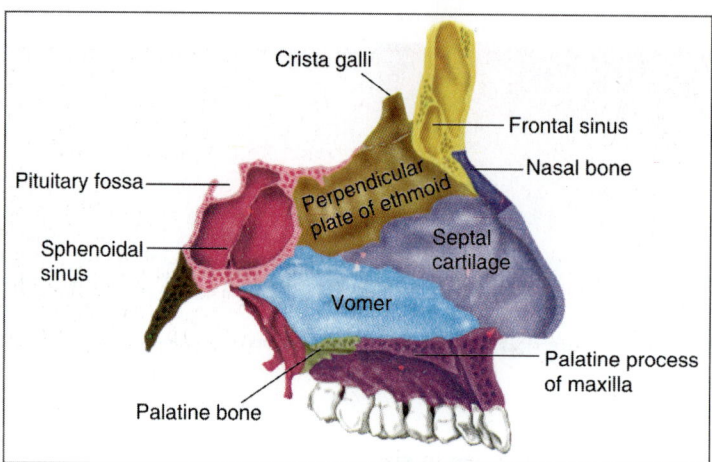

Fig. 32.2: Nasal Septum

- **Maxillary process** articulates with the maxilla and maxillary process of the bone and forms part of the medial wall of maxillary sinus.

Inferior border is thick.

Both ends are tapering.

OSSIFICATION

It ossifies from one centre which appears during 5th month in the foetal life in the lower border of the lateral wall of nasal capsule.

33

Nasal Bone

It is a small and oblong bone which varies in size and form. It is placed side by side between the frontal processes of the maxillae; jointly they form nasal bridge.

It presents

- Two surfaces
- Four borders

Outer surface is concavo-convex from above downwards while it is transversely convex. It is covered by the **procerus** and **nasalis**. In the centre it is perforated by a small venous foramen.

Inner surface is transversely concave. It is traversed by a longitudinal groove for the anterior ethmoidal nerve.

Superior border is thick and serrated which articulates with the frontal bone.

Inferior border is thin and notched. It is continuous with the lateral nasal cartilage.

Lateral border joins the frontal process of the maxilla.

Medial border is thick above. It joins its fellow and projects behind as a vertical crest - part of nasal septum. It articulates from above downwards with

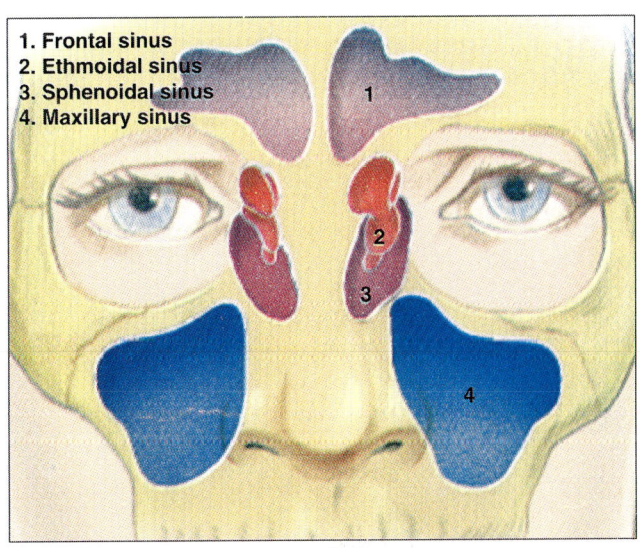

1. Frontal sinus
2. Ethmoidal sinus
3. Sphenoidal sinus
4. Maxillary sinus

Fig. 33.1: Paranasal Air Sinuses

- Nasal spine of the frontal bone
- Perpendicular plate of ethmoid
- Septal cartilage of nose

Relation between length and breadth of nasal bone in children and adults

- Children 1:1
- Adults 3:1

It ossifies from one centre which appears during 3rd month of intrauterine life in mesenchyme which overlies the cartilaginous anterior part of the nasal capsule.

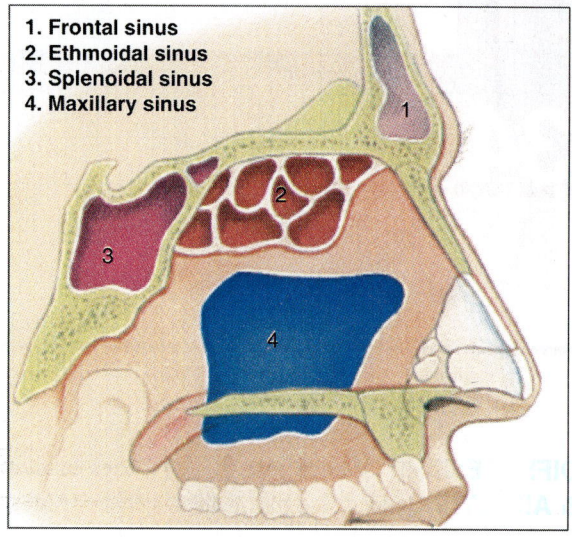

1. Frontal sinus
2. Ethmoidal sinus
3. Splenoidal sinus
4. Maxillary sinus

Fig. 33.2: Paranasal Air Sinuses: Lateral view

34

Foetal Skull

DIFFERENCES BETWEEN FOETAL SKULL & ADULT SKULL

SIZE

Large in proportion to the rest of the body

NORMA FRONTALIS

Compared to the adult the facial portion in a foetal skull is small. It is one eighth of the size of cranium while in adult it is one half.

FONTANELLES

The skull vault develops in membrane. The ossification in the skull bones starts from the centres more or less in the middle of the bone e.g. frontal eminence. Thus with the spread of ossification, the periphery of the membranous bone remains un-ossified for sometime. The un-ossified membranous intervals are seen at the angles of parietal bone. These are six in number.

NORMA BASALIS

In front and behind the occipital condyles the distance is equal.

FRONTAL & PARIETAL EMINENCES

Placed within or near the centre of the bone. These are sites of maximum convexity. They represent the areas where from ossification spreads.

THICKNESS OF BONE

The foetal skull bones do not show inner and outer tables. In foetal life the skull bones remain membranous/cartilaginous with process of ossification continuing. It is only later that bones grow and thicken by appositional growth on both surfaces.

FEATURES

FRONTAL BONE

Develops in two halves joined by metopic suture which disappears subsequently. Most of the bone develops in membrane except orbital plates which develop in cartilage.

PARIETAL BONE

This bone develops totally in membrane. The parietal eminences are well marked in the foetal life. This fact is utilized for relating foetal growth by measuring biparietal diameter (BPD) using USG.

FONTANELLES

These are six in number - Two in middle (anterior and posterior) and four in the sides.

- Anterior fontanalle (Bregma) -Diamond shaped

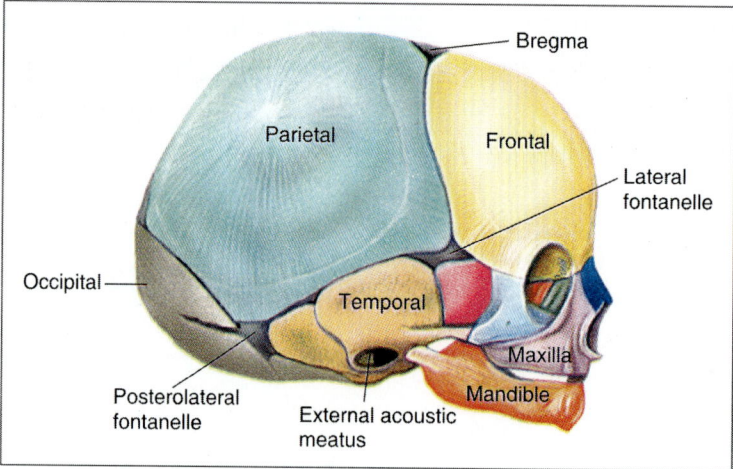

Fig. 34.1: Foetal skull: Lateral view

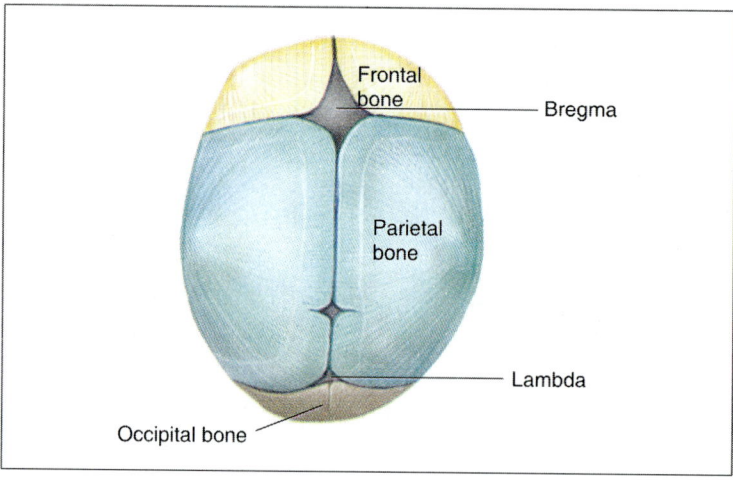

Fig. 34.2: Foetal skull: Superior view

- Posterior fontanalle (Lambda) – Triangular shaped
- Two anterolateral fontanalle
- Two posterolateral fontanalle.

TEMPORAL BONE

It is ossified by two processes

- **Ossified in membrane**: Squamous part
- **Ossified in cartilage**: Petromastoid, Tympanic plate and Styloid process

OCCIPITAL BONE

Ossifies in membrane (squamous part) and cartilage – condylar and basilar parts.

MANDIBLE

Ossifies from two sources (a) membrane covering the outer surface of Meckel's cartilage forms ramus and part of the body. The Meckel's cartilage gives rise to condyloid process, coronoid process and part of the ramus above the mandibular canal including the lingula.

GROWTH OF SKULL TO ADULT SIZE

HEAD CIRCUMFERENCE

- **In newborn**   **14 inches**
- **At 4 month**   **16 inches**
- **At 1 year**   **18 inches**
- **At 5 years**   **20 inches**
- **7-10 years**   **21 inches**

The height and other dimensions gained by the foetal skull are attributed to deposition of bone and other factors.

Maximum growth in 1st year

Usually stops by puberty

MECHANISM OF GROWTH

Sutural growth

The mesenchymal tissue permits the growth at the sutures

Endochondral growth

The cartilaginous part of foetal skull grows by ossification in all the dimensions.

Surface accretion: To meet the requirement of growing structures the capacity of skull has to increase steadily and gradually. This is possible by deposition (accretion) of bone on outer aspect and erosion on the inner aspect.

Other features influencing growth

- Appearance of dentition – growth of lower face
- Appearance of paranasal air sinuses
- Increase respiratory need in childhood associated with growth of upper face and nasal cavity
- Development of muscles of mastication
- General growth of the brain and eyes
- Sex may also have influence on the growth of an individual.

Growth in antero-posterior length

Takes place at the cartilaginous joints
- Body of sphenoid and ethmoid
- Basiocciput – basisphenoid

Growth in width

Takes place in:
- Sagittal suture
- Occipitomastoid suture
- Sutures around greater wing of sphenoid
- Petro occipital joint

Growth in height

It is attained at:
- Fronto-zygomatic suture
- Pterion
- Squamosal suture
- Asterion

CLOSURE OF SUTURES

Begins on the inner surface at around 30-40 years of age. At outer surface the process begins 10 years later. There is a sequence of sutural obliteration beginning with bregma and successively including sagittal, coronal and lambdoid sutures.

CRANIOMETRY

DEFINITION

Anthropologists make use of measurements of indices of skull to compare them. Anthropometry is a wider technique which deals with measurements of entire body. Hence craniometry is a part of anthropometry. For this certain bony landmarks are used.

$$\text{Cephalic index} = \frac{\text{Breath}}{\text{Length}} \times 100$$

- **BRACHYCEPHALIC:** 80.0 TO 84.9

- **MESATICEPHALIC:** 75.0 TO 79.9
- **DOLICHOCEPHALIC:** Up to 74.

Cranial capacity

A reasonable estimate of the volume of brain is 150 to 200 cc less than the cranial capacity. This is determined by filling the cranial cavity with millet seeds. In male the skull capacity on average is **1200 to 1800 cc**. In female the capacity is 10% less than male.

CLINICAL CONSIDERATIONS

Biparietal Diameter

It is the maximum distance between two parietal eminences. It is very important and reliable indicator of foetal growth – measured by ultrasound. This distance increases with the gestational age. In adults this parameter is used in craniometry.

Clinical importance of anterior fontanelle

- Abnormal bulging or depressed fontanalle indicates increased intracranial tension and dehydration.
- Sample of cerebrospinal fluid from the lateral ventricle can be obtained through it. The needle is passed downwards and laterally through its lateral angle.
- The superior sagittal sinus is accessed through it for intravenous injections.
- By PV examination during labour anterior fontanalle helps in determining presentation, position and attitude of the foetal head.

Fractures

The bones of skull in a child are highly elastic. Thin fracture is quire uncommon. However, in a localized blow depressed fracture may be seen termed "**pond fracture**"

35

Cervical Vertebrae

INTRODUCTION

Smallest amongst all vertebrae. They are seven in number and are identified by the presence of foramen transversarium. First, second and seventh cervical vertebrae are atypical in nature.

IDENTIFYING FEATURES OF TYPICAL VERTEBRAE

Body : Transversely kidney shaped with triangular vertebral foramen proportionately larger than the size of the body.

    Transverse process : Bears foramen transversarium

    Spine : It is bifid

TYPICAL CERVICAL VERTEBRA

PARTICULAR FEATURES
BODY

Anterior surface is convex from side to side. Posterior surface is flat with foramina for basivertebral veins. Superior surface is concave transversely with upward projecting lips. Inferior surface is concave from before backward. The anterior border of inferior surface projects downwards to conceal the intervertebral discs.

VERTEBRAL FORAMEN

It is triangular in outline and is wider in the lower cervical vertebrae to accommodate the cervical enlargement of the spinal cord.

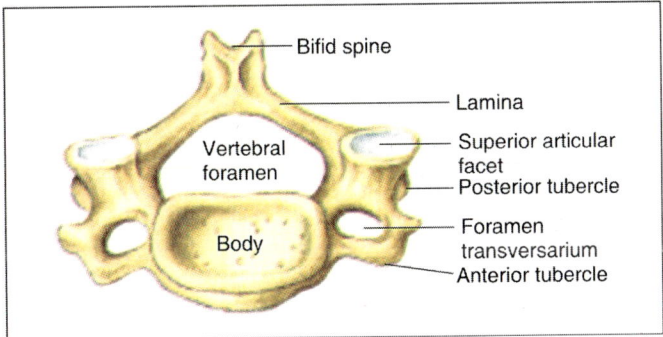

Fig. 35.1: Typical cervical vertebra: Superior view

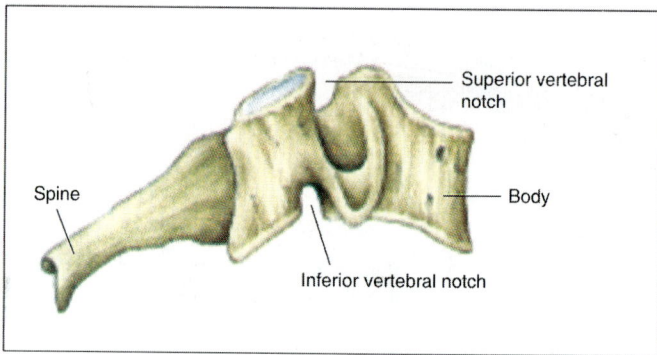

Fig. 35.2: Typical cervical vertebra: Lateral view

VERTEBRAL ARCH

Pedicles

Divergent presenting superior and inferior vertebral notches

Articular processes

Together they form articular pillar placed between pedicles and lamina

Spinous process

Short and bifid and cupped by tubercles. They give attachment to ligamentum nuchae and deep muscles of the back.

Transverse process

The foramen transversarium divides the transverse process into anterior and posterior roots. The costo-transverse bar connects the two roots lateral to foramen transversarium.

ATYPICAL CERVICAL VERTEBRAE

ATLAS

IDENTIFYING FEATURES

Body is absent as it is fused with the centrum of second cervical vertebra – odontoid process

It has **no spine.**

It has **two lateral masses** connected anteriorly and posteriorly corresponding anterior and posterior arches.

Along the superior aspect of posterior arch behind the lateral mass is the **groove for vertebral artery** (third part).

The first cervical nerve (**C-1**) is placed between the artery and the posterior arch. The anterior and posterior arches present on the external aspect in the midline the anterior and posterior tubercles.

Behind the anterior tubercle a circular facet is seen for the odontoid process.

LATERAL MASS

Placed obliquely with upper and lower surfaces bearing articular areas.

Superior articular facets

For occipital condyles. Hence it is elongated, concave and been shaped. This feature of the articular facet permits nodding movement (**Synovial – condylar variety**).

Inferior articular facets

For the convex facet on second cervical vertebra. Hence it is gently concave and circular.

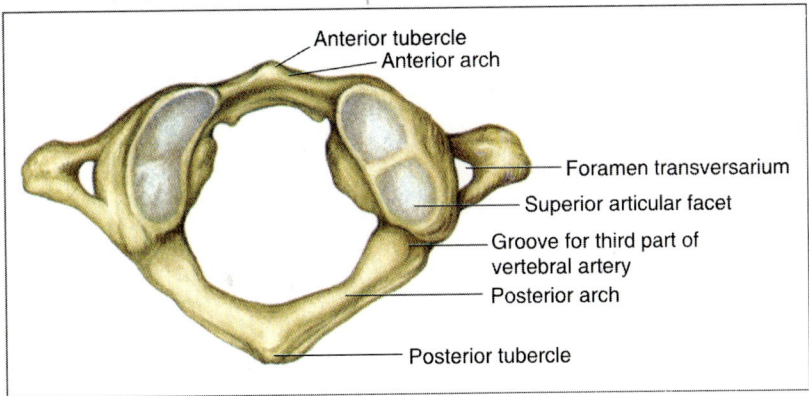

Fig. 35.3: Atlas: Superior view

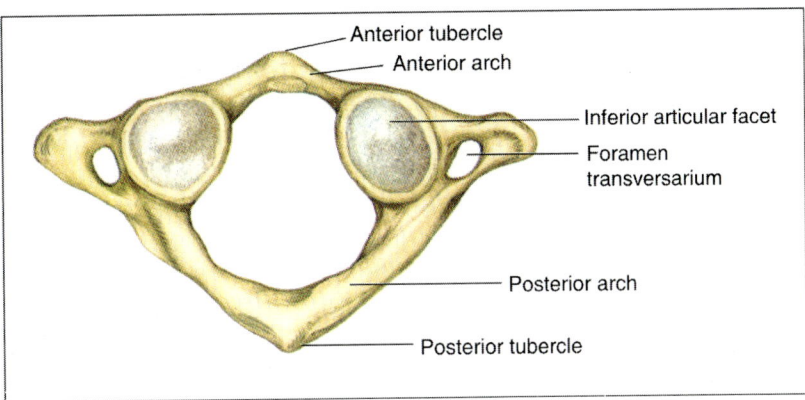

Fig. 35.4: Atlas: Inferior view

TRANSVERSE PROCESS

Longest in the first cervical vertebra except for seventh. This facilitates rotatory movement of the head around the pivot formed by odontoid process of second cervical vertebra.

AXIS

FEATURES

- The tooth like odontoid process makes it easy to be identified. The odontoid process articulates with anterior arch of atlas hence it has a small oval facet on its anterior surface and a groove posteriorly for the transverse ligament of the dens which keeps it in place. The apex of odontoid process superiorly gives attachment to apical ligament of dens. Below the apex on the sides are flattened impressions for alar ligaments.

- On each side of odontoid process superior articular surface is for articulation with atlas. This circular facet is placed over the upper surfaces of lateral part of body and adjoining part of the pedicle.

- The transverse process is very small with no distinction between anterior and posterior tubercles.

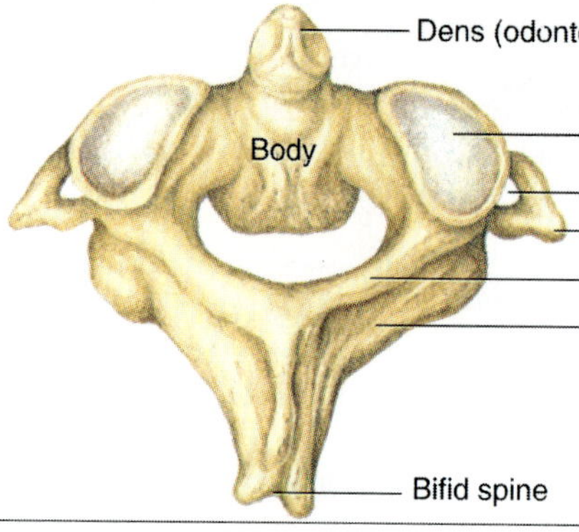

Fig. 35.5: Axis vertebra: Superior aspect

- Foramen transversarium is directed upwards and laterally.
- Laminae are thick and stout making the vertebral foramen large.
- Spine is large and very strong as it provides attachment to the muscles that extend and rotate the head.

The spinal nerves come out through intervertebral foramina below the corresponding vertebra exception being C-1 to C-7 which pass above the corresponding cervical vertebra. There are eight cervical spinal nerves while the vertebrae are seven. Thus the arrangement of nerves with respect to vertebrae to be considered:

- First cervical (C-1) nerve is above the first cervical vertebra
- Eighth cervical (C-8) nerve follows the other spinal nerves.

VERTEBRA PROMINENS – C 7

FEATURES

- The atypical feature of this vertebra is an elongated spine, the tip of which can be felt in midline near the lower end of nuchal groove. It is called vertebra prominence because of this feature.

- Transverse processes are bigger with large and prominent posterior part. A cervical rib is the manifestation of the anterior part of the transverse process (costal element).
- Foramen transversarium is smaller compared to other cervical vertebrae as the vertebral artery does not pass through it. The foramen may be doubled or absent.
- The shape of the body of seventh cervical vertebra is in the transition between cervical and thoracic vertebrae.

CLINICAL CONSIDERATIONS

Fracture of Cervical Vertebrae

This may result by a fall on the head with acute flexion of the neck. Dislocation results in automobile/aviation crashes. This is due to sudden forward jerk. The dislocation results as the intervertebral facets (zygogophyseal joints) are in a horizontal plane.

Prolapsed Intervertebral Disc

The relatively thin posterior part of annulus fibrous ruptures (trauma/degenerative changes). The nucleus pulposus protrudes posteriorly into the vertebral canal. The common sites are C5-C6 and C6-C7 intervertebral discs.

Fusion of Cervical Vertebrae (Klippel Feil Syndrome)

Congenital fusion of cervical vertebrae is one of the features of Klippel Feil syndrome. Fusion of cervical vertebrae result in grossly restricted movements of the neck.

Cervical Spondylosis

This is a degenerative condition of cervical vertebrae seen after 50 years of age. This is commonly seen in persons who are susceptible to neck strain (keeping the neck in one position) e.g. reading and writing.

The degeneration of disc results in reduction of disc space and peripheral osteophytes formation. The posterior intervertebral joints (articular facets) are also involved resulting pain in the neck. The osteophytes impinge on nerve roots – pain in the upper limb.

Cervical spondylosis is most commonly seen in lowest three intervertebral joints.

QUESTIONS: CERVICAL VERTEBRAE

- Which vertebrae lack body and spinous process?
- Which cervical vertebra is called vertebra prominence? Why?
- Yes gesture movement occurs at which joint?
- No gesture results from movement of which bones?
- Which part of axis makes a pivot for 'no' gesture movement?
- Which part of axis can cause death in a whiplash injury?
- Open mouth view X ray is taken for visualizing which vertebrae / part of vertebrae
- What is Jefferson's fracture?
- What is Hangman's fracture?
- What age does the fusion of cervical vertebrae begin and what age it is completed?

Section-III
Dissection & Text

CONTENTS

36. **Scalp and Temple**   149-153

37. **Cervical Fascia**   154-156

38. **Face**   157-169

39. **Posterior Triangle of Neck**   170-175

40. **Back**   176-180

41. **Anterior Triangle of Neck**   181-192

42. **Deep Dissection of Neck**   193-217

43. **Parotid Region**   218-221

44. **Temporal and Interatemporal Fossae**   222-236

45. **Submandibular Region**   237-240

46. **Mouth and Pharynx**   241-251

47. **Nasal Cavity**   252-258

48. **Tongue**   259-264

49. **Larynx**   265-272

50. **Orbit**   273-284

51. **Ear**   285-291

52. **Eye**   292-295

36

Scalp and Temple

A longitudinal incision is given in the skin of the scalp from the root of nose to the external occipital protuberance. Second incision is made at right angle (**in coronal plane**) from the middle of the first incision extending to both auricles. This incision is continued behind the auricle upto the mastoid process while in front to the root of the zygomatic arch. Avoid damage to blood vessels, nerves placed in the subcutaneous tissue. Reflect skin flaps outwards.

Identify

- Upper part of orbicularis oculi

Trace occipitofrontalis from below upwards.

- Branches of supratrochlear and supraorbital vessels and nerves
- Anterior part of epicranial aponeurosis and its extension into the temple

Identify

- Two temporal branches of the facial nerve – crosses zygomatic arch two cm in front of the auricle.

Trace these nerves upwards to the deep surface of orbicularis oculi.

- Zygomaticotemporal nerve – pierces temporal fascia just behind the frontal process of zygomatic bone.

Identify

- Superficial temporal vessels

- Superficial temporal nerve

Both cross the root of zygomatic arch, anterior to the auricle. Trace these to the scalp.

Identify

- Great auricular nerve
- Lesser occipital nerve
- Posterior auricular vessels and nerve

These are placed behind the root of auricle.

Trace their branches.

Identify

Terminal branches of the 3rd occipital nerve in the fascia over the external occipital protube-rance.

Divide the dense superficial fascia over the superior nuchal line about two to three cm lateral to the external occipital protuberance.

Identify

- Occipital vessels
- Greater occipital nerve

Trace these towards the vertex.

Identify

- Occipital belly of occipitofrontalis muscle

Make a small incision in the epicranial aponeurosis near the vertex. Put a blunt seeker through this incision into the loose areolar tissue under this aponeurosis and demonstrate the extent of the aponeurosis. Epicranial aponeurosis (**galea aponeurotica**) is attached to the periosteum at the temporal and nuchal lines.

149

SCALP: DESCRIPTION

Structurally, scalp differs from palm and sole in having hair and sebaceous glands. The blood vessels and nerves are placed superficially over aponeurotic layer. Scalp extends antero-posteriorly from eyebrows to highest nuchal lines. Forehead is thus common to face and scalp. Laterally it blends with superior temporal lines.

Scalp has five layers. Each letter of **SCALP** stands for the layers in sequence:

- **S – Skin**
- **C – Connective tissue** (dense)
- **A - Aponeurosis** (Galea aponeurotica)
- **L – Loose connective tissue**
- **P – Pericranium**

Abundant fibrous strands anchor skin to the aponeurotic layer. Thus dense connective tissue layer is practically inseparable. Like elsewhere in superficial fascia, this layer also has fat, blood vessels and nerves.

Scalp is richly supplied by branches of internal carotid artery (ICA) and external carotid artery (ECA). This is one of the sites of anastomosis between ICA and ECA.

- Ten nerves supply each half of scalp.
- Four sensory and one motor, each in front and behind the auricle.
- Motor branches of facial nerve (VII CN) are for fronto-occipitalis

OCCIPITOFRONTALIS

It is a broad, musculofibrous layer which covers the skull. It extands from the highest nuchal lines to the eyebrows. It consists of four parts. On either side it has occipital and frontal bellies which are connected by the epicranial aponeurosis.

The occipitalis arises by tendinous fibres from the lateral two-thirds of the highest nuchal line and the mastoid process and inserted in the aponeurosis.

The frontalis is adherent to the superficial fascia (without bony attachments) of the eyebrows. It is broader than the occipitalis.

- Medial fibres are continuous with procerus
- Intermediate fibres blend with corrugator supercilii and orbicularis oculi
- Lateral fibres blend with orbicularis over the zygomatic process

The muscles fibres ascend to get inserted in the epicranial aponeurosis in front of the coronal suture.

Between the medial margins of two occipital bellies there is a considerable gap which is occupied by an extension of the epicranial aponeurosis.

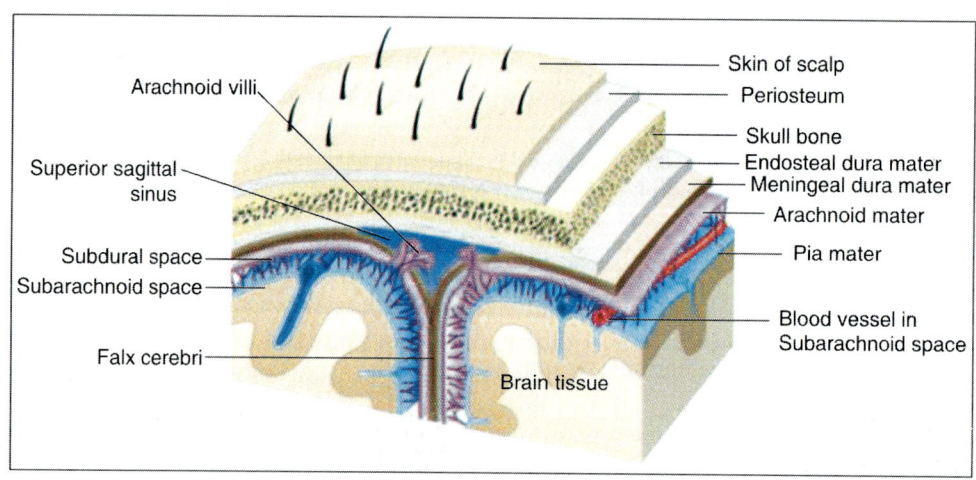

Fig. 36.1: Scalp and its layers

TEMPOROPARIETALIS

Temporoparietalis is a variably developed muscle that occupies the interval between the frontal parts of occipitofrontalis and the anterior and superior auricular muscles.

Nerve supply

- Occipital part - Posterior auricular branch of facial nerve
- Frontal part - Temporal branches of the facial nerve

Actions of frontalis

1. Acting from above, frontalis raise the eyebrows and the skin over the root of nose (expression of surprise, horror or fright)
2. Acting from below, frontalis draw the scalp forwards causing transverse wrinkles in the forehead

Actions of occipitalis

1. Draws the scalp backwards.
2. Acting alternately, occipital and frontal parts can move the entire scalp backwards and forwards

EPICRANIAL APONEUROSIS

It forms a continuous fibromuscular sheet which extends from the occiput to the eyebrows.

Attachments

Posteriorly - External occipital protuberance and highest nuchal line

Anteriorly - splits to enclose the frontal parts and sends a short narrow prolongation between them

On each side - anterior and superior auricular muscles are attached in it. Here it is thin and continues over the temporal fascia to get attached to the zygomatic arch.

Over the vault of skull it is intimately adherent to the skin by the fibrous septa but it is loosely attached to the pericranium by areolar tissue. This allows aponeurosis to move freely over pericranium along with the skin of the scalp.

CLINICAL CONSIDERATIONS

Scalp layers

The first three layers of scalp are considered as a single layer because when these are torn off in accidents, or turned down surgically, they remain firmly connected to each other.

The subcutaneous connective tissue is very dense. Thus any inflammatory swelling is slight but much painful because of rich innervation and a wound that does not involve epicranial aponeurosis does not gape. The dense nature of this tissue impedes contraction and retraction of arteries and therefore haemorrhage from scalp wounds is often profuse.

Subaponeurotic areolar tissue is surgically important. It is loose and lax. It can be easily torn. Hence it is avulsed when surgical exposures are made. The vessels are placed in the avulsed tissue. They anastomose freely therefore necrosis is rarely seen

Open wounds of scalp bleed profusely

Scalp has rich cutaneous blood supply with numerous anastomoses between various branches of ICA and ECA.

Cut ends of the vessels are prevented from retraction by the fibrous strands which anchor the vessel walls. The bleeding is stopped effectively by applying firm pressure against the underlying bone for same time.

Scalp swellings are painful

Fibrous stands of dense connective tissue layer restrict the expansion of swelling / subcutaneous haemorrhage. Hence the swelling is tensile and presses on the nerve endings.

Sebaceous cysts

Sebaceous glands are associated with hair follicles. Any blockade in the extrusion of secretions of sebaceous glands may lead to formation of sebaceous cyst. Thus scalp is the commonest site for sebaceous cyst.

Suturing of scalp

Interrupted sutures by non-absorbable material e.g. silk, are applied to approximate the cut ends of wounds of scalp.

Medico-legal importance of scalp wounds

Galea aponeurotica is involved / cut in grievous injuries inflicted with a blunt / sharp weapon. This wound has incised margins of galea aponeurotica.

Emissary veins

These connect intracranial dural venous sinuses to the subcutaneous veins of the scalp. These are valve-less and blood can flow in either direction. Infection of the scalp can spread via these veins to cause:

- Meningitis
- Dural venous sinus thrombosis

Scalp flaps

In opening of skull (craniotomy), the first three layers of the scalp are cut together and the line of cleavage is loose connective tissue layer. The scalp flaps are turned down so as to retain the blood vessels and nerves in the peripheral pedicles of the flops.

Black eye

Direct black eye is due to local blow to the eye causing blackish discolorations of both eyelids simultaneously within two hours due to subcutaneous haemorrhage.

Indirect black eye is due to grievous injury causing haemorrhage in the subaponeurotic layer. The haemorrhage fills subaponeurotic space up to the highest nuchal liner posteriorly and superior temporal line laterally. It slowly gravitates under frontalis to the upper eyelid first followed by lower eyelid causing their discoloration. This usually takes one to two days to appear.

Traumatic Cephalhydrocele

A grievous injury to the skull can cause fracture of ault and tearing of meninges. It leading to escape of cerebrospinal fluid (CSF) exteriorly resulting in a scalp swelling.

Cephalhaematoma

Pericranium is loosely attached to the bone. At sutural lines it dips and blends with the endosteum. Any collection of fluid beneath the pericranium will result in a swelling resembling the shape of the bone.

This swelling is caused by subcutaneous bleeding and accumulation of blood. It may form in the scalp of a foetus during difficult labour. It enlarges slowly in the first few days after birth.

It usually results from trauma or following forceps delivery. Large cephalhematoma may become infected which requires surgical drainage.

Caput succedaneum

It is a localized pitting oedema in the scalp of a foetus that may overlie sutures of the skull. It is usually formed during labour as a result of the circular pressure of the cervix on the foetal occiput.

On PV examination - swelling may be mistaken for unruptured membranes. If the caput enlarges appreciably during labour it may give an impression of foetal descent on successive examinations.

At birth the baby's head may appear markedly deformed. The swelling starts resolving immediately and in few days it disappears.

Moulding (shaping)

This is the natural process by which a baby's head is shaped during labour as it is squeezed into and through the birth canal during labour.

The head often becomes quite elongated. The skull bones may overlap slightly at the suture lines.

The biparietal diameter of the head may be compressed as much as 0.5 cm without intracranial damage. The changes caused by moulding resolve during the first few days of life.

Safely valve hematoma

In children dura and pericranium are intimately adherent to the skull bones than adults. The fracture of the vault may tear dura and pericranium. This results in collection of intracranial haemorrhage in sub-aponeurotic compartment of skull through the fracture line. No signs of brain compression develop until sub-aponeurotic space is filled with blood. After this signs of cerebral compression develop rapidly. This collection of blood is termed **safety valve hematoma**.

Clinical testing of facial nerve

Facial nerve is commonly affected in various neurological conditions. To assess the facial nerve involvement, the facial muscles are tested by asking the patient to perform some actions. These are:

- Frowning of forehead
- Closing of eyes
- Showing of teeth
- Whistling
- Smiling

Cephalopelvic disproportion (CPD)

This is an obstetric condition in which a baby's head is too large or a mother's birth canal too small to permit birth.

Relative CPD - Size of the baby's head is within normal limits but larger than average or the size of the mother's birth canal is within normal limits but smaller than average.

The relative CPD is overcome by

- Moulding of the head
- Forces of labour
- Use of forceps during delivery

Absolute CPD - Baby's head is abnormally enlarged or the mother's birth canal is abnormally contracted. This makes vaginal delivery impossible.

Fracture of skull base

Basilar fractures often involve the petrous part of temporal bone.

The most common type resulting from a temporal blow begins in the squamous part of temporal bone. This fracture often produces deformity of the external ear and or rupture of the lympanic membrane.

The adjacent dura mater is often torn resulting in leakage of cerebrospinal fluid (**CSF**) from the ear canal - **otorrhoea**. When the tympanic membrane remains intact, blood may collect behind the tympanic membrane (**hemotympanum**) or CSF may collect in the middle ear cavity and drain, through the eustachian tube, into the nose - **rhinorrhoea**.

Disruption of the ossicles may occur, producing a conductive hearing loss.

Injury to the facial nerve may produce **Bell's palsy**.

If the fracture extends to the sigmoid sinus with bleeding into the mastoid air cells and beneath the pericranium produces a post auricular swelling and hematoma -**Battle's sign.**

The anterior part of skull base is a common fracture site. The subarachnoid space and the external environment (via the nasal cavity and paranasal sinuses) are in close proximity, separated by thin bone, including cribriform plate of ethmoid bone. This is lined with mucous membrane and with the dura mater on the other surface.

Fractures commonly lacerate the dura mater. This causes CSF to drain into

- Paranasal sinuses
- Nasal cavity - **rhinorrhoea**

Damage to the anterior venous sinuses may cause leakage of blood into the periorbital tissue **Panda bear** sign. Absence of subconjunctival haemorrhage distinguishes this injury from direct ocular trauma. Indirect evidence of anterior basilar fractures includes:

- air-fluid level in one of the sinuses
- presence of intracranial air on skull radiographs or CT scans.

37

Cervical Fascia

SUPERFICIAL CERVICAL FASCIA

It is usually a thin fascia which covers platysma. It is hardly demonstrable as a separate layer and contains considerable amounts of adipose tissue, especially in females.

DEEP CERVICAL FASCIA

It consists of fibro-areolar tissue placed deep to platysma. It invests the muscles and other structures of the neck. In certain situations it forms well-defined fibrous sheets; elsewhere it is loosely arranged.

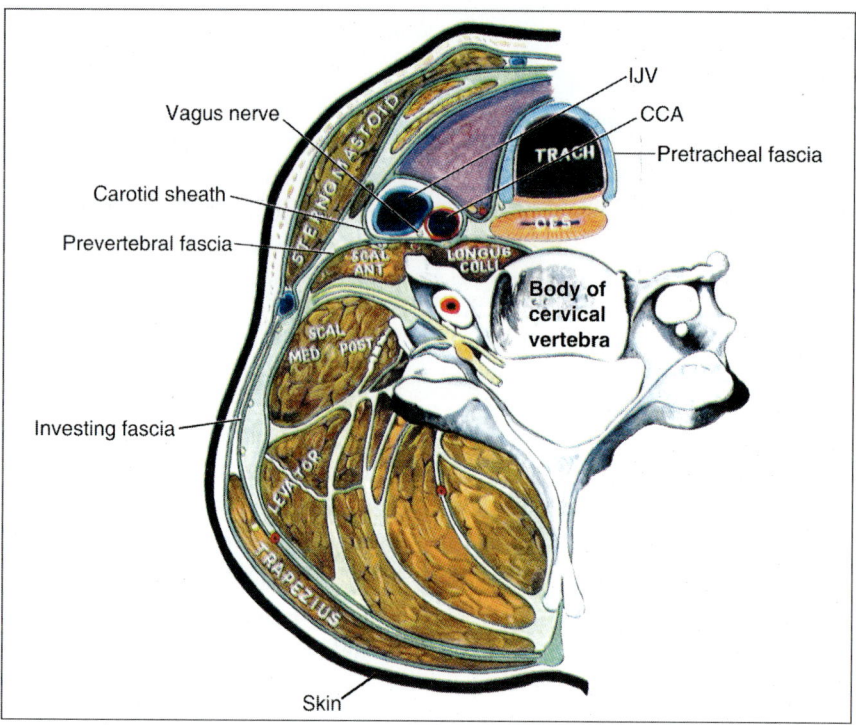

Fig. 37.1: Deep Cervical Fascia

It consists of following layers

1. INVESTING FASCIA

It is attached behind to the ligamentum nuchae and the spine of the 7th cervical vertebra. It covers trapezius and continues forwards from the anterior border of trapezius as a single layer over the posterior triangle (forms roof) to the posterior border of sternocleidomastoid. Here it splits and encloses sternocleidomastoid. At the anterior margin of SCM it becomes a single layer which covers the anterior triangle of the neck and reaches forwards to the midline where it meets the corresponding layer from the opposite side. In the midline it is attached to the symphysis menti and the body of the hyoid bone.

Above it is attached the superior nuchal line, mastoid process and the base of the mandible. Between the mandible and the mastoid process it encloses the parotid gland. The superficial layer over the gland extends upwards as the parotid fascia which is attached to the zygomatic arch. From the deep layer to the gland, stylomandibular ligament passes to the styloid process.

Below the investing fascia is attached to the acromion process, clavicle and manubrium sterni. Just above the manubrium it splits into superficial and deep layers. The superficial layer is attached to the anterior border of the manubrium while the deep layer is attached to its posterior border and the interclavicular ligament. Between these two layers is suprasternal space (**of Bern**).
This space contains

1. Small amount of areolar tissue
2. Lower parts of the anterior jugular veins
3. Jugular venous arch
4. Sternal heads of SCM muscles
5. Lymph node

In the lower part of the posterior triangle (between trapezius and SCM) the deep fascia again divides into superficial and deep layers.

Superficial layer - attached to the superior border of the clavicle

Deep layer - surrounds the inferior belly of omohyoid and its intermediate tendon. It blends with periosteum on the posterior surface of clavicle and anterior end of the 1st rib.

2. CAROTID SHEATH

It is the condensation of deep cervical fascia around the common and internal carotid arteries, internal jugular vein, vagus nerve and the constituents of the ansa cervicalis. It is thicker around the arteries than the vein. It is connected at the margins to adjacent layers by loose areolar tissue.

3. PREVERTEBRAL FASCIA

It covers the anterior vertebral muscles and extends laterally on scalenus anterior, scalenus medius and levator scapulae. It forms a fascial floor of the posterior triangle. As the subclavian artery and the nerves of the brachial plexus emerge from behind scalenus anterior muscle they carry a sleeve which is derived from the prevertebral fascia termed as the **axillary sheath**.

Laterally the prevertebral fascia is thin and areolar under cover of trapezius. Superiorly it is attached to the base of the skull. Inferiorly it descends in front of longus colli into the superior mediastinum where it blends with the anterior longitudinal ligament. Anteriorly the prevertebral fascia is separated from the pharynx and its covering buccopharyngeal fascia by a loose areolar tissue termed as **retropharyngeal space**. Laterally this loose connective tissue connects the prevertebral fascia to the carotid sheath and the fascia on the deep surface of sternocleidomastoid.

4. PRETRACHEAL FASCIA

This layer is very thin which provides a fascial sheath for the thyroid gland. Above it is attached to the arch of the cricoid cartilage and below it continues into the superior mediastinum with the inferior thyroid veins.

CLINICAL CONSIDERATION

The investing layer of deep cervical fascia opposes the spread of abscesses towards the surface and pus beneath it migrates laterally.

If the pus is present in the anterior triangle, it may go into the mediastinum, anterior to the pretracheal lamina. The fascia here is very thin thus it approaches the surface and 'points' above the sternum.

Pus behind the prevertebral lamina may extend laterally and point in the posterior triangle. It may perforate this layer and the buccopharyngeal fascia to bulge into the pharynx as a retropharyngeal abscess.

38

Face

Make an incision in the skin extending from the root of the nose to the chin. Give a transverse incision from the angle of the mouth to the posterior border of the mandible. Reflect the skin flaps out-wards. Avoid damage the muscles of face (**Penniculus carnosus**) and associated nerves and vessels.

Pull eyelids laterally and expose the medial palpebral ligament. Expose the outer part of orbicularis oculi. Follow its inner part to the margins of the eyelids.

Identify

- Palpebral branch of lacrimal nerve

This enters the lateral part of the upper eyelid through the orbicularis oculi.

- Levator labii superioris alaeque nasi at the side of the nose
- Facial vein lying on the surface of the muscle.

Trace it downwards until it passes deep to zygomaticus major.

- Infratrochlear nerve (above)
- External nasal nerve (below)

These are seen running down-wards on the side of the nose.

Expose zygomaticus major and levator labii superioris muscles. Follow levator labii superioris upward deep to orbicularis oculi.

Expose platysma at the lower border of the mandible. Note its structure like a broad, thin sheet. Trace it downwards into the neck. Its posterior fibres curve forwards towards the angle of the mouth form a part of risorius muscle.

Identify

- Depressor anguli oris
- Depressor labii inferioris

DEEP DISSECTION OF FACE

Separate risorius and reflect it to the corner of the mouth along with remnants of the platysma. Avoid injury to the underlying vessels and nerves.

Identify cut end of the great auricular nerve. Trace it upwards over the lower part of the parotid gland.

Identify

- Facial artery and vein at the anteroinferior angle of masseter

Divide the fascia over the parotid gland in front of the auricle, from the zygomatic arch to the angle of the mandible. Reflect it to the margins of the gland. The vessels, nerves, and duct of the gland emerge from its anterior border. The parotid duct appears at the anterior border, one cm below the zygomatic arch.

Identify (above parotid duct)

- Accessory parotid gland
- Transverse facial artery and vein
- Zygomatic branches of facial nerve

Identify

- Branches of the facial nerve emerging from the anterior border of parotid gland

Trace these branches forward and note their communications with the branches of the trigeminal nerve.

- Upper zygomatic branch of the facial nerve deep to the lateral part of orbicularis oculi
- Lower zygomatic branch of the facial nerve below the orbit and deep to zygomatic muscles

Divide zygomaticus major and minor, and levator labii superioris at their origins. Reflect them downwards and expose facial vessels.

Identify

- Buccal branch of the facial nerve at the anterior border of parotid gland

Trace this nerve forwards to the buccinator muscle through the buccal pad of fat.

- Marginal mandibular branch of facial nerve from lower border of parotid gland to the depressor anguli oris

Cut depressor anguli oris and identify its communication with the mental nerve which emerges through the mental foramen. Trace the branches of mental nerve to the lower lip and chin.

Identify (at upper border of parotid gland)

- Superficial temporal vessels
- Temporal branches of facial nerve (anterior to the vessels)
- Auriculotemporal nerve (behind superficial temporal vessels)

Identify (at lower border of parotid gland)

- Anterior and posterior divisions of retromandibular vein
- Cervical branch of facial nerve

Trace the facial vein downwards till it joins the anterior tributary of the retromandibular vein.

Identify

- Levator anguli oris
- Buccinator

Clear the buccal pad of fat from the buccinator avoid-ing damage to the buccal nerve. Excise the fascia over the buccinator and identify its attachments to the maxilla and mandible.

Remove mucous membrane over the inner surface of the lips by everting them.

Identify small labial glands under the mucosa.

Identify the **incisive muscles** near the bases of lips opposite the sockets of the incisor teeth. Remove them from the lower lip and expose mentalis.

Make a circular incision and separate the palpebral part of orbicularis oculi and turn it towards the palpebral fissure. Avoid damage to the palpebral fascia, vessels and nerves.

Identify

- Palpebral fascia and tarsi
- Medial palpebral ligament

Divide the superolateral part of the palpebral fascia and expose lacrimal gland. Elevate it and find its ducts.

Identify

- Lacrimal papillae at the medial ends of eyelids

Pass a fine bristle along the lacrimal canaliculi through the puncta.

Identify

- Lacrimal sac behind the medial palpebral ligament
- Lacrimal part of orbicularis oculi on the lateral aspect of the sac

Open the sac and put a probe in it and explore its extent. Then pass the probe downwards through the nasolacrimal duct into the nasal cavity.

Remove the skin and muscles from the nose and identify its cartilages.

FACE: DESCRIPTION

Topographically and functionally these muscles can be grouped as

(A) Epicranial

(B) Circumorbital and palpebral

(C) Nasal

(D) Buccolabial

These muscles are innervated by the branches of the facial nerve (**VII CN**).

(A) EPICRANIAL MUSCLES

- Comprises occipitofrontalis and temporoparietalis

These are considered in scalp.

(B) CIRCUMORBITAL AND PALPEBRAL MUSCLES

This group comprises
- Orbicularis oculi
- Corrugator supercilii
- Levator palpebrae superioris (LPS)

ORBICULARIS OCULI

This broad, flat elliptical muscle surrounds the circumference of the orbit. It spreads into

- Eyelids
- Anterior temporal region
- Infraorbital cheek
- Superciliary region

Its parts are
1. Orbital
2. Palpebral
3. Lacrimal

Orbital part arises from the nasal part of frontal bone, frontal process of maxilla and medial palpebral ligament between them. Its fibres form complete ellipses without interruption.

The upper fibres blend with frontalis and corrugator supercilii. Many of them are inserted into the skin and subcutaneous tissue of the eyebrow forming **depressor supercilii**.

Inferiorly, these ellipses blend with the attachments of levator labii superioris alequae nasi, levator labii superioris and zygomaticus minor.

Palpebral part is thinner than the orbital part. It arises from the medial palpebral ligament. It also arises from the bone immediately above and below

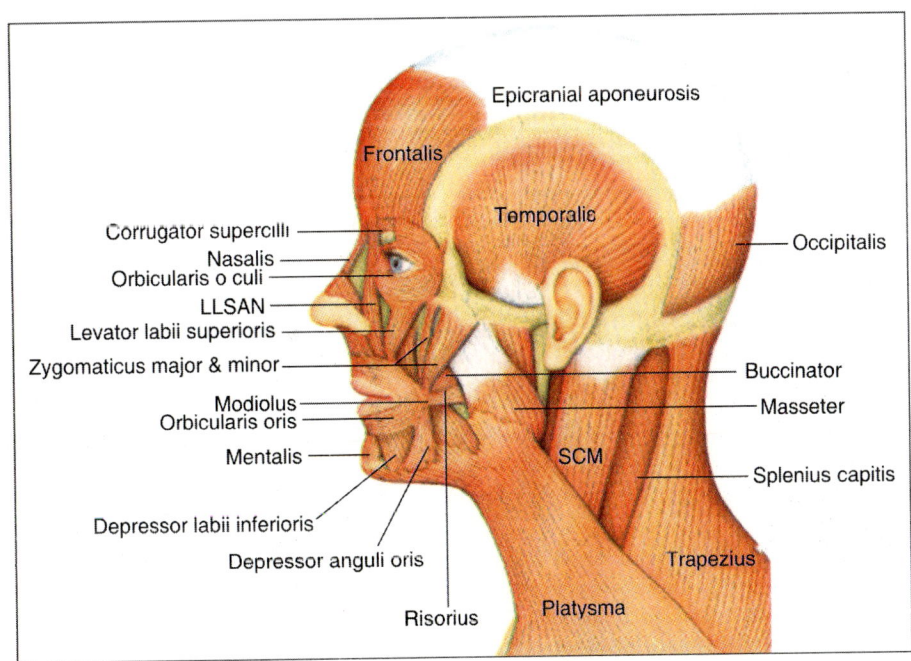

Fig. 38.1: Muscles of face and neck

the ligament. The fibres sweep across the eyelids anterior to the orbital septum. These interlace at the lateral commissure to form the lateral palpebral raphe.

Lacrimal part lies behind the lacrimal sac from which it is separated by the lacrimal fascia. It is attached to

- Lacrimal fascia
- Upper part of the crest of the lacrimal bone
- Adjacent lateral surface of the lacrimal bone

The muscle passes laterally behind the lacrimal sac and divides into upper and lower slips. Some fibres are inserted into the tarsal plate of the eyelids close to the lacrimal canaliculi. Most of the fibres continue across in front of the tarsal plate and interlace in the lateral palpebral raphe.

It is about 4 mm long and 2 mm broad. It is attached to the frontal process of the maxilla, anterior to the nasolacrimal groove. It crosses lacrimal sac, from which it is separated by lacrimal fascia. It divides into upper and lower parts. Both are attached to corresponding tarsus.

Lateral palpebral raphe

It is formed by the interlacing lateral ends of the palpebral fibres of orbicularis oculi. A small lobule of fat may lie between it and the deeply placed lateral palpebral ligament.

Nerve supply

Temporal and zygomatic branches of the facial nerve

Actions

1. **Sphincter muscle** of the eyelids
2. **Palpebral part** can be contracted voluntarily which closes the lids **gently** (in sleep) or **reflexly** (protectively in blinking).
3. **Orbital part** is activated under voluntary control.

   When the entire orbicularis oculi muscle contracts, the skin of the forehead, temple and cheek is drawn towards the medial angle of the orbit, and the eyelids are closed firmly and also displaced a little medially. The skin is thrown into folds which radiate from the lateral angle of the eyelids. In the middle aged people these

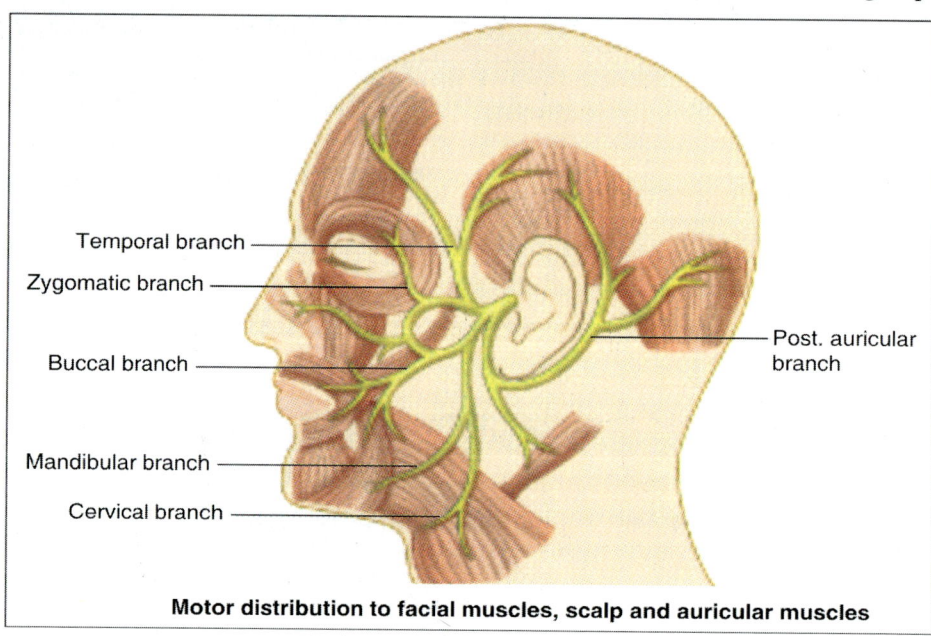

Temporal branch

Zygomatic branch

Buccal branch

Mandibular branch

Cervical branch

Post. auricular branch

Motor distribution to facial muscles, scalp and auricular muscles

Fig. 38.2: Facial nerve on face

wrinkles often become permanent termed as **crow's feet**.

4. **Transport of tears:** The lacrimal part of the muscle draws the eyelids and lacrimal papillae medially. This exerts traction on the lacrimal fascia and aid in drainage of tears by dilating the lacrimal sac.

   It may also influence pressure gradients within the lacrimal gland and ducts.

5. **Muscle of facial expression and ocular reflexes:** Narrowing of the palpebral fissure together with protrusion of the eyebrows reduces the amount of light to enter the eyes. This action of the upper orbital fibres produces vertical furrowing above the bridge of the nose.

CORRUGATOR SUPERCILII

It is a small pyramidal muscle. It is placed at the medial end of each eyebrow, deep to frontalis and orbicularis oculi. It is partially blended with these muscles.

It arises from the bone at the medial end of superciliary arch. It passes laterally and slightly upwards to exert traction on the skin above the middle of the supraorbital margin.

Nerve supply

Temporal branches of the facial nerve

Actions

1. Acts with orbicularis oculi in drawing the eyebrows medially and downwards (shield the eyes in bright sunlight)
2. Involved in frowning
3. Combined action of the two muscles produces vertical wrinkles on the forehead

(C) NASAL MUSCLES

This group comprises
- Procerus
- Nasalis
- Depressor septi

PROCERUS

Procerus is a small pyramidal muscle which partially blends with the medial side of frontalis. It arises from a fascial aponeurosis covering the lower part of nasal bone and upper part of lateral nasal cartilage. It is inserted into the skin over lower part of the forehead between the eyebrows. Its lower aponeurosis blends with the transverse part of nasalis.

Actions

1. Draws down medial angle of eyebrow and produces transverse wrinkles over the bridge of nose.
2. Active in frowning and 'concentration'.

NASALIS

It consists of transverse and alar parts which may be continuous at their origins.

Transverse part (Compressor naris) arises from the maxilla just lateral to nasal notch. Its fibres pass upwards and medially and expand into a thin aponeurosis. At the bridge of nose, aponeuroses of both muscles merge and with the aponeurosis of procerus.

Alar part (Dilatator naris) arises from the maxilla. It is attached to the cartilaginous ala nasi.

Actions

1. **Transverse part** of nasalis compresses the nasal aperture at the junction of the vestibule with the nasal cavity.
2. **Alar part** draws ala downwards and laterally and assists in widening the anterior nasal aperture. These actions accompany deep inspiration. These are thus associated with exertion but also with some emotional states.

DEPRESSOR SEPTI

It is considered as part of dilatator naris. It arises from the maxilla above the central incisor tooth and attached to the mobile part of the nasal septum. It is immediately deep to the mucous membrane of the upper lip.

Actions

Depressor septi acts with the alar part of nasalis to widen the nasal aperture.

Nerve supply

All the muscles of this group are supplied by the superior buccal branches of the facial nerve.

(D) BUCCOLABIAL MUSCLES

These include
Elevators, retractors and evertors of upper lip
- Levator labii superioris alaeque nasi
- Levator labii superioris
- Zygomaticus major and minor
- Levator anguli oris
- Risorius

Depressors, retractors and evertors of lower lip
- Depressor labii inferioris
- Depressor anguli oris
- Mentalis

Compound sphincter
- Orbicularis oris
- Incisivus superior and inferior

LEVATOR LABII SUPERIORIS ALAEQUE NASI

It arises from the upper part of the frontal process of the maxilla. It passes obliquely downwards and laterally and divides into medial and lateral slips.
Medial slip is inserted into the greater alar cartilage of the nose and the skin over it.
Lateral slip is prolonged into the lateral part of the upper lip and blends with levator labii superioris and orbicularis oris.

Actions

Lateral slip

1. Raises and everts upper lip
2. Raises, deepens and increases the curvature of the top of the nasolabial furrow

Medial slip

1. Dilates nostril
2. Displaces the circumalar furrow laterally and modifies its curvature

LEVATOR LABII SUPERIORIS

It arises from the maxilla and zygomatic bone above the infraorbital foramen. Its fibres converge into the muscular substance of the upper lip between the lateral slip of levator labii superioris alaeque nasi and zygomaticus minor.

Actions

1. Raises and everts the upper lip.
2. Acting with other muscles it modifies the nasolabial furrow

ZYGOMATICUS MINOR

It arises from the lateral surface of the zygomatic bone immediately behind the zygomaticomaxillary suture. It passes downwards and medially into the muscular substance of the upper lip.

Actions

1. Elevates upper lip and exposes upper teeth
2. Assists in deepening and elevating nasolabial furrow

LEVATOR ANGULI ORIS

It arises from the canine fossa, just below the infraorbital foramen and inserted into the modiolus (lateral to the angle of mouth). At modiolus its fibres mingle with the fibres of zygomaticus major, depressor anguli oris and other muscular bands, including orbicularis oris.

Actions

1. Raises the angle of mouth
2. Contributes in the depth and contour of nasolabial furrow

ZYGOMATICUS MAJOR

It arises from the zygomatic bone, in front of the zygomaticotemporal suture and inserted into the modiolus. It blends with the fibres of levator anguli oris, orbicularis oris and other deeply placed muscular slips.

Actions

Draws the angle of mouth upwards and laterally (as in laughing)

Nerve supply

Buccal branches of the facial nerve

MENTALIS

This is a small muscle. The fibres arise from the incisive fossa of mandible and descend to get attached to the skin of chin.

Actions

1. Raises lower lip and mentolabial sulcus
2. Wrinkles skin of chin
3. Helps in protruding and everting the lower lip (as in drinking and also in expressing doubt)

DEPRESSOR LABII INFERIORIS

This is a quadrilateral muscle. It arises from the oblique line of the mandible, between the symphysis menti and the mental foramen. It passes upwards and medially into the skin and mucosa of the lower lip. It blends with the paired muscle from the opposite side and with orbicularis oris.

Below and laterally it is continuous with platysma.

Actions

1. Draws lower lip downwards and little laterally in mastication.
2. Contributes to the expression of irony, sorrow and doubt.

DEPRESSOR ANGULI ORIS

It arises from the mental tubercle of the mandible and the oblique line, below and lateral to depressor labii inferioris. It converges and blends at the modiolus with orbicularis oris and risorius. Its some fibres continue into levator anguli oris.

It is continuous below with platysma and cervical fasciae.

Actions

1. Draws the angle of mouth downwards and laterally in opening the mouth.
2. Assists in expressing sadness

Nerve supply

Mandibular marginal branch of the facial nerve

BUCCINATOR

This thin quadrilateral muscle occupies the interval between the maxilla and the mandible in the cheek. It is attached to the outer surfaces of the alveolar processes of maxilla and mandible opposite the molar teeth and to the anterior border of pterygomandibular raphe. The raphe separates the muscle from the superior constrictor of pharynx.

The fibres converge towards the modiolus with following mode of attachment

- Central (**pterygomandibular**) fibres intersect each other; those from below crosses to the upper part of orbicularis oris and those from above crosses to the lower part
- Highest (**maxillary**) and lowest (**mandibular**) fibres enter their corresponding lips without decussation.

Relations

Posteriorly – covered by buccopharyngeal fascia.
Superficially – fat separates its posterior part from the ramus of the mandible, masseter and part of temporalis.

Anteriorly - superficial surface is related to zygomaticus major, risorius, levator and depressor anguli oris and parotid duct.

The duct pierces it opposite the third upper molar tooth. The duct is crossed by the facial artery, facial vein and branches of the facial and buccal nerves.

Deep surface - related to buccal glands and mucous membrane of the mouth

Nerve supply

Lower buccal branches of the facial nerve

Actions

1. Compresses cheeks against the teeth and gums.
2. During mastication, assists tongue in directing food between the grinding molar teeth
3. Buccinators expel air from the cheeks between the lips (**blowing muscle**)

PTERYGOMANDIBULAR RAPHE

It extends from the pterygoid hamulus to the posterior end of the mylohyoid line. Medially it can be easily palpated where it is covered by the mucous membrane of the mouth while laterally it is separated from the ramus of the mandible by adipose tissue.

It provides attachments to

Posteriorly - Superior constrictor of pharynx
Anteriorly - Central part of buccinator

MODIOLUS AND ITS ROLE IN FACIAL MOVEMENTS

On each side of the face a number of muscles converge towards a point just lateral to the buccal angle where they interlace to form a compact fibromuscular mass termed as the **modiolus**.

- In the modiolus the muscles radiate from a central point.
- The muscles lie in different planes and their modiolar stems are spiralized.

- There are nine muscles attached to each modiolus.
- The shape and dimensions of the modiolus varies.

Structure

It resembles a blunt cone. The base of the cone (**basis moduli**) is adherent to the mucosa. It is elliptical and extends vertically about 20 mm above and 20 mm below a horizontal line through the buccal angle and 20mm laterally from the angle.

The blunt apex of the cone (**apex moduli**) is about 4 mm across and about 12 mm lateral to the buccal angle.

It is divided into basal, central and apical parts.

Central body has an oblique fibrous cleft which transmits the facial artery.

The apex of the modiolus is adherent to the panniculus fibrosus. There its free border forms a crescentic subcutaneous fibro-elastic cord that accommodates the various expressions of the modioli, lips, mouth and jaws.

Modiolar Muscles

Muscles radiate from the modiolus. Some muscles are almost closed and strap-like while others are widely open and their planes vary.

Most of the muscle stems rotate as they approach the modiolus.

Peripherally the attachment of the depressor lies in the plane of the body of mandible, whereas at the modiolus it lies in an apicobasal direction. The orbicular is in the free lip lie in a roughly coronal plane, but the stem thickens dorsoventrally and attaches at the modiolus from apex to base.

Cruciate modiolar muscles

- Zygomaticus major
- Levator anguli oris
- Depressor anguli oris
- Platysma (pars modiolaris)

These muscles resemble a compound X.

Transverse modiolar muscles

- Buccinator

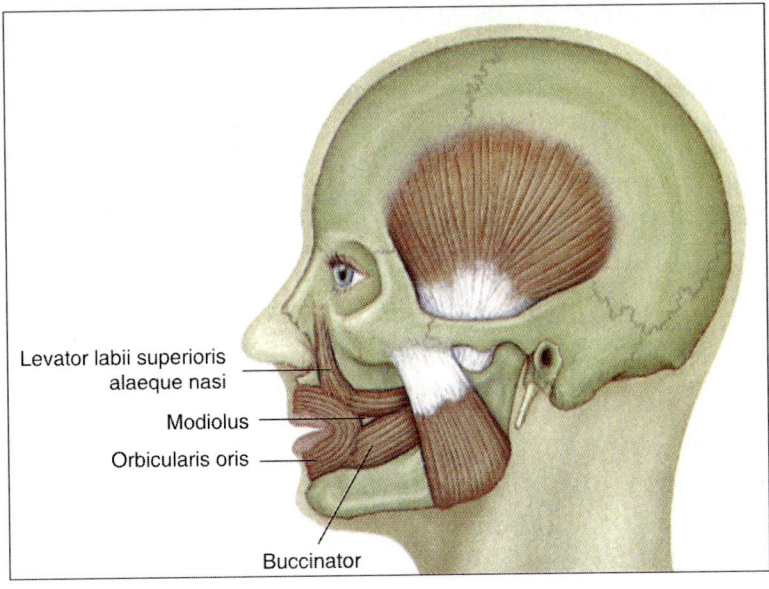

Levator labii superioris
alaeque nasi

Modiolus

Orbicularis oris

Buccinator

Fig. 38.3: The Modiolus

- Risorius
- Various parts of orbicularis oris
- Incisivus superior and inferior

The attachment of these muscles at the modiolus consists of interdigitation, partly with neighbouring bundles but mainly with antagonists. Most fibres terminate after attachment within the modiolus.

Modiolar movements

Mobility of the modioli integrate the activities of

- Cheeks
- Lips
- Oral fissure
- Oral vestibule
- Jaws

These activities include

1. Biting
2. Chewing
3. Drinking
4. Sucking
5. Swallowing
6. Changes in vestibular contents and pressure
7. Variations in speech
8. Modulation of musical tones
9. Production of sounds as in shouting
- Facial expressions

Activities take place in three phases

- Particular modiolar muscle group becomes dominant over its antagonists and the modiolus is relocated
- Modiolus is transiently fixed by simultaneous contraction of modiolar muscles (cruciate muscles).
- Acting from this fixed base the main effectors (**Buccinator** and **Orbicularis oris**) carry out their specific actions.

These actions are integrated with partial separation or closure of the jaws. This determine the positions of the lips and oral fissure from moment to moment. Modiolar movements may be

- Bilaterally symmetrical
- Unilateral
- Asymmetrical

ORBICULARIS ORIS

It consists of four independent quadrants (upper, lower, left and right). Each part contains larger pars peripheralis and pars marginalis.

These parts are apposed along lines that correspond to the junction between the red-lip and the skin. Thus orbicularis oris is composed of eight segments.

Pars peripheralis

Its lateral stem is attached to the labial side of the modiolus from apex to base. These fibres are reinforced by the fibres from

In the upper lip
- Buccinator (upper fibres and decussating lower central fibres)
- Depressor anguli oris

In the lower lip
- Buccinator (lower fibres and decussating upper central fibres)
- Levator anguli oris
- Superficial part of zygomaticus major

The fibres of orbicularis oris enter their respective superior and inferior labial areas and diverge to form triangular muscular sheets. These are thickest at the junctions between skin and red-lip.

The greater part of each sheet enters free lip, where its fibres aggregate into cylindrical bundles which are orientated parallel to the red-lip margin.

In the upper lip, the highest fibres run near the nasolabial sulcus.

In the lower lip, the lowest fibres reach and attached to the mentolabial sulcus. Most fibres continue towards the median plane and cross about five mm into the opposite half-lip.

Pars marginalis

It consists of a single band of narrow muscle fibres which are lodged within the tissues of each red-lip margin. At their medial end, the marginal fibres meet and interlace with their contralateral fellows. At their lateral ends, the fibres converge and are attached to the deepest part of the modiolar base.

Nerve supply

Lower buccal and mandibular marginal branches of the facial nerve

INCISIVUS LABII SUPERIORIS

It is an accessory muscle of the orbicular is oris complex. It arises from the floor of incisive fossa of maxilla above the eminence of lateral incisor tooth. It arches laterally. As it approaches the modiolus, it divides into superficial and deep parts.

Superficial part blends partially with levator anguli oris and attached to the body of the modiolus

Deep part is attached to the superior cornu and base of the modiolus.

INCISIVUS LABII INFERIORIS

It is an accessory orbicular muscle. It is attached to the floor of the incisive fossa of mandible. It curves laterally and upwards and blends partially with orbicularis oris before reaching the modiolus.

PLATYSMA

It has following components:

Pars mandibularis is attached to the lower border of the body of mandible.

Pars labialis is placed in the interval between depressor anguli oris and depressor labii inferioris.

Pars modiolaris consists of the remaining fibres posterior to pars labialis. Pars modiolaris is placed posterolateral to depressor anguli oris.

RISORIUS

It is a highly variable muscle that ranges from fascicles to a wide and thin muscle.

Peripheral attachments include
- Zygomatic arch
- Parotid fascia
- Fascia over masseter (anterior to parotid)

- Fascia enclosing pars modiolaris of platysma
- Fascia over mastoid process

Its fibres converge to apex of modiolus.

It helps in various facial activities other than laughter.

Nerve supply

Buccal branches of the facial nerve

DIRECT LABIAL TRACTORS

These pass directly into the tissues of the lips and not via the modioli. Their action cause

- Elevate and/or evert whole or part of the upper lip
- Depress and/or evert whole or part of the lower lip

From medial to lateral

In the upper lip

- Labial part of levator labii superioris alaeque nasi
- Levator labii superioris
- zygomaticus minor

In the lower lip

- Depressor labii inferioris
- Platysma pars labialis

In both upper and lower lips the tractors blend into a continuous sheet which enters the free lip.

Sheets are divided into three groups

Superficial group comprises a fibre bundles that curve anteriorly a short distance before attaching to the dermis between the hair follicles, sebaceous glands and sweat glands.

Intermediate group is attached to the dermis of the modified skin of red lip.

Deep group is closely applied to the anterior surface of pars peripheralis of orbicularis oris. It sends fine tractor fibres posteriorly to get attached on the submucosa.

MOVEMENTS OF THE LIPS

Various groups of direct labial tractors may act together or individually.

Partial contraction of the superior labial tractors can result in localized elevation of a segment of the upper lip (**canine snarl**).

The activity of the tractors is modified by the superimposed activity of orbicularis oris and the modiolar muscles.

Lip protrusion is passive in its initial stages. It may be suppressed by powerful contraction of the whole of orbicularis oris.

Lip movements accommodate separation of the teeth caused by depression of the mandible.

Contraction of pars marginalis alters the cross-sectional profile of the red-lip rim. It is involved in the production of some consonantal sounds.

ACTION OF FACIAL MUSCLES

All facial muscles arise from the bone and except few, are inserted on to the skin. Thus wounds of the face gape and require stitching. These muscles can be classified anatomically in to following groups:

- Circumorbital
- Nasal
- Buccolabial

Each group consists of **sphincter** and **dilator** muscles.

Actions of the facial muscles are primarily to regulate the openings of the three regions, orbit, nose and mouth. Their names convey the actions that most of these muscles perform.

In addition the facial muscles are also termed as **mimetic group of muscles** or **muscles of facial expression**. By virtue of their insertion on to the skin these cause various facial expressions.

CUTANEOUS INNERVATION OF FACE – EMBRYOLOGICAL BASIS

The face develops from above downwards by three process: frontonasal, maxillary and mandibular process. The cutaneous innervation for the components for these three processes is derived from the branches of Trigeminal nerve (V-CN). These branches are ophthalmic, maxillary and mandibular nerves, respectively.

CLINICAL CONSIDERATIONS

Bleeding from the face

The arterial supply to the face is very rich because of anastomoses between the branches of the two facial arteries in the midline as well as anastomoses of posterior branches with branches that run along the various branches of trigeminal nerve namely supratrochlear, supraorbital, infraorbital and uccal. Because of these extensive anastomoses any arterial cut would lead to bleeding from both the cut ends.

Palpation of the facial artery

Facial artery enters the face at the anteroinferior angle of masseter. This is made prominent by asking the individual to clinch his teeth. Due to easy accessibility the anesthetists prefer to palpate the facial artery here.

Clinical testing of facial nerve

Facial nerve is commonly affected in various neurological conditions. To assess the facial nerve involvement, the facial muscles are tested clinically by asking the patient to perform some actions. They are:

- Frowning of forehead
- Closing of eyes
- Showing of teeth
- Whistling
- Smiling

Suturing of facial wounds

Facial wounds require suturing because of tendency to gape. Since the blood supply of face is profuse, the healing of facial wounds is early and leave very minimal scan. The sutures are continuous and subcuticular in nature.

Dangerous area of face

It includes upper lip and septum of the nose. Any infection in this area may cause spread of infection to the cut ends of venules. Following factors facilitate the spread of infection:

1. Unlike other parts of the body it is difficult to immobilize this part.
2. Absence of deep fascia fails to restrict infection.
3. Veins here do not have valves. Once the infection enters anterior facial vein it initiates thrombus formation. This may occlude the facial vein and open up alternative passage of venous return namely:
   - Via superior ophthalmic vein draining in the cavernous sinus.
   - Via infra-orbital vein which joins inferior ophthalmic vein to drain in cavernous sinus
   - Via deep facial vein to join pterygoid venous plexus which is connected to cavernous sinus by emissary vein.

Along these alternative pathways the infection may enter cavernous sinus and can cause cavernous sinus thrombosis. The cavernous sinus is close to pituitary and cranial nerves II, III, IV, V-1 & V-2 of V CN and VI CN, the clinical picture appears as ophthalmo-plegia along with pituitary dysfunctions. It may prove fatal.

Trigeminal Neuralgia

The sudden onset of excruciating pain, characterizes trigeminal neuralgia - **tic douloureux**. It is a common condition affecting the sensory component of the trigeminal nerve (V CN). Pain may occur in the sensory zone of any division of the nerve. It is most common in the maxillary nerve but rare in the ophthalmic territory.

Pain may often be initiated by touching sensitive **trigger zones** in the skin.

There are no signs of trigeminal nerve dysfunction.

Exploration may show an aberrant loop of one of the cerebellar arteries impinging on the sensory root.

Facial Paralysis

This is characterized by the partial or total loss of the functions of facial muscles or the loss of sensations in the face.

It may be caused by disease or trauma. The degree of paralysis depends on the nerves affected.

Brain injury above the facial nerve nucleus does not block the innervation of the forehead muscles. Injury to the nucleus of the facial nerve or injury to its peripheral neurons paralyzes all the ipsilateral facial muscles.

Bell's Palsy

It is the paralysis of the facial nerve. This may result from

- Trauma to the nerve
- Nerve compression by a tumour
- Infection

Any or all branches of the nerve may be affected. The person may not be able to close an eye or control salivation on the affected side. The condition is generally unilateral. The palsy can be transient or permanent.

Fractures of facial bones

Signs includes:

- Deformity
- Ocular displacement
- Abnormal movement
- Malocclusion of teeth.

Fractures of nasal bones are usually the result of direct violence. Most of these are simple fractures.

Fractures of the maxilla are also a result of direct violence as seen in road traffic injuries. Following will be noted

- Malocclusion of teeth
- Enophthalmos
- Anaesthesia of cheek and upper lip

The zygomatic arch fracture may be due to violence to the side of the skull.

Fractures of mandible are the most common fractures of facial bones. The fractures are usually bilateral. The neck, body, angle, symphysis and ramus are common sites of fracture.

39

Posterior Triangle of Neck

Reflect skin of the posterior triangle of the neck. Avoid damage to the supraclavicular nerves and accessory nerve.

Make an incision in the skin between the mastoid process and sternal end of clavicle. Do not cut the superficial fascia to avoid damage to

- Great auricular nerve
- Transverse nerve of neck
- Anterior external jugular vein

Extend this incision along the clavicle to its lateral end. Reflect the skin flap towards trapezius.

Reflect platysma upwards and forwards from the clavicle and expose

- Supraclavicular nerves
- External jugular vein

These lie underneath the platysma. Trace EJV downwards until it pierces the deep fascia, and upwards to the point it is joined by posterior auricular vein.

Identify

- **Lesser occipital nerve -** runs upwards along the posterior border of SCM
- **Great auricular nerve** - crosses SCM obliquely towards the auricle
- **Transverse nerve of the neck** - passes horizontally forwards across SCM

These nerves pierce the deep fascia at the middle of the posterior border of SCM

Identify

- Medial, intermediate & lateral supraclavicular nerves

These nerves pass downwards across the front of the clavicle.

Divide the investing layer of deep cervical fascia above the clavicle along the posterior border of SCM and expose its deep layer.

Identify

- External jugular vein
- Transverse cervical vein
- Supraclavicular vein

These are placed between the two layers of fascia. Trace them to their union.

Identify

- **Nerve to subclavius** lateral to external jugular vein
- **Anterior jugular vein** entering into external jugular vein
- **Suprascapular artery** deep to clavicle

Trace suprascapular vessels deep to trapezius.

Identify

- Cutaneous nerves at the middle of the posterior border of SCM

- Lesser occipital nerve - hooks around the Accessory nerve

Clear fat and fascia from posterior triangle and note

- Occipital artery at the apex of the triangle
- Accessory nerve
- Branches from 3rd and 4th cervical nerves to trapezius

Cut and clean fascia over inferior belly of omohyoid. Turn it forwards to expose the nerve entering its deep surface.

Clean the upper part of the brachial plexus.

Identify

- Suprascapular nerve: runs posteroinferiorly under omohyoid, just above the brachial plexus
- Dorsal scapular nerve: placed above suprascapular nerve which runs posteroinferiorly deep to trapezius.
- Roots of long thoracic nerve: seen arising from the back of the plexus and which descend behind the roots of the plexus

Identify

- Transverse cervical artery at the upper border of omohyoid

Trace this artery across the posterior triangle and to its origin.

Identify

- Nerve to subclavius
- Subclavian vessels

Divide clavicular attachment of SCM and reflect it forwards. Clean the underlying fat and ex-pose

- Scalenus anterior
- Brachial plexus

Identify

- Omohyoid
- Transverse cervical artery
- Anterior jugular vein
- Internal jugular vein
- Phrenic nerve
- Subclavian vein

POSTERIOR TRIANGLE OF NECK: DESCRIPTION

Boundaries

- **In front** - Posterior border of SCM
- **Below** - Middle third of the of the clavicle
- **Behind** - Anterior border of trapezius

Its apex (between the attachments of SCM and trapezius) is blunt

Inferior belly of the omohyoid crosses about 2.5 cm above the clavicle divides posterior triangle into

- Upper larger occipital triangle
- Lower smaller supraclavicular triangle

OCCIPITAL TRIANGLE

Boundaries

- **In front** - Posterior border of SCM
- **Below** – Inferior belly of omohyoid
- **Behind** - Anterior border of trapezius

Floor (from above downwards)

- Semispinalis capitis
- Splenius capitis
- Levator scapulae
- Scalenus medius and posterior.

It is covered by the skin, superficial and deep fasciae and below by the platysma. The accessory nerve pierces the sternocleidomastoid and crosses the levator scapulae obliquely downwards and backwards to enter the deep surface of the trapezius.

- Cutaneous and muscular branches of the cervical plexus emerge at the posterior border of the SCM.
- Below, supraclavicular nerves, transverse cervical vessels and the upper part of the brachial plexus cross the triangle.
- Lymph nodes are arranged along the posterior border of the SCM extending from the mastoid process to the root of the neck.

SUPRACLAVICULAR TRIANGLE

Boundaries

- **In front** - Posterior border of SCM
- **Below** – Middle third of clavicle
- **Behind** – Inferior belly of omohyoid

It corresponds to the supraclavicular fossa.

Floor contains

- 1st rib
- Scalenus medius
- First slip of serratus anterior

The triangle is covered by the skin, superficial and deep fasciae and platysma. It is crossed by supraclavicular nerves.

Just above the clavicle the third part of the subclavian artery curves inferolaterally from the lateral margin of the scalenus anterior, across the first rib to enter axilla. The subclavian vein is behind the clavicle and does not appear in the triangle.

The brachial plexus is placed partly above and behind the subclavian artery, closely related to it. The trunks of the brachial are palpated here.

The suprascapular vessels pass transversely behind the clavicle and at a higher level the transverse cervical vessels are seen.

The external jugular vein descends behind the posterior border of the SCM to terminate in the subclavian vein. It receives the transverse cervical and suprascapular veins.

The nerve to subclavius crosses this triangle.

CLINICAL CONSIDERATIONS

Torticollis (Wryneck)

In this condition the head is inclined to one side as a result of the contraction of the sternocleidomastoid muscle on that side of the neck. It may be congenital or acquired.

Spasmodic torticollis

It is a type of torticollis which is characterized by episodes of spasms of the neck muscles. The condition is generally transient in nature. In most cases no cause could be found. In some cases it may be due to severe stress and muscular spasm.

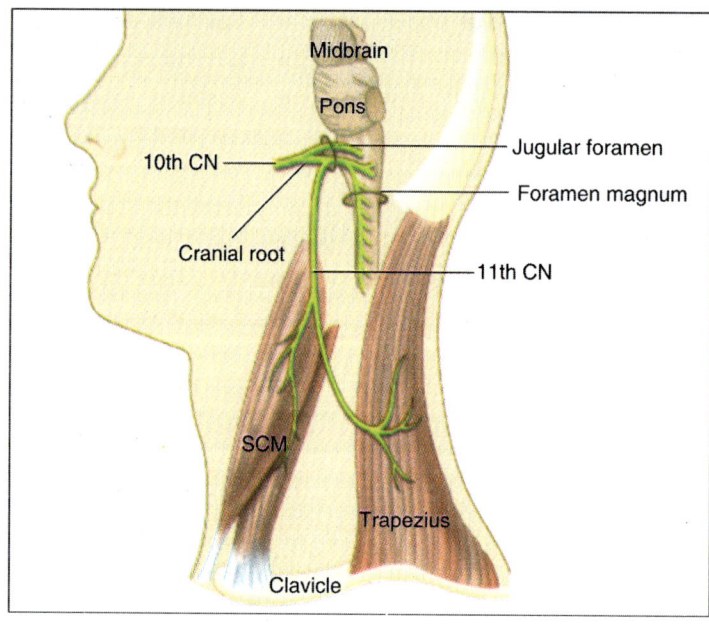

Fig. 39.1: Accessory Nerve

Enlargement of lymph nodes along the Accessory nerve (XI CN) in the posterior triangle would lead to stimulation of the nerve causing spasm of sternocleidomastoid and trapezius resulting in wry neck. Birth injuries resulting in damage to SCM fibers would give rise to **congenital torticollis**.

Management depends on the cause and the severity of the condition. It include

- Surgery
- Support
- Immobilization

Injuries to accessory nerve (XI CN) during surgery

Being superficial accessory name in the posterior triangle is liable to be injuries during any surgical intervention in this region.

Air Embolism

External jugular vein (EJV) enters subclavian vein by piercing the general investing layer of deep cervical fascia an inch above the medial end of clavicle. A cut here would prevent the vein from collapsing leaving its opening patent where from air may be sucked in during inspiration. This may cause air embolism.

Central Venous Pressure (CVP)

It is the blood pressure in the large veins of the body which is distinguished from peripheral venous pressure in an extremity.

It is measured with a water manometer that may be attached to the head side of patient's bed and to a central venous catheter inserted into the vena cava.

Central Venous Pressure (CVP) Monitor

It is a device for measuring and recording the venous blood pressure by means of an indwelling catheter and a pressure manometer.
It is used to evaluate

- Right ventricular function
- Right atrial filling pressure
- Capacity of the blood vessels

CVP Line

To monitor central venous pressure, emergency venous access or long term intravenous feeding central venous line is inserted into the subclavian vein. This procedure is performed in the omo-clavicular triangle.

Brachial Plexus Injuries

Roots

These are likely to be compressed when intervertebral foramen are narrowed by osteo-arthritic changes with advancing age.

Trunks

Upper trunk is stretched and injured when the angle between the head and the shoulder is increased. This may happen when the traction is applied during forceps delivery. In adults, fall on the shoulder may cause this injury. This injury would affect the muscles those are supplied by C5 and C6 segments of brachial plexus. The upper limb is adducted and medially rotated at shoulder joint, extended at elbow joint and pronated at radio-ulnar joints. This deformity is termed as **waiter's tip hand.**

Lower trunk is stretched and injured during childbirth (**breech presentation**). In adults, the injury may result when person falling from a height tries to hold an object with his out stretched upper limb by the hand.

Branches

Long thoracic nerve - Winging of scapula
Axillary nerve in arm – Dropping of shoulder
Radial nerve in arm - Wrist drop
Ulnar nerve in hand – Ulnar claw hand
Median nerve at wrist

- Carpal tunnel syndrome
- Median claw hand
- Ape thumb deformity

Horner's Syndrome

A syndrome is a set of symptoms and signs peculiar to a particular disease. In Horner's syndrome, a set of symptoms are observed due to involvement of sympathetic innervation to the eyeball and face. This is usually after cervical sympathectomy performed for improving blood flow to the distal parts of upper limbs (**Reynard's disease**). These symptoms are also seen in **klumpke's paralysis** where the lower trunk of brachial plexus is affected. Sympathetic innervation for the smooth muscles of blood vessels, sweat glands and arrector pilorum muscle of the upper limb is carried in the brachial plexus and thereafter via the blood vessels to the effector organ. Symptoms of Horner's syndrome are:

Flushing of face – dilatation of cutaneous blood vessels

Anhidrosis – loss of secretions of sweat glands of face

Ptosis – upper eyelid droops marginally because of paresis of smooth muscle component of LPS.

Enophthalmos – The sinking of eyeball in the orbit is known as enophthalmos. The inferior orbital fissure is bridged by a smooth muscle – Muller's muscle – supplied by sympathetic fibers. Thus the paresis/paralysis of this muscle cause the eyeball to slink in the orbit. It is termed as an optical illusion due to narrowing of the palpable fissure.

Miosis – Constriction of the pupil is known as miosis. It is due to interruption in the nerve supply to the dilator pupillae muscle.

Horner's syndrome is an unavoidable aftermath of **cervico-thoracic ganglionectomy** as all pre-ganglionic sympathetic fibers to the head region course upwards through the part of the sympathetic chain that is excised. All the symptoms observed in Horner's syndrome are unilateral

Cervical Rib

The costal element of seventh cervical vertebra at times enlarges to form various grades of cervical rib. A fully formed cervical rib is usually anchored close to the anterior end of the first rib. In such a situation the lower trunk of brachial plexus overrides

the cervical rib causing its stretching. This would lead to a group of neurological symptoms. Subclavian artery is also likely to be compressed due to a long cervical rib. This causes various vascular symptoms with positive **Adam's test**.

Cold Abscess

It is the name given to a swelling which does not shows classical signs of inflammation. Tubercular abscess (**cold abscess**) of cervical vertebrae may gravitate under the prevertebral fascia to reach axilla along the axillary sheath.

Spinal Cord Lesion

It is suspected in a patient with numbness or weakness of one or more limbs especially when associated with pain in the neck or back. The motor dysfunction depends on the extent of the lesion.

Complete spinal cord lesions destroy all function below the affected level. Incomplete lesions cause partial weakness, atrophy, and weak reflexes at the affected level.

- C-3 and C-4 segments innervate the diaphragm - thus a high cervical lesion affects respiration
- Shoulder abduction (deltoid and supraspinous) is a test of C-5 function
- Weak elbow flexion (especially biceps) in the presence of normal deltoid function indicates a C-6 lesion
- Elbow and wrist extensors (triceps and extensor carpi muscles) are innervated by C-7 – tested by these actions
- Lesions at C-8 and T-1 affect intrinsic muscles of the hand (abduction and adduction of fingers)
- Level of a lesion of the thoracic part of the spinal cord can be determined by assessing abdominal muscles. If the lower abdominal musculature is weaker than the upper musculature, producing a positive **Beevor's sign**, the lesion is below the T-9 or T-10 level

- Hip flexors (iliopsoas and rectus femoris) and adductors are supplied by the L-2 and L-3 segments
- Knee extension (quadriceps) indicates L-4 function
- Standing on the heels (dorsiflexion) tests L-5 function
- Standing on the toes (plantar-flexion) tests S-1 and S-2 segements
- Lowest segments of the spinal cord (S-2 to S-4) control anal sphincter

Cervical Disc Disease

It is a common disorder, which is generally not associated with trauma. As the intervertebral disc degenerates, tears or defects developing in the annulus fibrosus of the disc may cause herniation of nucleus pulposus - **ruptured disc.**

Compression the spinal cord or nerve root

- Directly by ruptured disc
- Bony spurs (**osteophytes**) - develop in response to the degeneration of the disc

Only ruptured discs or osteophytes which are directed posteriorly compress nervous structures and produce symptoms.

Cervical radiculopathy with symptoms and signs of compression of a specific cervical nerve root is the first manifestation of cervical disc disease.

The cervical nerve roots exit above the vertebral body of the same number, with the exception of C-8, which emerges between C-7 and T-1 intervertebral space. Thus, a lesion of the C-5 and C-6 disc produces C-6 radiculopathy.

Spondylosis causes cervical nerve root compression. It most frequently involves the C-6 and C-7 nerve roots. C-5 and C-8 are less commonly involved. The T-1 root is involves rarely. Cervical and unilateral upper limb pain is a common symptom of cervical disc disease.

Patients complain of numbness or weakness in the involved limb. The hyperextension and rotation of the neck (**Spurling's maneuver**) causes tension on cervical nerve roots. This further decreases the size of the intervertebral foramina thus increasing the radicular symptoms.

Dislocation of facet (Zygapophyseal joints)

Dislocation of one of the facet joints is called **unilateral locked facet**. The inferior facet of the upper vertebra is displaced anterior to the superior facet of the lower vertebra and locked in position. **Mechanism of injury** is rotation with associated flexion. Continuation of the rotation-flexion would dislocate both facet joints termed **bilateral locked facets**. Unilateral and bilateral locked facet dislocations are distinguished on the basis of the degree of displacement of a vertebral body in relation to that of the adjacent vertebra (**spondylolisthesis**) seen in lateral radiographs.

Management

- Reduction with cervical traction
- If the injury is a facet joint dislocation, then reduction and fixation with a cervical collar orthosis.
- If the dislocation is unstable after reduction, then a posterior fusion at the level of injury is necessary

40

Back

Give a longitudinal skin incision between external occipital protuberance and the spine of C-7 vertebra. Make a transverse incision from the spine of C-7 to the acromion. Reflect the skin flaps outwards.

Identify

- Occipital belly of occipitofrontalis and the
- occipital branch of the posterior auricular nerve

This runs across it near its attachment.

- Cutaneous nerves over the upper part of trapezius
- Branch of occipital artery
- Branch of grater occipital nerve

These are seen on the back of the scalp.

- Third occipital nerve between the grater occipital nerve and midline

Trace this nerve where it pierces the trapezius and deep fascia close to midline.

Remove fascia over trapezius. Separate it from superior nuchal line and divide it vertically one cm from the vertebral spines. Reflect it laterally and expose

- Accessory nerve
- Branches from C-3 and C-4 nerves
- Superficial branch of transverse cervical artery

Note the attachments of levator scapulae.

Trace and identify

- Deep branch of transverse cervical artery
- Dorsal sca-pular nerve

Reflect serratus posterior superior and note the nerves entering its deep surface. Excise thoracic part of thoracolumbar fascia and identify under it the erector spinae muscles with the splenius curving superolaterally across it above the mid-thoracic region. Note the attachment of splenius capitis and the nerves piercing it. Separate the muscle from vertebral spines and reflect it superolaterally without damaging the nerves.

Identify

- Semispinalis
- Erector spinae
- Obliquus capitis superior

Excise fascia over semispinalis capitis and longissimus. Avoid damage to the nerves which pierce semispinalis capitis close to midline. Note attachments of these muscles.

Separate longissimus capitis from the skull and reflect it away.

Identify

- Occipital artery

This is seen deep to the mastoid process over superior oblique capitis. Note its attachments.

Separate semispinalis capitis from occipital bone and reflect it laterally. Avoid damage to the nerves which pierces it.

Identify

- Suboccipital muscles
- Semispinalis cervicis
- Deep cervical artery

Note the attachments of semispinalis cervicis.

Branch of dorsal ramus of C-1 nerve which enters semispinalis capitis is retained by cutting a piece of the muscle with the nerve. Follow this branch to the ramus and the other branches from there are traced. Trace communicating branch to greater occipital nerve. Clear fascia from suboccipital triangle and study the area including the muscles.

SUBOCCIPITAL TRIANGLE

Boundaries

- **Above and medially** - Rectus capitis posterior major
- **Above and laterally** – Superior oblique capitis
- **Below and laterally** – Inferior oblique capitis

Floor is formed by

- Posterior atlanto-occipital membrane
- Posterior arch of the atlas

Medially it is covered by a layer of dense adipose tissue, deep to semispinalis capitis.

Laterally, it is placed under longissimus capitis and sometimes splenius capitis, both overlap superior oblique capitis

Contents

1. Vertebral artery (3rd part)
2. Dorsal ramus of the C-1

COMMUNICATIONS OF SUB OCCIPITAL VENOUS PLEXUS

In and around the sub-occipital triangle, the venous plexus is placed. The plexus receives venous return from:

- Muscles
- Internal vertebral venous plexus
- Condylar emissary vein

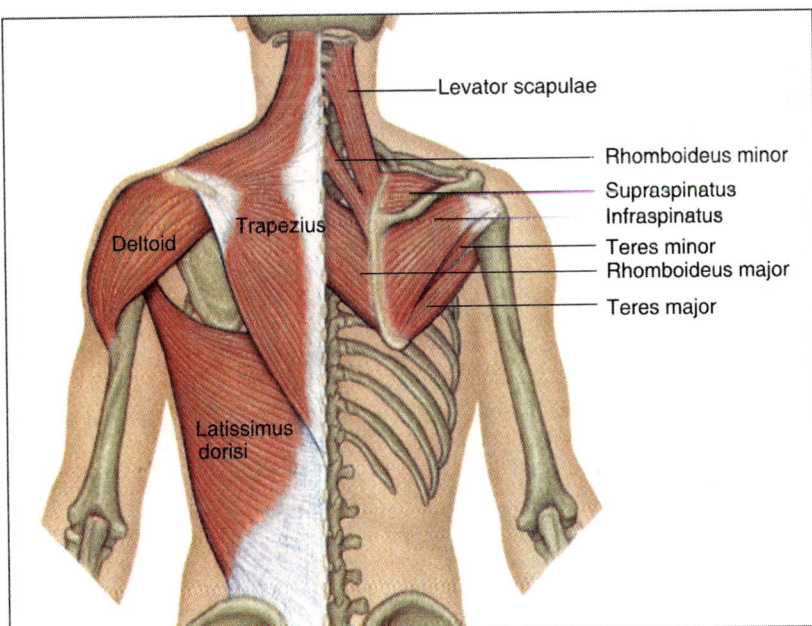

Fig. 40.1: Muscles of back

Labels: Levator scapulae, Rhomboideus minor, Supraspinatus, Infraspinatus, Teres minor, Rhomboideus major, Teres major, Deltoid, Trapezius, Latissimus dorisi

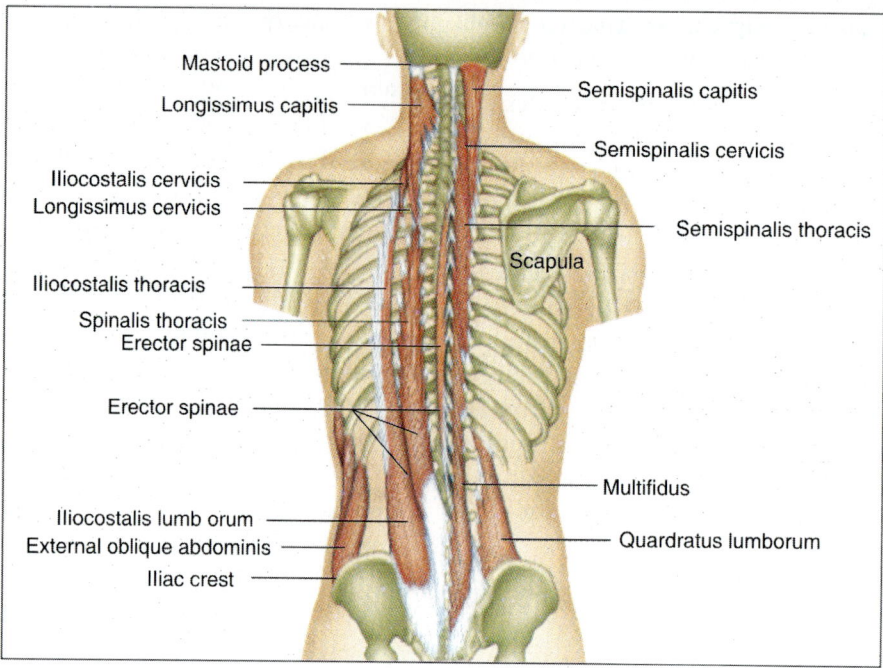

Mastoid process

Longissimus capitis

Iliocostalis cervicis
Longissimus cervicis

Iliocostalis thoracis
Spinalis thoracis
Erector spinae

Erector spinae

Iliocostalis lumb orum
External oblique abdominis
Iliac crest

Semispinalis capitis

Semispinalis cervicis

Semispinalis thoracis
Scapula

Multifidus

Quardratus lumborum

Fig. 40.2: Muscles of back

- Plexus of veins around vertebral artery

It drains into

1. Vertebral venous plexus
2. Deep cervical vein

Thus it presents a number of alternative routes for the venous drainage

SUBOCCIPITAL MUSCLES

These include
- Rectus capitis posterior major and minor
- Superior oblique capitis
- Inferior oblique capitis

These small muscles **cause**

1. **Extension** of the head at the atlanto-occipital joints
   - Recti capitis posterior major
   - Rectus capitis posterior minor
2. **Rotation** of the head and atlas on the axis
   - Superior oblique capitis
   - Inferior oblique capitis

Blood supply

- Vertebral artery
- Deep descending branches of the occipital artery

Nerve supply

All are supplied by the dorsal ramus of the C-1 spinal nerve

RECTUS CAPITIS POSTERIOR MAJOR

It arises from the spine of the axis (C-2) and inserted to the lateral part of the inferior nuchal line and the occipital bone immediately below it.

As the muscles of the two sides pass upwards and laterally, triangular space between them contains parts of the recti capitis posterior minor.

Actions

Extension of the head with rotation of the face towards the same side

RECTUS CAPITIS POSTERIOR MINOR

It arises from the tubercle on the posterior arch of the atlas and inserted on the medial part of the inferior nuchal line and also the occipital bone between the line and the foramen magnum.

Action

Extension of the head

INFERIOR OBLIQUE CAPITIS

This passes laterally and slightly upwards. It arises from the lateral surface of the spine and the adjacent upper part of the lamina of the axis and inserted to the inferoposterior aspect of the transverse process of the atlas.

Action

Rotation of the face towards the same side

SUPERIOR OBLIQUE CAPITIS

It arises from the upper surface of the transverse process of the atlas and inserted to the occipital bone between the superior and inferior nuchal lines, lateral to semispinalis capitis. It overlaps the insertion of rectus capitis posterior major.

Actions

Flexion of the head backwards and to the same side

CLINICAL CONSIDERATIONS

This region is clinically important for
- Neurosurgeon
- Physician
- Orthopedic surgeon

To approach the posterior cranial fossa, neurosurgeon gives "**cross bow incision of *Cushing***". This gives an access to cerebellum, cerebellopontine angle (commonest site of brain tumour), fourth ventricle, medulla, upper part of spinal cord and other structures in posterior cranial fossa.

Neck Rigidity in Meningitis

It is due to spasm of extensor muscles caused by irritation of nerve roots as they pass through infected subarachnoid space.

Symptoms of vertebro-basilar insufficiency

These can be alleviated by surgical removal of the bony ring in Atlas vertebra.

Cisternal puncture

In this procedure a needle is inserted into the **cerebellomedullary cistern** to withdraw cerebro-spinal fluid (CSF) for examination

Subarachnoid space of cerebello-medullary cistern can be tapped by inserting a needle in the sub-occipital region. It is placed in midline just above the spine of axis and is pushed forwards and upwards, parallel to the line joining external acoustic meatus with nasion. The needle pierces in its course, the posterior

Atlanto-occipital membrane and enters the cerebello-medullary cistern. To avoid injury to medulla, the needle should not be pushed more than an inch after it has pierced the posterior atlanto-occipital membrane. The procedure is carried out with the patient sitting or lying on one side with the head flexed forward.

Fracture of 1st Cervical Vertebra

A burst fracture of the C-1 vertebra (**atlas**) is called **Jefferson fracture**. The arch of C-1 may be broken at one or more places. Jefferson fractures usually result from axial loading of the cervical part of the vertebral column (blow to the skull vault).

In most patients with Jefferson fracture, neurological function is intact. The fracture site is stable after bone healing.

Management

Cervical tong traction followed by immobilization with a brace for three months.

Fracture of 2nd Cervical Vertebra

Fractures of the C-2 vertebra (**axis**) usually nvolve the odontoid process (dens).

1. **Type I** – avulsion of the tip of the dens. This is a stable injury that heals when immobilized with a cervical orthosis.

2. **Type II fracture** – occurs at the junction of the base of the dens with the body of C-2 vertebra. These are unstable and reduced with cervical traction and immobilized with a brace for three months.

Nonunion is a serious and quite common complication of these fractures treated with conservative measures.

Criteria to identify patients at risk for nonunion include:

- Age more than 65 years
- Posterior translation of the dens
- Displacement of the dens greater than 5 mm.

These patients are treated by primary posterior fusion (**arthrodesis**) of C-1to C-2.

3. **Type III fractures** - extend into the body of C-2 vertebra. They axe managed with immobilization with brace after reduction with cervical traction.

Bilateral fracture of the Pedicles or Laminae of C-2

A bilateral fracture of the pedicles or laminae of C-2 is called the **hangman fracture**. It is caused by the sudden distraction of the cervical part of the vertebral column (occurs in hanging).

The majority of patients remain neurologically intact.

Management of hangman fracture

- Reduction with cervical traction and immobilization with brace for three months. It usually results in spontaneous fusion of C-2 and C-3.
- If nonunion of the fractured pedicles of C-2 occurs, surgical fusion (**arthrodesis**) of C-2 and C-3 is required.

41

Anterior Triangle of Neck

Make a skin incision from chin to sternum in the midline. Reflect skin flap inferolaterally. Do not damage platysma in the posterosuperior part. Reflect platysma upwards and cut nerves which enter it.
Identify
- Branches of transverse nerve of the neck crossing SCM

Trace these branches forward to their termination.
- Cervical branch of facial nerve at the lower border of parotid gland

Trace this nerve anteroinferiorly.
- Anterior jugular vein near midline

Follow it inferiorly where it pierces deep fascia two cm above sternum.

Cut the investing layer of deep fascia transversely just above the sternum. Continue the incision upwards along the anterior border of SCM. Open the suprasternal space by reflecting the fascia upwards. Follow anterior jugular vein and deeper layer of the fascia deep to SCM. Trace the fascia upwards till it fuses with the superficial layer midway between the sternum and thyroid cartilage. Trace it downward till it fuses with the back of the sternum.

Clean SCM without damaging nerves and vessels around it. Displace the parotid gland forwards to expose the accessory nerve and its

accompanying artery entering the anterior border of SCM. Lift the muscle and observe structures placed deep to it.

Clear the fascia from the anterior bellies of both digastric muscles and the area between them.
Identify
- Mylohyoid muscles
- Median raphe formed by mylohyoids

Remove fascia below the hyoid and expose **infrahyoid muscles**.

Separate these in midline and expose the **pretracheal fascia**. Remove it below the isthmus of thyroid gland to expose the **trachea**.
Identify
- Inferior thyroid veins seen descending on the trachea
- Thyroidea ima artery which ascends on trachea

Identify
- Median thyrohyoid ligament
- Anastomosis of infrahyoid arteries

The anastomosis is seen between the thyroid cartilage and hyoid bone.
Identify
- Facial vessels at the lower border of the mandible

Divide the deep fascia below the mandible and reflect it downwards.

Identify

- Submandibular gland
- Two bellies of the digastric muscle

Trace facial vein posteroinferiorly, superficial to the gland and the posterior belly of the muscle.

Identify

- Submental branch of facial artery at the lower border of the mandible
- Mylohyoid nerve

Remove fat and lymph nodes from the submandibular gland and push it to a side.

Identify

- Intermediate tendon of digastric
- Stylohyoid muscle

Trace stylohyoid and posterior belly of digastric to the angle of the mandible.

Expose the posterior border of mylohyoid by pulling submandibular gland backwards. Note the hypoglossal nerve and a vein of the tongue passing above the muscle.

Identify

- Hyoglossus muscle deep to the hypoglossal nerve

Clean mylohyoid and hyoglossus and study the area.

Remove fat and fascia from the carotid triangle. This is bounded by the posterior belly of digastric and supe-rior belly of omohyoid.

Identify (from lateral to medial)

- Internal jugular vein (IJV)
- Common carotid artery (CCA)
- Internal carotid artery (ICA)
- External carotid artery (ECA)

Identify

- Facial vein
- Lingual vein

Trace these veins to their entry into the IJV in the upper part of carotid triangle.

Identify

- Superior thyroid vein entering IJV in the lower part of carotid triangle
- Hypoglossal nerve between IJV and ICA

Trace hypoglossal nerve forwards across the ECA and note its following branches

- **Superior root of ansa cervicalis** - arises at the site where nerve hooks the occipital artery to enter carotid triangle
- **Thyrohyoid branch** arise near the exit of the nerve from the carotid triangle

Remove superficial part of the carotid sheath. Avoid damage to the superior root of ansa cervicalis placed anterior to the IJV and the inferior root which lies lateral to the vein.

Identify

External carotid artery and its branches

- Lingual artery
- Facial artery
- Occipital artery
- Superior thyroid artery

Identify

- Internal laryngeal nerve in the thyrohyoid interval.

Follow the nerve posterosuperiorly deep to the carotid arteries to the superior laryngeal branch of vagus. Trace the external laryngeal nerve downwards deep to the superior thyroid artery.

Identify

- Thyrohyoid muscle

Push superior thyroid and carotid arteries posteriorly. Clear fat from the external laryngeal nerve and expose

- Inferior constrictor muscle – passes backwards from the side of the thyroid cartilage

Identify

- **Vagus nerve** placed between and behind IJV on one side, and ICA and CCA on the other.

Pull the arteries anteromedially and expose the sympathetic trunk.

Expose anterior jugular vein by pushing the sternal head of SCM aside.

Identify

- Intermediate tendon of omohyoid

Raise superior belly of omohyoid and expose its nerve - traced to ansa cervicalis.

Clean fascia over infrahyoid muscles without damaging their nerves and attachment of **sternohyoid** is noted. Divide the muscle in its lower part and reflect it upwards to expose the muscles underneath. Note their attachments.

ANTERIOR TRIANGLE OF THE NECK: DESCRIPTION

MIDLINE STRUCTURES IN THE NECK

The midline structures in the neck can be divided as suprahyoid structures and infrahyoid structures

Suprahyoid structures

In submental triangle: submental lymph nodes and the raphe to which mylohyoid muscle of the two sides are attached.

Infrahyoid structures

- Hyoid bone – C-3
- Thyrohyoid membrane
- Notch of thyroid cartilage – C-4
- Cricothyroid cartilage – C-6
- Tracheal rings
- Isthmus of thyroid gland in front of 2nd, 3rd, 4th tracheal rings
- Suprasternal notch – disc between T-1 and T-2

Sternocleidomastoid (SCM) divides the side of the neck into two triangles

- Anterior triangle
- Posterior triangle

Boundaries of anterior triangle

In front - Midline structures of neck

Above - Base of the mandible

Behind - Anterior border of the SCM

It is subdivided into

1. Muscular triangle
2. Carotid triangle
3. Digastric triangle
4. Submental triangle

MUSCULAR TRIANGLE

Boundaries

- **Median line** from the hyoid bone to the sternum
- **Inferoposteriorly** - Anterior margin of the sternocleidomastoid
- **Posterosuperiorly** - Superior belly of the omohyoid

CAROTID TRIANGLE

Boundaries

- **Posteriorly** - SCM
- **Anteroinferiorly** - Superior belly of the omohyoid
- **Superiorly** - Stylohyoid and posterior belly of the digastric

Roof is formed by the skin, superficial fascia, platysma and deep fascia containing branches of facial and cutaneous cervical nerves.

Hyoid forms its anterior angle and adjacent floor; its position can be located immediately on inspection, verified by palpation.

Floor is formed by

- Parts of thyrohyoid
- Hyoglossus
- Inferior and middle constrictors of pharynx

Contents

1. CCA and its division into ECA and ICA
2. **Branches of the ECA**
   – Superior thyroid passing anteroinferiorly
   – Lingual artery running anteriorly with its upward loop
   – Facial artery coursing anterosuperiorly
   – Occipital artery runs posterosuperiorly
   – Ascending pharyngeal artery is placed medial to the ICA
3. Corresponding veins ending in the internal jugular vein (IJV)
4. Hypoglossal nerve (XII CN) crossing both carotid arteries
5. Internal laryngeal nerve (medial to the external carotid and below the hyoid)
6. External laryngeal nerve (internal laryngeal nerve)
7. Internal jugular vein (IJV)
8. Deep cervical lymph nodes
9. Vagus nerve

DIGASTRIC TRIANGLE

Boundaries

Above - Base of the mandible
Posteroinferiorly - Posterior belly of the digastric and stylohyoid
Anteroinferiorly - Anterior belly of digastric
Roof - skin, superficial fascia, platysma and deep fascia containing branches of facial and transverse cutaneous cervical nerves.
Floor - mylohyoid and hyoglossus muscles

Contents

In anterior region
1. Submandibular gland
2. Facial vessels
3. Submental artery
4. Mylohyoid artery and nerve
5. Submandibular gland
6. Submandibular lymph nodes

In posterior region
1. Lower part of the parotid gland
2. External carotid artery, passing deep to the stylohyoid. It curves above the muscle and overlaps its superficial surface where it ascends deep to the parotid gland to enter it.

The external carotid artery is superficial to the internal carotid and crosses it posterolaterally. ICA, IJV and 10th cranial nerve (vagus) are deeply placed and separated from ECA by styloglossus and stylopharyngeus.

SUBMENTAL TRIANGLE

The submental triangle is unpaired.

Boundaries
Anterior bellies of both digastric muscles
Apex - At chin
Base - Body of the hyoid
Floor - mylohyoid muscles

Contents
1. Lymph nodes
2. Small veins uniting to form the anterior jugular

ANTEROLATERAL MUSCLES OF THE NECK

Following groups are noted
- Superficial and lateral cervical muscles
- Suprahyoid muscles
- Infrahyoid muscles
- Anterior vertebral muscles
- Lateral vertebral muscles

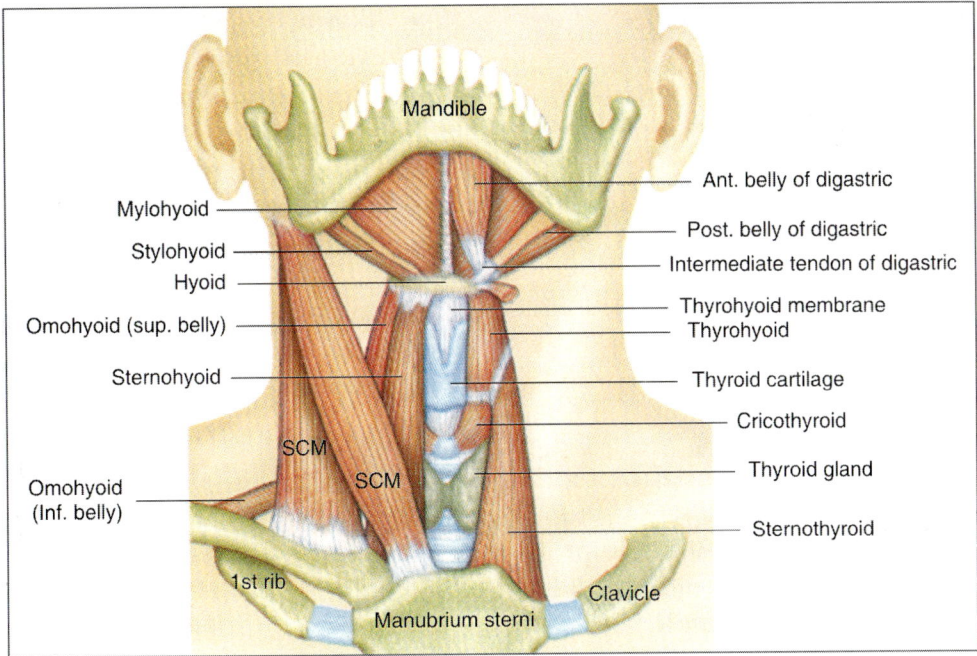

Fig. 41.1: Anterior triangle of neck

SUPERFICIAL AND LATERAL CERVICAL MUSCLES

These include platysma, trapezius and sterno-cleidomastoid (SCM).

PLATYSMA

This broad sheet of muscle arises from the fascia covering the upper parts of pectoralis major and deltoid. Its fibres ascend medially in the side of the neck.

Anterior fibres interlace across the midline with the muscle fibres of the opposite side below and behind the symphysis menti.

Intermediate fibres are attached to the lower border of the body of mandible which passes upwards and medially, deep to depressor anguli oris, to get attached in the lateral half of the lower lip.

Posterior fibres cross the mandible and the anterolateral part of masseter to get attached to the skin and subcutaneous tissue of the lower face. Many fibres blend with modiolar muscles near the buccal angle.

Variations

Varies in extent and it may be absent on one side or both.

Nerve supply

Cervical branch of the facial nerve

Actions

It is not important functionally.

Anterior part (thickest part) may assist in depressing the mandible.

Through its labial and modiolar attachments it can draw down the lower lip and corners of the mouth in expressions of horror or surprise.

Electromyographic studies - active in sudden deep inspiration

STERNOCLEIDOMASTOID (SCM)

It descends obliquely across the side of the neck and forms a prominent surface landmark. It forms the common boundary of triangles of neck.

It arises by two heads:

Sternal head - upper part of the anterior surface of the manubrium sterni

Clavicular head - superior surface of the medial third of the clavicle

The two heads are separated at their origin by a triangular interval - **lesser supraclavicular fossa**. As the muscle ascends, the clavicular head spirals behind the sternal head forming a rounded belly. The muscle is inserted into the lateral surface of the mastoid process and into the lateral half of the superior nuchal line. The clavicular fibres are directed mainly to the mastoid process. The sternal fibres are more oblique and superficial and extend to the occiput. The direction of pull of the two heads is different. The muscle is **cruciate and spiralized**.

Relations

Superficial surface is related to
- Skin and platysma
- External jugular vein
- Great auricular nerve
- Transverse cervical nerve
- Investing layer of deep cervical fascia
- Parotid gland near the insertion

Deep surface is related to
- Sternoclavicular joint
- Sternohyoid
- Sternothyroid
- Omohyoid
- Anterior jugular vein (crossing deep)

Posterior part is related to
- Splenius
- Levator scapulae
- Scaleni
- Cervical plexus
- Supraclavicular part of brachial plexus
- Phrenic nerve
- Transverse cervical artery
- Suprascapular artery
- Occipital artery (crossing deep to muscle)

The accessory nerve (XI CN) passes deep to sternocleidomastoid. It pierces (and supplies) the muscle and reappears just above the middle of the posterior border.

Nerve supply

- Spinal accessory nerve (XI CN)
- Branches from the ventral rami of the 2nd to 4th cervical spinal nerves

Actions

- **Acting alone**, one SCM tilts the head towards the same shoulder and simultaneously rotates the head so that the face turns towards the opposite side (sideways glance).
- **Acting together from below**, the muscles draw the head forwards, helping the longus colli to flex the cervical part of the vertebral column (common in feeding).
- **Two muscles** are used to raise the head when the body is supine.
- **When the head is fixed**, they help to elevate the thorax in forced inspiration.

Clinical Relevance

Torticollis (or wryneck)

This postural deformity of the neck is due to a permanent contracture of the sternocleidomastoid.

Spasmodic torticollis

- Can develop in adult life
- Begins with tonic spasm of one SCM
- Followed by a spasm of trapezius

SUPRAHYOID MUSCLES

These include digastric, stylohyoid, mylohyoid and geniohyoid

DIGASTRIC

It consists of two bellies which are joined by a central tendon. It is placed below the mandible. It extends from the mastoid process to the chin.

Posterior belly is attached to the mastoid notch of the temporal bone. It slopes downwards and forwards.

Anterior belly is attached to the digastric fossa on the base of the mandible close to the midline. It slopes downwards and backwards.

The two bellies meet in an intermediate tendon, which runs in a fibrous sling that is attached to the body and greater cornu of the hyoid bone.

Variations

The intermediate tendon is absent and the muscle is attached midway along the body of the mandible.

Superficial relations

- Platysma
- Sternocleidomastoid
- Splenius and longissimus capitis
- Mastoid process
- Stylohyoid muscle
- Retromandibular vein
- Parotid and submandibular salivary glands
 Medial to the anterior belly mylohyoid is placed.

Medial to the posterior belly

- Superior oblique capitis
- Rectus capitis lateralis
- Transverse process of the atlas (C-1)
- Accessory nerve (XI CN)
- Internal jugular vein (IJV)
- Occipital artery
- Hypoglossal nerve (XII CN)
- Internal carotid artery (ICA)
- External carotid artery (ECA)

- Facial artery
- Lingual artery
- Hyoglossus muscle

Nerve supply

Anterior belly - Mylohyoid branch of the inferior alveolar nerve

Posterior belly - Facial nerve

Actions

1. Depresses the mandible
2. Elevates the hyoid bone
3. Paired digastric muscles always act together. These are secondary to and causes lateral pterygoids depression of mandible

STYLOHYOID

It arises from the posterior surface of the styloid process near its base. It passes downwards and forwards and inserted into the body of the hyoid bone at its junction with the greater cornu. Near its insertion it is perforated by the intermediate tendon of digastric.

Variations

The muscle may be absent or double occasionally.

Nerve supply

Facial nerve (VII CN)

Actions

Elevates the hyoid bone and draws it backwards to elongate the floor of the mouth

STYLOHYOID LIGAMENT

This extends from the tip of the styloid process to the lesser cornu of the hyoid bone. It provides attachment to the highest fibres of the middle constrictor of pharynx. It is intimately related to the lateral wall of the oropharynx. Below, it is overlapped by hyoglossus.

It is derived from the cartilage of the second branchial arch. It may be partially ossified.

MYLOHYOID

It lies superior to the anterior belly of digastric. Two mylohyoid muscles forms muscular floor of the oral cavity.

It is flat and triangular muscle. It is attached to the mylohyoid line of the mandible. It consists of three sets of fibres.

Posterior fibres pass medially and slightly downwards to the front of the body of the hyoid bone near its lower border.

Middle and anterior fibres from each side decussate in a median fibrous raphe which stretches from the symphysis menti to the hyoid bone.

Variations

The median raphe may be absent and where the two muscles form a continuous sheet.

Relations

Inferior surface is related to
- Platysma
- Anterior belly of digastric
- Superficial part of the submandibular gland
- Facial vessels
- Submental vessels
- Mylohyoid vessels
- Nerve to mylohyoid

Superior surface is related to
- Geniohyoid
- Part of hyoglossus
- Styloglossus
- Hypoglossal nerve
- Lingual nerve
- Submandibular ganglion
- Sublingual gland
- Submandibular gland (deep part) and its duct
- Lingual vessels

Nerve supply

Mylohyoid branch of the inferior alveolar nerve

Actions

1. Elevates the floor of the mouth in the first stage of deglutition
2. Elevates the hyoid bone
3. Depresses the mandible

GENIOHYOID

This narrow muscle lies above the medial part of mylohyoid. It arises from the lower genial tubercle. It runs backwards and slightly downwards to get attached to the anterior surface of the body of the hyoid bone. The paired muscles are contiguous and may fuse with each other or with genioglossus.

Nerve supply

1st cervical spinal nerve through the hypoglossal nerve

Actions

1. Elevates the hyoid bone and draws it forwards
2. Depresses the mandible (when the hyoid is fixed)

INFRAHYOID MUSCLES

These are sternohyoid, sternothyroid, thyrohyoid and omohyoid.

These are antagonists to the suprahyoid muscles (depress hyoid bone). The suprahyoid and infrahyoid muscles also act together to stabilize the hyoid bone - serves as a fixed base for the action of muscles of the tongue attached to hyoid.

STERNOHYOID

This thin, narrow strap muscle arises from the posterior surface of the medial end of the clavicle, posterior sternoclavicular ligament and the upper posterior aspect of the manubrium sterni. It ascends medially and is attached to the inferior border of the body of the hyoid bone.

Variations

It may be absent or double.

Nerve supply

Branches from the ansa cervicalis (C-1, 2, 3)

Action

Depresses the hyoid bone after it has been elevated in deglutition

STERNOTHYROID

It is placed deep and medial to it. It arises from the posterior surface of the manubrium sterni and the posterior edge of the cartilage of the first rib. Above it is attached to the oblique line on the lamina of the thyroid cartilage.

Nerve supply

Branches from the ansa cervicalis (C-1, 2, 3)

Action

Draws the larynx downwards after it has been elevated for swallowing or vocal movements

THYROHYOID

This is a small, quadrilateral muscle – upward continuation of sternothyroid. It extends from the oblique line on the lamina of the thyroid cartilage to the lower border of the greater cornu and adjacent part of the body of the hyoid bone.

Nerve supply

A branch of the hypoglossal nerve (this branch contains fibres of the C-1 first cervical spinal nerve)

Actions

1. Depresses the hyoid bone

2. When hyoid is stabilized, it pulls the larynx upwards

OMOHYOID

It consists of two bellies which are united by an intermediate tendon.

Inferior belly arises from the upper border of the scapula (near scapular notch). This inclines forwards and slightly upwards across the lower part of the neck. It passes behind sternocleidomastoid and ends in the intermediate tendon. The inferior belly divides the posterior triangle into upper larger **occipital triangle** and lower smaller **supraclavicular triangle**.

Superior belly begins at the intermediate tendon. It passes vertically upwards near the lateral border of sternohyoid and attached to the lower border of the body of the hyoid bone lateral to the insertion of sternohyoid.

Intermediate tendon varies in length and form. The angulated course of the muscle is maintained by a band of deep cervical fascia which is attached to the clavicle and the 1st rib - ensheathes the tendon.

Variations

- Either belly may be absent or double
- Inferior belly may be attached directly to the clavicle
- Superior belly is sometimes fused with sternohyoid

Nerve supply

Superior belly - Branches from the superior ramus of the ansa cervicalis (C-1)

Inferior belly- Ansa cervicalis itself (C-2 & 3)

Actions

1. Depresses hyoid bone after it has been elevated

2. Tenses lower part of the deep cervical fascia in prolonged inspiratory efforts.

ANTERIOR VERTEBRAL MUSCLES

These includes longus colli, longus capitis and recti capitis anterior and lateralis

LONGUS COLLI

It is placed on to the anterior surface of the vertebral column. It extends from the atlas (C-1) to the T-3 vertebra.

Divided into three parts

- Inferior oblique
- Superior oblique
- Vertical

Inferior oblique part is smallest. It runs upwards and laterally from the front of the bodies of the first two or three thoracic vertebrae to the anterior tubercles of the transverse processes of C-5 & C-6 vertebrae.

Superior oblique part passes upwards and medially from the anterior tubercles of the transverse processes of C-3 to C-5 vertebrae. It is attached by a narrow tendon to the anterolateral surface of the tubercle on the anterior arch of the atlas.

Vertical intermediate part ascends from the front of the bodies of the upper three thoracic and lower three cervical vertebrae to the front of the bodies of the C-2 to C-4 vertebrae.

Nerve supply

Branches from the ventral rami of the C-2 to C-6 spinal nerves

Actions

Longus colli flexes the neck forwards; Oblique parts flex it laterally.

Inferior oblique part rotates it to the opposite side. Its main antagonist is longissimus cervicis.

LONGUS CAPITIS

Longus capitis is broad and thick above, where it is attached to the inferior surface of the basilar part of the occipital bone, and narrow below, where it is attached by tendinous slips to the anterior tubercules of the transverse processes of the C-3 to C-6 vertebrae.

Variations

Both longus capitis and longus colli vary chiefly in the number of their vertebral slips.

Nerve supply

Branches from the ventral rami of the C-1 to C-3 cervical spinal nerves

Actions

Longus capitis flexes the head.

RECTUS CAPITIS ANTERIOR

It is a short, flat muscle situated behind the upper part of longus capitis. It arises from the anterior surface of the lateral mass of the atlas and the root of its transverse process. It ascends vertically to the inferior surface of the basilar part of the occipital bone immediately anterior to the occipital condyle.

Nerve supply

Branches from the loop between the ventral rami of the C-1 & 2 spinal nerves

Action

Rectus capitis anterior flexes the head at the atlanto-occipital joints.

RECTUS CAPITIS LATERALIS

This short, flat muscle arises from the upper surface of the transverse process of the atlas and inserted into the inferior surface of the jugular process of the occipital bone.

It is homologous with the posterior intertransverse muscles.

Nerve supply

Branches from the loop between the ventral rami of C-1 and C-2 spinal nerves

Action

Rectus capitis lateralis flexes the head laterally to the same side.

LATERAL VERTEBRAL MUSCLES

These include scaleni- Anterior, Medius and Posterior.

These muscles extend obliquely between the upper two ribs and the transverse processes of cervical vertebrae.

SCALENUS ANTERIOR

It is placed at the side of the neck deep (posteromedial) to SCM. Above, it is attached to the anterior tubercles of the transverse processes of the C-3 to C-6 vertebrae. These origins converge, blend and descend vertically. Below it is attached by a narrow, flat tendon to the scalene tubercle on the inner border of the first rib.

Anterior relations
- Clavicle
- Subclavius
- Sternocleidomastoid
- Omohyoid
- Lateral part of the carotid sheath
- Transverse cervical artery
- Suprascapular artery
- Ascending cervical artery
- Subclavian vein
- Prevertebral fascia
- Phrenic nerve

Posterior relations
- Suprapleural membrane
- Pleura
- Roots of the brachial plexus
- Subclavian artery

The medial border of the muscle is separated from longus colli in which vertebral artery and vein ascend

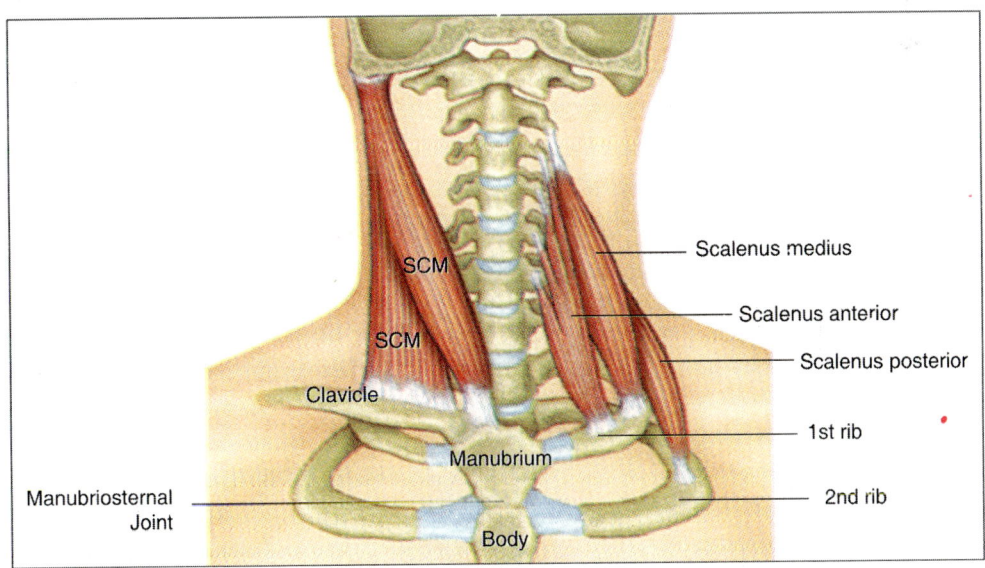

Fig. 41.2: Scaleni Muscles

to reach foramen transversarium of the C-6 vertebra.

- The inferior thyroid artery crosses the interval from the lateral to the medial side near its apex.
- The sympathetic trunk and its cervicothoracic ganglion are closely related to the posteromedial side of the vertebral artery.
- On the left side the thoracic duct crosses this triangular interval at the level of the C-7 vertebra and comes in contact with the medial border of scalenus anterior.

Nerve supply

Branches from the ventral rami of the C-4 to C-6 nerves

Actions

Acting from below – bends cervical part of the vertebral column forwards and laterally and rotates it towards the opposite side

Acting from above – elevates the 1st rib

Clinical relevance

The proximity of the muscle to the lower part of brachial plexus, subclavian artery and vein can give rise to compression syndromes.

SCALENUS MEDIUS

It is the largest and longest scalenus muscle. It is attached to the transverse process of the axis (C-1) and the front of the posterior tubercles of the transverse processes of the C-4 to C-8 vertebrae. Below it is attached to the upper surface of the 1st rib (between the tubercle of rib and the groove for subclavian artery).

Relations

- Anterolateral surface of the muscle is related to SCM.
- It is crossed by the clavicle and omohyoid.

- Anteriorly it is separated from scalenus anterior by the subclavian artery and ventral rami of the cervical spinal nerves.
- Posterolateral to it levator scapulae and scalenus posterior are placed.
- Upper two roots of the nerve to serratus anterior and the dorsal scapular nerve (nerve to rhomboids) pierce the muscle and appear on its lateral surface.

Nerve supply

Branches from the ventral rami of the C-3 to C-8 spinal nerves

Actions

Acting from below - bends the cervical part of the vertebral column to the same side

Acting from above - helps to raise the first rib. Scalene muscles are active during inspiration

SCALENUS POSTERIOR

It is the smallest and most deeply situated scalenus. Above it is attached to the posterior tubercles of the transverse processes of the C-4 to C-6 vertebrae and below to the outer surface of the 2nd rib (behind the tubercle for serratus anterior).

Nerve supply

Branches from the ventral rami of the C-6 to C-8 spinal nerves

Actions

1. When the 2nd rib is fixed, it bends lower end of cervical part of the vertebral column to the same side.
2. When its upper attachment is fixed, it helps in elevation of 2nd rib.

SCALENUS MINIMUS (PLEURALIS)

Scalenus minimus (pleuralis) is associated with the suprapleural membrane and cervical pleura.

42

Deep Dissection of Neck

Push SCM and superior belly of omohyoid laterally. Divide SCM near its lower end and turn it upwards and note its nerve supply.

Identify
- Inferior thyroid veins in front of the trachea
- Extension (if present) of thymus

Remove fascia from the surfaces of the trachea and oesophagus. **Note** recurrent laryngeal nerve in the groove between the two.

Identify thoracic duct on the left of the oesophagus. Pull the upper part of the thyroid gland laterally and find the external branch of the superior laryngeal nerve going to cricothyroid muscle.

Identify the lower part of the inferior constrictor muscle arising from a fibrous arch crossing the cricothyroid muscle.

Divide the isthmus of thyroid and vessels of one lobe. Excise the lobe and study the cut surface with a magnifying glass.

Identify
- Anastomosis between the superior and inferior thyroid arteries
- On the medial aspect of the posterior surface – Yellowish-brown parathyroid glands

Remove fat, lymph nodes and carotid sheath from around the CCA and IJV.

Identify
- Vagus nerve between CCA & IJV
- Right recurrent laryngeal nerve

This nerve arises from the vagus as it crosses the subclavian artery and trace it to the groove between trachea and oesophagus
- Thoracic duct on the left side,

This duct enters the junction of IJV and subclavian vein.
- Cervical part of the brachiocephalic vein and its tributaries
- Phrenic nerve behind the IJV and prevertebral fascia

Push the IJV medially and identify sub-clavian artery above it and cervical pleura below it.

Identify
- Internal thoracic artery
- Thyrocervical trunk and its branches

Push scalenus anterior laterally and expose costocervical trunk which arises from the subclavian artery at the medial border of the muscle. Trace it over the cervical pleura to the neck of the first rib.

Identify
- Vertebral artery behind CCA & IJV

Trace vertebral artery upwards in front of the transverse process of C-7 vertebra. Clear the fat behind this artery and expose the ventral ramus of the C-7 nerve above the transverse process of C-7 vertebra.

Identify

- Sympathetic trunk posteromedial to CCA
- Cervicothoracic ganglion between the neck of first rib and transverse process of C-7 vertebra behind the vertebral artery
- Middle cervical ganglion on the inferior thyroid artery near the transverse process of C-6 vertebra
- Grey rami communicantes connecting these ganglia to the ventral rami of the spinal nerves

Separate the right greater occipital nerve from the scalp and turn it downwards. Cut the descending branch of the occipital artery. Divide great auricular, occipital and transverse nerve of neck on sternocleidomastoid (SCM). In the suboccipital triangle, separate superior oblique, rectus capitis posterior major and minor muscles from their attachments. Remove them and expose posterior atlanto-occipital membrane. Cut it close to the skull. Avoid damage to the vertebral arteries on the posterior arch of the atlas. Separate longissimus muscle from the skull. Avoid damage to the occipital artery on or deep to the muscle.

Reflect SCM upwards up to the skull. Cut the accessory nerve in the posterior triangle, leaving its upper part with the muscle.

Separate pharynx and carotid sheath from prevertebral fascia and sympathetic trunk up to the superior cervical ganglion.

Cut the mandible in midline with a saw. Cut the tongue and epiglottis in midline with a knife. Continue the cut through the hyoid bone, larynx, pharynx, and trachea up to the inferior border of the isthmus of the thyroid gland. Cut the right halves of trachea, oesophagus and neurovascular bundle transversely. Avoid damage to the sympathetic trunk, phrenic nerve, and scalenus anterior muscle. Separate the divided structures from the posterior structures.

Saw through the skull longitudinally a little on the right of the midline, leaving the nasal septum with the left half. Continue the cut to the foramen magnum without damaging atlas. Detach dura and membrana tectoria from the anterior margin of foramen magnum. Turn them downwards and expose the alar ligaments and longitudinal fibres of the cruciate ligament.

Divide the right alar ligament. Flex the right half of the head on the vertebral column and divide the posterior part of the capsule of the atlanto-occipital joint. Take out the occipital condyle out of the joint.

Separate the vertebral artery and the C-1 nerve from the posterior arch of atlas. Divide the artery near its exit from the transverse process of the atlas. Divide rectus capitis lateralis and anterior, longus capitis and the anterior atlanto-occipital membrane.

Cut the remaining portion of the soft palate and posterior pharyngeal wall in the midline. Separate the right half of the skull and the structures attached to it. Divide the nerve fibres passing from the superior cervical ganglion to ICA and to the cranial nerves in the neurovascular bundle, leaving the ganglion and sympathetic trunks on the vertebral column.

Identify

- Internal laryngeal nerve on the thyrohyoid membrane

Trace this nerve up to the superior laryngeal nerve medial to the ECA & ICA

- Pharyngeal branch of vagus above the origin of the superior laryngeal nerve. Trace it to the pharynx

Divide the posterior belly of digastric on the left side, close to its attachment. Pull it anteroinferiorly and expose stylopharyngeus muscle.

Identify

- Glossopharyngeal nerve curving on the lateral aspect of stylopharyngeus
- IX, XI and XII nerves in the upper part of the neurovascular bundle

Trace these nerves distally. Trace stylo-pharyngeus to styloid process and pharynx between superior & middle constrictor muscles. Clean the upper border of middle constrictor and trace stylopharyngeus forwards to the hyoid bone.

Identify

- Ascending pharyngeal branch of ECA

Trace this artery to the pharynx medial to the ICA

- Carotid sinus nerve between ECA & ICA

Lift left neurovascular bundle from the sym-pathetic trunk. Trace the latter upwards to the superior cervical ganglion.

Identify

- Branches of the ganglion to ECA & ICA and cranial nerves
- Branches of the right ganglion to the upper four cervical ventral rami (**grey rami communicantes**)
- Longus capitis

Trace longus capitis to its attachment to the transverse processes of cervical vertebrae.

Identify

- Right occipital artery from occiput to its origin from ECA
- Hypoglossal nerve hooking around the origin of occipital artery
- Ventral ramus of C-1 nerve forwards along with the vertebral artery on the base of the skull

Expose the cervicothoracic ganglion of the sympathetic trunk by displacing the vertebral artery laterally.

Identify

- Branches of cervicothoracic ganglion
- Branches of middle and superior cervical ganglia
- Prevertebral muscles and cervical plexus

Trace the ventral rami of the cervical nerves and their branches.

- Attachments of the scalene muscles.

Trace the lower cervical and first thoracic ventral rami medially.

PREVERTEBRAL AREA

Remove scalenus anterior and identify

- Anterior intertransverse muscles
- Posterior intertransverse muscles

These muscles are separated by the ventral rami of the cervical nerves.

- Dorsal rami of cervical nerves

Dorsal rami pass posteriorly medial to the posterior intertransverse muscles.

Remove the anterior intertransverse muscles and expose vertebral artery. Remove anterior tubercles and costal processes of 3rd, 4th, 5th and 6th cervical vertebrae and expose related part of the vertebral artery.

THYROID GLAND

It is a highly vascular gland weighing about 30 grams. It consists of two lateral lobes connected in the middle by a narrow isthmus. It is slightly heavier in women than in men and enlarges during pregnancy. The thyroid gland secretes thyroxin directly into the blood. It is part of the endocrine system of ductless glands. It is essential for normal body growth in infancy and childhood. Its removal significantly reduces the oxidative processes of the body, producing a lower metabolic rate characteristic of **hypothyroidism**.

It is situated in the lower part of front of neck. This gland surrounds trachea and sides of larynx. It is enclosed in **pretracheal fascia**, which anchors it to

- Oblique line of thyroid cartilage
- Arch of cricoid cartilage

This forms outer false capsule of the gland, which makes it move up and down with deglutition.

The outer condensation of the gland forms the true capsule. There are networks of anastomosing arteries and venous plexus under the true capsule.

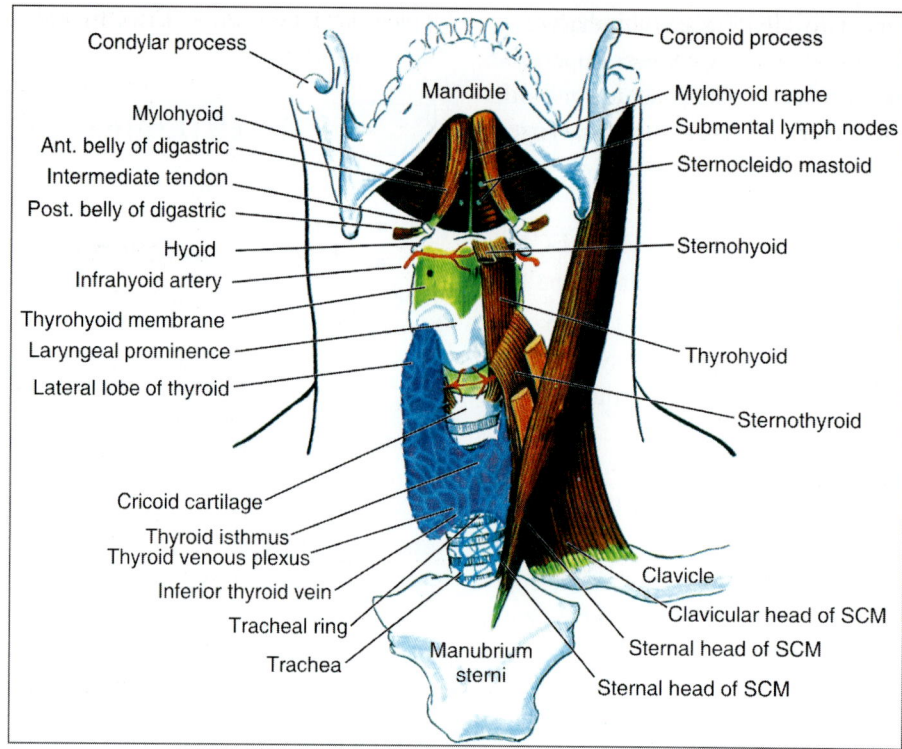

Fig. 42.1: Deep structures of neck

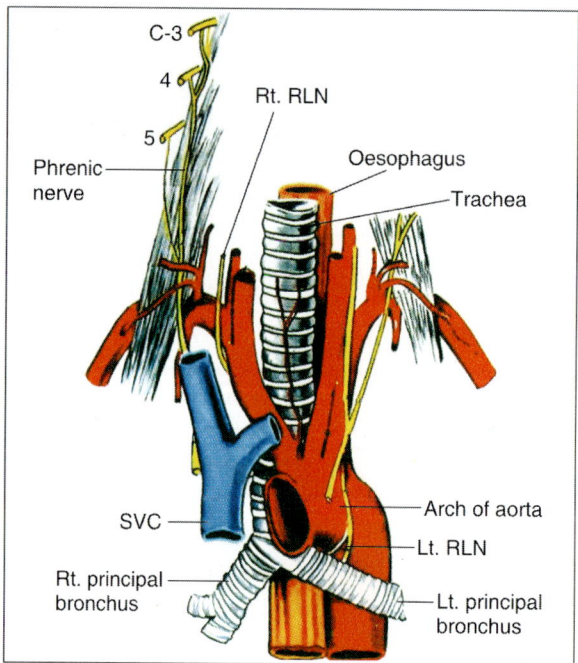

Fig. 42.2: Deep structures of neck

The gland has two lateral lobes joined by an isthmus. The isthmus overlies second, third and fourth tracheal rings. The gland presents a pyramidal lobe (15-30% cases) from the upper border of the isthmus or close to the left lobe. The apex of pyramidal lobe is may be connected to hyoid bone by a fibrous / fibro muscular band – **levator glandulae thyroidae**.

Each lateral lobe is pyriform in shape with apex upwards. Its dimensions are 2 × 1 × 1 inches.

Each lobe extends superiorly up to oblique line on the thyroid cartilage under sternothyroid muscle. Thus enlargement of the gland is restricted superiorly by the attachment of sternothyroid.

Important relations of lateral lobe:

Anterolateral – infrahyoid strap muscles and SCM
Posterior– carotid sheath and its contents
Medial
- Two cartilages – Thyroid and Cricoid

- Two muscles – Cricothyroid and Cricopharyngeus
- Two tubes – Trachea and Oesophagus
- Two nerves – External and recurrent laryngeal nerves

Arterial supply

1. **Superior thyroid artery** (branch of ECA)
2. **Inferior thyroid artery** (branch of thyrocervical trunk)
3. **Thyroidea ima** (occasionally) from (brachiocephalic or aortic arch)

The arteries of the thyroid are remarkably large and form numerous anastomoses.

Venous return

Features of thyroid veins are
1. Short in course
2. Wide lumen
3. Absence of valve
4. Do not accompany the arteries

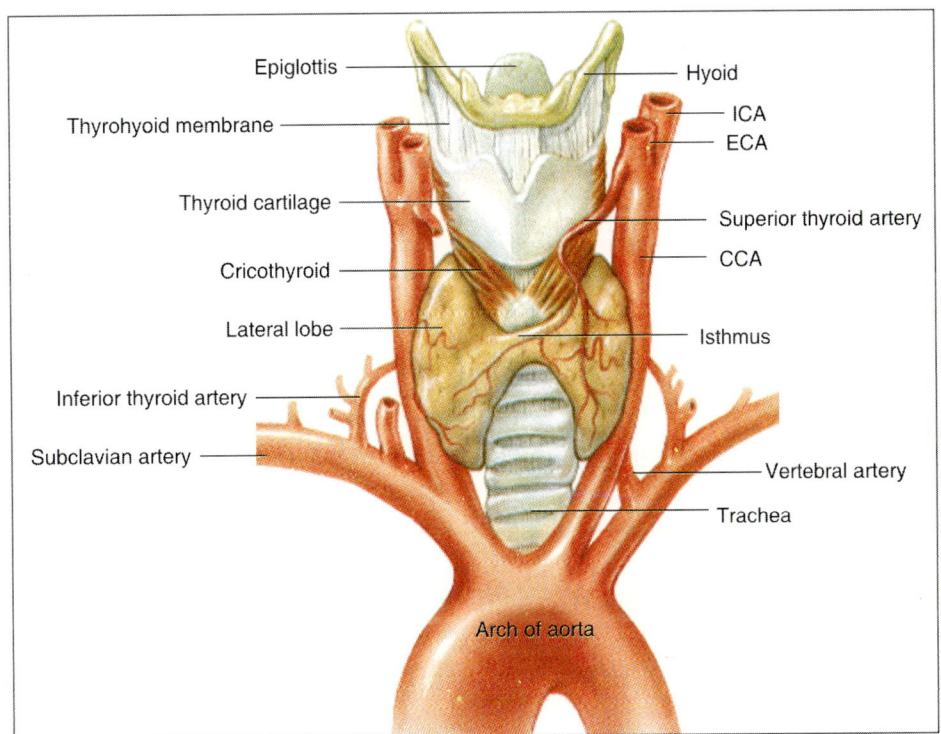

Fig. 42.3: Thyroid Gland

Three pairs of veins usually with occasional fourth thyroid vein (**vein of Kocher**)

Superior and middle thyroid veins open into internal jugular vein

Inferior thyroid vein opens into brachiocephalic vein

Lymphatics

The thyroid gland is drained by following nodes
1. **Pre-laryngeal nodes** – upper half of isthmus joint parts of lateral lobes
2. **Pre-tracheal nodes** – lower half of isthmus and adjoining parts of lateral lobes
3. **Anterosuperior group** (deep cervical nodes) – upper lateral half of lateral lobe
4. **Posteroinferior group** (deep cervical nodes) – lower lateral half of lateral lobe

LYMPHATIC DRAINAGE OF HEAD AND NECK

The lymph nodes draining head and neck and face region are arranged in two sets, namely:
- Superficial set/group
- Deep set/group

Superficial group

In this group, the lymph nodes are arranged in a circular manner.
1. **Pre auricular node** are situated in front of tragus
2. **Parotid lymph nodes** are embedded in the parotid gland
3. **Submental lymph nodes** are located in the submental triangle
4. **Submandibular lymph nodes** are placed the in submandibular triangle
5. **Superficial cervical nodes** lie on outer surface of SCM around EJV.
6. **Anterior cervical nodes** are placed near midline in front of larynx and trachea
7. **Occipital lymph nodes** are situated between mastoid process and external occipital protuberance.
8. **Posterior auricular nodes** – situated over mastoid process behind the pinna.

Deep group

In this group, a large number of big lymph nodes are placed vertically along the carotid sheath. They are
1. **Jugulo- digastric nodes**
2. **Jugulo-omohyoid nodes**

These lymph nodes get enlarged in pathological conditions of the region that they drain. Thus clinical conditions of tongue, larynx or stomach can be confirmed by palpation of these nodes.

THORACIC DUCT IN NECK

It is the largest lymph duct starting from cisterna chyli in the upper lumbar region.

It drains
- Left half of the body above diaphragm
- Both halves between the diaphragm **except** right lobe of the liver and upper right quadrant of anterior abdominal wall.

It enters thorax through aortic opening. It then ascends in the posterior mediastinum along the oesophagus. It enters the root of neck on the left side to reach transverse process of C-7. It then turns laterally between vertebral artery system posteriorly and carotid artery system anteriorly. Before termination it runs across the apex of left pleura and crosses the first part of left subclavian artery superficially. To prevent regurgitation of blood into the duct it has a set of valves close to its opening. It terminates by opening into the **jugulo-subclavian junction**.

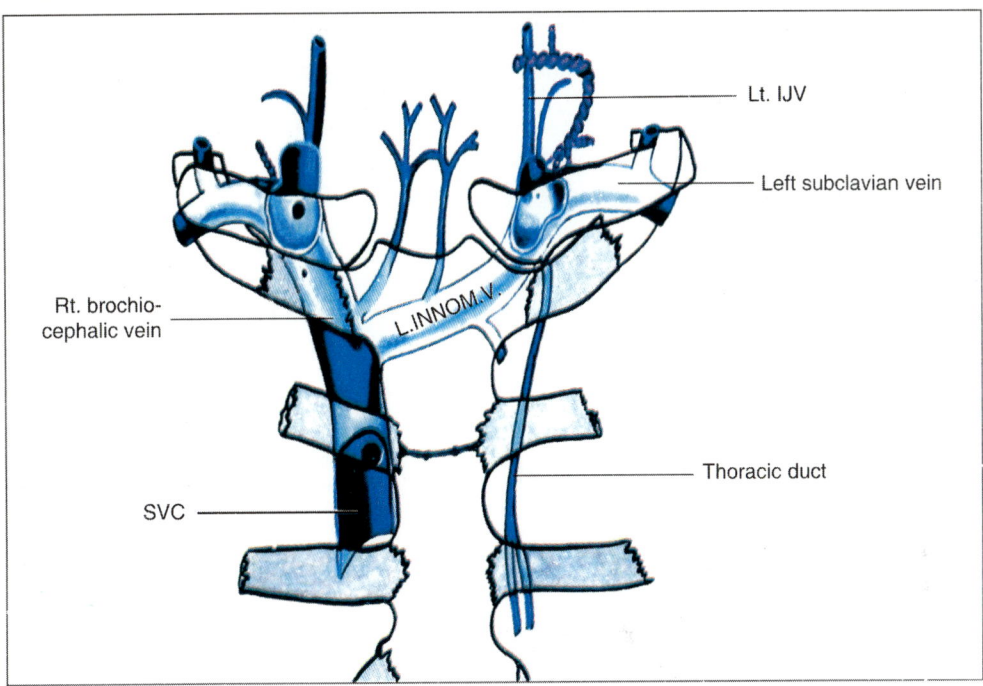

Fig. 42.4: Thoracic Duct in Neck

CLINICAL CONSIDERATIONS

Thyroid Swellings

Thyroid disorders – hyposecretions and hyper secretions lead to a set of complex symptoms but invariably they present as thyroid swelling. The line of least resistance for the thyroid swelling to grow is along its posteromedial border. These swellings compress the structures that are in close proximity namely trachea, oesophagus and recurrent laryngeal nerves. The presenting symptoms for these involvements would range from dyspnoea, dysphagia and hoarseness of voice.

All thyroid swellings move with deglutition as **ligament of *Berry*** (a slip of pre-tracheal fascia) attaches each lateral lobe to cricoid cartilage.

Anatomical considerations during Thyroidectomy

1. *Ligation of thyroid arteries*

The arteries should be ligated first. To avoid accidental ligation of superior laryngeal nerve, the superior thyroid artery should be ligated close to the upper pole. The inferior thyroid artery is ligated away from the gland to avoid accidental ligation of recurrent laryngeal nerve.

Ligation of external laryngeal nerve leads to

- Weak voice
- Monotonous voice
- Temporary hoarseness of voice

Ligation of recurrent laryngeal nerve leads to hoarseness of voice.

2. Mobilization of gland

Cutting of ligament of Berry releases the gland.

3. Thyroid capsules

The thyroid gland has two capsules. The outer or false capsule is derived from pretracheal fascia white inner or true capsule is the condensation of the peripheral part of the gland tissue. The thyroid venous plexus is placed deep to true capsule. In thyroidectomy, the gland is removed along with both capsules to avoid bleeding from the venous plexus which is situated deep to true capsule. This is contrary to prostatectomy where both capsules are retained to keep the venous plexus intact (placed between both capsules)

4. Preservation of parathyroid gland

Thyroidectomy is never total unless absolutely indicated. It is subtotal in which a part of thyroid gland is preserved in order to avoid post-operative hypothyroidism. In thyroidectomy, the parathyroid glands are always preserved which are placed along the posterior border of the thyroid gland.

Thyroidectomy

It is the surgical removal of the thyroid gland. **Indications** include
- Colloid goiter
- Thyroid tumors
- Hyperthyroidism not responding to iodine therapy and antithyroid drugs

About 5% to 10% of the gland is left behind. The growth of the gland begins shortly after surgery and the thyroid function may return to normal.

For thyroid carcinoma the entire gland is removed, along with surrounding structures from neck in a radical dissection.

Before surgery, the basal metabolism rate is lowered to normal by giving iodine and antithyroid drugs.

After surgery the patient is most comfortable in **semi-Fowler's position**. Postoperatively the patient is observed for

- Haemorrhage
- Respiratory difficulty caused by glottic oedema
- Muscular twitching of tetany from accidental removal of a parathyroid gland

Plunging Goitre

In short necked persons long standing retro-sternal swelling may be indicative of retro-sternal thyroid enlargement. It is a potential space in which this swelling can descend. The associated symptoms are related to intra-thoracic pressure exerted on the neighboring structures especially great veins. This manifest as engorgement of superficial veins of the region.

Graves' Disease

It is also called exophthalmic goiter, thyrotoxicosis or toxic goiter.

It is characterized by pronounced hyperthyroidism associated with an enlarged thyroid gland and exophthalmos (abnormal protrusion of eyeball).

The disease is familial and may be autoimmune. Antibodies to thyroglobulin are present in more than 60% of patients.

It is about five times more common in women, occurs most frequently between 20 and 40 years of age.

Clinical features

- Nervousness
- Fine tremor of the hands
- Weight loss
- Fatigue
- Breathlessness
- Palpitations
- Increased heat intolerance
- Increased metabolic rate

There may be associated
- Enlarged thymus

- Generalized hyperplasia of the lymph nodes
- Blurred or double vision
- Localized oedema
- Atrial dysrhythmias
- Osteoporosis

Management

- Subtotal thyroidectomy
- Antithyroid drugs
- Radioactive iodine

Hyperthyroidism

This condition is characterized by hyperactivity of the thyroid gland. The gland is enlarged. It secretes greater amounts of thyroid hormones with increased metabolic processes of the body.

Clinical features

- Nervousness
- Exophthalmos
- Tremor
- Constant hunger
- Weight loss
- Fatigue
- Heat intolerance
- Palpitations

Management

- Antithyroid drugs
- Radioactive iodine in certain cases.
- Surgical ablation of the gland

Untreated hyperthyroidism may lead to death because of cardiac failure.

Thyroid Crisis (Thyrotoxic crisis)

There is sudden exacerbation of the symptoms of thyrotoxicosis. It is characterized by

- Fever
- Sweating
- Tachycardia
- Extreme nervous excitability
- Pulmonary oedema

It is usually seen in patients, with inadequate treatment of thyrotoxicosis. If untreated this may prove fatal.

Carcinoma of Thyroid

This is characterized by slow growth and a prolonged clinical course. Nontoxic colloid goiters and follicular adenomas may be the precursors of malignant tumours.

Clinical presentation

- Increase in size of the gland
- Palpable nodule
- Hoarseness of voice
- Dysphagia
- Dyspnoea
- Pain on pressure

Diagnostic measures include

- X ray examination
- Radioisotope scanning
- Needle aspiration biopsy
- Ultrasound examination

Classification of thyroid tumours

- One half: papillary carcinoma
- One third: follicular carcinomas
- Rest consists of anaplastic carcinomas, medullary carcinomas and metastatic lesions from primary tumours in the breast, kidneys or lungs

Management

- Total or subtotal thyroidectomy with excision of involved lymph nodes
- Radioactive iodine (postoperatively)
- High doses of exogenous thyroid to suppress TSH.

Cancer of the thyroid is twice as common in women, most frequently between thirty and fifty years of age. It may occur in children and elderly individuals.

Compressions of structures in carcinoma of thyroid

Carcinoma of thyroid may appear as symptoms due to compression of related structures that are likely to be involved:

- **Dyspnoea** - compression of trachea
- **Dysphagia** – compression of esophagus
- **Hoarseness of voice** – involvement of recurrent laryngeal nerve
- **Horner's syndrome** – involvement of cervical sympathetic chain
- **Haemorrhage** – erosion of carotid sheath

COMMON CAROTID ARTERY

These are two in number, one on each side of neck.

The right and left carotid arteries differ in length and origin.

Right common carotid artery – Has cervical part only and arises from the brachiocephalic trunk behind the right sternoclavicular joint.

Left common carotid artery - Has both thoracic and cervical parts and originates directly from the aortic arch immediately posterolateral to the brachiocephalic trunk.

THORACIC PART OF LEFT CCA

It ascends till left sternoclavicular joint where it enters the neck. It is 2 to 2.5 cm long. At first it is placed in front of the trachea, and then it inclines to the left.

Relations

Anterior relations
- Sternohyoid and sternothyroid
- Anterior parts of the left pleura and lung
- Left brachiocephalic vein
- Remains of thymus

Posterior relations
- Trachea

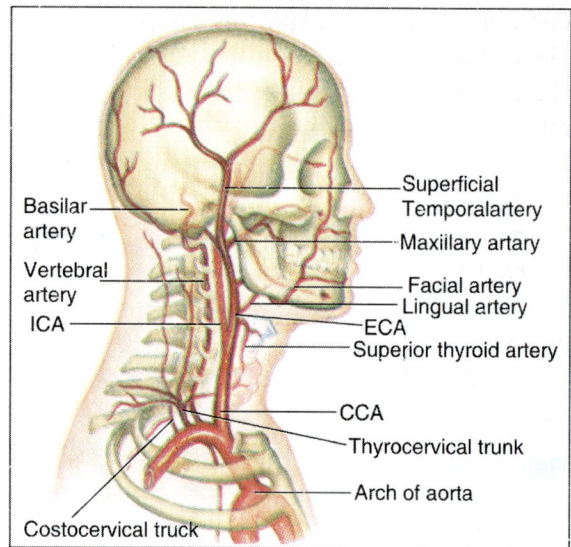

Fig. 42.4: Carotid Arteries

- Left subclavian artery
- Left border of the oesophagus
- Left recurrent laryngeal nerve
- Thoracic duct

To the right
- Brachiocephalic trunk (below)
- Trachea(above)
- Inferior thyroid veins
- Remains of thymus

To the left
- Left vagus
- Left phrenic nerve
- Left pleura and lung

CERVICAL PART OF COMMON CAROTID ARTERIES

Both have a similar course.

This part ascends up to the upper border of thyroid cartilage, where it divides into external and internal carotid arteries.

At its division the artery shows a dilatation - **carotid sinus**. Here the tunica media is thinner and the tunica adventitia is relatively thick which contains many receptor endings of the glossopharyngeal nerve. The sinus is responsive to changes in arterial blood pressure which leads to reflex haemodynamic modification. It acts as a baroreceptor for control of intracranial pressure.

Carotid body is a small, reddish-brown structure situated behind the common carotid artery bifurcation. It acts as a **chemoreceptor**.

CCA is contained in carotid sheath. This sheath also encloses the internal jugular vein (IJV) and vagus nerve (vein lies lateral to the artery, nerve between them and posterior to both).

Relations

Anterolaterally at the level of cricoid cartilage the artery is crossed by the intermediate tendon of the omohyoid.

Anterior relations below omohyoid

- Skin and superficial fascia
- Platysma
- Deep cervical fascia
- Sternocleidomastoid
- Sternohyoid
- Sternothyroid

Above the omohyoid the artery is superficial. It is covered by skin, superficial fascia, platysma, deep cervical fascia and the medial border of sternocleidomastoid. It is crossed obliquely from its medial to lateral side by the sternocleidomastoid branch of the superior thyroid artery.

In front of carotid sheath the superior root of the ansa cervicalis joins inferior root derived from the C-2 & C-3 spinal nerves.

- Superior thyroid vein crosses the artery near its termination.
- Middle thyroid vein crosses just below the cricoid cartilage.
- Anterior jugular vein crosses it above the clavicle.

Posterior relations

- Transverse processes of C-4 to C-6
- Longus colli and longus capitis
- Tendinous slips of scalenus anterior
- Sympathetic trunk
- Ascending cervical artery

Below C-6 vertebra the artery is placed in an angle between the scalenus anterior and longus colli. It is placed anterior to the vertebral vessels, inferior thyroid and subclavian arteries, sympathetic trunk. On the left thoracic duct is located.

Medial relations

- Oesophagus
- Trachea
- Inferior thyroid artery
- Recurrent laryngeal nerve
- Larynx and pharynx (at higher level)

Thyroid gland overlaps it anteromedially.

Lateral relation

- Internal jugular vein, which in the lower neck is also anterior to the artery;

Posterolaterally in the angle between artery and vein the vagus nerve (X CN) is placed.

On the right

- Recurrent laryngeal nerve crossing obliquely behind the artery
- Right internal jugular vein

Variations

- In about 12% right CCA arises above the level of the sternoclavicular joint.
- Right CCA may be a separate branch from the aorta.
- Left CCA may arise from the brachiocephalic trunk.
- Division of the common carotid may occur at higher level near the level of the hyoid bone.

- Very rarely it ascends without division, either the ECA or ICA being absent. Rarely CCA is replaced by separate external and internal carotid arteries arising directly from the aorta.
- CCA does not gives branches but the vertebral, superior thyroid, ascending pharyngeal, inferior thyroid or occipital artery may arise from it.

EXTERNAL CAROTID ARTERY

This begins lateral to the upper border of thyroid cartilage (disc between C-3 and C-4). It first ascends slightly forwards and then inclines backwards and slightly laterally. It passes midway between the tip of mastoid process and the angle of mandible. In the parotid gland it divides into the superficial temporal and maxillary arteries (behind the neck of mandible).

At its origin it is placed in the carotid triangle, anteromedial to the internal carotid artery. It becomes anterior and then lateral to ICA as it ascends. At mandibular level the styloid process and its attached structures intervene between the vessels, ICA being deep and the ECA superficial to the styloid process. A finger tip placed at the carotid triangle perceives arterial pulsation. Beneath the finger lie:

- Termination of common carotid
- Origins of external and internal carotids
- Stems of the external carotid's initial branches.

Relations

In the carotid triangle the artery is covered by the skin, superficial fascia, loop between the cervical branch of facial nerve and the transverse cutaneous nerve of the neck, deep fascia and the anterior border of SCM. It is crossed by the hypoglossal nerve, lingual (common), facial and the superior thyroid veins. After it leaves the triangle it is crossed by the posterior belly of the digastric and stylohyoid.

It ascends between stylohyoid and the posteromedial surface of the parotid gland. It enters the parotid gland and placed medial to the facial nerve.

Structures medial to ECA

- Pharyngeal wall
- Superior laryngeal nerve
- Ascending pharyngeal artery

At a higher level the ICA is separated from ECA by

- Styloid process,
- Styloglossus and stylopharyngeus
- Glossopharyngeal nerve
- Pharyngeal branch of vagus nerve
- Part of the parotid gland

Branches

These include

1. Superior thyroid artery
2. Ascending pharyngeal artery
3. Lingual artery
4. Facial artery
5. Occipital artery
6. Posterior auricular artery
7. Superficial temporal artery
8. Maxillary artery

SUPERIOR THYROID ARTERY

This arises from the front of the ECA just below the greater cornu of the hyoid bone. It divides into terminal branches at the apex of the lateral lobe of thyroid gland.

Relations

It descends forwards in the carotid triangle along the lateral border of the thyrohyoid muscle. It is covered by skin, platysma and fasciae. It is deep to the omohyoid, sternohyoid and sternothyroid. Medially it is related to inferior constrictor of pharynx and external laryngeal nerve.

Branches

It supplies adjacent muscles and the thyroid gland. It anastomoses with opposite artery and the inferior thyroid artery.

Glandular branches

Anterior ascending – along the medial side of the upper pole of the lateral lobe. Supplies mainly the anterior surface. A branch crosses above the isthmus to anastomose with its fellow:

Posterior descending – on the posterior border. These branches supply medial and lateral surfaces, anastomosing with the inferior thyroid artery.

Named branches are

1. Infrahyoid branch
2. Superior laryngeal branch
3. Sternocleidomastoid branch
4. Cricothyroid branch

Infrahyoid artery

This small artery runs along the lower border of the hyoid deep to thyrohyoid. It anastomoses with its opposite fellow.

Sternocleidomastoid artery

It descends laterally across the carotid sheath and supplies SCM.

Superior laryngeal artery

It accompanies internal laryngeal nerve deep to the thyrohyoid. It pierces lower part of the thyrohyoid membrane. It supplies larynx. It anastomoses with opposite artery and the inferior laryngeal branch of the inferior thyroid.

Cricothyroid artery

This small artery crosses cricothyroid ligament and anastomoses with opposite artery.

ASCENDING PHARYNGEAL ARTERY

This is the smallest branch of the ECA.
It ascends between the internal carotid artery and pharynx to the base of cranium. It is crossed by the styloglossus and stylopharyngeus.

It anastomoses with the ascending palatine branch of facial artery.

Named branches are

1. Pharyngeal arteries
2. Inferior tympanic artery
3. Meningeal branches

Various small branches supply

- Longus capitis and longus colli
- sympathetic trunk
- IX, X and XII CN

It anastomoses with the branches of the ascending cervical and vertebral arteries.

Pharyngeal arteries

These (three or four) supply constrictors of pharynx and stylopharyngeus. These also supply palate. It descends forwards between the upper border of superior constrictor and levator veli palatini. It gives minute branches to the tonsil and one to the auditory tube.

Inferior tympanic artery

This small branch traverses the canaliculus for the tympanic branch of the glossopharyngeal nerve. It supplies the medial wall of tympanic cavity.

Meningeal branches

These small vessels enter cranium through the foramen lacerum, jugular foramen and hypoglossal canal. They supply the nerves in these passages and their surrounding tissues. Posterior meningeal artery reaches the cerebellar fossa via the jugular foramen – terminal branch of ascending pharyngeal artery.

LINGUAL ARTERY

This is the chief supply to the tongue and buccal floor of the mouth. It arises opposite the tip of greater cornu of hyoid bone between the superior thyroid and facial arteries.

It ascends medially at first, loops downwards and forwards. It passes medial to the posterior border of hyoglossus and horizontally forwards deep to it. It ascends again almost vertically. It courses sinuously forwards on the inferior surface of tongue up to its tip.

Relations

The artery has three parts

First part is placed in the carotid triangle. It ascends medially, and then descends to the level of the hyoid bone. Its loop is crossed by the hypoglossal nerve.

Second part passes along the upper border of hyoid bone deep to hyoglossus, tendons of digastric and stylohyoid, lower part of the submandibular gland and posterior part of mylohyoid. Hyoglossus separates it from the hypoglossal nerve. Here its medial aspect adjoins the middle constrictor and crosses the stylohyoid ligament. It is accompanied by lingual veins.

Third part (arteria profunda linguae) turns upwards near the anterior border of the hyoglossus and passes forwards close to the inferior surface of tongue near the frenulum. It is accompanied by the lingual nerve. Near the tip of tongue it anastomoses with opposite artery.

Named branches are

1. Suprahyoid artery
2. Dorsal lingual arteries
3. Sublingual artery

Suprahyoid artery

This small artery runs along the upper border of hyoid bone. It anastomoses with the opposite artery.

Dorsal lingual arteries

These (two or three) small arteries arise medial to the hyoglossus. These ascend to the posterior part of the dorsum of tongue.

These supplies

- Mucous membrane of tongue
- Palatoglossal arch
- Tonsil

- Soft palate
- Epiglottis

They anastomose with the opposite vessels.

Sublingual artery

It arises at the anterior margin of hyoglossus. It passes forward between the genioglossus and mylohyoid to the sublingual gland.

It supplies

- Sublingual gland
- Mylohyoid muscle
- Buccal and gingival mucous membranes

FACIAL ARTERY

It (**external maxillary**) arises anteriorly in the carotid triangle above the lingual artery, immediately above the greater cornu of the hyoid bone.

It arches upwards and grooves the posterior aspect of the submandibular gland. It then turns down again between the gland and the medial pterygoid. It reaches the surface of the mandible where it curves round its inferior border, anterior to the masseter, to enter the face.

On the face it ascends forwards across the mandible and buccinator to traverse a cleft in the modiolus near the buccal angle. It then ascends the side of the nose and ends at the medial palpebral commissure. It ends by supplying the lacrimal sac and joins the dorsal nasal branch of the ophthalmic artery.

The artery is very sinuous throughout its course:

In the neck – to adapt to the movements of the pharynx during deglutition.

On the face – to adapt to the movements of the mandible, lips and cheeks.

Facial artery pulsation is taken at the base of mandible at the anteroinferior angle of masseter.

Relations

In the neck it is crossed by the hypoglossal nerve. It runs up and forwards, deep to the digastric and the stylohyoid and posterior part of the submandibular gland. At first on the middle constrictor of pharynx, it may reach the lateral surface of the styloglossus. Then it descends to the lower border of the mandible in a lateral groove on the submandibular gland.

On the face it is superficial and placed beneath the platysma. It is covered by skin, fat of the cheek and near the buccal angle by superficial modiolar muscles. Buccinator and levator anguli oris are deep to it. The facial vein is placed posterior to the artery having a direct course over the face. At the anterior border of the masseter both are in contact while in the neck the vein is superficial.

Branches are both cervical and facial.

A. Cervical branches

1. Ascending palatine artery

It ascends between styloglossus and stylopharyngeus to the side of the pharynx. Along pharynx it ascends between the superior constrictor and the medial pterygoid muscle towards the base of cranium. Near the levator veli palatini it bifurcates.

One branch winds over the upper border of the superior constrictor and supplies soft palate and anastomoses with opposite artery and the greater palatine branch of the maxillary artery.

Other branch pierces the superior constrictor and supplies tonsil and pharyngotympanic tube. It joins tonsillar and ascending pharyngeal arteries.

2. Tonsillar artery

It is the main supply to the tonsil. It ascends between medial pterygoid and styloglossus. At the upper border of styloglossus it pierces superior constrictor and ramifies in the tonsil and posterior musculature of tongue.

3. Glandular branches

These (three or four) supply submandibular salivary gland and adjacent muscles and skin.

4. Submental artery

It is the largest cervical branch. It arises below the mandible. It supplies the surrounding muscles and anastomoses with a sublingual branch of the lingual and mylohyoid branch of the inferior alveolar arteries. At the chin it ascends over the mandible and divides into superficial and deep branches. These anastomose with the inferior labial and mental arteries which supply the chin and lower lip.

B. Facial branches

1. Inferior labial artery

It arises near the buccal angle. It passes upwards and forwards under depressor anguli oris. It pierces orbicularis oris and runs sinuously near the lower margin of lip between the muscle and mucous membrane.

It supplies inferior labial glands, mucous membrane and muscles. It anastomoses with the opposite artery and the mental branch of the inferior alveolar artery.

2. Superior labial artery

It is larger and more tortuous branch. It has a similar course along the superior margin of lip between the mucous membrane and orbicularis oris. It anastomoses with the opposite artery.

It supplies upper lip. It gives a septal branch, which ramifies antero-inferiorly in the nasal septum, and an alar branch.

3. Lateral nasal artery

It ascends the side of the nose. It supplies ala of nose. It anastomoses with the opposite artery, septal and alar branches of the superior labial, dorsal nasal branch of the ophthalmic and infraorbital branch of the maxillary artery.

FACIAL ANASTOMOSES

These are numerous.

In the neck
- Sublingual branch of the lingual artery
- Ascending pharyngeal artery
- Palatine branch of the maxillary artery

On the face

- Mental branch of the inferior alveolar artery
- Transverse facial branch of the superficial temporal artery
- Infraorbital branch of the maxillary artery
- Dorsal nasal branch of the ophthalmic artery

Variations of facial artery

1. May arise with the lingual, as a linguo-facial trunk
2. May end as the submental artery

OCCIPITAL ARTERY

It arises from the posterior aspect of ECA.

Course and relations

At its origin it is crossed by the hypoglossal nerve. It turns backwards, upwards deep to the posterior belly of digastric. It crosses ICA, IJV, XII CN, X CN and XI CN.

Between the transverse process of the atlas (C-1) and mastoid process it reaches the lateral border of the rectus capitis lateralis. It then runs in the occipital groove of temporal, medial to the mastoid process. It lies successively on the rectus capitis lateralis, superior oblique and semispinalis capitis. Along greater occipital nerve, it turns upwards and pierces the fascia connecting the cranial attachments of the trapezius and SCM. It ascends tortuously in the dense superficial fascia of the scalp and divides into many branches.

Its branches are

1. Sternocleidomastoid branches

These are two branches.

Lower branch arises near the origin of the occipital artery. It descends backwards over the XII CN and IJV and enters SCM. It anastomoses with the sternocleidomastoid branch of the superior thyroid artery.

Upper branch arises as the occipital artery crosses XI CN. It runs downwards and backwards, superficial to the IJV. It enters deep surface of SCM with XI CN.

2. Mastoid artery

This small artery enters the cranial cavity via mastoid foramen. It supplies mastoid air cells and dura mater.

3. Stylomastoid artery

This artery is seen in two-thirds of subjects.

4. Auricular branch

It supplies medial aspect of the auricle. It anastomoses with the posterior auricular artery.

5. Muscular branches

These supply the digastric, stylohyoid, splenius, longissimus capitis and neighbouring muscles.

6. Descending branch

This artery divides into superficial and deep branches.

Superficial branch passes deep to the splenius. It anastomoses with the superficial branch of the transverse cervical artery.

Deep branch descends between semispinalis capitis and cervicis. It anastomoses with vertebral and the deep cervical arteries (costocervical trunk).

7. Meningeal branches

These branches enter the cranium through jugular foramen and condylar canal. These supply dura mater and bone of the posterior cranial fossa and the last four cranial nerves.

8. Occipital branches

These tortuous terminal branches are distributed to the scalp upto the vertex. These run between the skin and the occipital belly of the occipitofrontalis. These anastomose with opposite occipital, posterior auricular and temporal arteries. These supplies

- Occipital belly of the occipitofrontalis
- Skin and pericranium

POSTERIOR AURICULAR ARTERY

This is a small artery which arises from the posterior aspect of ECA just above the digastric and stylohyoid muscles. It ascends between parotid gland and styloid process to the groove between the auricular cartilage and mastoid process. It divides into auricular and occipital branches. It supplies digastric, stylohyoid, sternocleidomastoid, and parotid gland.

Named branches are

1. Stylomastoid artery

It enters the stylomastoid foramen and supplies

- Facial nerve
- Tympanic cavity
- Mastoid antrum and air cells
- Semicircular canals

Its posterior tympanic branch forms a circular anastomosis with the anterior tympanic artery.

2. Auricular branch

It ascends deep to auricularis posterior muscle. It ramifies on the cranial aspect of the auricle and supplies its lateral aspect.

3. Occipital branch

It passes laterally across the mastoid process. It turns backwards over the SCM to supply occipital belly of occipitofrontalis and scalp above and behind the ear. It anastomoses with the occipital artery.

SUPERFICIAL TEMPORAL ARTERY

It is the smaller terminal branch of the ECA. It is given in the parotid gland behind the neck of mandible. It crosses the posterior root of the zygomatic process of the temporal and about five cm above it divides into anterior and posterior branches.

Relations

In the parotid gland it is crossed by temporal and zygomatic branches of the facial nerve.

In the scalp the auriculotemporal nerve lies posterior to it.

This artery supplies

- Parotid gland
- Temporomandibular joint
- Masseter

Named branches are

1. Transverse facial artery

It arises within the parotid gland. It traverses the gland and crosses masseter between the parotid duct and zygomatic arch. It divides into numerous branches supplying the parotid gland and duct, masseter and skin. It anastomoses with facial, masseteric, buccal, lacrimal and infraorbital arteries.

2. Anterior auricular branches

These are distributed to the ear lobule, anterior part of the auricle and the external acoustic meatus.

3. Zygomatico-orbital artery

It skirts the upper border of the zygomatic arch between two layers of temporal fascia to the lateral orbital angle. It supplies orbicularis oculi. It anastomoses with the lacrimal and palpebral branches of the ophthalmic artery.

4. Middle temporal artery

It arises just above the zygomatic arch. It pierces temporal fascia and supplies the temporalis. It anastomoses with the deep temporal branches of the maxillary artery.

5. Frontal (anterior) branch

It passes towards the frontal tuberosity and supplies muscles, skin and pericranium here. It anastomoses with the opposite artery and supraorbital and supratrochlear arteries.

Parietal (posterior) branch

This larger branch curves upwards and backwards, superficial to the temporal fascia. It anastomoses with opposite artery, posterior auricular and occipital arteries.

CLINICAL CONSIDERATIONS

- Superficial temporal artery is palpable through skin and fascia as it crosses the zygomatic process. This artery is compressed above the zygomatic process to control bleeding.
- Superficial temporal and other arteries supplying the scalp from below are well protected by dense connective tissue.
- In craniotomy, incisions should be convex upwards to include the superficial temporal artery in the flap.
- In carotid angiograms, branches of superficial temporal and middle meningeal arteries are superimposed. This is distinguished by the straighter course, lack of anastomoses and narrower calibre in the meningeal branches.

VEINS OF THE NECK

Veins of the neck are superficial or deep to the deep fascia. The superficial veins drain smaller volume of tissue while the deep veins drain all except the subcutaneous structures, mostly into the internal jugular vein and also the vertebral vein.

EXTERNAL JUGULAR VEIN

It drains the scalp and face. It is formed by the union of posterior division of retromandibular vein and posterior auricular vein near the angle of mandible, just below the parotid gland.

It descends from the angle to the mid-clavicle. It passes obliquely and placed superficial to SCM. In the subclavian triangle it pierces the deep fascia to terminate in the subclavian vein.

It is covered by platysma, superficial fascia and skin and separated from SCM by the deep cervical fascia.

It crosses the transverse cervical nerve and is parallel with the great auricular nerve.

It contains valves at its entrance into the subclavian vein and about 4 cm above the clavicle. Between the two valves it is dilated - **sinus**. The valves do not prevent regurgitation.

Tributaries

- Posterior external jugular vein
- Transverse cervical vein
- Suprascapular vein
- Anterior jugular vein

Posterior external jugular vein

It starts in the occipital region. It drains skin and superficial muscles in the region. It joins middle part of the external jugular.

Anterior jugular vein

It starts near the hyoid bone by the union of superficial submandibular veins. It descends between midline and anterior border of SCM. It turns laterally and in the lower part of neck it joins lower end of external jugular vein. It may join subclavian vein directly.

It communicates with IJV and receives laryngeal veins.

There are two anterior jugular veins which are united just above the manubrium by transverse jugular venous arch - receives the inferior thyroid tributaries.

Surface anatomy

EJV is visible where it crosses the sterno-cleidomastoid. It can be made prominent by expiring against resistance (**Valsalva's manoeuvre**) or by gentle supraclavicular digital pressure.

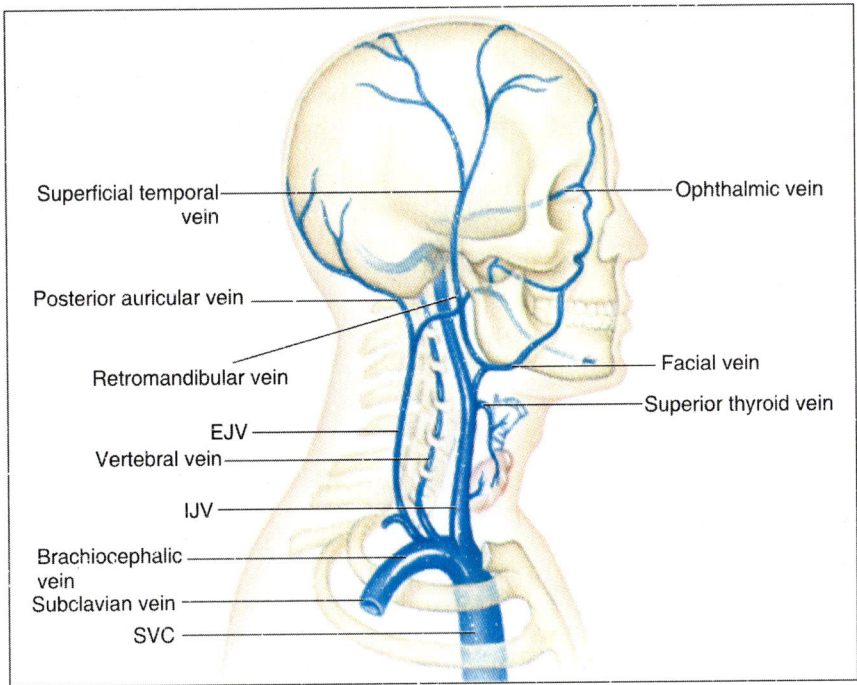

Fig. 42.6: Veins of Head and Neck

INTERNAL JUGULAR VEIN

This is a large vein which collects blood from

- Skull
- Brain
- Superficial parts of face
- Neck

It begins at the base of cranium in the posterior part of the jugular foramen by the continuation of sigmoid sinus.

At the commencement its upper end is called **superior bulb** which is placed below the posterior part of the floor of tympanic cavity.

The vein descends in carotid sheath and joins with subclavian vein, (posterior to the sternal end of the clavicle) to form brachiocephalic vein.

Its lower end is also dilated - **inferior bulb**, above which it contains valves.

Relations

Posterior relations from above are

- Rectus capitis lateralis
- Transverse process of C-1
- Levator scapulae
- Scalenus medius
- Cervical plexus
- Scalenus anterior
- Phrenic nerve
- Thyrocervical trunk
- Vertebral vein
- First part of subclavian artery

On the left it crosses anterior to the thoracic duct Medial to the vein following structures are placed

- Internal carotid artery
- Common carotid artery
- Vagus nerve (between vein and arteries but posterior to them)

Superficially the vein is overlapped by SCM. It is crossed by the posterior belly of digastric and superior belly of omohyoid.

Superior to digastric - Parotid gland and styloid process are superficial while, XI CN, posterior auricular and occipital arteries cross the vein.

Between digastric and omohyoid - Inferior root of ansa cervicalis crosses it.

Below omohyoid - it is covered by infrahyoid muscles and SCM and crossed by anterior jugular vein.

Deep cervical lymph nodes are placed along the vein.

Tributaries

1. Inferior petrosal sinus
2. Facial vein
3. Lingual vein
4. Pharyngeal vein
5. Superior and middle thyroid veins
6. Occipital vein (sometimes)

IJV may communicate with EJV. Thoracic duct opens near the union of the left subclavian vein and IJV.

Inferior petrosal sinus

It leaves cranium through the anterior part of jugular foramen and opens into superior bulb of IJV.

LINGUAL VEINS

Dorsal lingual veins drain dorsum and sides of the tongue and join the veins accompanying lingual artery between hyoglossus and genioglossus. Near the greater cornu of the hyoid bone they join IJV.

Deep lingual vein begins near the tip of tongue and runs backwards near the mucous membrane on the inferior surface of tongue. Near the anterior border of hyoglossus it joins sublingual vein (from sublingual gland) to form **vena comitans nervi hypoglossi**. It runs backwards between mylohyoid and hyoglossus to join facial vein, IJV or lingual vein.

PHARYNGEAL VEINS

These start in a pharyngeal plexus. These receive meningeal veins and a vein from the pterygoid canal. These end in IJV. These may terminate in facial, lingual or superior thyroid vein.

SUPERIOR THYROID VEIN

After formation it accompanies the artery and receives superior laryngeal and cricothyroid veins. It terminates in IJV or facial vein.

MIDDLE THYROID VEIN

It drains lower part of the gland and receives veins from the larynx and trachea. It crosses anterior to common carotid artery to end in IJV behind the superior belly of omohyoid.

VERTEBRAL VEIN

In the suboccipital triangle many small tributaries from internal vertebral plexuses and leave the vertebral canal above the posterior arch of atlas. These join small veins from the surrounding deep muscles. This formed vein enters foramen transversarium in the transverse process of atlas and forms a plexus around the vertebral artery.

This terminates as the vertebral vein which exit from the C-6 transverse foramen. During it descent it is anterior then anterolateral to the vertebral artery. It opens into the brachiocephalic vein. The opening has valve.

The vertebral vein descends behind IJV but in front of the first part of the subclavian artery.

Tributaries

1. Occipital vein
2. Veins from prevertebral muscles
3. Internal and external vertebral plexuses

It is connected to sigmoid sinus by an emissary vein which passes through the posterior condylar canal.

It is joined by anterior vertebral and deep cervical veins.

Anterior vertebral vein

It starts in a venous plexus around the upper cervical transverse processes. It descends near ascending cervical artery between the attachments of scalenus anterior and longus capitis. It opens into the terminal part of the vertebral vein.

Deep cervical vein

It begins in the suboccipital region from
- Communicating veins of the occipital veins
- Veins from the suboccipital muscles
- Venous plexuses around the cervical spines

It passes forwards between transverse process of C-7 and neck of the first rib. It opens in the lower part of vertebral vein.

Clinical relevance

- In superior jugular bulb thrombosis (in otitis media), IX, X and XI cranial nerves may be affected.
- IJV may be endangered during removal of neoplastic lymph nodes.
- Venous pulsation may be visible in the EJV at the root of the neck. As there are no valves in the brachiocephalic vein or SVC; the right atrial systole causes a wave of distension up in EJV. This may be seen as a feeble flicker. This atrial systolic impulse is increased when the right atrium is abnormally distended or hypertrophied (diseases of mitral valve).

Surface projection of IJV

- From the ear lobule to the medial end of the clavicle
- The inferior bulb is placed in the depression between the sternal and clavicular heads of the SCM in the lesser supraclavicular fossa.

VEINS OF THE HEAD AND NECK

These are subdivided into three groups:
- Veins of the exterior of head and face
- Veins of neck
- Diploic, meningeal, intracranial veins and dural venous sinuses

At cranial level the veins are arranged as a three-layered system:
- Veins of the scalp
- Dural venous sinuses
- Cerebral and cerebellar veins
- Veins of scalp and dura are variable and intercommunicate extensively through emissary veins
- Dural venous sinuses share drainage to internal jugular vein which is also common to veins of the cerebrum and cerebellum.
- Diploic veins constitute a fourth venous tier.
- Intracranial veins communicate at many places with extracranial vessels via the emissary and other veins.

EXTERNAL VEINS OF THE HEAD AND FACE

SUPRATROCHLEAR VEIN

This starts on the forehead from a venous network. This forms a single trunk which descends near the midline parallel with the opposite vein. The veins then diverge; each joins by supraorbital vein to form the facial vein near the medial canthus.

SUPRAORBITAL VEIN

It begins near the zygomatic process of the frontal bone which passes medially above the orbital opening under orbicularis oculi. It pierces orbicularis oculi to form the facial vein by joining the supratrochlear near the medial canthus.

FACIAL VEIN

It is formed by the union of supraorbital and supratrochlear veins near the medial canthus of eye.

After formation it descends obliquely near the side of the nose. It turns posterolaterally below the orbital opening and passes downwards and backwards behind the facial artery.

It passes under zygomaticus major, risorius and platysma. It then descends on to the anterior border and then the surface of the masseter. It crosses body of the mandible and runs obliquely backwards under the platysma but superficial to submandibular gland, digastric and stylohyoid.

At antero-inferior angle of mandible it joins anterior division of retromandibular vein to form **common facial vein**. It passes downwards superficial to the loop of lingual artery, hypoglossal nerve and external and internal carotid arteries.

It enters internal jugular vein (IJV) near the greater cornu of hyoid bone (superior angle of the carotid triangle). Its upper part above the drainage of superior labial vein is termed as **angular vein**.

Tributaries

Near its commencement the facial vein is connected to the superior ophthalmic vein

Via supraorbital vein it is connected to the cavernous sinus.

It receives following veins
1. Ala of nose
2. Deep facial vein from the pterygoid venous plexus
3. Inferior palpebral vein
4. Superior and inferior labial veins
5. Buccinator vein
6. Parotid vein

7. Masseteric vein

Below the mandible following veins join it
1. Submental vein
2. Tonsillar vein
3. External palatine (paratonsillar) vein
4. Submandibular veins

Clinical relevance

The facial vein has no valves. It is connected to the cavernous sinus by two routes:
- Through the ophthalmic vein
- By deep facial vein to pterygoid venous plexus and thus to the cavernous sinus

Infection may thus spread from the face to the intracranial venous sinuses.

SUPERFICIAL TEMPORAL VEIN

This begins in a venous network joined across the scalp to the contralateral vein and to the supratrochlear, supraorbital, posterior auricular and occipital veins of the same side.

The anterior and posterior tributaries unite above the zygoma to form the superficial temporal vein which is joined by the middle temporal vein. It crosses posterior root of the zygoma and enters parotid gland. In the gland it joins maxillary vein to form **retromandibular vein**.

Tributaries

1. Parotid veins
2. Vein from temporomandibular joint
3. Anterior auricular veins
4. Transverse facial vein

MIDDLE TEMPORAL VEIN

After receiving orbital vein it passes backwards between the layers of temporal fascia. After piercing temporal fascia it joins superficial temporal vein.

PTERYGOID VENOUS PLEXUS

It is placed between
- Temporalis and lateral pterygoid muscle
- Pterygoids

Tributaries

1. Sphenopalatine vein
2. Deep temporal veins
3. Pterygoid veins
4. Masseteric vein
5. Buccal vein
6. Dental vein
7. Greater palatine vein
8. Middle meningeal vein
9. Branch from inferior ophthalmic vein

This plexus is connected to
- **Facial vein** by the deep facial vein
- **Cavernous sinus** through
  1. Sphenoidal emissary foramen
  2. Foramen ovale
  3. Foramen lacerum

MAXILLARY VEIN

This short vein accompanies the first part of the maxillary artery. It is formed by the pterygoid venous plexus. It passes backwards between spheno-mandibular ligament and the neck of mandible. It joins superficial temporal vein to form retromandibular vein.

RETROMANDIBULAR VEIN

After formation it descends in the parotid gland, between ECA and facial nerve. It divides into:

Anterior branch – joins facial vein to form common facial vein

Posterior branch – joins posterior auricular vein to form EJV

POSTERIOR AURICULAR VEIN

It begins in parieto-occipital venous network. It descends behind the auricle to join posterior division of retromandibular vein in or just below the parotid glands, to form EJV.

It receive :

1. Stylomastoid vein
2. Tributaries from cranial surface of auricle

OCCIPITAL VEIN

It begins in a posterior venous network in the scalp. It pierces cranial attachment of trapezius and appears in the suboccipital triangle. Here it joins deep cervical and vertebral veins. It terminates in IJV.

Sometimes it may join posterior auricular vein. Through parietal and mastoid emissary veins it is connected with the superior sagittal and transverse sinuses.

CLINICAL CONSIDERATIONS

Carotid Pulse

Arterial pulsations can be felt in the carotid triangle by placing the fingertips in front of anterior border of SCM at the level of laryngeal prominence. The carotid sinus is likely to be stimulated if this maneuver is not performed gently.

Carotid Body

The carotid body contains chemoreceptors that are activated primarily by

1. Low oxygen levels in arterial blood
2. Low blood pH
3. High levels of carbon dioxide in the blood

It is located at the bifurcation of common carotid artery into internal and external carotid branches.

It has its own arterial and venous connections.

Innervation of carotid body: via carotid sinus nerve. This contains afferent fibers that join glossopharyngeal nerve (IX CN) and autonomic efferent fibers derived from vagus nerve (X CN).

The afferent fibers from the carotid body play an important role in increasing respiration in response to a drop in blood oxygen levels.

The **carotid sinus** is a thin-walled, elastic section of the internal carotid artery, the wall of which contains stretch receptors. These receptors are mechanoreceptive endings of afferent nerve fibers that reach the sinus via the glossopharyngeal nerve (IX CN) and carotid sinus nerves.

The carotid sinus receptors function as baroreceptors, informing the central nervous system about blood pressure within the artery.

Strong stimulation (pressure) on these receptors results in reflex bradycardia and a marked fall in blood pressure. This may lead to loss of consciousness (carotid sinus syncope).

Since the more sensitive baroreceptive endings are active even at normal blood pressure levels, this reflex is constantly acting to restrict the heart rate and blood pressure.

Jugular Venous Pressure

The pressure in the right atrium with which these vessels are usually in direct communication affects the pressure in the jugular veins. In conditions of the heart where there is venous stasis in the right atrium, the jugular venous pressure rises which can be observed clinically as engorged neck veins.

Maintenance of a patent airway

Maintenance of a patent airway is a primary supportive and resuscitative maneuver.

Loss of consciousness is associated with relaxation of the pharyngeal muscles. This causes a retracted position and occlude the oropharynx. Asphyxiation follows soon. Correction is done by:

- Proper positioning of the head and jaw (neck extended, mandible supported)
- Displacement of the tongue to clear the air passages.

Patency of the air passages is maintained by passage of an oropharyngeal or nasopharyngeal tube. For sustained ventilatory support, an endotracheal tube is placed.

Outside the hospital, tracheostomy or cricothyrotomy may be necessary.

Endotracheal intubation

For sustained ventilatory support, endotracheal intubation is the most rapid method of obtaining and maintaining an adequate airway.

Outside a hospital setting this is not possible. The alternatives are

- Tracheostomy
- Cricothyrotomy

Cricothyrotomy can be readily performed. The prominence of thyroid cartilage (**Adam's apple**) is palpated. From there, the palpating finger is moved inferiorly in the midline until an indentation is felt. The cricothyroid membrane is identified which extends from the thyroid cartilage above to the cricoid cartilage below.

A transverse stab incision is made in the midline with the point of the blade directed inferiorly to avoid injury to the larynx.

Patency is maintained by a tube.

This carries the risk of permanent damage to the larynx. It is performed by skilled personnel in an extreme emergency.

Endotracheal intubation is a lifesaving procedure.

Proper positioning of the patient is essential to provide a straight line from the oral cavity into the trachea.

The patient's neck is flexed forward and the head tilted slightly backward. The laryngoscope is inserted into the mouth to displace the tongue and expose the larynx. The endotracheal tube should not be introduced unless the larynx is adequately exposed.

Nasotracheal intubation is preferred when it is to be continuing for a period of days.

Advantages of nasal tubes

1. Anchored more securely

2. Better tolerated
3. Permit swallowing
4. Not bitten off by teeth

Nasotracheal intubation

The procedure is similar to that for the oral tube except that the larger nostril is selected for tube passage. Once the tube reaches pharynx, it is grasped with a curved (**Magill**) forceps. It is then guided into the larynx and trachea.

When the patient is breathing during intubation, it is done during inspiration.

Once the tube has passed the vocal cords, it is advanced to a point midway between the cords and carina. The low-pressure cuff is inflated with air to overcome any leak during forced ventilation. Auscultation for breath sounds is then carried out over both lungs. After the tube is correctly positioned, it is secured by tape.

Tracheostomy

It is a surgical operation to establish airway.

It is a surgical opening into the trachea through which an indwelling tube may be inserted. In this procedure, trachea is opened and a tube is inserted.

Indications

1. Laryngeal obstruction
2. For prolonged continuous artificial respiration

To avoid damage to neighboring vascular structures (carotid system) and recurrent laryngeal nerve, the incision should always be given in the midline.

Vertical incision – extends downwards from the lower margin of cricoid cartilage in the first tracheal ring.

Horizontal incision – a transverse incision is placed low above the suprasternal notch. This incision is given for cosmetic reason.

After tracheostomy, patient's chest is auscultated for breath sounds.

The tube is suctioned frequently to keep it free from tracheobronchial secretions.

Complications include

1. Pneumothorax
2. Respiratory insufficiency
3. Obstruction of the tracheostomy tube
4. Pulmonary infection
5. Atelectasis
6. Tracheoesophageal fistula
7. Haemorrhage
8. Mediastinal emphysema

The tracheostomy is closed after normal breathing is restored.

When the tracheostomy is permanent (with laryngectomy) the patient is taught self-care.

43

Parotid Region

Clean and expose parotid gland. Trace its duct to buccinator muscle. Trace a branch of the facial nerve back through the gland to the parent trunk. **Identify** and trace the other branches of the nerve away from it. **Identify** communicating branches from the auriculotemporal nerve.

Follow facial nerve back to the stylomastoid foramen.

Identify

- Posterior auricular branch
- Branch to posterior belly of digastric
- Branch to stylohyoid
- Posterior auricular artery

Remove part of the parotid gland and expose

- Retromandibular vein
- External carotid artery

PAROTID REGION : DESCRIPTION

It is placed in front of the auricle, below the zygomatic arch the posterior part of lower part of face up to the angle of mandible. It lodges largest salivary gland – parotid gland. The shape of the gland is uneven (inverted pyramid to fit in the parotid space.

PAROTID SPACE

Superficial extent

Antero-posteriorly – overlapping masseter anteriorly and sternocleidomastoid (SCM) posteriorly

Supero-inferiorly – from lower surface of external auditory meatus to below and behind the angle of mandible

Structures forming parotid bed

Postero medial structures

- Mastoid process – SCM and posterior belly of digastric
- Stylomastoid foramen – emerging facial nerve
- Styloid apparatus with three muscles and two lipaments
- Carotid sheath with its contents
- Spine of sphenoid with middle meningeal artery
- Foramen ovale and its contents
- Scaphoid fossa with tensor palati

Antero-medial structures

- Rumus of mandible with masseter.

On surface, the parotid space is a hollow **bounded anteriorly** by posterior margin of ramus of mandible and **posteriorly** by anterior border of sternocleidomastoid

PAROTID GLAND

It is the largest salivary gland. It is placed at the side of the face just below and in front of the external ear.

The gland has two parts – superficial and deep

The main part of the gland is superficial which is flattened and quadrilateral. It lies between the ramus of mandible, mastoid process, temporal bone and sternocleidomastoid muscle. It is wide superiorly and reaches up to the zygomatic arch while inferiorly it tapers near the angle of mandible.

The rest of the gland is wedge-shaped and extends deeply toward the pharyngeal wall.

The gland is enclosed in a capsule which is continuous with the deep cervical fascia.

The parotid duct starts at the anterior border of the gland and opens in the vestibule of mouth opposite the crown of upper second molar tooth.

PAROTID DUCT (Stenson's duct)

This is about 7 cm long. It extends from the anterior border of parotid gland to the vestibule of mouth. After leaving the parotid gland it lies over masseter, pierces buccinator, runs for a short distance obliquely forward between the buccinator and the mucous membrane of the mouth. It opens in the vestibule of mouth through a small opening opposite the second upper molar tooth. The duct has a thick wall. It is about 4 mm in diameter. which narrows at the opening into the mouth.

As the parotid duct crosses masseter, it receives duct from the accessory part of parotid gland.

COURSE OF PAROTID DUCT

The parotid duct (**Stenson's**) appears at the anterior border of parotid gland. It courses forwards on the masseter muscle where it can be palpated. At the anterior border of masseter, parotid duct terns medially to pierce following structures (from superficial to deep):

1. Buccal pad of fat
2. Bucco-pharyngeal fascia
3. Buccinator muscle
4. Pharyngo-basilar fascia
5. Mucous membrane of cheek

It pierces the mucous membrane to open obliquely in the vestibule of mouth opposite the crown of upper second motor toot.

SECRETO-MOTOR PATHWAY FOR PAROTID GLAND

Pre-ganglionic parasympathetic impulses arise in inferior salivatory nucleus and are carried subsequently in:

*   Glossopharyngeal (IX CN) nerve
*   Recurrent branch of IX CN (**Jacobson's nerve**)
*   Tympanic plexus
*   Lesser petrosal nerve, to end in otic ganglion.

Post-ganglionic parasympathetic impulses reach parotid gland through the posterior root of auriculotemporal nerve.

The auriculotemporal nerve is related to the spine of sphenoid. It is liable to be injured when the spine is fractured. Patient complain of dryness of mouth, which may be accompanied by loss of sensations from anterior two third of the tongue as chorda tympani is also likely to be affected because this nerve is also related to the spine of spheroid.

CLINICAL CONSIDERATIONS

Incisions in parotid surgery

The facial nerve on entering the substance of parotid gland divides into zygomatico-temporal and cervico-facial trunks. They issue branches which form an extensive anastomosis (Pes anserinus). Terminal branches arise from this anastomosis. These emerge along the superior and anterior borders of the parotid gland. During its course in the parotid gland, nerve plexus / branches divide the gland into superficial and deep lobes.

Surgical intervention of parotid swelling requires adequate care to avoid injury to branches of facial nerve as well as parotid duct. Hence, horizontal incisions are given. A vertical incision is likely to cut branches of facial nerve and parotid duct

Parotid Swellings

MUMPS

It is an acute viral infection which is characterized by swelling of the parotid gland. Children between five and fifteen years of age are affected more but it may occur at any age. Passive immunity from maternal antibodies usually prevents this disease in children under one year of age. The incidence of mumps is highest during late winter and early spring.

Symptoms include

- Anorexia
- Headache
- Malaise
- Fever

These are followed by

- Earache
- Parotid gland swelling
- Patient experiencing pain while drinking or chewing

The parotid swelling (in **mumps**) is very painful as it causes stretching of parotido-masseteric fascia where the nerve endings are stimulated. This is because of unyielding nature of parotido-masseteric fascia (deep fascia).

The prognosis in mumps is good.

Complications include

1. Arthritis
2. Pancreatitis
3. Myocarditis
4. Oophoritis
5. Nephritis

Mumps-induced orchitis result in some atrophy of the testicles.

Epididymoorchitis and mumps meningitis may develop.

About 25% of the postpubertal mumps develop epididymoorchitis.

Mumps meningitis develops in 10% of the patients with mumps.

Sialolith and Sailograply

Parotid calculi or sailolith occur less commonly compared with submandibular salivary gland. The calculus is deeply placed within the parotid duct systems. It leads to painful swelling of gland especially at meal times. The diagnosis is established by **sialography.** At times the stone can be palpated from within the mouth.

Bell's Palsy

The facial nerve is a mixed nerve consisting of several types of fibers:

- Branchial - motor fibers to ipsilateral facial muscles
- Autonomic (secretomotor) fibers to the lacrimal, submandibular and sublingual glands
- Special sensory fibers for taste from the anterior two-thirds of the tongue
- Somatosensory component supplying the anterior aspect of the ear canal.

Acute lesions of the facial nerve (VII CN) are the most common of the mononeuropathies affecting cranial nerves. As it emerges from the stylomastoid foramen it consists mainly of motor fibers to ipsilateral facial muscles.

The most common disorder of the facial nerve seen at or distal to the stylomastoid foramen is **Bell's palsy**.

It is a unilateral lesion that is usually idiopathic (exposure to cold weather) and occurs acutely. The idiopathic lesion resolves in 75% to 80% of patients. It may also be caused by

- Trauma
- Parotid gland tumour
- Iatrogenic injury during parotidectomy

Manifestations include

- Partial or complete unilateral facial paralysis
- Marked facial asymmetry

Levator palpebrae superioris (LPS) is unopposed:

1. Upper lid rises higher when the eye is open
2. Patient is unable to wink on the affected side

Lower eyelid and lacrimal puncta fall away from the surface of the eye

1. Exposure of the lower conjunctiva
2. Complete closure does not occur
3. Tears tend to run down the cheek
4. Eye become dry
5. Increased corneal irritation result

Buccinator and orbicularis oris muscles are unable to work with the tongue to keep food between the teeth while chewing

1. Food accumulates in the vestibule of oral cavity
2. Lips cannot be held together tightly to keep food from falling out of the mouth during eating
3. Constant drooling from the corner of the mouth

When facial nerve lesions occur within the facial canal:

1. Loss of taste and decreased salivation on the affected side – involvement of chorda tympani
2. Hyperacusia – paralysis of stapedius

3. Lesions at geniculate ganglion – pain in ear canal

Herpes zoster infections may involve the geniculate ganglion - the herpes rash occurs on the tympanic membrane and adjacent auditory canal.

Frey's syndrome

This syndrome is a sequel of an incision for **suppuartive parotitis** causing injury and subsequent anastomosis of auriculotemporal nerve to great auricular nerve. It is characterized by:

- Unilateral facial flushing
- Unilateral gustatory sweating on the parotid region
- Hyperesthesia over the cutaneous distributions of auriculotemporal nerve
- Attacks of pain in the area supplied by the nerve

Herpes Zoster

It is an infectious disease. It affects the peripheral nervous system. It is also known as **shingles**. Herpes zoster is an acute neuralgia confined to the distribution of a specific spinal nerve root or cranial nerve. It is associated with characteristic vesicular rash. It occurs more often in immunocompromised people.

Primary site of infection is

- Sensory ganglion
- Dorsal root
- Trigeminal ganglion

Generally a single sensory ganglion is affected. Although the rash occurs most often in the distribution of the lower thoracic dermatomes, any spinal segment or trigeminal nerve division may be involved.

The Herpes zoster infections may involve the geniculate ganglion of VII CN; herpes rash occurs on the eardrum and adjacent auditory canal.

44

Temporal and Interatemporal Fossae

Cut zygomatic arch in front of and behind the attachments of masseter. Turn it down with masseter muscle. Cut the neurovascular structures which enters deep surface of masseter.

Separate masseter from the angle of mandible and turn it downwards and identify **temporalis**. Cut the coronoid process of the mandible. Avoid damage to the buccal nerve and artery. Turn the coronoid process and temporalis upwards. Separate the fibres of temporalis from the temporal fossa.

Identify

- Deep temporal vessels
- Deep temporal nerves

These are placed between the muscle and skull.

- Middle temporal artery

It passes upwards on squamous part of temporal bone.

- Zygomaticotemporal nerve

Divide the mandible horizontally through its neck and also just above the mandibular foramen. Avoid damage to the underlying structures. Study the exposed muscles, vessels, and nerves.

Trace **maxillary artery** anterosuperiorly until it passes through pterygomaxillary fissure.

Identify

- Maxillary nerve

It passes towards the inferior orbital fissure. Its following branches are noted:

- Zygomatic nerve – passes through the inferior orbital fissure
- Posterior superior alveolar nerve

Trace the branches of the posterior superior alveolar nerve - pass through small openings in the posterior surface of the maxilla.

Separate two heads of lateral pterygoid muscle. Avoid damage to the buccal nerve - placed between them. Detach the upper head from the capsule of temporomandibular joint and also remove it from the infratemporal fossa. Avoid damage to the deep temporal nerves between it and the skull. Detach the lower head of the muscle from the lateral pterygoid plate and reflect it backwards.

Disarticulate the head of the mandible from the articular disc. Remove it along with the lower head of the lateral pterygoid. Avoid damage to the auriculotemporal nerve. Trace auriculotemporal nerve towards mandibular nerve – branch of mandibular nerve.

Identify

- Branches of the mandibular nerve
- Chorda tympani nerve

Trace chorda tympani to the spine of sphenoid. Trace it lower down till it joins the lingual nerve.

Identify

- Otic ganglion

It is placed medial to the mandibular nerve.

- Tensor palati

It is seen medial to the middle meningeal artery and mandibular nerve.

- Zygomatic nerve - between the floor and lateral wall of the orbit

Separate periosteum from the floor of the orbit.

Identify

- Infraorbital groove
- Infraorbital nerve and vessels

These are seen over infraorbital groove.

Remove the outer table of the mandible with a chisel and bone forceps and expose the mandibular canal.

INFRATEMPORAL REGION

It is placed under the base of skull, behind the maxilla and between the lateral wall of the pharynx and ramus of mandible.

Boundaries

Anterior – Posterior surface of body of maxilla

Posterior – Styloid process and tympanic plate

Lateral – Muscles (Temporalis and Masseter) attached to coronoid process and ramus of mandible.

Medial – Lateral pterygoid plate and muscles of upper part of pharynx (superior constrictor) and tensor and levator palati.

Superior (roof) – Infratemporal surface of greater wing of sphenoid

Inferior – Continues with the sides of pharynx

Communications

Superiorly – with temporal fossa

With cranial cavity

- Foramen ovale
- Foramen spinosum

Anteriorly – with Pterygo-palatine fossa through pterygomaxillary fissure

Superficial contents

Muscles: Medial and lateral pterygoids

Vessels:

- Pterygoid venous plexus
- Maxillary artery and branches of its first and second parts

Ligament: Sphenomandibular ligament

Deep contents

Muscles – Tensor veli palati

Nerves

- Mandibular and its branches
- Chorda tympani
- Maxillary nerve and its branches

Ganglion – Otic ganglion with its roots and branches

V CRANIAL NERVE (TRIGEMINAL NERVE)

It is a mixed nerve having motor and sensory roots.

Nerve components

Branchial efferent

- Nerve of the first arch
- Supplies muscles of mastication and anterior belly of digastric (ABD) and mylohyoid (MH)

Somatic afferent

Pain and temperature sensations

From skin of

- Face
- Scalp

From mucous membrane of

- Nose and paranasal air sinuses (PNS)
- Oral cavity
- Gums and teeth
- Anterior two third of tongue

Discriminatory touch from

- Face

Proprioceptive impulses from

- Muscles of mastication
- Extrinsic muscles of eye
- Facial muscles
- Gums and teeth

Nuclei

Branchial efferent

- Motor nucleus is in Pons

Somatic afferent

- Spinal nucleus for pain and temperature is located in pons and medulla
- Main sensory nucleus for discriminatory touch is located in the pons
- Mesencephalic nucleus for proprioception is located in the whole length of midbrain

Course

Intraneural course

Axons from various nuclei ascend / descend to come out in the middle of anterolateral aspect of basilar part of pons.

Intracranial course

The motor and sensory roots together pass below the tentorium cerebelli to the mouth of the trigeminal cave.

Tubular prolongation of arachnoid and dura mater are present around the sensory and motor roots.

The nerve crosses the upper border of petrous temporal near its apex and enters middle cranial fossa

Extracranial course

The extracranial course of the three divisions of trigeminal nerve is covered at appropriate dissection schedules

DISTRIBUTIONS OF MANDIBULAR NERVE

Mandibular nerves enters infratemporal region through foramen ovale. Here it is placed between lateral pterygoid muscle laterally and tensor palati and auditory tube medially. In the infratemporal

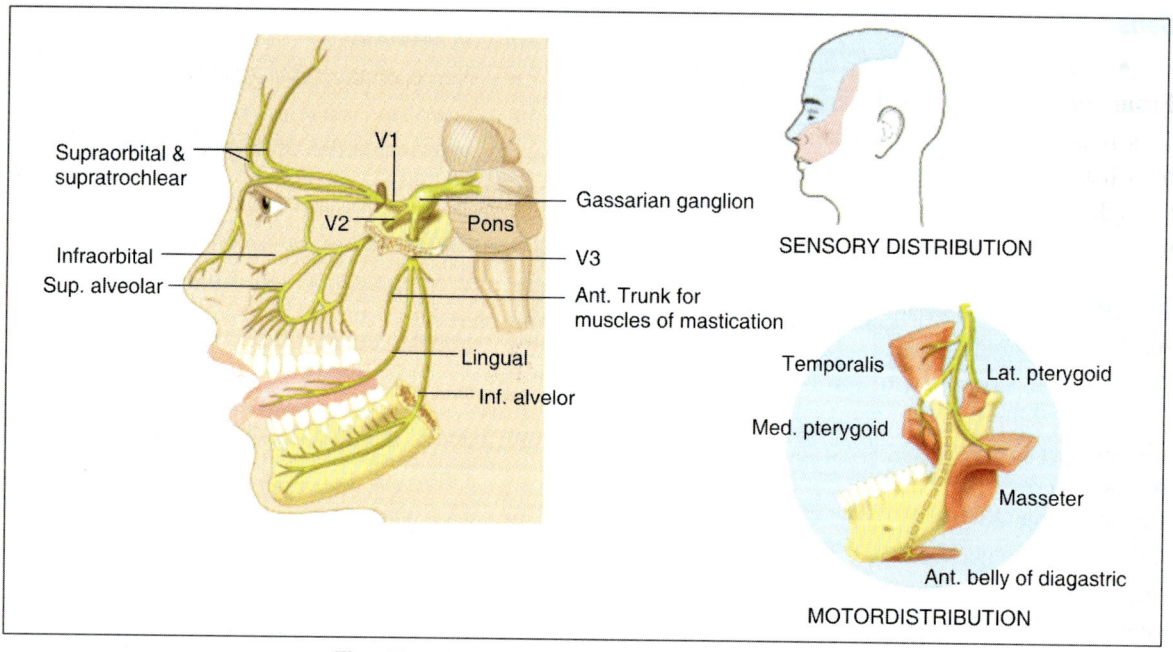

Fig. 44.1: Trigeminal nerve & its distribution

region, the trunk divides into anterior and posterior divisions.

Branches and distribution

From the trunk – One motor and one sensory branch

    Motor – Nerve to medial pterygoid. The nerve to medial pterygoid gives branches to tensor tympani and tensor palati after passing through pterygopalatine ganglion.

    Sensory - Nervous spinosus, which enters middle cranial fossa through foramen spinosum. It supplies due mater in the middle cranial fossa.

From the anterior division

This is predominantly motor division with three motor / muscular branches (for remaining muscle of mastication) and one sensory branch.

Motor branches

- Deep temporal nerves for temporalis
- Masseteric branch for masseter
- Nerve to lateral pterygoid

Sensory branch

- Buccal nerve.

From the posterior division

This is predominantly sensory with three sensory branches and one motor branch. **Motor fibers** (nerve to mylohyoid) are contained in inferior alveolar nerve.

Sensory branches

Auriculo-temporal nerve (ATN) has two roots, which encloses middle meningeal artery. ATN innervates skin of scalp, temple and pinna.

Lingual nerve is a mixed nerve that carries general and taste sensations from the anterior two third of tongue and secretomotor impulses to submandibular and sublingual glands

Inferior alveolar nerve before entering mandibular foramen issues motor branches to mylohyoid and anterior belly of digastric. Its sensory component

is for the gum and teeth of lower jaw. Its terminal branch (mental nerve) emerges through mental foremen to supply adjoining skin.

DISTRIBUTION OF CHORDA TYMPANI

This is a mixed nerve which arises arising from the geniculate ganglion of facial nerve (VII CN) within the petrous part of temporal bone. It comes out through the petrotympanic fissure and joins posterior aspect of lingual nerve at an acute angle in the infratemporal region. It carries secretomotor impulses to the submandibular ganglion. It carries taste sensations from the anterior two third of the tongue excluding circumvallate papillae. This is carried in peripheral process of geniculate ganglion represented by:

    – Lingual nerve

    – Chorda tympani

The central process of geniculate ganglion (**nervous intermedius**) carries taste sensation to nucleus of **tractus solitarius** situated in the open part of medulla.

MAXILLARY ARTERY

This is one of the terminal branch of the external carotid artery, other being superficial temporal artery. This larger terminal branch arises behind the neck of mandible. Initially it is embedded in the parotid gland. It then passes medial to the neck of mandible, either superficial or deep to the lower head of the lateral pterygoid to reach the pterygopalatine fossa. It passes between the two heads of lateral pterygoid.

It has three parts

- First (**mandibular**) part
- Second (**pterygoid**) part
- Third (**pterygopalatine**) part

First part is horizontal and passes between the neck of mandible and sphenomandibular ligament. It is parallel and slightly below the auriculo-temporal nerve crossing the inferior alveolar nerve.

Second part ascends obliquely forwards medial to the temporalis and superficial to the lower head of lateral pterygoid.

Third part passes through pterygomaxillary fissure into pterygopalatine fossa. Here it is situated anterior to the pterygopalatine ganglion.

Distribution

The maxillary artery is distributed to

1. Mandible
2. Maxilla
3. Teeth
4. Muscles of mastication
5. Palate
6. Nose
7. Cranial dura mater

Branches of First Part

- Gives five branches
- Branches pass through bony foramina

1. Deep auricular artery

It arises with anterior tympanic artery. It ascends in the parotid gland behind temporomandibular joint. It pierces osseous wall of external acoustic meatus and supplies its cuticular lining, exterior of tympanic membrane and TM joint.

2. Anterior tympanic artery

It ascends behind temporomandibular joint and enters tympanic cavity through the petrotympanic fissure. It ramifies on the interior of tympanic membrane. It forms a vascular circle around the membrane with posterior tympanic branch of stylomastoid artery.

3. Middle meningeal artery (MMA)

This largest meningeal artery ascends between sphenomandibular ligament and lateral pterygoid. It passes between two roots of auriculotemporal nerve. It enters cranial cavity through foramen spinosum.

In the cranium it runs in a groove on the squamous part of temporal bone. It divides into frontal and parietal branches.

Frontal (anterior) branch crosses greater wing of sphenoid and reaches a groove in the sphenoidal angle of parietal bone. Here it divides into branches between dura mater and cranium.

Parietal (posterior) branch curves back on the squamous temporal bone and reach of anferior to mastoid angle of parietal bone. It supplies posterior parts of dura mater and cranium.

These branches anastomose with their fellows and with the anterior and posterior meningeal arteries.

Branches of MMA in cranial cavity

- **Ganglionic branches** supply trigeminal ganglion and its roots
- **Petrosal branch** enters hiatus for greater petrosal nerve and supplies facial nerve, geniculate ganglion and tympanic cavity. It anastomoses with stylomastoid artery
- **Superior tympanic artery** traverses canal for tensor tympani. It supplies tensor tympani and mucosa of the canal.
- **Temporal branches** pass through minute foramina in greater wing of sphenoid and anastomose with deep temporal arteries.

Anastomotic branch enters orbit through superior orbital fissure and anastomoses with recurrent branch of lacrimal artery.

Surface anatomy

Middle meningeal artery enters skull medial to the midpoint of zygoma and 2 cm above this divides into two branches.

Frontal branch runs first up and forwards to the pterion and then upwards and backwards towards a point midway between the inion and nasion.

Parietal branch runs upwards and backwards towards the lambda.

Clinical anatomy

Middle meningeal artery may be torn in

- Fractures of temporal bone
- Injuries separating dura mater from the bone, followed by haemorrhage between them

Trephining may be required to reduce cerebral compression.

4. Accessory meningeal artery

This may arise from the maxillary or middle meningeal artery. It enters cranial cavity through foramen ovale. It supplies trigeminal ganglion, dura mater and bone. Its main distribution is extracranial and supplies

- Medial and lateral pterygoids
- Tensor veli palatini
- Sphenoid bone
- mandibular nerve and otic ganglion

5. Inferior alveolar (dental) artery

It passes posterior to the inferior alveolar nerve and enter mandibular foramen. At the foramen sphenomandibular ligament is medial to it.

Its mylohyoid branch pierces sphenomandibular ligament and descends with the mylohyoid nerve in the groove on the ramus of mandible.

The inferior alveolar artery traverses mandibular canal with the inferior alveolar nerve and divides into **incisor and mental branches** near the first premolar. The incisor branch continues below the incisor teeth towards the midline, where it anastomoses with the artery of opposite side.

In the mandibular canal the arteries supply mandible, tooth sockets and teeth with branches entering the minute hole at the apex of the root to supply the pulp. The mental branch exit through mental foramen and supplies chin. It anastomoses with submental and inferior labial arteries.

Near its origin the inferior alveolar artery has a lingual branch, which descends with lingual nerve to supply the buccal mucous membrane.

Branches of Second Part

- Gives four branches
- Distributed to the muscles of mastication

1. Deep temporal branches

These anterior and posterior branches ascend between temporalis and the bone to supply temporalis. They anastomose with middle temporal artery.

2. Pterygoid branches

These branches supply pterygoid muscles.

3. Masseteric artery

This small artery along with masseteric nerve passes behind the tendon of temporalis through the mandibular notch to the deep surface of masseter. It anastomoses with masseteric branches of facial and transverse facial arteries.

4. Buccal artery

It runs obliquely forwards with buccal nerve between medial pterygoid and the attachment of the temporalis. It supplies external aspect of buccinator. It anastomoses with branches of facial and infraorbital arteries.

Branches of Third Part

- Gives six branches
- Pass through bony foramina

1. Posterior superior alveolar (dental) artery

It descends on the infratemporal surface of maxilla. It then divides into various branches which enter alveolar canals to supply molar and premolar teeth and maxillary air sinus. Other branches continue over the alveolar process to supply the gingivae.

2. Infraorbital artery

It enters orbit through inferior orbital fissure. It runs in the infraorbital groove and canal with the infraorbital nerve and both structures emerge on the face through infraorbital foramen.

It has following branches in the canal

Orbital branches - Supply the inferior rectus, inferior oblique and lacrimal sac

Anterior superior alveolar (dental) branches - supply the upper incisor, canine and the mucous membrane of the maxillary sinus.

On the face some branches ascend to the medial canthus and lacrimal sac which anastomose with the terminal branches of the facial artery

Other branches anastomose with a dorsal nasal branch of the ophthalmic artery. Some branches descend between the levator labii superioris and levator anguli oris and anastomose with the facial, transverse facial and buccal arteries.

3. Descending palatine artery

The artery descends in the palatine canal. It gives off two or three lesser palatine arteries which pass through lesser palatine canals to supply the soft palate and tonsil, anastomosing with the ascending palatine artery. The main vessel continues as greater palatine artery and emerges on the palate's oral surface by passing through greater palatine foramen. It runs in a curved groove near the alveolar border of the hard palate to the incisive canal. It anastomoses with a branch of the sphenopalatine artery.

It supplies

- Gingivae
- Palatine glands
- Mucous membrane of hard palate

4. Pharyngeal artery

This very small artery runs backwards through the palatovaginal canal with the pharyngeal branch of the pterygopalatine ganglion.

It supplies

- Mucosa of the roof of nose
- Nasopharynx
- Sphenoidal air sinus
- Auditory tube

5. Artery of pterygoid canal

It passes backwards in the pterygoid canal with the corresponding nerve. **It supplies**

- Mucous membrane of the upper pharynx
- Pharyngotympanic tube
- Tympanic cavity

6. Sphenopalatine artery

This is the continuation of the maxillary artery. It passes through the sphenopalatine foramen into the walls of the nasal cavity.

Posterior lateral nasal branches ramify over the conchae and meatuses. These anastomoses with the ethmoidal arteries and nasal branches of greater palatine artery supplying frontal, maxillary, ethmoidal and sphenoidal sinuses. It crosses anteriorly on the inferior sphenoid surface and terminates on the nasal septum as posterior septal branches. These branches anastomose with the ethmoidal arteries. One branch descends on vomer to the incisive canal to join greater palatine artery and septal branch of superior labial artery of facial artery.

Collateral Circulation

After interruption of one common carotid artery the collateral circulation is established by the connections across the midline between the carotid arteries (intra- and extracranial anastomoses) and by enlargement of the branches of subclavian artery. Main extracranial connections include:

- Between superior and inferior thyroid arteries
- Between deep cervical artery and descending branch of occipital artery

After interruption of the external carotid artery the circulation is maintained by

- Anastomoses of branches of ECA with branches of ICA
- Anastomosis between occipital artery with branches of subclavian artery.

TEMPOROMANDIBULAR JOINT

BONES TAKING PART

From above - Articular tubercle and anterior part of mandibular fossa of temporal bone

From below - Head of the mandible

The articular surfaces are covered by white fibrocartilage

CLASSIFICATION

Synovial of condylar variety

Right and left joints form bicondylar articulation. An articular disc divides the joint into upper and lower compartments

- Upper or Meniscofemoral compartment
- Lower or Meniscomandibular compartment

LIGAMENTS

Fibrous capsule

The joint is surrounded by short capsular fibres which stretch from the condyle to the articular disc and from the disc to the temporal bone.

Longer bands extend from the condyle to the temporal bone. These are reinforcing fibres. True capsular fibres are present only on the lateral side of the joint. Posteriorly, anteriorly and medially the upper and lower laminae of the articular disc are attached separately either to the temporal bone or mandibular condyle.

Above the capsule is attached to the articular tubercle and to the lips of the squamotympanic fissure. Between these the capsular fibers are attached to the edges of the mandibular fossa.

Below it is attached to the neck of the mandible.

Above the articular disc the capsule is loose while below it is taut.

Lateral ligament

It is attached above to the tubercle on the root of zygoma and below to the lateral surface and posterior border of the neck of mandible. Its fibres are directed downwards and backwards deep to the parotid gland.

Sphenomandibular ligament

This is placed medially and separated from the capsule. It is a flat and thin band. It extends from the spine of sphenoid to the lingula of mandibular foramen.

- Lateral pterygoid and auriculotemporal nerve are superolateral to it.
- It is separated from the neck of mandible by maxillary vessels,
- It is separated from the ramus of mandible by inferior alveolar vessels and nerve.
- At its lower end nerve and vessels to the mylohyoid pierce the ligament.
- Near its upper end it is crossed by the chorda tympani.
- It is separated from the pharynx by fat and pharyngeal veins.

The role of this vestigial ligament in mandibular mechanics is negligible.

Stylomandibular ligament

It is a thickening of deep cervical fascia. It extends from the apex and adjacent anterior aspect of the styloid process to the angle of mandible and posterior border. It is an accessory ligament to the joint.

Articular disc

This fibrocartilaginous oval plate completely divides the joint. Its upper surface is sagittally concavo-convex to fit the articular tubercle and fossa while its inferior concave surface is applied to the head of mandible. Its circumference blends with the fibrous capsule. Anteromedially the tendon of lateral pterygoid is attached to it.

From its medial and lateral aspects short, strong bands pass from its margins to the medial and lateral aspects of the mandibular condyle.

Posteriorly in the disc a venous plexus separates its upper and lower layers. The disc is thickest behind its centre.

The disc consists of two thick regions (anterior and posterior bands) with thinner zones between. The anterior and posterior thickened bands are continuous medially and laterally with the mandibular condyle.

From the fifth decade it often shows macroscopic degeneration (fraying, thinning and perforation). This is normal ageing process. The disc is variably perforated.

SYNOVIAL MEMBRANE

This lines the capsule, above and below the disc (but does not cover the disc). On each side it lines the non-articular surfaces of both superior and inferior synovial compartments. Below the disc, synovial membrane is reflected upwards along the neck of mandible and lateral pterygoid tendon.

BLOOD SUPPLY

- Superficial temporal artery
- Maxillary artery

NERVE SUPPLY

- Auriculotemporal nerve
- Masseteric branches of mandibular nerve

MOVEMENTS

The movements are
- Depression and elevation
- Protrusion and retraction
- Rotation (around a vertical axis)

These actions involve gliding, spin, roll and angulation.

Position of rest - upper and lower teeth are slightly apart

Closure position – upper and lower teeth are apposed (occlusal position)

Opening of mouth:

Mandibular condyles rotate on a horizontal axis and also glide forwards and downwards on the inferior surfaces of their articular discs. The disc slides in the same direction on the temporal bones

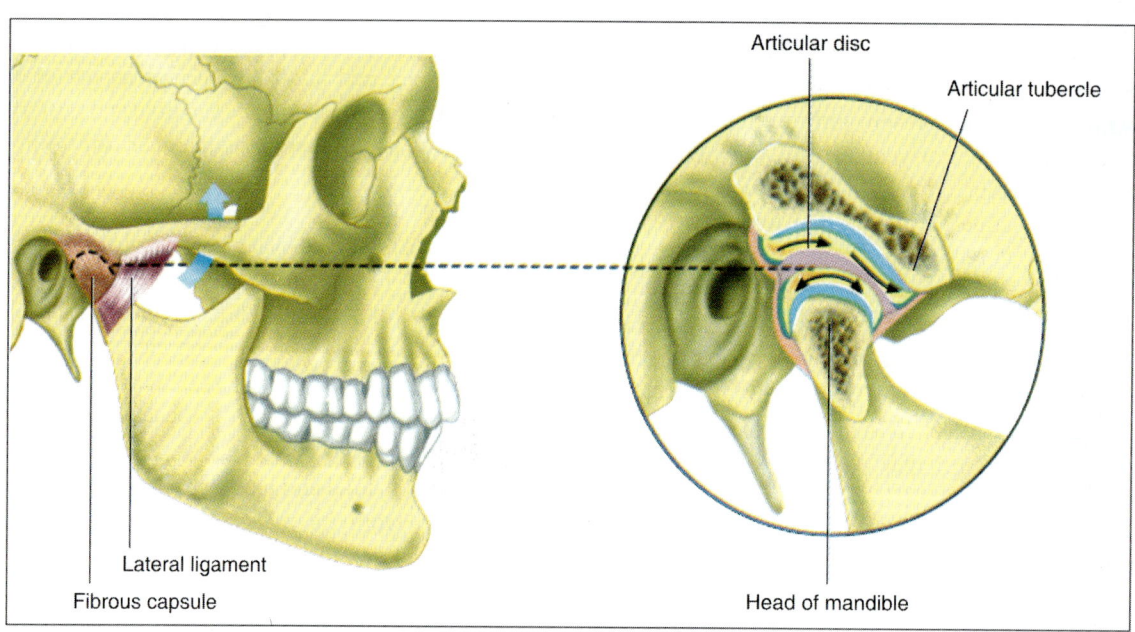

Articular disc

Articular tubercle

Lateral ligament

Fibrous capsule

Head of mandible

Fig. 44.2: Temporomandibular joint

due to their attachments to the mandibular heads. The contraction of the lateral pterygoids draws the heads and discs on to the articular tubercles. Sliding of the disc ceases when their posterior attachments to the temporal bones are stretched to their limit. Further hinging and gliding of the condyles brings them into articulation with the most anterior parts of the discs as the mouth opens fully.

Closure of mouth:

The movements are reversed. The head glides back and hinges on its disc, still held by the lateral pterygoid, which relaxes to allow the disc to glide back and up into the mandibular fossa.

In protrusion the teeth are parallel to the occlusal plane but variably separated. The lower, teeth are carried forwards by both lateral pterygoid muscles.

In retraction the mandible is returned to the position of rest.

In rotatory movements, one head with its disc glides forwards, rotating around a vertical axis immediately behind the opposite head. Then it glides backwards rotating in the opposite direction, as the opposite head comes forward in turn. This alternation swings the mandible from side to side.

Measurement of mandibular movements

- In adults incisors may separate by 50 to 60 mm
- Maximal lateral displacement is 10 mm
- Protrusion is 10 mm

Adult range is reached earlier in females than in males

Adult form is reached between six and twelve years

Muscles causing movements

Protrusion
- Lateral and medial pterygoids

Retraction
- Temporalis (posterior fibres)
- Middle and deep parts of masseter

- Digastric
- Geniohyoid

Elevation
- Temporalis
- Masseter
- Medial pterygoid of both sides

Depression
- Lateral pterygoids
- Digastric
- Geniohyoid
- Mylohyoid

Lateral movements
- Medial and lateral pterygoid of each side, acting alternately

MASTICATION

In this process the food is held, chewed, and moved within the oral cavity for swallowing (**deglutition**). Masticatory apparatus consists of
- Teeth
- Upper and lower jaws
- Muscles acting on them

Tongue with hyoid and its musculature, buccinator are important in placing and holding food for chewing.

Function of chewing - to increase the surface area of food items available to the action of the digestive juices by crusting the food.

Chewing comprises

- **Opening and closing stroke** in which the jaws close towards the food
- **Power stroke** in which the food is reduced

In primates the power stroke is divided into two phases

1. **Buccal phase -** lower teeth move upward and medially into maximal intercuspation.
2. **Lingual phase** - buccal cusps of the lower teeth slide downwards and medially against the palatal cusps of the upper teeth.

Muscles of Mastication

The muscles of mastication are

- Masseter
- Temporalis
- Medial pterygoid
- Lateral pterygoid

MASSETER

This quadrilateral muscle consists of three layers.

Superficial layer (largest) arises by a thick aponeurosis from the maxillary process of zygomatic bone and from anterior two-thirds of the inferior border of zygomatic arch. Its fibres pass downwards and backwards and inserted into the angle and lower half of the lateral surface of the ramus of mandible.

Middle layer arises from the medial aspect of anterior two-thirds of zygomatic arch and from the lower border of posterior third and inserted into the central part of mandibular ramus.

Deep layer arises from the deep surface of the zygomatic arch and inserted into the upper part of the ramus of mandible and coronoid process.

The middle and deep layers together constitute **deep part of masseter.** They form a cruciate muscle. The muscle is easily palpated when it contracts (clenching the teeth).

Superficial relations

- Skin
- Platysma
- Risorius
- Zygomaticus major
- Parotid gland

Deep relations

- Temporalis
- Ramus of mandibular ramus. Fat separates it from buccinator and buccal nerve
- Masseteric nerve and artery

The posterior margin is overlapped by the parotid gland.

The anterior margin is crossed below by the facial vein.

The muscle is crossed by

1. Parotid duct
2. Branches of facial nerve
3. Transverse facial vessels

Nerve supply

Branch of the anterior trunk of mandibular nerve

Actions

- Elevates mandible to occlude teeth in mastication
- Small effect in side-to-side movements, protraction and retraction

Temporal fascia

It is a strong aponeurosis which covers temporalis. The superficial temporal vessels and auriculo-temporal nerve ascend over it. Above it is single layered which is attached to superior temporal line. Below it has two layers - one attached to the lateral and the second to the medial margin of the upper border of the zygomatic arch. Between these layers following structures are placed

1. Zygomatic branch of superficial temporal artery
2. Zygomaticotemporal branch of maxillary nerve
3. Small amount of fat

The deep surface of fascia provides attachment to the superficial fibres of temporalis.

TEMPORALIS

It arises from the temporal fossa and the deep surface of the temporal fascia. Its fibres converge and descend into a tendon. The tendon passes through the gap between the zygomatic arch and the side of the skull. It is attached to the medial surface, apex, anterior and posterior borders of coronoid process and the anterior border of the ramus of mandible up to the last molar tooth.

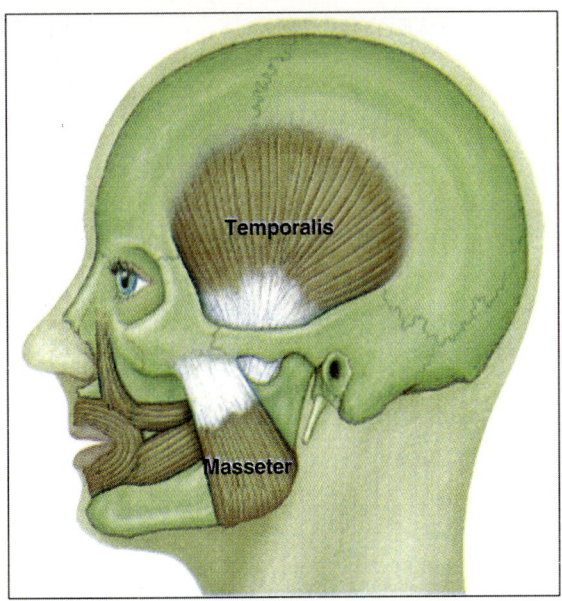

Fig. 44.3: Temporalis & Masseter

- **Anterior fibres** are orientated vertically
- **Most posterior fibres** are almost horizontal
- **Intervening fibres** are oblique

The muscle is difficult to palpate, but its contraction can be felt.

Superficial relations
- Skin
- Auricular anterior and superior muscles
- Temporal fascia
- Superficial temporal vessels
- Auriculotemporal nerve
- Temporal branches of facial nerve
- Zygomaticotemporal nerve
- Epicranial aponeurosis
- Zygomatic arch
- Masseter

Deep relations
- Temporal fossa
- Lateral pterygoid
- Superficial head of medial pterygoid
- Small part of buccinator
- Maxillary artery and its deep temporal branches

- Deep temporal nerves
- Buccal nerve and vessels

Nerve supply

Deep temporal branches of anterior trunk of mandibular nerve

Actions

- Elevates mandible (closes the mouth and approximates the teeth). This movement requires both the upward pull of the anterior fibres and the backward pull of the posterior fibres
- Side-to-side (grinding) movements
- Posterior fibres retract the mandible

LATERAL PTERYGOID

This short and thick muscle has two heads.

Upper head arises from the infratemporal surface and infratemporal crest of the greater wing of sphenoid bone.

Lower head arises from the lateral surface of lateral pterygoid plate.

The fibres pass backwards and laterally to get inserted into a depression on the front of the neck of mandible (**pterygoid fovea**), articular capsule and articular disc of the temporo-mandibular joint.

Superficial relations
- Ramus of mandible
- Maxillary artery
- Tendon of temporalis
- Masseter

Deep relations
- Upper part of medial pterygoid
- Sphenomandibular ligament
- Middle meningeal artery
- Mandibular nerve

Upper border is related to
- Temporal and masseteric branches of mandibular nerve

Lower border is related to

- Lingual nerve
- Inferior alveolar nerve

The buccal nerve and the maxillary artery pass between the two heads

Nerve supply

Branch from anterior trunk of mandibular nerve

Actions

1. Opening of the mouth by pulling forward the condylar process of mandible and articular disc
2. With medial pterygoid of same side, lateral pterygoid advances the condyle of that side so that the jaw rotates about a vertical axis through the opposite condyle
3. Medial and lateral pterygoids of the two sides - protrusion of the mandible

MEDIAL PTERYGOID

This thick, quadrilateral muscle has two heads.

Deep head arises from the medial surface of lateral pterygoid plate and grooved surface of the pyramidal process of palatine bone.

Superficial head arises from the lateral surfaces of the pyramidal process and maxillary tuberosity. The fibres descend posterolaterally to get attached to the postero-inferior part of medial surfaces of the ramus and angle of mandible extending up to mandibular foramen and upto mylohyoid groove.

Relations of lateral surface

It is related to the ramus of mandible from which it is separated by

- Lateral pterygoid
- Sphenomandibular ligament
- Maxillary artery
- Inferior alveolar vessels and nerve

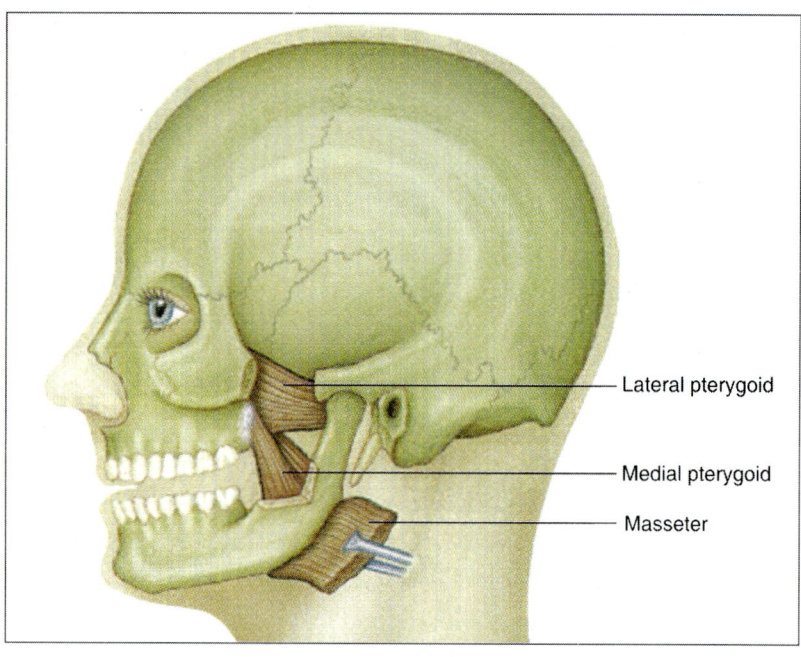

Fig. 44.4: Pteregoid Muscles

- Lingual nerve
- Process of parotid gland

Relations of medial surface

- Tensor veli palatini

This is separated from the superior constrictor by styloglossus and stylopharyngeus.

Nerve supply

Branch from the mandibular nerve

Actions

1. Elevation of the mandible
2. With lateral pterygoids - protrusion of jaw
3. Medial and lateral pterygoids of same side acting together - corresponding side of the mandible is rotated forwards and to the opposite side.
   - With opposite lateral pterygoid - side-to-side movements

ACTIONS OF MUSCLES OF MASTICATION

As a prerequisite the bolus of food has to be chewed properly. This is achieved by the movements of lower jaw by the muscles of mastication. These movements are:

- Elevation and depression of lower jaw
- Protraction and retraction of lower jaw
- Side to side movement of lower jaw

All these movements take at both temporal-mandibular joints.

Opening of mouth (**depression**) is brought about by lateral pterygoids by virtue of their attachment. This is assisted by supra hyoid muscles. **Closure of mouth** (**elevation**) is caused by medial pterygoids, masseter and temporalis. For this movement, the transverse axis passes through mandibular foramen which minimizes stretching of nerves and vessels entering the mandibular foramen.

Protraction of lower jaw is performed by medial and lateral pterygoids of both sides. The retraction is caused by posterior fibers of temporalis and deep fibers of masseter

Side to side movements (chewing) is performed by medial and lateral pterygoid of both sides acting alternately. The axis is a vertical axis passing behind the neck of the mandible and shifts from one side to the other.

CLINICAL CONSIDERATIONS

Dislocations of T.M. joint

The dislocation of temporomandibular joint may be unilateral or bilateral. It may results from

- Blow
- Fall
- Excessive yawning

In direct blow to the lower jaw as well as convulsive yawning, there could be dislocation of head of mandible. It comes to lie in the infra temporal region.

On examination the mandible appears in an open position. If the mandible seen deviated to one side, the dislocation involves only one side.

The patient presents with inability to close the mouth.

The dislocation is reduced manually.

- Place the thumbs in the oral cavity and press last molars of lower jaw down.
- This releases the muscle spasm.
- At the same time the chin is pushed backwards and upwards. Thus the dislocated head of mandible fits back in the mandibular fossa.

Derangement of Articular Disc

This may be seen in

- Following trauma
- Overclosure with backward displacement of a condyle
- Malocclusion

In such conditions clicking sound and pain during movement occur.

Referred pain from diseased tooth

The teeth of lower jaw are supplied by inferior alveolar nerve, which is a branch of mandibular nerve. Thus it is not uncommon to experience pain from the diseased tooth referred mostly to the external acoustic meatus - innervated by auriculo-temporal nerve (branch of mandibular nerve).

TM joint: Pain Dysfunction Syndrome

This is characterized by facial pain and mandibular dysfunction caused by malfunctioned or dislocated temporomandibular joint.

Clinical features include

1. Clicking of the joint during jaw movement
2. Limitation of jaw movement
3. Subluxation
4. Temporomandibular dislocation

Pterion

It is an important bony landmark where **four bones meet** namely anteroinferior angle of **parietal**, squamous part of **temporal**, greater wing of **sphenoid** and **frontal** bone. It is placed approximately two fingers breath above the zygomatic arch and two-finger breath behind the orbital margin. Deep to it in the cranium, anterior branch of middle meningeal vessels are related. This site is preferred for cerebral decompression by making a trephine hole.

45

Submandibular Region

Extend the neck and flex the head on the left. Turn the larynx and pharynx medially on the right. Divide the facial artery and vein at the lower border of the mandible. Detach the anterior belly of the digastric from the mandible.

Identify

- Posterior belly of digastric
- Stylohyoid muscle
- Mylohyoid muscle
- Deep part of submandibular gland

The deep part hooks around the free posterior border of the mylohyoid muscle.

Separate the facial artery from the deep surface of the gland and identify its branches.

Identify **mylohyoid nerve** on the mylohyoid muscle.

Identify

- Hypoglossal nerve

It is seen on the hyoglossus muscle just above the greater cornu of hyoid bone.

- Lingual nerve

It is seen crossing the muscle at a higher level.

- Submandibular ganglion - suspended from lingual nerve
- Submandibular duct

This duct passes forwards from the deep part of the gland.

Push the submandibular gland and the sub-mental vessels backwards. Divide the mylohyoid

nerve. Turn the anterior belly of digastric downwards. Study the attachments of the mylohyoid muscle.

Separate mylohyoid from geniohyoid muscle. Separate geniohyoid from genioglossus.

Pull the tongue to one side and cut the mucous membrane between it and the mandible. Separate the mucosa from the floor of the mouth and mandible.

Expose and identify

- Sublingual gland
- Submandibular duct
- Lingual nerve

Trace the lingual nerve backwards and **identify** its branches to the sublingual gland and submandibular ganglion. Note that the nerve passes close to the last molar tooth.

Identify

- Lower edge of the superior constrictor
- Hyoglossus muscle
- Styloglossus muscle

It is seen on the posterior aspect of hyoglossus, mingling with it.

- Lingual artery

This artery appears at the anterior margin of the hyoglossus.

Trace styloglossus to the styloid process.

Identify

- Stylohyoid ligament
- Stylopharyngeus

Trace stylohyoid ligament to the lesser cornu of the hyoid bone.

Identify

- Glossopharyngeal nerve

It curves around stylopharyngeus and passes forwards deep to the hyoglossus.

- Upper border of the middle constrictor

Trace this muscle to the hyoid bone and stylohyoid ligament, lateral to the stylopharyngeus.

Separate hyoglossus from the hyoid bone. Turn it upwards and expose

- Lingual artery
- Dorsal branches of lingual artery
- Lingual veins
- Posterior part of genioglossus
- Middle constrictor of pharynx
- Attachment of stylohyoid ligament

SUBMANDIBULAR REGION AND SUBMANDIBULAR GLAND

SUBMANDIBULAR REGION

It is situated between the mandible and hyoid bone under cover of body of mandible. Its lower part includes:

- Submental triangle
- Digastric triangle
- Various structure there in

Contents

The structures are related to two key muscles e.g., **Hyoglossus** and **Mylohyoid**.

Structures in superficial fascia

- Fat
- Platysma
- Cervical branch of facial nerve
- Anterior cutaneous nerve of neck
- Submental lymph nodes
- Anterior jugular vein

Structures deep to investing layer of deep cervical fascia

Muscles

- Digastrics and intermediate tendon
- Stylohyoid
- Mylohyoid
- Geniohyoid
- Genioglossus ⎤
- Styloglossus ⎬ Muscles of tongue
- Hyoglossus ⎦

Ligament: Stylohyoid ligament

Salivary glands

- Submandibular gland
- Sublingual gland

Arteries

- Facial artery and its branches
- Lingual artery and its branches

Nerves

- Nerve to mylohyoid
- Lingual with submandibular ganglion
- Glossopharyngeal nerve
- Hypoglossal nerve

Lymph nodes: Submandibular lymph nodes.

SUBMANDIBULAR GLAND

This walnut-sized mixed salivary gland (secretes both mucus serous fluid) is placed in the submandibular triangle. It reaches anteriorly to the anterior belly of digastric and posteriorly to the stylomandibular ligament (ligament lies between submandibular and parotid gland). The gland extends superiorly under the inferior border of mandible and extends as a deep process anteriorly above the mylohyoid muscle. The upper part of superficial surface of the gland lies partly against the submandibular depression on the inner surface of mandible and partly on the medial pterygoid muscle.

The lower part is covered by skin, superficial fascia, platysma, and deep cervical fascia.

The submandibular duct (**Wharton's duct**) is about five cm long. It starts at the deep surface of the gland. It runs between the sublingual gland and genioglossus. It opens on a small papilla at the side of the frenulum linguae.

SUBLINGUAL GLAND

This paired salivary gland is situated under the mucous membrane of the floor of the mouth, beneath the tongue. It is narrow and almond-shaped. It weighs about two grams. The alveoli of sublingual gland secrete mucus.

Important relations include:

Mylohyoid - inferiorly

Submandibular gland - posteriorly

Mandible - laterally

Genioglossus - medially from which it is separated by the lingual nerve and submandibular duct

It has about eight to twenty ducts which join to form the sublingual duct which opens in the flour of the mouth.

The major duct of the sublingual salivary gland is called **Bartholin's duct**.

The minor sublingual duct is called duct of **Rivinus**.

SUBMANDIBULAR GANGLION

It is a parasympathetic ganglion for secretomotor innervation to:

- Submandibular gland
- Sublingual gland
- Anterior lingual glands

Topographically it is related to lingual nerve (V-3) while functionally it is related to VII CN. It lies over hyoglossus muscle.

Preganglionic parasympathetic impulses arise from **superior salivatory nucleus.** These are carried successively in nervous intermedius, chorda tympani and lingual nerve. The post-ganglionic parasympathetic impulses are carried to the submandibular gland via direct branches from the ganglion. For the sublingual gland, the impulses run in one of the roots of lingual nerve.

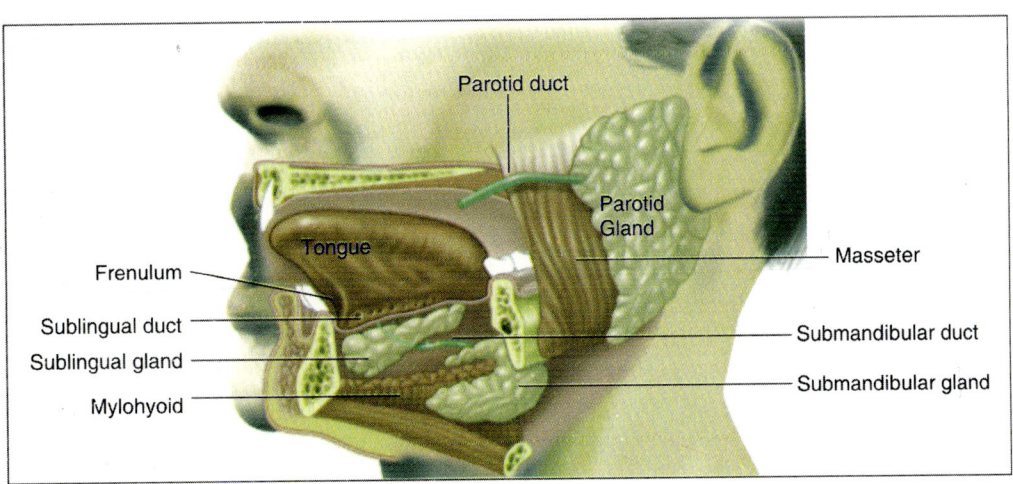

Fig. 45.1: Submandibular & Sublingual Glands

STYLOMANDIBULAR LIGAMENT

It is a modification of deep cervical fascia which forms an accessory ligament of the temporomandibular joint. It extends from the styloid process of temporal bone to the ramus of mandible. It is placed between masseter and pterygoid muscles. It separates parotid gland and submandibular gland.

FACIAL ARTERY

This tortuous artery arises from the external carotid artery in the carotid triangle. It divides into four cervical and five facial branches.
The cervical branches include
1. Ascending palatine
2. Tonsillar
3. Glandular
4. Submental

MYLOHYOID MUSCLE

It is a flat triangular muscle. Muscles of both sides form the floor of the cavity of the mouth (**diaphragm of oral cavity**). It is placed immediately superior to the anterior belly of digastric. It arises from the mylohyoid line of mandible and inserted into the hyoid bone. It is supplied by the mylohyoid nerve (branch of mandibular nerve).
Its action is to raise hyoid bone and tongue.

DIGASTRIC MUSCLE

This muscle comprises two parts - anterior and posterior belly.
Anterior belly arises from the digastric fossa of mandible and inserted into the body and great cornu of hyoid bone. It is a suprahyoid muscle. It is supplied by nerve to mylohyoid (branch of mandibular nerve of trigeminal nerve). It helps in

to opening the jaw and to draw the hyoid bone forward.
Posterior belly arises from the mastoid notch of temporal bone and inserted in the body and great cornu of hyoid bone. It is supplied by the facial nerve. It draws back and raise hyoid bone

GENIOHYOID MUSCLE

This is one of the four suprahyoid muscles. It arises from the symphysis menti of mandible and inserted into the body of hyoid bone. It is a narrow muscle. It is supplied by a branch of the C-1 nerve. It draws hyoid bone and tongue forward.

STYLOHYOID MUSCLE

This is one of four suprahyoid muscles which lie anterior and superior to the posterior belly of digastric. It is a slender muscle. It arises from the styloid process and inserted into the hyoid bone. Near its insertion it is pierced by the tendon of the digastric. It is supplied by the facial nerve. It draws hyoid bone up and back.

CLINICAL CONSIDERATIONS

Submandibular Salivary Calculi

Submandibular salivary gland is a mixed gland. Its mucoid secretion causes sluggish flow in the duct. This together with course of the duct may result in formation of calculi. The calculi in the duct can be felt in the floor of the mouth bimanually.

Submandibular Lymph Nodes

Their involvement in oral carcinoma necessitates section of submandibular gland along with removal of lymph nodes. This is because these nodes are embedded in the superficial part of the gland.

46

Mouth and Pharynx

Remove buccopharyngeal fascia from the surface of pharyngeal muscles on the right side and expose plexus of nerves and veins underneath. Remove the plexus.

Identify

- Stylopharyngeus muscle

It is seen on the posterior surface of the pharynx between the superior and middle constrictor muscles.

Note **glossopharyngeal nerve** winding around the posterior surface of stylopharyngeus and identify its branch to the muscle.

Define the upper border of the **inferior constrictor muscle**. Turn it downwards and expose the lowest fibres of **middle constrictor** arching up towards the hyoid bone.

Detach the right medial pterygoid muscle from the pterygoid plate and turn it downwards and expose superior constrictor.

Study the interior of the pharynx from the left side. Remove its mucosa and study its muscle coat from inside.

Detach the medial pterygoid muscle from the lateral pterygoid plate and turn it down and note the superior constrictor.

Remove the mucous membrane from the **palatopharyngeus and palatoglossal arches** and from the **salpingopharyngeal fold** and expose the muscles within.

Remove the mucous membrane, submucosa and pharyngobasilar fascia from the pharyngeal wall in front of and behind the opening of the auditory tube.

Identify

- Levator palati - posterior to auditory tube
- Ascending palatine artery - beside levator palati
- Tensor palati
- Superior constrictor - lateral to levator palati.

Remove the mucous membrane from medial surface of superior constrictor which is not covered by the palatal muscles. Expose the anterior part of the superior constrictor by dissecting out the palatine tonsil.

Identify

- Palatopharyngeus
- Pterygoid hamulus with the tendon of tensor palati
- Pterygomandibular raphe - connecting hamulus and mandible

Follow the superior constrictor anteriorly to the pterygomandibular raphe.

Strip the mucous membrane from the inner surface of the **buccinator** anterior to the pterygomandibular raphe and identify its attachments and the **opening of parotid duct**.

Remove the mucous membrane from the medial surface of the middle constrictor without disturbing the palatopharyngeus on its medial aspect. Trace palatopharyngeus to the posterior border of the lamina of the thyroid cartilage.

Identify

- Stylopharyngeus

It is placed anterior to the palatopharyngeus, which enters pharynx between superior and middle constrictor muscles. The muscle spreads anteroposteriorly so that its anterior fibres pass to the lateral aspect of the epiglottis, while its posterior fibres are attached along with those of the palatopharyngeus. Its intermediate fibres form a thin layer medial to the superior part of the thyrohyoid membrane.

Identify

- Glossopharyngeal nerve

It is seen anterolateral to the stylopharyngeus at its entry into the pharynx. Trace the nerve to the tongue.

Remove the mucous membrane from the medial surface of the inferior constrictor, the upper part of the oesophagus and the piriform recess.

Identify

- Medial surface of thyroid membrane in the recess
- Superior laryngeal vessels
- Internal branch of superior laryngeal nerve

The vessels and nerve pierce thyrohyoid membrane.

Separate the opening of the auditory tube from the medial pterygoid plate and turn it posteriorly. Free the cartilaginous part of the tube from the base of skull and tensor palati.

Identify

- Tensor tympani

It is attached to the petrous temporal bone superomedial to the tube and passes posterolaterally with it.

Separate tensor palati from the base of the skull and turn it inferiorly. Remove the underlying fascia and expose **mandibular nerve** and the **otic ganglion**

on its anteromedial aspect.

Identify

- middle meningeal artery

It is placed posterior to the mandibular nerve. Trace the branches of the nerve.

PHARYNX AND SOFT PALATE

PHARYNX

It is a fibromuscular tube which is lined with mucous membrane. It extends from the base of skull to the lower border of cricoid cartilage (**C-6**). It is 12-14 cm long. It is situated in front of the cervical vertebrae. At the lower border of cricoid, it continues as oesophagus.

The pharynx serves as a passage for the respiratory and digestive tracts.

It is composed of muscles (circular and longitudinal) with mucous membrane lining. Pharynx is divided into

- Nasopharynx
- Oropharynx
- Laryngopharynx

It presents

1. Openings of auditory tubes
2. Openings of two posterior nares
3. Opening into larynx
4. Opening into esophagus

It also contains

- Pharyngeal tonsils
- Palatine tonsils
- Lingual tonsils

NASOPHARYNX

It is situated behind the nasal cavity above and behind the soft palate. It is a part of respiratory tract. It communicates through pharyngeal isthmus with oropharynx. In the lateral wall, it receives the opening of pharyngotympanic tube half inch behind

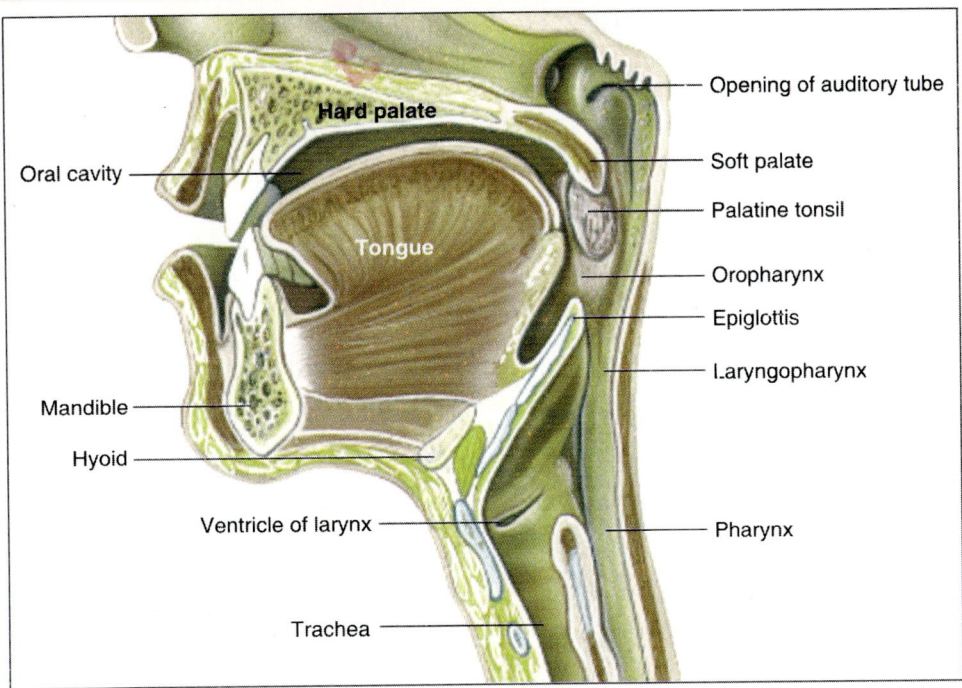

Fig. 46.1: Sagittal section of head & neck

at the level of inferior nasal concha. The opening is guarded by a curved prominence – **tubal elevation. Salpingopharyngeal fold** is a ridge of mucous membrane, which extends from the posterior margin of tubal elevation to side wall of pharynx downwards. Salpingopharyngeus lies in this fold. Behind the salpingopharyngeal fold is a narrow vertical depression – **pharyngeal recess.** The roof and the posterior wall form a continuous slope. Under the mucous membrane of it lymphoid tissue is placed called **nasopharyngeal tonsil.**

OROPHARYNX

It is placed behind the mouth and tongue. Oropharyngeal isthmus communicates it with oral cavity. This is common to both respiratory and digestive systems. Its posterior wall is smooth and the lateral walls have **palatine tonsils** placed in a triangular space placed (above and back of tongue and below soft palate) between palatoglossal and palatopharyngeal arches.

LARYNGOPHARYNX

It lies behind the larynx. Its upper part is common to digestive and respiratory tracts. Its lower part, which is the narrowest part of the pharynx, is continuous with oesophagus. It is anterior and posterior walls are approximated except when food is passing. Posterior wall and lateral are smooth. Anterior wall from above downwards presents

- Epiglottis
- Arytenoids and cricoid cartilages
- Aryepiglottic folds
- Inlet of larynx
- Pyriform fossa

Thus, the anterior wall forms the back of larynx.

ARRANGEMENT OF CONSTRICTORS

The musculature of pharynx differs from the rest of the musculature of gastrointestinal tract in the following:

- Muscles are skeletal
- Longitudinal muscles are placed inside
- Circular muscles (**constrictors**) are incomplete anteriorly. These muscles are arranged in three layers overlapping each other.

Constrictors of pharynx are

- Superior constrictor
- Middle constrictor
- Inferior constrictor

Superior constrictor

It has four parts from above downwards, namely:

1. Pterygopharyngeus
2. Buccopharyngeus
3. Mylopharyngeus
4. Glossopharyngeus

The highest fibers are attached to the pharyngeal tubercle while the lowest fibers reach up to the level of vocal cords. The space between the base of skull and the upper fiber (space of **Morgagni**) is occupied by auditory tube surrounded by tensor and levator palati.

Middle constructor

It arises from stylohyoid ligament, lesser and greater cornu of hyoid bone. The fibers overlap superior constrictor. The lowest fibers reach up to the level of vocal cords. Stylopharyngeus and Glosso-pharyngeal nerve (IX CN) enter deeper plane by traversing space along the lower border of superior constrictor and upper border of middle constrictor.

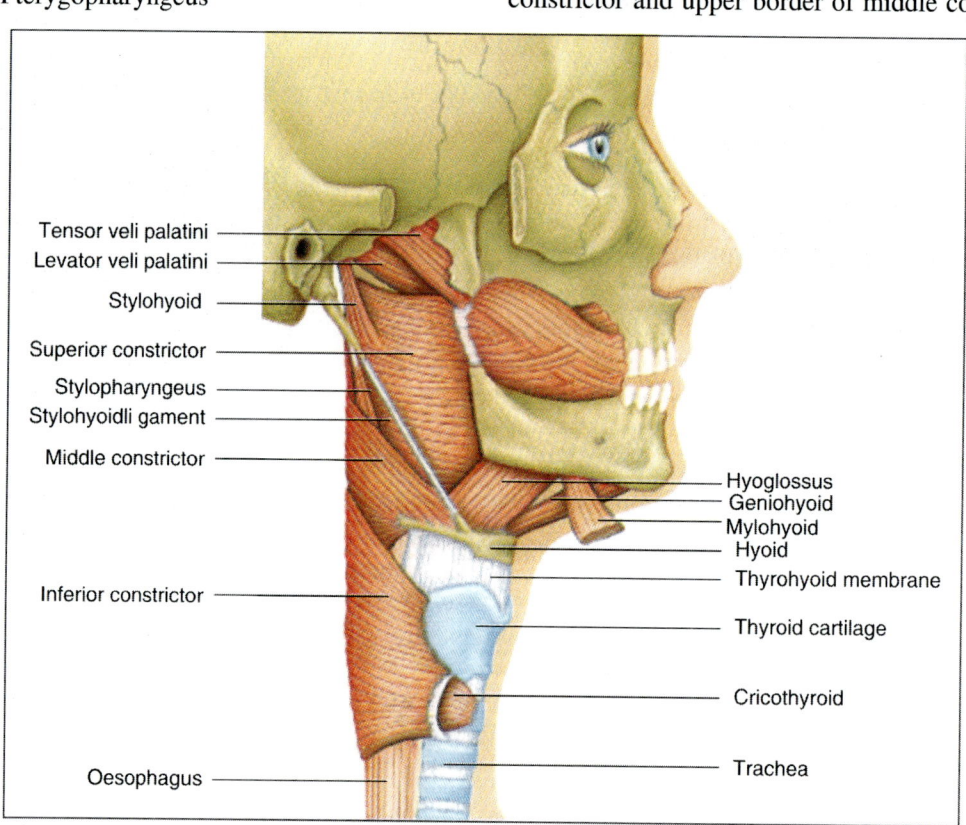

Fig. 46.2: Constrictors of pharynx

Inferior constrictor

It has two parts
- **Thyropharyngeus**
- **Cricopharyngeus**

Thyropharyngeus overlaps middle constrictor. Cricopharyngeus forms a sling below the level of vocal cords by becoming continuous with the other side. It has no attachment of the pharyngeal raphe.

Superior laryngeal nerve and vessels appear in the space between lower border of middle constrictor and upper border of inferior constrictor. The space between the lower border of inferior constrictor and oesophagus is occupied by **recurrent laryngeal and inferior laryngeal vessels**.

The longitudinal muscles are
1. Stylopharyngeus
2. Salpingopharyngeus
3. Palatopharyngeus

These muscles are attached to the posterior border of thyroid cartilage. These muscles help in second stage of deglutition by lifting the pharynx.

PASSAVANT'S RIDGE

The upper fibers of palatopharyngeus along with the mucous membrane of pharynx form crescentric elevation at the level of hard palate. During second stage of deglutition, the soft palate is raised and is supported by this ridge.

SOFT PALATE

It is a musculo-membranous structure which separates nasopharynx from oropharynx. Anteriorly it is continuous with hard palate while its posterior border is free. It has seromucous glands. In the middle from its posterior border, uvula hangs as a protrusion. It moves during speech. Laterally it blends with the sidewalls of pharynx.

Structure

From oral surface to pharyngeal surface
- Mucous membrane with stratified squamous epithelium
- Mucous glands forming the thickest layer
- Layer of muscle – Palatoglossus
- Palatine aponeurosis
- Layer of muscles – Levator palati and palatopharyngeus
- Mucous membrane (respiratory type)

The oropharyngeal isthmus is bounded by
- **Above** - Soft palate
- **Below** - Tongue
- **Sides** - Palatoglossal arch

PALATINE ARCH

This is the vault-shaped muscular structure forming the soft palate between the mouth and the nasopharynx. An opening in the arch connects the mouth with the oropharynx. It has uvula (containing musculus uvulae) which is suspended from the middle of the posterior border of the arch.

PHARYNGEAL TONSIL

These are two large masses of lymphoid tissue situated on the posterior wall of the nasopharynx behind the posterior nares.

During childhood these masses often enlarge and block the air passage from the nasal cavity into the pharynx. This prevents the child from breathing through the nose.

PALATINE TONSIL

These are paired almond-shaped masses of lymphoid tissue situated between the palatoglossal and palatopharyngeal arches on each side. They are covered with mucous membrane and contain numerous lymph follicles and various crypts.

Blood supply of palatine tonsil

The palatine tonsil has rich blood supply from the neighboring arteries. These are the branches entering the tonsil from the various aspects as under:

Anteriorly – Dorsal lingual

Inferiorly – Facial

Posteriorly – Ascending pharyngeal

Superiorly – Lesser palatine

Laterally – Facial

The venous return is by a venous plexus placed on the capsule laterally. The veins drain into the lingual vein while some are connected to pharyngeal venous plexus. **Paratonsillar vein** (external palatine vein) runs down from the soft palate, pierces superior constrictor muscle in the tonsillar bed and joins the pharyngeal plexus. This vein is embedded in the capsule, which gets thickened due to repeated infections. It may be the chief source of bleeding in tonsillectomy.

DEGLUTITION

Swallowing or deglutition is completed in three stages:

1st stage: It is voluntary. The intrinsic muscles of the tongue help in pushing the bolus against the hard palate towards the oropharynx.

2nd stage: The later part of this stage is involuntary in nature. To prevent regurgitation of the food into nasopharynx:

- **Nasopharyngeal isthmus is narrowed** by the raising of soft palate. The muscles involved are tensor palati and levator palati; climbing on the palatopharyngeal fold (**Passavant's ridge**).

- **Oropharyngeal isthmus is narrowed** by raising of posterior part of tongue by styloglossus and palatoglossus

- **Closure of laryngeal inlet** – it is not a complete closure. The epiglottis is raised and bends to prevent the descent of bolus into the posterior part of laryngopharynx. Aryepiglotticus and the longitudinal muscles of the pharynx bring about the change in the position of epiglottis.

3rd stage: It is involuntary in nature. It permits food bolus to enter oesophagus. This is brought about by gradual rhythmic contractions of constrictions of pharynx. Propulsive action of thyropharyngeus helps in entry of bolus into oesophagus.

IX CRANIAL NERVE (GLOSSOPHARYNGEAL NERVE)

It is a mixed cranial nerve

Nerve components

Branchial efferent

This is the nerve of III branchial arch and thus supplies stylopharyngeus

General visceral efferent

Through Otic ganglion it supplies parotid gland

General visceral afferent

Carries general sensation from

- Palate
- Tongue
- Tonsil
- Oropharynx
- Carotid sinus

Special visceral afferent

Carries taste sensation from

- Posterior 1/3 of tongue including circumvallate papillae

Somatic afferent

Carries sensations from tympanic membrane

NUCLEI

Branchial efferent

Nucleus Ambiguus – in the open part of medulla

General visceral efferent

Inferior salivatory nucleus – in the open part of medulla

General visceral afferent

Dorsal nucleus of vagus – in the open part of medulla

Special visceral efferent

Nucleus of tractus solitarius – in the open part of medulla

Somatic afferent

Spinal nucleus of trigeminal – in the open part of medulla and lower pons

COURSE

Intraneural course

Axons from various nuclei run laterally

    Emerge at the postero-lateral sulcus between olive and inferior cerebellar peduncle

Intracranial course

3-4 rootlets join to form trunk under the flocculus of cerebellum

    Rests on jugular tubercle

    Bends sharply

    Enters central part of jugular foramen – making a deep notch in the inferior border of petrous bone.

Extracranial course

Under styloid apparatus

Passes forwards between internal jugular vein (IJV) and internal carotid artery (ICA)

Descends over and in front of ICA upto lower border of stylopharyngeus

Curves forwards over stylopharyngeus

Runs deep to external carotid artery (ECA) and stylohyoid ligament

Ascends under hyoglossus to enter the tongue

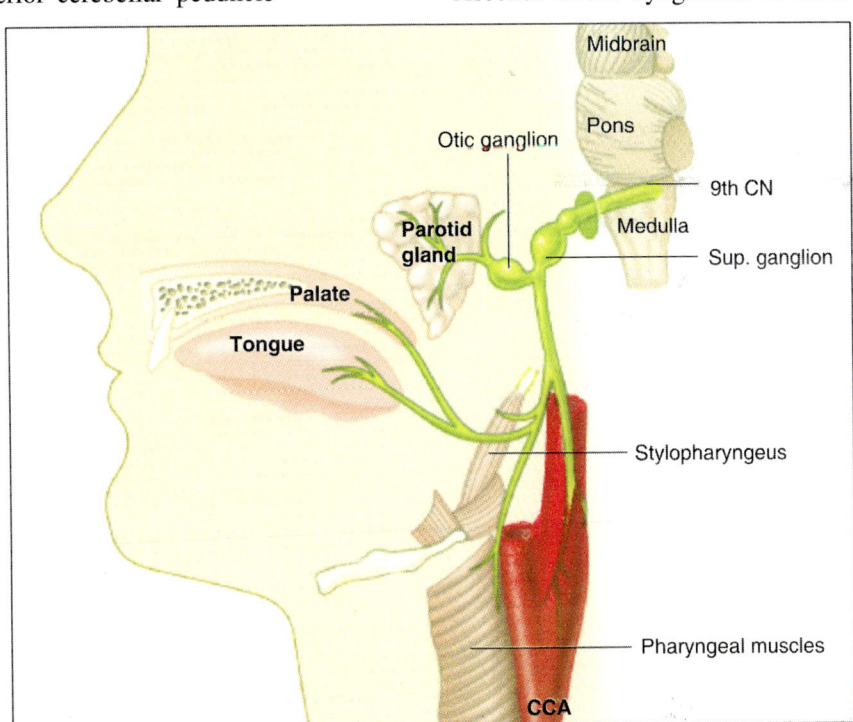

Fig. 46.3: Glossopharyngeal Nerve

BRANCHES

Tympanic branch - Parotid gland

Motor - Stylopharyngeus

Superior ganglion of X

- Carotid sinus - C S
- Tonsillar -Tonsil
- Pharyngeal - Oropharynx
- Lingual - Posterior 1/3 of tongue including circumvallate papillae
- Auricular -Tympanic membrane

CLINICAL CONSIDERATIONS

GAG REFLEX (Pharyngeal reflex)

It is a normal neural reflex elicited by touching the soft palate or posterior pharynx. The normal response will be

- Symmetrical elevation of the palate
- Retraction of the tongue
- Contraction of the pharyngeal muscles

The reflex is used to test

- Vagus nerve (X CN) and
- Glossopharyngeal nerve (IX CN)

Pharyngitis

It is the inflammation of the pharynx which causes symptoms of sore throat. Important causes include

- Diphtheria
- Herpes simplex virus
- Infectious mononucleosis
- Streptococcal infection

Symptoms may be relieved by analgesics, drinking warm liquids or saline irrigation of the throat.

Sore Throat

It is an infection of the oropharynx and palatine tonsils generally caused by streptococcus bacteria. The infection is characterized by

- Sore throat
- Chills

- Fever
- Swollen lymph nodes in the neck
- Nausea and vomiting (sometimes)

The symptoms usually begin abruptly a few days after exposure to airborne droplets or after direct contact with an infected person.

Dysphagia

Difficulty in swallowing is termed as **dysphagia**. It may have intrinsic or extrinsic causes. Important causes of dysphagia include:

Extrinsic – Thyroid swellings, aortic aneurysm

Intrinsic – Carcinoma of oesophagus.

Difficulty in swallowing is commonly associated with obstructive or motor disorders of the oesophagus.

Patients with obstructive disorders like oesophageal tumour can not swallow solids but can tolerate liquids.

Persons with motor disorders (achalasia) can not swallow solids or liquids. Diagnosis of the underlying condition is by

- Barium studies
- Clinical signs
- Evaluation of the patient's symptoms

Dyspepsia

It is a vague feeling of epigastric discomfort which is felt after eating. There is an uncomfortable feeling of fullness, heartburn, bloating, and nausea.

It may be a sign of underlying intestinal disorder

- Peptic ulcer
- Gall bladder disease
- Chronic appendicitis

Peritonsillar abscess

It is also called **quinsy**.

It is an infection of tissue between the tonsil and pharynx. It results usually after acute follicular tonsillitis.

Symptoms include

- Dysphagia

- Pain radiating to the ear
- Fever

Redness and swelling of the tonsil and adjacent soft palate is observed.

Management includes antibiotics, warm saline irrigation, incision and drainage with suction. Quinsy (**paratonsillar abscess**) is drained by an incision in the most prominent part of the abscess where softening can be felt.

In most cases it is treated by tonsillectomy.

Embryological basis of cleft palate

The development of palate is completed by fusion of:

- Two horizontal plates of maxillary process
- Frontonasal process

Any derangement in this fusion can lead to different grades of cleft lip and cleft palate. The cleft palate could be anterior or posterior to incisive fossa. It may be complete. Cleft palate presents with difficulty in swallowing and phonation. This is more common in female.

This congenital defect is characterized by a fissure in the midline of the palate. This results from the failure of the two sides to fuse during embryonic development.

The fissure may be complete which extends through both hard palate and soft palate into the nasal cavities.

There may be incomplete or partial cleft. This condition occurs approximately once in every 2500 live births. It is often associated with upper cleft lip. Together these abnormalities are the most common of the craniofacial malformations. These account for half of the total number of defects.

Surgical repair of the defect is not done until the first or second year of life and performed in steps.

Long-term postoperative problems include

- Speech impairment
- Hearing loss

- Improper tooth development and alignment
- Chronic respiratory and ear infections

Cleft lip (Hare lip)

It is a congenital anomaly consisting of one or more clefts in the upper lip. This results from the failure of fusion of the maxillary and median nasal processes in the embryonic life.

Treatment – surgical repair in early childhood.

Killian's dehiscence and pharyngeal diverticulum

Posteriorly between thyropharyngeus and cricopharyngeus of inferior constrictor there is a gap – **killian's dehiscence**. Through this gap the mucosa of pharynx may protrude posterolaterally – pharyngeal diverticulum. This diverticulum is because of neuromuscular incoordination. Pharyngeal plexus supplies thyropharyngeus while cricopharyngeus is supplied by recurrent laryngeal nerve. In addition to this disparity, the muscular incoordination is enhanced by difference in their action. Normally the propulsive contraction of thyropharyngeus is accompanied by relaxation of cricopharyngeus to permit easy descend of food bolus. The incoordination between two components of inferior constrictor leads to strain at Killian's dehiscence. Repeated episodes of this incoordination would lead to appearance of a pharyngeal diverticulum from this site.

Retropharyngeal abscess

Acute retropharyngeal abscess arise from enlarged retropharyngeal lymph nodes. The bucco-pharyngeal fascia enters the posterior wall of pharynx in the midline to the prevertebral fascia. Hence acute abscess that is in front of the prevertebral fascia, would appear as paramedian swelling. **Chronic retropharyngeal abscess** usually originates from tuberculosis of cervical vertebrae. The swelling is behind the prevertebral fascia. Initially it appears as midline swelling.

Subsequently the abscess gravitates and may be seen in under the prevertebral fascia in:

- Posterior triangle
- Superior mediastinum
- Axilla (along axillary sheath)

The axillary swelling is restricted by the fusion of axially sheath with adventitial lining of the axillary artery. The swelling in the superior mediastinum does not descend into posterior mediastinum, because at T-4 vertebra prevertebral fascia blends with anterior longitudinal ligament.

Adenoids

At the junction of roof and posterior wall of naso-pharynx, collection of lymphoid tissue in the midline is termed as pharyngeal tonsil. It is a part of **Waldayer's ring**. Its enlargement in children causes obstruction of posterior nasal aperture. This is reflected as **adenoid facies.** This is characterized by:

- Open mouth with protruded tongue
- Pinched nose

Adenoidal speech

It is an abnormal speech caused by hypertrophy of the adenoidal lymphoid tissue that normally exists in the nasopharynx of children. It is characterized by a muted, nasal quality. It is corrected by surgical removal of the adenoids.

Adenoidectomy

It is the surgical removal of the lymphoid tissue in the nasopharynx. The surgical procedure is performed because the adenoids are enlarged which cause obstruction or chronic infection.

Adenoids are excised as a prophylactic measure during tonsillectomy. This is performed under general anesthesia in children. After removal of the adenoids, bleeding is checked. In some cases vessels may be ligated.

Tonsillitis

It is an infection or inflammation of a tonsil. Acute tonsillitis is frequently caused by streptococcus infection. It is characterized by

- Severe sore throat
- Fever, headache and malaise
- Difficulty in swallowing
- Earache
- Enlarged and tender lymph nodes in the neck

Management includes systemic antibiotics, analgesics and warm saline gargles. **Tonsillectomy** is done for recurrent tonsillitis or tonsillar abscess.

Tonsillectomy

Infections of tonsil (**tonsillitis**) – acute and chronic, are commonly seen in children. Repeated episodes of tonsillitis may lead to **paratonsillar abscess**, which is known as **quinsy**.

Tonsillectomy is indicated in chronic tonsillitis. Tonsils can be removed by

- **Guillotine method**
- **Dissection method**

In Guillotine method: Guillotine is applied to the tonsil held in the ring of the instrument. Thus entire tonsil is removed intact.

In dissection method: Along the anterior pillar of tonsil an incision is made and the gland is dissected out by blunt dissection. Glands held only by the pedicle of the vessels near the lower pole. Important precaution – irrigate tonsillar bed thoroughly because superior constrictor may not contract effectively in presence of a clot.

Lesions of X CN

Unilateral lesion of the vagus nerve (X CN) at or near the skull base results in

- **Dysphonia** – altered voice production – **hoarseness**
- **Dysphagia** – difficulty in swallowing

The dysphagia results from an inability of levator palati to elevate the soft palate sufficiently to seal the pharyngeal isthmus. Thus, food passes into the nasopharynx.

Examination

- Arch of the soft palate is sagged on the affected side.
- Uvula is drawn to the nonparalyzed side as the patient says **Aaah**. This is due to the unopposed pull of the intact muscles acting on the soft palate.

The **hoarseness** is due to the uncompensated unilateral loss of function of the intrinsic muscles of the larynx.

Lesions of the recurrent laryngeal nerve are more common. They are often an iatrogenic (physician-caused) consequence of neck surgery

- Thyroidectomy
- Carotid endarterectomy
- Procedures on or near the aortic arch

In such cases the nerve may be severed or traumatized by clamping or stretching.

A left unilateral lesion may also result from

- Aortic aneurysm
- Metastatic carcinoma involving the paratracheal lymph nodes in lung or breast cancer
- Extension of carcinoma of the thyroid or oesophagus

Paralysis of all the intrinsic laryngeal muscles innervated by the vagus/recurrent laryngeal nerve on one side leaves the affected cord fixed in the paramedian position.

Though the paralyzed cord rests close to the midline, the glottis cannot be closed completely for phonation.

The decrease in cord tension causes reduction of vocal intensity and range.

Bilateral paralysis results in difficult or distressful respiration (**dyspnoea**). Both cords are adducted to the paramedian position with a glottic gap of only 2 mm to 3 mm. The voice is weak. Since these cords do not abduct for inspiration, the airway is inadequate. The slightest exertion produces dyspnoea and stridor.

Permanent relief is obtained by

- Tracheostomy
- Intralaryngeal surgery (arytenoidectomy)

47

Nasal Cavity

Excise the nasal septum piecemeal without damaging the mucous membrane on the other side. Separate the nerves from the mucous membrane and then excise the membrane to open the nasal cavity.

Remove the anterior part of the inferior concha and expose the **opening of nasolacrimal duct**. Pass a probe up the duct into the lacrimal sac. Remove the thin plate of bone over the duct and expose the duct and the sac.

Follow the nasopalatine nerve from the nasal septum, across the roof of the nose to the sphenopalatine foramen.

Identify
- Sphenopalatine artery

Reflect the mucous membrane over the medial pterygoid plate anteriorly and expose **nasal branches of greater palatine nerve** as they pierce the perpendicular plate of palatine bone.

Identify
- Greater palatine nerve
  It is seen through perpendicular plate of the palatine bone.
- Descending palatine artery - accompanies the nerve

Remove perpendicular plate of the bone and expose the nerve and artery. Open the entire canal by removing the remaining lamina lying medial to the canal. Note that the nerve passes up to join **pterygopalatine ganglion** at the level of sphenopalatine foramen.

Identify
- Nasopalatine nerve

Remove a transverse strip of the hard palate near the lower end of the canal and open the palatine foramen through which the **greater palatine nerve** reaches the hard palate. Excise the fibrous sheath of the nerve to expose **lesser palatine nerves** along its upper part. Trace them as they enter separate bony canals in the lower part. Open these canals and trace the nerves to the soft palate.

Excise three nasal conchae. Remove thin medial walls of the ethmoidal air cells. Remove the mucous membrane lining these cells, and the bony walls between them and expose the medial surface of the orbital lamina of ethmoid.

Remove the medial wall of maxillary sinus from the greater palatine canal to the nasolacrimal duct. Study the sinus from inside. Remove the orbital process of palatine bone and posterior part of the roof of the sinus.

Expose
- Maxillary nerve in the pterygopalatine fossa
- Pterygopalatine ganglion
- Terminal part of the maxillary artery

Remove the sphenoid bone medial to the ganglion. Avoid damage to the pharyngeal branch of the ganglion and the **nerve of the pterygoid canal** entering its posterior surface.

Chip away the floor of the infraorbital groove and canal. Trace the **infraorbital nerve** anteriorly. Identify its **anterior superior alveolar branch** and trace it through its bony canal below the opening of the naso-lacrimal duct, into the anterior part of the floor of the nose above the incisor teeth. Lift it out of the canal and identify its branches to the upper teeth, gums and mucosa of the maxillary sinus.

NASAL CAVITY

NASAL SEPTUM

It is formed by bones and cartilages.
Bones
- Perpendicular plate of ethmoid
- Vomer

Cartilages – Septal cartilages

Cuticular part – Fibrofatty tissue
The epithelium in the upper part is olfactory in nature and the remaining is respiratory (**pseudo-stratified**)

Nerve supply

Olfactory region –Olfactory nerve

Antero-superior part – Anterior ethmoidal nerve → nasociliary → V-1

Postero-inferior part
- Sphenopalatine nerve.
- Nerve of pterygoid canal
- Greater palatine nerve.

All are the branches of V-2.

Antero-inferior part – Infraorbital branch of V-2
Thus branches of maxillary nerve predominantly supply the nasal septum.

Blood supply

Antero-superior part – Anterior ethmoidal artery
Antero-inferior part – Septal branches of facial artery

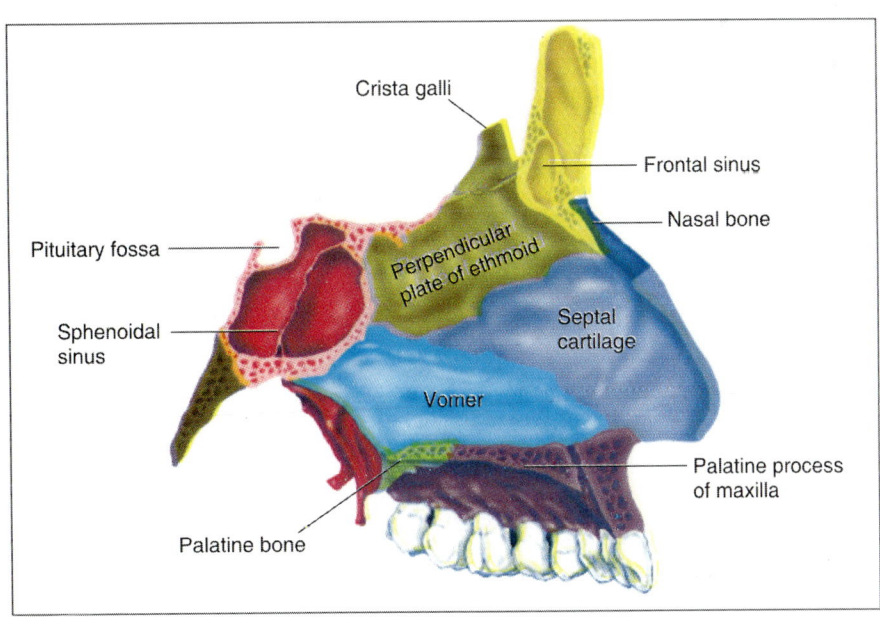

Fig. 47.1: Nasal Septum

Postero-inferior part – Greater palatine and sphenopalatine arteries

LATERAL WALL OF NOSE

It is formed by bones, cartilage and fibro fatty tissue.

Bones – Maxilla, ethmoid with superior and middle nasal conchae and inferior nasal concha.

Cartilages – Upper and lower nasal cartilage and alar cartilage.

Cuticular part by fibrofatty tissue

This wall is covered by mucoperiosteum.

The mucosa is highly vascular to

- Humidity the air
- Warm the inspired air

The **conchae** are also termed as turbinate bones. They help to regulate the flow of air. They reduce the force of inhaled air. The serous glands in the mucosa help in moistening the inspired air. The mucosa is similar to cavernous tissue and in females it shows changes during the menstrual cycle (more in menstrual phase). The lateral wall has following components from anterior to posterior.

- Vestibule
- Atria
- Region of meati

Nerve supply

Above the superior concha – Olfactory nerve

Antero-superiorly – Anterior ethmoidal → nasociliary → V-1

Antero-inferiorly – Anterior superior alveolar → V-2

Postero-superiorly – Branches from Pterygo-palatine ganglion

Posteroinferiorly – Branches from Pterygo-palatine ganglion

Blood supply

The four quadrants of lateral wall receive blood supply predominantly from the branches of maxillary artery.

Antero-superior – Anterior ethmoidal → Ophthalmic artery

Antero-superior

- Alar branch of facial artery
- Branch from greater palatine

Postero-superior – Sphenopalatine artery → Maxillary (third part)

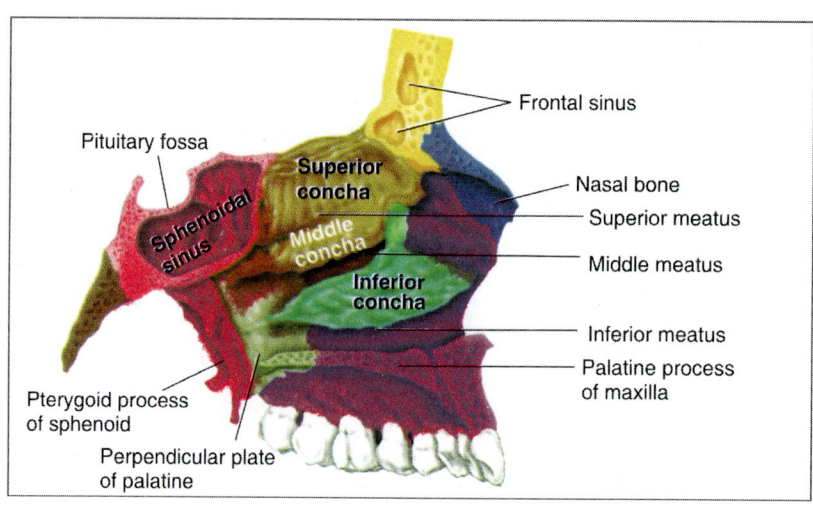

Fig. 47.2: Lateral wall of nose

Postero- inferior – Greater palatine artery →
Maxillary (third part)

The venous plexus lies over inferior and middle
conchae and is connected to:

- Cerebral vein via ethmoidal vein
- Pterygoid venous plexus
- Anterior facial vein

FUNCTIONAL ASPECTS OF PARANASAL SINUSES

Developmentally, the paranasal sinuses are the out
pouches from the lateral wall of nose. Hence all
these sinuses open in the lateral wall of nose. These
sinuses are:

- Frontal sinus
- Sphenoidal sinus
- Ethmoidal group of sinuses
- Maxillary sinus

These sinuses are absent / rudimentary at birth. The
maxillary sinus (largest) is present at birth (all these
sinuses start appearing / growing after 6th year of
life. Only after puberty these sinuses enlarge in
dimension and attain maximum size in old age.
These sinuses are bilateral but asymmetrical. They
are lined by mucous membrane, which is not as
firmly attached as that of lateral wall of nose. Among
the functions, no definite roll can be ascribed to
them. However they:

1. Impart resonance to voice
2. Act as insulators to regulate the temperature
   of inhaled air
3. May contribute in reducing the weight of
   the skull
4. They also contribute in humidifying the
   inspired air.

The openings of paranasal sinuses are placed in a
definite manner. From posterior to anterior in three
meati:

- **Sphenoidal air sinus** – Sphenoethmoidal
  recess

- **Posterior ethmoidal sinus** – Superior
  meatus
- **Middle and anterior ethmoidal sinuses**
  – Middle meatus under cover of bulla
  ethmoidale
- **Maxillary sinus** – Hiatus semilunaris of
  middle meatus
- **Frontal sinus** – Infundibulum of middle
  meatus.

In addition to these, the inferior meatus receives
nasolacrimal duct.

PTERYGOPALATINE GANGLION (SPHENOPALATINE GANGLION)

It is a parasympathetic ganglion to carry
secretomotor fibers from superior salivary and
lacrimatory nuclei to:

- Lacrimal gland
- Palatine glands
- Nasal glands
- Pharyngeal glands

It is situated in the pterygopalatine fossa. It has
three roots

Sensory root – Two in number connecting to
maxillary nerve

Parasympathetic / secretomotor root

This is termed as nerve of pterygoid canal. Two
nerves form it, namely:

1. **Greater superficial petrosal nerve**
   (mixed) which carries secretomotor
   impulses to the gland and afferent of taste
   sensation
2. **Deep petrosal nerve** carries postganglionic
   sympathetic impulses.

Sympathetic root

Formed by the plexus around internal carotid artery.
Deep petrosal nerve arises from this plexus to join
greater superficial petrosal nerve to form the nerve
of pterygoid canal (**Vidian's nerve**)

The nerve enters pterygopalatine fossa to reach
pterygopalatine ganglion.

Branches from the ganglion:

- Nasal
- Palatine
- Pharyngeal

The branch to lacrimal gland runs in zygomatico-temporal branch of maxillary nerve to join lacrimal nerve (ophthalmic nerve: V-1) to innervate lacrimal gland.

Taste sensations from the palate are carried in the peripheral process of geniculate ganglion. These peripheral processes are represented by palatine branch → pterygopalatine ganglion (without relay) → Vidian's nerve → greater superficial petrosal nerve. The central process of geniculate ganglion carries the taste sensations to nucleus of tractus solitaries.

OLFACTORY NERVE

The olfactory nerve is the first cranial nerve. It is composed of numerous fine filaments that ramify in the mucous membrane of the olfactory area of lateral wall of nose and nasal septum. It is the nerve of smell.

The fibers of the olfactory nerve are non-medullated and unite into fasciculi that form a plexus under the mucous membrane and pass through the cribriform plate of ethmoid bone.

The fibers pass into the skull and form synapses with the dendrites of the mitral cells. The area in which the olfactory nerves arise is situated in the most superior portion of the mucous membrane that covers the superior nasal concha. The olfactory sensory endings are modified epithelial cells. These are least specialized of the special senses. The olfactory nerves connect with the olfactory bulb and the olfactory tract. These are components of the part of the brain associated with the sense of smell.

CLINICAL CONSIDERATIONS

Little's area and epistaxis

Little's area (**Kieselbach's area**) lies at the anteroinferior part of nasal septum, lies.

This area is highly vascularized having a rich anastomosis. This anastomosis is formed by:

- Anterior ethmoidal artery
- Sphenopalatine artery
- Septal branch of superior labial branch of facial artery
- Greater palatine artery

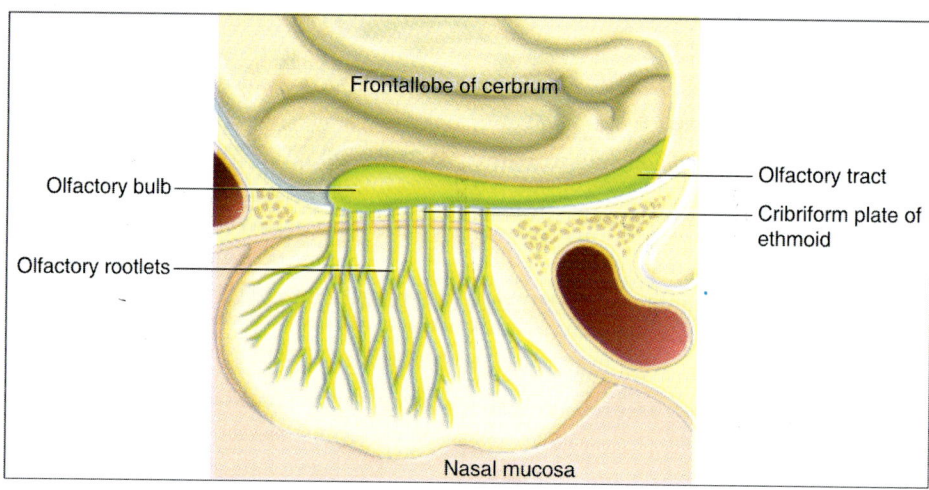

Fig. 47.3: Olfactory Nerve

This area is also known as **Little's area of epistaxis.** The bleeding through nose – epistaxis results because of rupture of vessels due to various causes, namely

1. Sudden rise in blood pressure
2. High temperature
3. High attitude

Sinusitis

Inflammation of mucosal lining of paranasal sinuses is termed as **sinusitis**. Frontal sinusitis or maxillary sinusitis is common after common cold. Frontal sinusitis causes heaviness and pain in the forehead as the patient bends his head.

It may be a complication of

1. Upper respiratory infection
2. Dental infection
3. Allergy
4. Change in atmosphere
5. Structural defect of the nose

The resultant swelling of nasal mucous membrane blocks the openings of the sinuses to the nasal cavity. This results in an accumulation of sinus secretions. This causes pressure, pain, headache, fever, and local tenderness.

Complications
- Cavernous sinus thrombosis
- Spread of infection to brain or meninges

Management includes steam inhalations, nasal decongestants and analgesics. Antibiotics are given when infection is present.

Surgery is done to improve drainage in chronic sinusitis.

Maxillary sinusitis requires surgical intervention to drain the stagnated inflammatory exudates by making an opening through the incisive fossa-**Caldwel Luc operation**. This procedure is carried out when the usual method of drainage of maxillary sinus does not give desired result. The drainage of maxillary sinus is via its opening eg. Hiatus semilunaris or by enlarging this opening – **Antrum puncture**. The **disadvantage** in this procedure is repeated maxillary sinusitis due to enlarged and exposed opening.

Deviated Nasal Septum

It may be congenital or acquired. Most individuals have mild degree of DNS but are asymptomatic

Here there is a shift in the partition (nasal septum) of the nasal cavity.

The nasal septum more commonly shifts to the left during normal growth. This deflection may be aggravated by a blow to the nose or by other injuries.

Severe deflection of the septum significantly obstructs the nasal passage and may result in
- Infection
- Sinusitis
- Breathlessness
- Headache
- Recurrent epistaxis

Severe deviated septum deviation is corrected by
- Rhinoplasty
- Septoplasty

Nasal Obstruction

This may reduce the breathing capacity. This is caused by
- Irregular septum
- Nasal polyps
- Foreign bodies
- Enlarged turbinates

Sinusitis is a common complication of nasal obstruction.

Nasal Polyp

It is a rounded and elongated mucosal mass projecting into the nasal cavity. It is an important cause of nasal obstruction.

Dacrystitis

The opening of nasolacrimal duct may be obstructed – congenital or acquired. This would lead to overflowing of tears. It can also lead to dacryocystitis – inflammation of lacrimal sac.

It is the infection of the lacrimal sac caused by obstruction of the nasolacrimal duct.

This is characterized by tearing and discharges from the eye. In the acute phase the lacrimal sac becomes inflamed and painful.

This is normally unilateral and usually occurs in infants.

Surgical treatment - dacryocystorhinostomy

- **Dacryocystorhinostomy** – surgical procedure for restoring drainage into the nose from the lacrimal sac when the nasolacrimal duct is obstructed
- **Dacryocystectomy** – Partial or total excision of the lacrimal sac

Rhinoplasty

It is a surgical procedure (plastic surgery) in which the structure of the nose is changed where bone or cartilage may be removed, tissue grafted from another part of the body or synthetic material implanted to alter the shape.

Rhinoscopy

This is the examination of the nasal cavity to inspect the mucosa and detect inflammation, deformities or asymmetry - deviation of the septum.

Nasal cavity may be examined anteriorly by introducing a speculum into the nostrils or posteriorly by introducing a rhinoscope through the nasopharynx.

Nasogastric intubation

This is the placement of a nasogastric tube through the nose into the stomach

- To relieve gastric distention by removing gas or gastric secretions
- To give medication, food or fluids
- To obtain a specimen for investigation

This is used in any condition in which the person is able to digest food but not able to eat. The tube is introduced and left in place for tube feeding until the ability to eat is restored.

CSF Rhinorrhoea

The fracture of cribriform plate of ethmoid leads to copious leakage of cerebrospinal fluid. This fluid discharge is too thin to be pure blood.

48

Tongue

Study the cut surface of the tongue.

Identify

- Genioglossus
- Geniohyoid

Note the positions and attachments of these muscles. Separate buccinator, pterygomandibular raphe and superior constrictor from their attachments to the mandible on the right side. Turn the body of the mandible downwards and expose the lateral surface of the tongue.

Identify

- Lingual nerve
- Palatoglossus

Remove mucous membrane from the lateral aspect of the tongue and trace extrinsic muscles of the tongue into its substance.

Identify

- Anterior lingual gland

These glands are seen as small, oval glandular mass on the undersurface of the tongue.

TONGUE

A thin median fibrous septum divides the tongue into right and left halves. Together they are composed of

- **Muscles** – Extrinsic and intrinsic
- **Fat**
- **Glands**
  - Mucous at the side and back
  - Serous near vallate papillae
  - Seromucous, e.g., anterior lingual gland

These are placed among the muscle

- **Covering of mucous membrane**

Components of tongue include

- Root
- Tip
- Body

The root is formed by the muscles and mucous membrane. It is fixed to hyoid bone, mandible, pharynx, epiglottis and palate.

Body has two parts – pharyngeal and oral. **Oral part** has rough mucous membrane caused by various types of papillae. **Sulcus terminalis** - V shaped groove separates it from the pharyngeal part. The apex of the groove is pointed backwards and has foramen caecum. The inferior surface of the free part of tongue has smooth mucous membrane. Frenulum connects it to the floor of the mouth in midline. On either side of frenulum, deep lingual vein is seen through the mucous membrane. Still laterally fringed fold - fimbriated fold is seen under which deep lingual artery is located.

Pharyngeal part is directed backwards into the

pharynx. Its mucous membrane is smooth and presents pitted nodes - **lingual tonsil**. It is connected to epiglottis by a median fold of mucous membrane - **median glosso-epiglottic fold**. Apex and margins of tongue are free and are in contact with the teeth. The extrinsic muscles move the tongue in different directions. These are:

- **Styloglossus**
- **Hyoglossus**
- **Genioglossus**
- **Palatoglossus**

The intrinsic muscles alter the shape of the tongue. These are:

- Superior longitudinal
- Inferior longitudinal
- Vertical muscle
- Transverse muscle

Papillae of tongue

The sulcus terminalis divides dorsum of tongue into anterior two third and posterior one third. The anterior two third (oral part) presents following papillae:

Filiform – These are in large number, arranged posteriorly in rows parallel to sulcus terminalis. They are irregularly placed anteriorly.

Foliate – These are five or six vertical folds along the margins in front of palatoglossal arch. These are studded with taste buds.

Fungiform – These are more numerous, bright red in appearance. Each has a rounded head with a narrow base. These are found chiefly at apex and margins. These have taste buds.

Circumvallate – About ten in number. These are placed anterior and parallel to sulcus terminalis. A circular trench, outer wall of which is raised as a collar, surrounds each. Serous glands (**Von Ebor's glands**) drain their secretion into the trench. The taste buds line its walls.

Blood Supply

Lingual artery is the chief source. This artery arises from external carotid artery (ECA) in the carotid

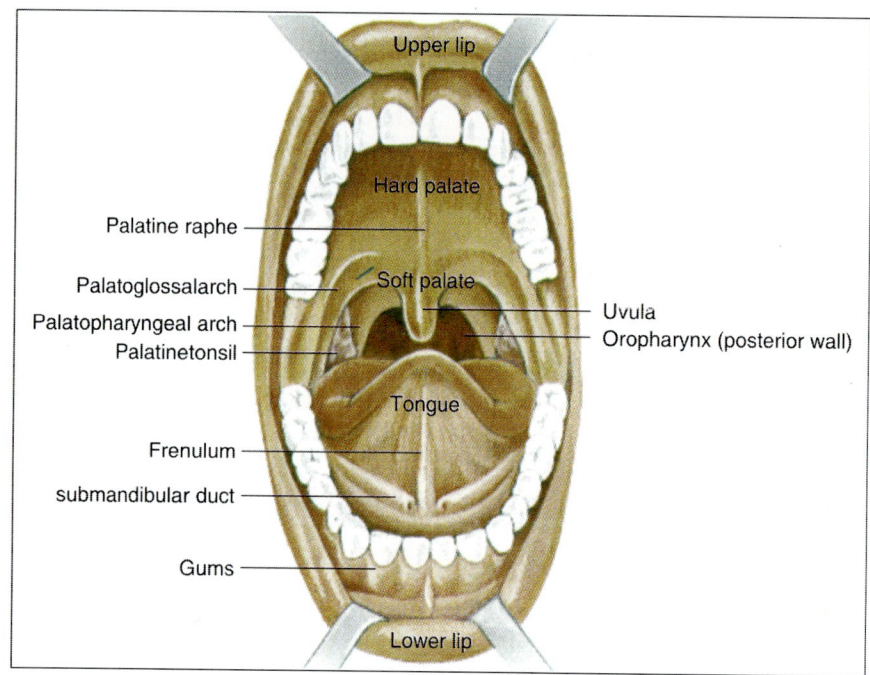

Fig. 48.1: Tongue and Palate

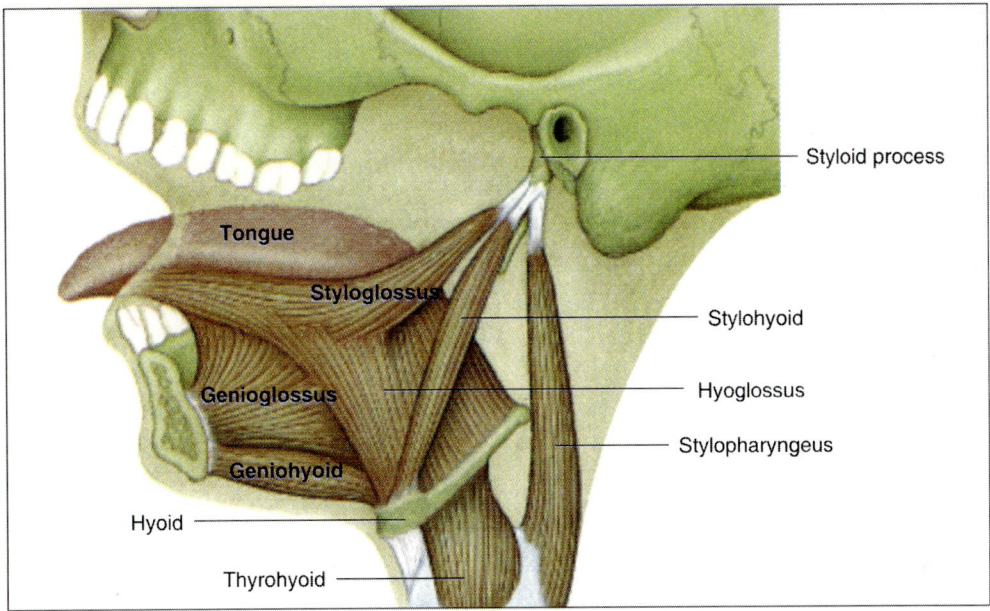

Fig. 48.2: Extrinsic muscles of Tongue

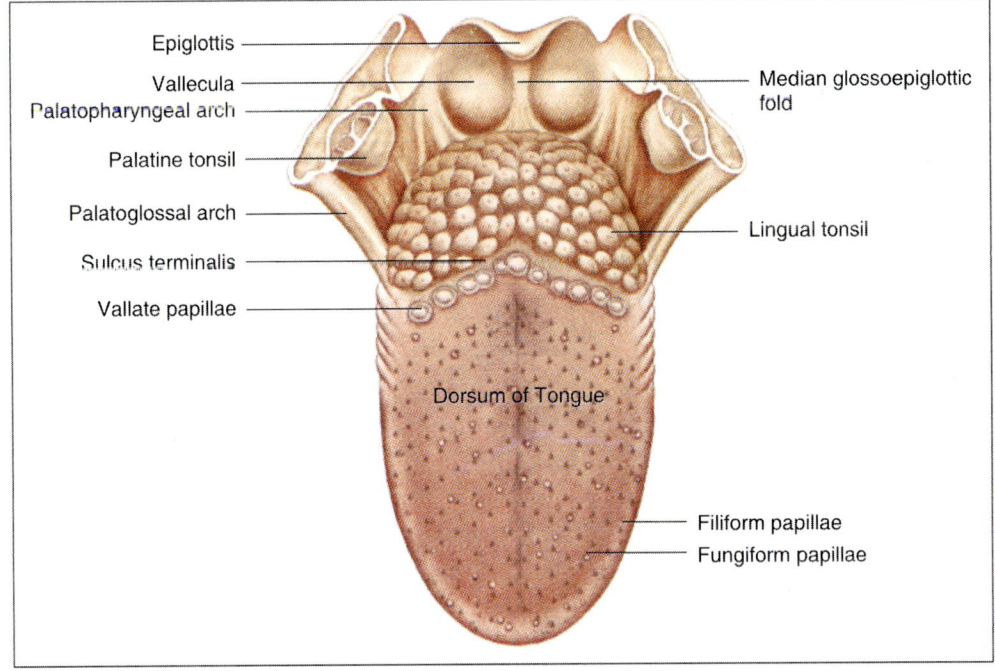

Fig. 48.3: Dorsum of Tongue

triangle. There is very little anastomosis across the **median plane. The lingual artery runs deep to hyoglossus.**

It divides into four branches, and supplies the tongue and surrounding muscles.

Branches of the lingual artery include
- Suprahyoid
- Dorsal lingual
- Sublingual
- Deep lingual

Deep lingual vein is formed by dorsal lingual veins, which drain into internal jugular vein (IJV).

LYMPHATIC DRAINAGE

Lymph vessels go the nearest lymph nodes
- From tip and lower surface – **Submental nodes**
- From margins – **Submandibular lymph nodes**
- From posterior one third, the lymph vessels pierce superior constrictor to drain into **Jugulo-digastric** group of lymph nodes
- From dorsum of tongue, the lymph vessels criss-cross to drain into **Submandibular nodes**

The **jugulo-omohyoid** lymph nodes receive lymphatics from submandibular lymph node, which in turn receives lymph from submental lymph nodes.

NERVE SUPPLY

Motor - All muscles of the tongue (**except palatoglossus**) are supplied by hypoglossal nerve (XII CN).

Sensory - From the anterior two third, general sensations are carried in lingual nerve and the taste sensation are carried by chorda tympani. From the mucous membrane of posterior one third of tongue including the circumvallate papillae, the general and taste sensations are carried in glossopharyngeal nerve (IX CN). Posterior most part of the tongue near epiglottis is innervated by internal laryngeal branch of superior laryngeal nerve which is a branch of vagus (X CN).

XII CRANIAL NERVE (HYPOGLOSSAL NERVE)

It is a motor nerve (? Mixed)

Supplies all muscles of tongue **except**
- Palatoglossus – Vago-Accessory complex
- Geniohyoid : C-1
- Thyrohyoid : C-1

Proprioceptive impulses from the tongue are carried in
- 12th nerve – (**Frorep's ganglion**)
- 5th nerve – to mesencephalic nucleus

NERVE COMPONENT
Somatic efferent

It is in the line with nuclei of 3rd, 4th & 6th cranial nerves

Nucleus

It is placed in the open part of medulla in the floor of IV ventricle – hypoglossal triangle

Course
Intraneural course

Fibers run anterolaterally to come out at the anterolateral sulcus between Pyramid and Olive

Intracranial course

Ten to twelve rootlets join to form 2 roots which form a trunk that pierces the dura mater to enter the hypoglossal canal

Extracranial course

Comes out of condylar canal
- Runs laterally
- Spirals around inferior ganglion of X nerve under cover of styloid apparatus

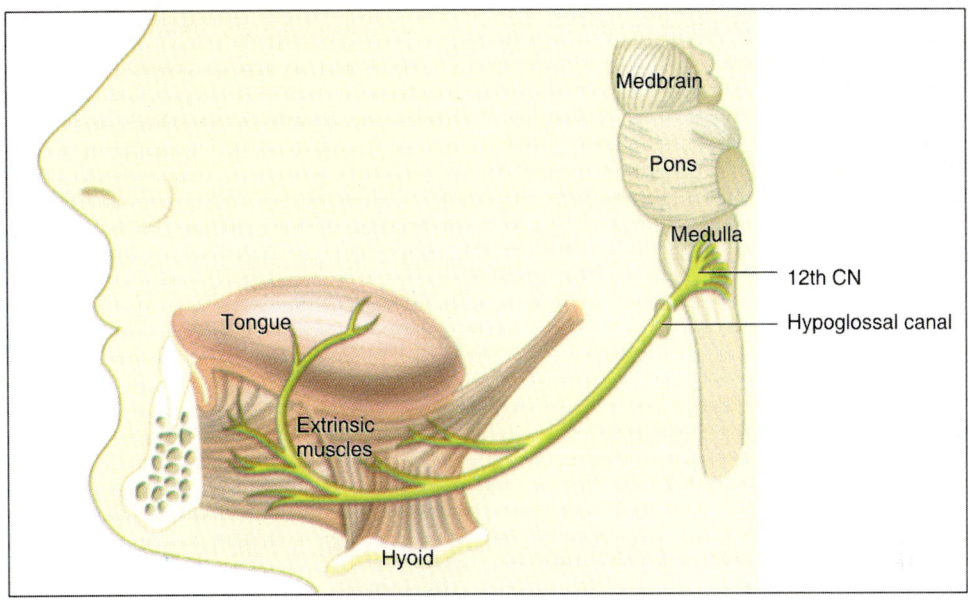

Fig. 48.4: Hypoglossal Nerve

– Descends along vagus over internal carotid artery and reaches lower border of posterior belly of digastric under cover of IJV

Runs forwards successively over

- Internal carotid artery (ICA)
- External carotid artery (ECA)
- Middle constrictor
- Hyoglossus

The nerve runs under cover of

- Posterior belly of digastric
- Stylohyoid
- Mylohyoid

The nerve ends end in genioglossus

Branches

Meningeal

Branch of C-1

Supplies dura of posterior cranial fossa

Muscular

- Styloglossus
- Hyoglossus
- Genioglossus

- Geniohyoid through C-1
- Thyrohyoid
- Omohyoid (superior belly)
- Sternohyoid
- Sternothyroid
- Omohyoid (inferior belly)

Last four muscles are supplied by descends hypoglossi through C-2, 3

CLINICAL CONSIDERATIONS

Clinical aspects of tongue

1. **Dorsal surface** of the tongue is an indicator of some clinical conditions. **For example:** in pernicious anemia, the tongue appears smooth and red while in central cyanosis it will appear bluish.

2. **In unconscious patient**, the tongue should be pulled out manually to prevent choking.

3. **Bleeding** from the tongue can be stopped temporarily by pulling the tongue out. In this first aid maneuver, the lingual artery is

compressed against the tip of greater cornu of hyoid bone.

Paralysis of Tongue

The tongue moves to the paralyzed side during protrusion of tongue. This is due to hemiatrophy of the tongue and unopposed action of normal genioglossus.

Carcinoma of tongue

It is fairly common in Indians due to tobacco chewing. Surgically it necessitates:

- Resection of affected part of tongue
- Block dissection of lymph nodes
- Hemi-mandibulectomy

This extensive operation is known as **Commando's operation**

Thromboses of anterior spinal artery

This may involve

12th nerve nucleus

- LMN type ipsilateral paralysis

Medial lemniscus

- Loss of conscious proprioceptive sensations on the contralateral side

Pyramid

- UMN paralysis on the contralateral side

Paralysis of XII CN

The tongue receives its motor innervation from the hypoglossal nerve (XII CN). It can protrude straight out and be held in the midline. This action is primarily the result of balanced bilateral contraction of

- Genioglossus muscles
- Vertical and transverse intrinsic muscles

Unilateral lesion of the hypoglossal nerve

The action of the contralateral, unparalyzed genioglossus muscle is unopposed, and the ipsilateral paralyzed muscle acts like an anchor holding the inactive side back. Thus, the tongue deviates toward the side of the nerve lesion.

Unilateral peripheral lesions of the nerve are usually due to

1. Traumatic wounds
2. Fractures base of skull

Complete bilateral paralysis is due to

- Lead, arsenic or alcohol poisoning

The tongue cannot protrude and lies flat in the mouth.

Unilateral or bilateral flaccid paralysis associated with atrophy is indicative of peripheral nerve involvement. In such cases

- Articulation is impaired
- Difficulty with chewing and swallowing

Supranuclear lesions result from

1. Medullary haemorrhage
2. Poliomyelitis
3. Bulbar palsies
4. Brain tumours
5. Brain abscesses

An upper motor neuron lesion (**UMN lesion**) results in fasciculation without atrophy of the tongue muscles. In such cases, the tongue deviates to the opposite side of the lesion.

49

Larynx

Reflect sternothyroid muscle upwards. Note its attachment to the thyroid cartilage. Define the attachments of inferior constrictor to thyroid, cricoid and the fascial arch crossing the cricothyroid muscle. Divide the arch and reflect the two parts of inferior constrictor and expose **cricothyroid muscle**.

Identify
- Articulation between inferior horn of the thyroid cartilage and cricoid cartilage
- Cricothyroid ligament

Divide thyrohyoid muscle and expose **thyrohyoid membrane** and the nerve and vessels piercing it. Note the attachments of the membrane.

Identify
- Epiglottis
- Thyroepiglottic ligament
- Hyoepiglottic ligament,

These are seen on the cut surface of the larynx.

Cut vestibular fold away from the upper part of arytenoid cartilage. Strip it away from the larynx. Avoid damage to the underlying **thyroepiglotticus muscle**. Separate it from the thyroid cartilage and open the saccule.

Separate the mucosa from the undersurface of the vocal fold and expose **conus elasticus** and **vocal ligament**. Separate conus elasticus from the upper border of the cricoid cartilage. Turn it up and dissect it away from the muscle lateral to it. Separate the mucous membrane from the upper surface of the vocal fold and expose upper surface of **thyroarytenoid muscle**. Note the continuity of the muscle with thyroepiglotticus.

Identify
- Recurrent laryngeal nerve

It enters larynx deep to inferior constrictor muscle. Remove the mucous membrane from the back of the arytenoid and cricoid cartilages. Find the attachment of the longitudinal fibres of the oesophagus in the form of a tendon to the median part of the cricoid lamina.

Identify
- Posterior cricoarytenoid
- Transverse arytenoid
- Oblique arytenoid muscles

Oblique arytenoid muscle is continuous with the aryepiglottic muscle.

Excise cricothyroid muscle. Excise on one side the lower part of the lamina and inferior horn of the thyroid cartilage and open the cricothyroid joint. Avoid damage to the recurrent laryngeal nerve which lies behind the cartilage.

Identify
- Thyroarytenoid muscle - in the vocal fold
- Lateral cricoarytenoid muscle

LARYNX

It is the organ of voice production. It is part of the air passage which connects pharynx with trachea. Thus functionally,

1. Passage of air
2. Phonation
3. Third stage of deglutition

Its thyroid cartilages forms laryngeal prominence called **Adam's apple** (larger in men than in women).

The larynx forms the lower part of the anterior wall of pharynx. It is lined with mucous membrane that is continuous with that of the pharynx and the trachea. The larynx extends vertically to the C-4 to C-6 cervical vertebrae. It is higher in the female and during childhood.

The larynx is broad above, narrow and cylindrical below.

Situation

– **Below** the hyoid bone and tongue
– **Between** carotid sheaths

– **In front** of C3-C6 vertebrae
    • Prevertebral muscles
    • Laryngo-pharynx

Anterolaterally it is related to

• Thyroid gland
• Infrahyoid strap muscles

Its position is variable

• **In foetus** – opposite C-3 and C-4 vertebrae
• **Till puberty** – extends gradually downwards till C-6 vertebra
• **Adult** – with movements of head and during deglutition and vocalization, its position changes

Structure of larynx

Cartilages form the framework of larynx. Membranes and ligaments join cartilages. They joints permit movement, which are carried by laryngeal muscles. It is lined with mucous membrane.

Cartilages

Three unpaired
• Epiglottis

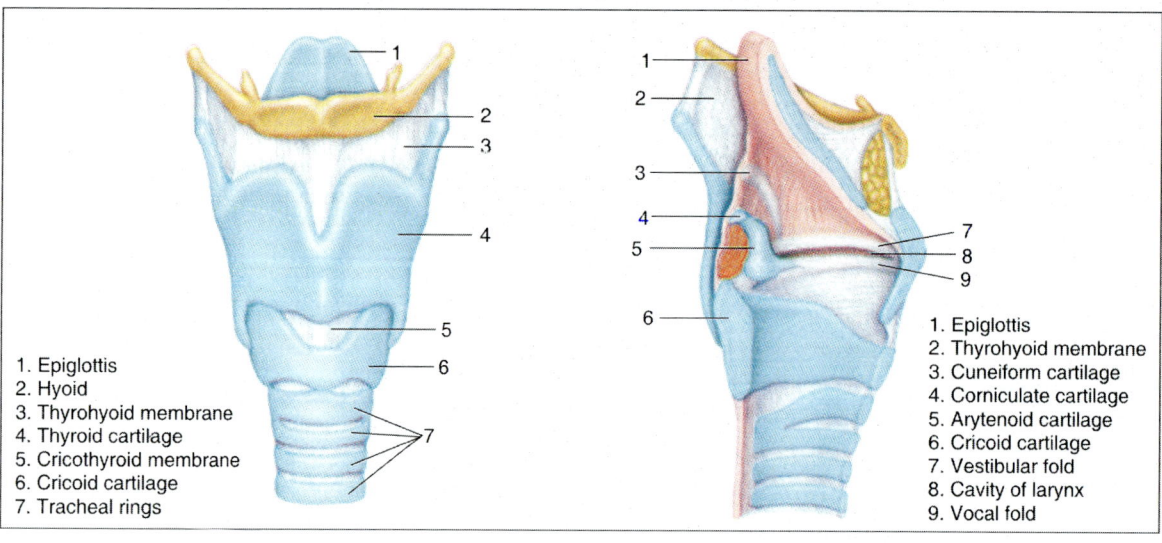

1. Epiglottis
2. Hyoid
3. Thyrohyoid membrane
4. Thyroid cartilage
5. Cricothyroid membrane
6. Cricoid cartilage
7. Tracheal rings

1. Epiglottis
2. Thyrohyoid membrane
3. Cuneiform cartilage
4. Corniculate cartilage
5. Arytenoid cartilage
6. Cricoid cartilage
7. Vestibular fold
8. Cavity of larynx
9. Vocal fold

Fig. 49.1: Larynx

- Thyroid
- Cricoid

Three paired
- Arytenoid
- Corniculate
- Cuneiform

Ligaments and membranes

Ligaments are both extrinsic and intrinsic.

Extrinsic ligaments are condensations - Thyrohyoid membrane and cricothyroid membrane.

Intrinsic ligaments are quadrate ligament and conus elasticus

- **Quadrate ligament** - Aryepiglottic fold and vestibular fold bound it. Anterolaterally it is attached to margins of epiglottis and posteriorly to the arytenoid cartilage. It bounds the vestibule of larynx laterally.
- **Conus elasticus** - It extends between the vocal folds and the upper margin of cricoid cartilage inferiorly. It is anchored anteriorly to the thyroid cartilage and cricothyroid membrane and posteriorly, to the base of arytenoid cartilage. It is covered by mucous membrane. Internally it bounds the cavity of larynx proper. Together, right and left conus elasticus constitute a sloping cone having vocal cords in its truncated apex.

Interior of larynx

It shows two pairs of shelf like projections
- Upper pair of vestibular folds
- Lower pair of vocal folds

Components

Vestibule – Above vestibular folds (**supra-glottic**)

Ventricle (glottic) – It is a narrow space between vestibular and vocal folds. It extends laterally as sinus of larynx.

Cavity of larynx proper (**infra-glottic**) - This lies below the vocal folds

Rima glottidis is the space between two vocal folds. Its parts are:
- Inter membranous
- Inter cartilaginous

Rima vestibuli is the space between two vestibular folds.

MUSCLES OF LARYNX

These are classified into
- Extrinsic muscles
- Intrinsic muscles

Extrinsic muscles move larynx as a whole

Those which pull up the hyoid bone and thyroid cartilage
- Digastric (both bellies)
- Mylohyoid
- Geniohyoid
- Thyrohyoid
- Stylohyoid

Those pull up thyroid cartilage
- Thyrohyoid
- Stylopharyngeus
- Palatopharyngeus
- Salpingopharyngeus

Those which depress the larynx
- Sternohyoid
- Sternothyroid
- Superior belly of omohyoid

Intrinsic muscles bring change in position of vocal cords

Lengthening of vocal cords
- Cricothyroid
- Vocalis

Abduction of vocal cords
- Posterior cricoarytenoid

Adduction of vocal cords
- Thyroarytenoid
- Lateral cricoarytenoid

These muscles reduce the inter-membranous part of rima glottidis while the inter- cartilaginous part of rima glottidis is widened.

- Inter-arytenoids (Transverse and oblique)

This reduces inter-membranous and inter-cartilaginous parts of rima glottidis

Depression of epiglottis

- Aryepiglotticus
- Thyroepiglotticus

Vocal cords (True vocal cord)

These are two strong bands of yellow elastic tissue in the larynx enclosed by membranes called vocal folds and attached ventrally to the angle of the thyroid cartilage and dorsally to the vocal process of the arytenoid cartilage.

False vocal cords

These are two thick folds of mucous membrane in the larynx separating the ventricle from the vestibule. Each fold encloses a narrow band of fibrous tissue (ventricular ligament).

CRICOTHYROID AND CRICOARYTENOID JOINTS

Developmentally cricothyroid is an extrinsic muscle of larynx and thus supplied by external laryngeal nerve.

Cricothyroid joint is between inferior horn of thyroid cartilage and lateral aspect of cricoid cartilage. It is a synovial joint of hinge variety. Movements occur in transverse axis passing through both joints. There is tilting of cricoid cartilage backwards. This is primarily caused by cricothyroid muscle, which is the principal tensor of the vocal cord.

Cricoarytenoid joint is between the base of arytenoid cartilage and facet on the superior aspect of lamina of cricoid cartilage. It is a synovial of plane variety. The movements are:

In vertical axis

Rotation of arytenoid cartilage causes change in the dimension of inter-cartilaginous part of rima glottidis. Muscles for this movement are posterior and lateral cricoarytenoids.

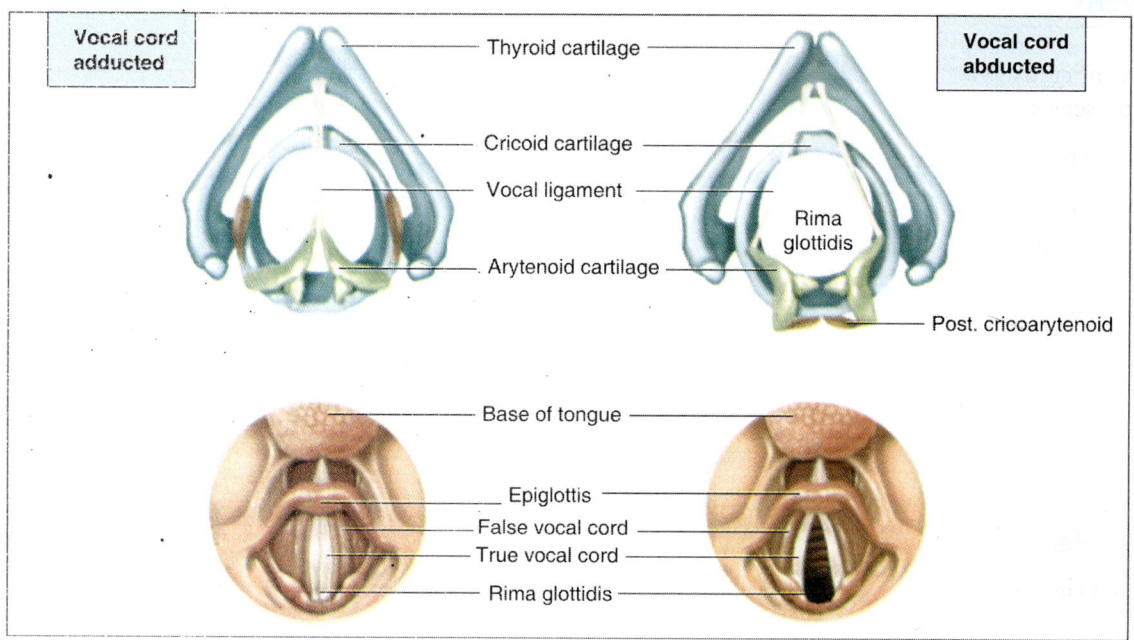

Fig. 49.2: Interior of Larynx

Gliding / sliding of arytenoids cartilage over lamina of cricoid cartilage

This causes tensing of vocal cords. This is caused by vertical fibers of posterior cricoarytenoid muscle, which pulls the muscular process of arytenoid cartilage. The arytenoid cartilages are approximated by the inter-arytenoids to reduce the inter-cartilaginous gap of rima glottidis (**adduction**).

PIRIFORM FOSSA

It is a depression of mucosa lateral to the vestibule of larynx. It is bounded laterally by thyroid cartilage and thyro-hyroid membrane. Medially aryepiglottic fold and epiglottis separate it from laryngeal orifice. This fossa is a potential space for lodging of foreign bodies. An attempt to remove foreign body from this fossa can cause damage to internal laryngeal nerve, which is deep to it. Damage to internal laryngeal nerve may predispose to aspiration pneumonia, as the sensations are lost in the supraglottic part of larynx.

NERVE AND BLOOD SUPPLY

Vocal cords demarcates the area of arterial supply and sensory nerve supply

A. Above the vocal folds

Arterial supply

- Superior laryngeal artery (branch of superior thyroid artery)

Venous return

- Superior laryngeal vein (tributary of superior thyroid vein)

Nerve supply

- Internal laryngeal nerve (superior laryngeal nerve branch of XCN)

B. Below the vocal folds

Arterial supply

- Inferior laryngeal artery (inferior thyroid artery from thyrocervical artery)

Venous return

- Inferior laryngeal vein (tributary of superior thyroid vein)

Nerve supply

- Recurrent laryngeal nerve branch of Vagus (X CN)

All the intrinsic muscles of larynx are supplied by recurrent laryngeal nerve except **cricothyroid** which is innervated by external laryngeal nerve. The vocal cords are made tense before they can be adducted or abduction. For this, the cricothyroid has to act first.

LYMPHATIC DRAINAGE

This is also demarcated by vocal folds

Above the vocal folds

- The lymphatics travel along superior laryngeal artery, through thyro-hyroid membrane to drain into anterosuperior group of deep cervical nodes.

Below the vocal folds

- The lymphatics pierce thyro-hyroid membrane and cricotracheal ligaments to drain into posteroinferior group of deep cervical nodes.

CLINICAL CONSIDERATIONS

VOCAL CORDS

For normal phonation, the vocal cords meet with each other. In respiration, they abduct to allow flow of air.

An adequate airway is provided by abduction of only one cord. Therefore, true dyspnoea is not seen where paralysis is unilateral.

When both cords are fixed near the midline, dyspnoea is a distressing symptom.

In most cases, paralysis is due to peripheral involvement of the recurrent laryngeal nerve (RLN).

There are fifteen muscles in larynx (seven paired and one unpaired). All are supplied by the RLN except cricothyroid which is supplied by the superior laryngeal nerve (SLN).

Superior laryngeal nerve has a shorter and less vulnerable course. Thus Injury to the SLN is rare.

Left RLN crosses under arch of the aorta, where it may be stretched by

- Aneurysm
- Enlargement of the left auricle secondary to mitral stenosis

RLN may become involved by bronchogenic carcinoma.

In the neck, the recurrent laryngeal nerves may be invaded by thyroid cancer. Either nerve may be inadvertently severed during thyroidectomy.

The RLN divide into several branches before entering the larynx. The different position in which a paralyzed cord may be found is thus explained by selective damage to one or more branches.

Unilateral Paralysis

- Affected cord in the paramedian position
- Glottis cannot be closed completely for phonation
- Hoarseness of voice
- Reduction of vocal intensity and range
- Paralyzed cord becomes fixed in midline

Bilateral Paralysis

- Both cords are adducted
- Glottal chink of only two mm to three mm
- Weak voice
- Inadequate airway
- Slightest exertion produces dyspnoea
- Stridor with noisy respiration

Simon's Law

In gradually advancing organic lesions of recurrent laryngeal nerve (RLN), the clinical stages of involvement of intrinsic muscles of larynx follow a sequence.

In first stage - only abductors are affected. Adduction is still possible.

In second stage - vocal cords are immobilized in median position due to addition contraction of adductors

In third stage - vocal cords assume cadaveric position. This is because the adductors are paralyzed.

The explanation of this sequence is:

1. Abductor are peripherally placed, hence they get affected first.
2. Abductors lie in a separate bundle and developed later. Hence these are more vulnerable. This view is not accepted any longer.

Thus the **Simon's law** states that in the lesions of recurrent laryngeal nerve there is preferential involvement of abductor. These are also last to recover.

Laryngeal Oedema (Glottic Oedema)

It is the swelling caused by fluid accumulation in the soft tissues of the larynx. This is usually inflammatory in nature which may result from an infection, injury, or inhalation of toxic gases.

In infections (**diphtheria**), there is accumulation of inflammation exudates, under the mucous membrane of vestibular folds. This oedema does not involve the vocal folds because the mucous membrane is firmly adherent here. This oedema can approximate vestibular folds and cause difficulty in breathing. Tracheostomy may be required.

Vocal Cord Palsy

The lesion of recurrent laryngeal nerve causes paralysis of intrinsic muscles of larynx. This may be unilateral or bilateral.

In unilateral palsy, affected vocal cord is pulled towards the healthy side while the arytenoid cartilage remains in place. Thus the rima glottidis is asymmetrical: **cadaveric position** of vocal cord. This is seen when both recurrent laryngeal nerve are affected. The rima glottidis appears as a minute slit / gap since vocal cords are in semi-abducted position.

Safety Muscle of Larynx

Three functions are ascribed to larynx

1. Air passage
2. Voice production
3. During swallowing acting as a valve

These functions are achieved by different sets of muscles

- For patent airway, the vocal cords have to be abducted. This is caused by **posterior cricoarytenoid**.

- For voice production, the vocal cords have to made tense and the dimensions of rima glottidis have to vary. This is possible by the contributions from almost all muscles of larynx.

- In third stage of deglutition, the bolus / liquid glides over epiglottis to enter the laryngo-pharynx. Tip of epiglottis is brought down as a flap to partial cover the laryngeal orifice by the contraction of **aryepiglotticus**. This "fold is further shortened by the contraction of **thyro-epiglotticus**.

Out of all the intrinsic muscles of larynx, **posterior cricor-arytenioid** being the only abductor of vocal cords should be considered as the **safety muscle** of larynx.

Laryngoscopy

To view the interior of larynx is termed **laryngoscopy**. This is required to assess the interior of larynx. This interior examination is done by

- Indirect laryngoscopy
- Direct laryngoscopy

Indirect laryngoscopy

It is an OPD procedure. Here the image of larynx is seen in a mirror indirectly. Structures visualized from above downwards are:

1. Posterior 1/3 of tongue
2. Valleculae
3. Epiglottis
4. Laryngeal inlet
5. Interior of larynx
6. Piriform fossa
7. Posterior pharyngeal wall

Direct laryngoscopy

This is done by an instrument called laryngoscope. It is usually performed under general anesthesia. Apart from visualizing interior of larynx, this procedure is indicated for diagnostic and therapeutic purposes.

Cafe Coronary Phenomenon

Eating and talking at the same time can cause entry of food bolus into the larynx. It leads to choking symptoms like coughing and difficulty in breathing. It may prove fatal. Since such an episode is commonly seen at an eating-place – **cafe coronary phenomenon.** It is a misnomer as there is no primary cardiac lesion. In postmortem that shows presence of a food bolus in the larynx.

Singer's Nodule (Vocal Cord Nodule)

SINGER'S NODULE (VOCAL CORD NODULE)

This is also called Teacher's nodule or Screamer's nodule.

It is a small inflammatory or fibrous growth that develops on the vocal cords of people who constantly strain their voices.

Misuse or over use of voice leads to hyper-keratosis of the free edges of vocal cords. These are bilateral and usually affect singers.

Heimlich Maneuver

Foreign bodies may get lodged in the rima glottidis to cause laryngeal obstruction. The individual gets asphyxiated. It requires an emergency procedure to dislodge the foreign body. Compression of abdomen raises the diaphragm, which in turn compresses the lungs, thereby expelling air from the lungs up the trachea to dislodge the foreign body from the rima glottidis. This is termed as Heimlich maneuver.

Laryngocele

It is an abnormal air-containing cavity connected to the laryngeal ventricle. It is caused by an evagination of the mucous membrane of the ventricle and may displace and enlarge the false vocal cord, resulting in hoarseness and airway obstruction. A laryngocele is a potential reservoir of infection. It is usually excised.

Larynitis

It is the inflammation of the mucous membrane lining the larynx, accompanied by oedema of the vocal cords with hoarseness of voice. It occurs as an acute disorder caused by

- Cold
- Sudden temperature changes
- Chronic condition resulting from excessive use of the voice
- Heavy smoking
- Exposure to irritating fumes

In acute laryngitis there may be a cough, and the throat is scratchy and painful.

Acute laryngitis may cause severe respiratory distress in children less than 5 years of age because of the relatively small larynx of the young child which is subjected to spasm when irritated.

Laryngeal Cancer

It is a malignant disease, characterized by a tumour arising from the epithelium of the larynx. Laryngeal tumors are almost 20 times more common in men than in women. Chronic alcoholism and tobacco increase the risk of developing the cancer.

Clinical features include

- Persistent hoarseness
- Sore throat
- Dyspnoea
- Dysphagia
- Unilateral cervical lymphadenopathy

Diagnostic measures

- Direct laryngoscopy
- Biopsy
- Radiological examination

Radiation is done for small lesions.

Total laryngectomy combined with radiotherapy is indicated for extensive lesions.

Laryngectomy

It is the surgical removal of the larynx. It is performed for the treatment of carcinoma of larynx. Under regional or general anesthesia, the trachea is sutured to the skin to ensure an adequate airway.

Partial laryngectomy - only the vocal cords are removed, and the tracheostomy is closed subsequently.

Complete laryngectomy - entire larynx is removed along with the thyroid cartilage and epiglottis. Here the tracheostomy is permanent, and a laryngectomy tube is left in place. It is done when the malignancy is extensive. The laryngectomy tube is removed three to six weeks after surgery.

50

Orbit

The bony walls of the orbit form a four-sided pyramid. The medial walls are parallel to each other while the lateral walls are at right angle.

The boundaries are

Base - Towards the face. It is bounded by orbital margin having contributions from following bones: frontal, zygomatic and maxilla.

Apex – In the depth and medial to superior orbital fissure.

Roof – formed by the orbital plate of frontal and lesser wing of sphenoid

Lateral wall – Greater wing of sphenoid and frontal process of zygomatic bone

Medial wall – Composite, having contributions from:

Frontal process of maxilla

Lacrimal

Orbital plate of ethmoid

Side of body of sphenoid

Openings in the orbit

1. **Inferior orbital fissure** – between lateral wall and floor
2. **Superior orbital fissure** – between roof and lateral wall
3. **Optic canal** – between roof and medial wall

Contents

1. **Eyeball** with its extra-ocular muscles and associated nerves and vessels
2. **Nerves:** II, III, IV and VI cranial nerves
3. **Vessels:** ophthalmic artery and its branches, superior & inferior ophthalmic vein
4. **Fat**
5. **Fascial sheath**, cheek ligaments and suspensory ligaments
6. **Lacrimal apparatus**
7. **Ciliary ganglion**

ACTIONS OF EXTRA OCULAR MUSCLES

Extra-ocular muscles include **four recti, two obliqui** and **levator palpabrae superioris**. The eyeball moves in three axes. All muscles except medial rectus (MR) and lateral rectus (LR) act on all the three axes. Medial and lateral recti act only in vertical axis.

Abductors of the eyeball are MR, superior rectus (SR) and inferior rectus (IR).

Abductors are LR, superior oblique (SO) and inferior oblique (IO). Except MR and LR, remaining muscles (SR, IR, SO and IO) are directed obliquely to act in the vertical axis.

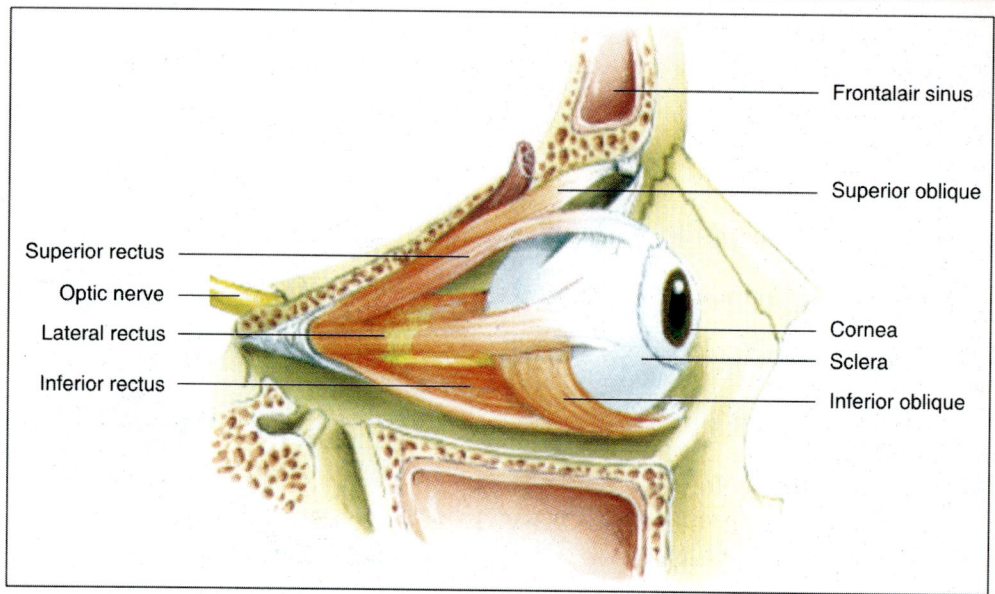

Fig. 50.1: Extraocular Muscles

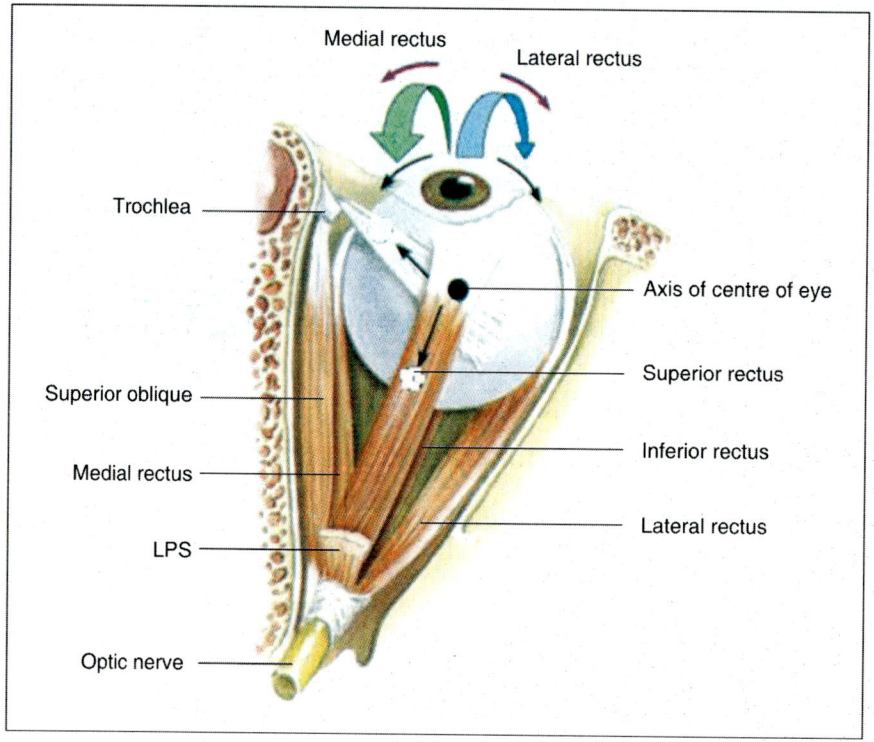

Fig. 50.2: Extraocular Muscles

The movements of elevation and depression take place in horizontal axis. The **elevators** are SR and IO. The inferior oblique is inserted in the upper part of postero-inferior quadrant of the eyeball behind the equator. Hence it pulls posteroinferior quadrant down and medially towards its origin. The **depressors** are IR and SO. The superior oblique is inserted in the lower part of postero-superior quadrant behind the equator. Thus it pulls posterosuperior quadrant down and medially towards its functional pull e.g., trochlea.

The movements of **intorsion and extorsion** take place in anteroposterior axis. In the movement of intorsion cornea rotates from 12 O'clock position to 3 O'clock and its opposite movement is termed as extorsion. Intorsion is brought about by superior oblique and superior rectus since they are attached on the upper and lateral aspect of the eyeball while extorsion is caused by inferior oblique and inferior rectus.

PARASYMPATHETIC GANGLIA

Introduction

All smooth muscles except that of blood vessels are supplied by parasympathetic nerves

- All glands except sweat glands are supplied by parasympathetic nerves
- Excluding head, neck and face, the parasympathetic supply to the body is by vagus nerve and sacral parasympathetic for pelvis and perineum
- Parasympathetic innervation of head, neck and face is by cranial nerves – 3rd, 7th, and 9th through peripheral ganglia. These ganglia are
    1. Ciliary
    2. Pterygo palatine
    3. Otic
    4. Submandibular

All ganglia have following roots
1. Secretomotor
2. Sensory
3. Sympathetic

All ganglia give off branches that are mixed which carry following impulses
1. Postganglionic parasympathetic
2. Postganglionic sympathetic
3. Sensory / motor

Ciliary ganglion is placed on nasociliary nerve, which is a branch of ophthalmic division of V cranial nerve. It is functionally connected to Oculomotor nerve (III CN).

Otic ganglion is placed on mandibular division of Trigeminal nerve (IX CN)

Pterygopalatine ganglion (*Spheno-palatine ganglion*) is placed on the maxillary division of Trigeminal nerve and functionally related to Facial nerve (VII CN).

Submandibular ganglion is placed on Lingual nerve (mandibular division of V CN) and functionally connected to Facial nerve (VII CN)

CILIARY GANGLION

It is a pinhead-sized ganglion placed between optic nerve and lateral rectus close to the apex of orbit. It has three roots, namely:

Sensory – connected to nasociliary nerve

Sympathetic – sympathetic plexus around ophthalmic artery

Parasympathetic – Arises from nerve to inferior oblique (branch of inferior division of III N).

Arising from the ganglion are about 8 to 10 branches (**short ciliary nerves**). These nerves pierce the sclera around the entrance of optic nerve. These branches carry sensory, post ganglionic sympathetic and post-ganglionic parasympathetic impulses. From cornea and conjunctiva the sensory impulses are carried in short and long ciliary nerves. The post-ganglionic sympathetic impulses supply **dilator pupillae**. The post-ganglionic parasympathetic impulses are carried to **sphincter pupillae** and **ciliaris**.

OPTIC NERVE

It is the second cranial nerve – nerve of sight. It consists mainly of coarse, myelinated fibers that arise in the ganglion layer of retina, and connected visual cortex.

At the optic chiasm a the fibres from the inner (**nasal half**) of the retina cross to the optic tract of the opposite side. The fibres from the outer (**temporal**) half of each retina are uncrossed and pass to the visual cortex on the same side.

The visual cortex functions in the perception of

- Light and shade
- Objects

Optic radiations conduct impulses from the lateral geniculate bodies in the cerebral hemispheres to the visual cortices.

The optic nerve is divided into parts within the bulb, orbit, optic canal, and cranial cavity.

Intraocular part of the nerve is about 1 mm long and contains unmyelinated fibers that become myelinated after passing through the lamina cribosa.

Orbital part of the nerve is about 3.5 mm in diameter and about 25 mm long. It is invested by the dura, arachnoid and pia mater (menings).

Within optic canal the nerve lies superior to the ophthalmic artery. The three miningeal sheaths are fused to each other, to the nerve and to the periosteum of the bone. This secures the nerve and prevents it from being forced back and forth in the foramen.

Intracranial part of the nerve is placed on the anterior portion of the cavernous sinus in close proximity with the internal carotid artery.

The optic nerve develops from a diverticulum of the lateral portion of the forebrain. The optic nerve fibers therefore correspond to a tract of fibers within the brain.

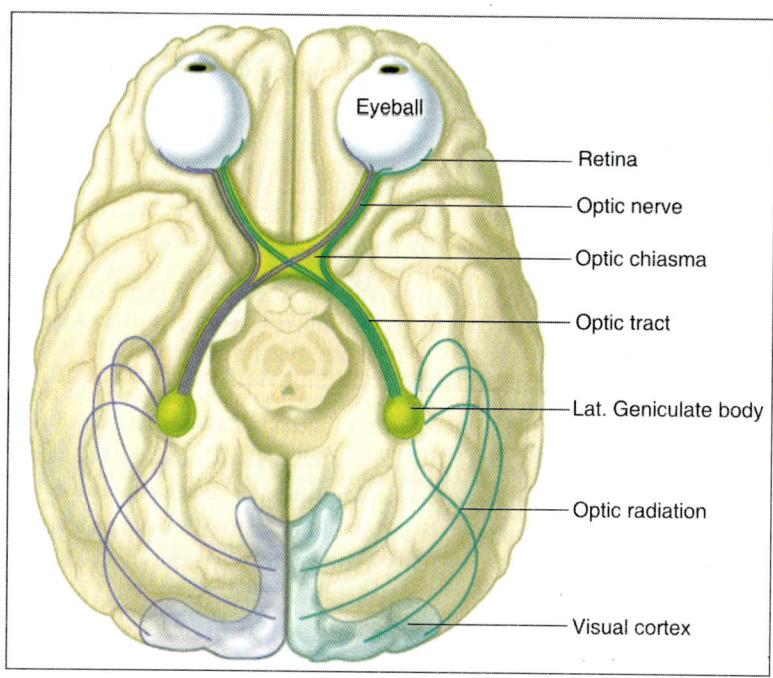

Eyeball

Retina

Optic nerve

Optic chiasma

Optic tract

Lat. Geniculate body

Optic radiation

Visual cortex

Fig. 50.3: Optic Pathway

III CRANIAL NERVE (OCULOMOTOR NERVE)

It is a mixed nerve

Nerve components
Somatic efferent

All extrinsic muscles of eyeball are supplied except lateral rectus (LR) and superior oblique (SO).
Eye lid - levator palpabrae superioris (LPS)

General visceral efferent

- – Constrictor pupillae
- – Ciliaris

Nuclei
Somatic efferent

Motor nucleus is in the midbrain (in superior colliculus) with subdivisions for each muscle

- – Dorsal nucleus for inferior rectus (IR)
- – Intermediate nucleus for inferior oblique (IO)
- – Ventral nucleus for medial rectus (MR)
- – Ventromedial nucleus for (SR)
- – Central caudal nucleus for levator palpabrae superioris (LPS) skeletal part

General visceral efferent

This is called Edinger Westphal nucleus
Through ciliary ganglion it supplies

- Constrictor pupillae
- Ciliaris

Course
Intraneural course

Axons from the nuclei run through the red nucleus
Descend to reach the lower level of crus cerebri.

Intracranial course

Nerve comes out in interpeduncular cistern
Runs laterally between posterior cerebral artery and superior cerebellar arteries
Reaches the free margin of tentorium cerebelli
Runs under the free margin and pieces it to enter the cavernous sinus
Runs along the lateral wall, close to the roof of cavernous sinus
Runs forwards to enter the superior orbital fissure where it divides into two divisions

- – Upper division
- – Lower division

Nasociliary nerve is placed in between the two divisions.

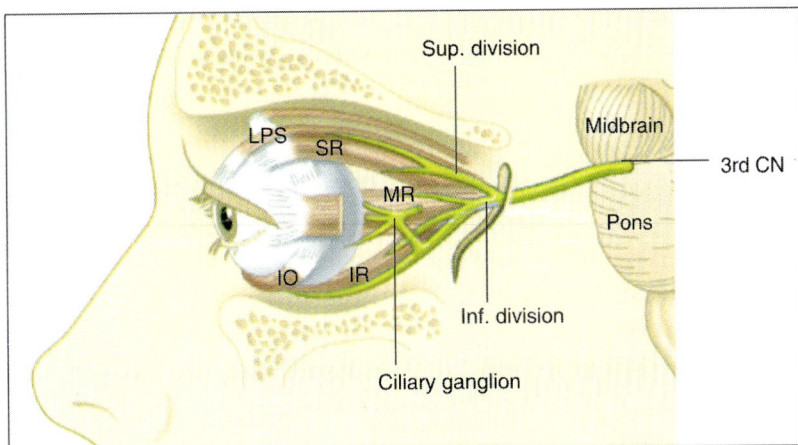

Fig. 50.4: Oculomotor Nerve

Extracranial course

The upper division gives off branches to LPS and SR

The lower division supplies MR, IR and IO

All these branches reach the muscles along their inner surface.

ACCOMMODATION REFLEX

This requires two actions

1. Convergence of eyeball by contraction of medial rectus
2. Constriction of pupil

To elicit this reflux the individual is asked to look at a distant object and thereafter he is asked to look at an object / finger placed close to the eyes. The afferent impulses are carried in three sets of neurons as:

I **Rods and cones**

Optic nerve

Optic chaisma
↓

Optic tract

II **Lateral geniculate body (LGB)**

Optic radiation (retro-lentiform part of internal capsule)

III **Occipital cortex**

By superior longitudinal fasciculus to the frontal eye field

The efferents start from the frontal eye field and are carried in corticonuclear fibers that pass through

- Genu of internal capsule
- Middle 3/5 of crus cerebri in midbrain

The impulses relay in

- Eginder Westphal nucleus
- Motor nucleus of III CN

The lower motor neuron (**LMN**) from III-CN nucleus runs in the superior division of Oculomotor nerve to reach the medial rectus.

The pre-ganglionic parasympathetic fibers from the Edinger Westphal nucleus run in branch to inferior oblique (inferior division of III CN) to reach the ciliary ganglion. The post-ganglionic parasympathetic impulses reach constrictor pupillae and ciliaris by short ciliary nerves.

IV CRANIAL NERVE (TROCHLEAR NERVE)

It is a motor nerve with certain peculiarities

1. Only CN to arise from dorsal aspect of brain
2. Only CN to cross / decussate
3. Most slender CN
4. Has longest intracranial course

Nerve component

Somatic efferent

- For superior oblique (SO)

Nucleus

It is placed at the level of inferior colliculus in the central grey matter

Course

Intraneural course

It runs laterally and then backwards to decussate within the substance of inferior colliculus.

It comes out at the lower border of inferior colliculus

Intracranial course

From the lower pole of inferior colliculus it winds round the midbrain.

Reaches cisterna Interpeduncularis immediately superior to pons.

Runs forwards under the free margin of tentorium cerebelli.

Pierces the arachnoid and dura to enter the middle cranial fossa.

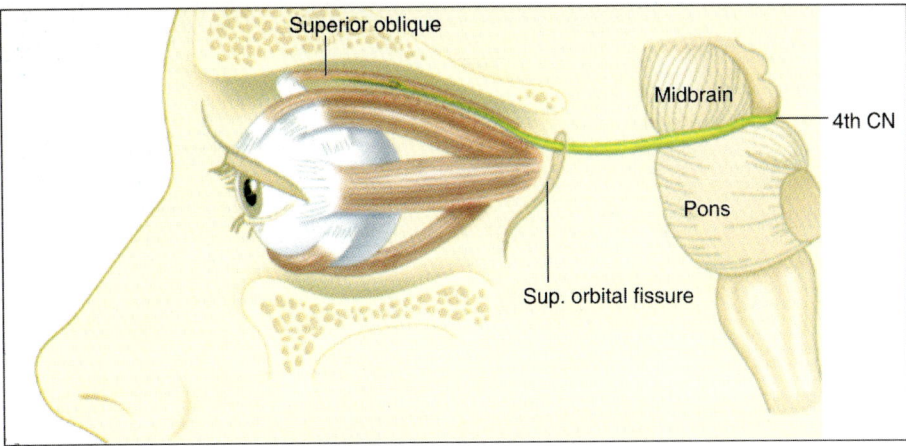

Fig. 50.5: Trochlear Nerve

Runs along the lateral wall of cavernous sinus to reach superior orbital fissure.

Extracranial course

It is placed outside the tendinous ring of Zinn
It runs medially over SR and LPS to supply SO along its outer surface.

VI CRANIAL NERVE (ABDUCENT NERVE)

It is a motor nerve which supplies lateral rectus (LR)

Nerve component

Somatic efferent
- For lateral rectus (LR)

Nucleus

It is placed in lower pons which is surrounded by fibers of VII CN, causing an elevation called **facial colliculus**. This elevation is seen in the floor of fourth ventricle

Course

Intraneural course

The nerve axons run downwards to reach the junction of pons and medulla

Intracranial course

Emerges at lower border of pons

Enters cisterna pontis

Turns upwards between anterior inferior cerebellar artery (AICA) and pons or labyrinthine artery

Pierces arachnoid and dura mater on the clivus

Runs up and lateral between the two layers of dura mater

Reaches apex of petrous temporal

Bends forwards under petro-clenoid ligament (**Dorello's canal**) to enter cavernous sinus (floor and medial wall)

Runs straight, lateral to internal carotid artery (ICA) to reach superior orbital fissure

Enters the tendinous ring below the inferior division of III CN

Extracranial course

Passes within the cone of the muscles to enter the ocular surface of lateral rectus (LR)

VENOUS DRAINAGE OF ORBIT

It bears clinical relevance as superior and inferior ophthalmic veins are connected to cavernous sinus

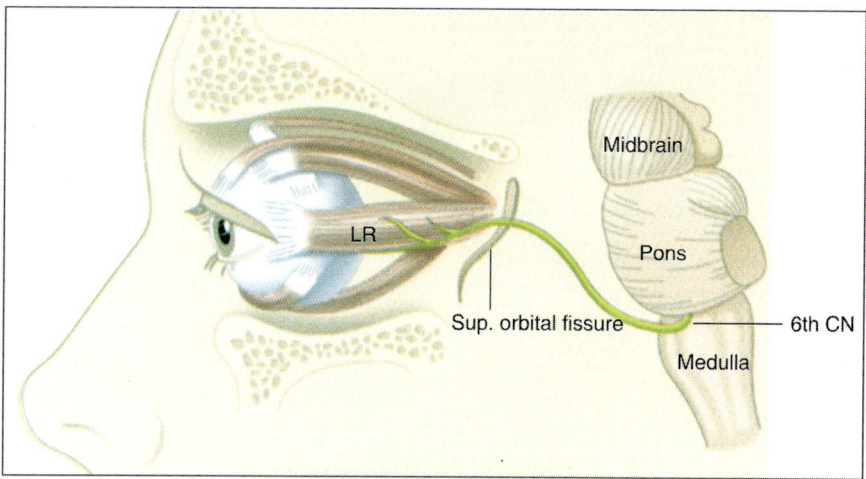

Fig. 50.6: Abducent Nerve

in the cranium. On the face they receive superficial veins namely supra-orbital, supra-trochlear and angular vein. Thus these act as emissary veins, capable of transmitting superficial infection of the face to cavernous sinus causing **cavernous sinus thrombosis** which may prove fatal.

CLINICAL CONSIDERATIONS

Functional aspects of movement eyeball

While seeing a thing, the image has to fall on the central fovea of retina. It requires positioning of the two eyeballs very precisely. Any incoordination would affect the vision causing blurring. Thus finely graded movements of the eye are necessary

The conjugate movements of the eye require contraction of synergist muscles of the two eyes as well as relaxation of the antagonists

E.g. Right lateral rectus and left medial rectus **contract**

- Right medial rectus and Left lateral rectus **relax**

This causes abduction of the eye to the right.

Voluntary movements of eyeballs are brought about reflexly by

1. Visual impulses

2. Vestibular impulses via medial longitudinal bundle

Cortical impulses from occipital cortex to frontal cortex (Area no. 8) by corticonuclear fibers to these cranial nerve nuclei (III, IV and VI)

The finely coordinated conjugate movements of the eyes require that each neuron in the CN nucleus should supply few muscle fibers

- IV CN has 3400 fibers for one muscle (SO)
- VI CN has 6600 fibers for one muscle (LR)
- III CN has 24000 fibers for five muscles (LPS, SR, MR, IR and IO)

In addition, rich blood supply ensures proper functioning of the muscles of eyeballs

Squint: Deviation of the eyeball which the subject cannot overcome

Convergent squint - "Your eyes are very attractive. They attract each other"

Divergent squint - "Looking London talking Tokyo"

Nystagmus: Involuntary movements of the eyeball which may be horizontal or vertical

The embarrassment and the anguish to live on with such a problem is immeasurable

How do these conditions result?

Supranuclear causes

Lesion is in the frontal and occipital lobes

Both eyes are involved

Nuclear causes

Poliomyelitis

Infranuclear causes

Fracture of skull leads to haematoma that pushes the temporal lobe causing stretching of III cranial nerve

Increased intracranial tension affects VI nerve first

Other conditions that can affect these CN include:

- Meningitis
- Tumours
- Aneurysm

Squint (Strabismus)

It is a condition when one eye deviates away from the fixation point. This condition may affect both the eyes together.

In **convergent squint** the unopposed action of medial rectus causes cornea to direct medially. In **divergent squint** unopposed action of lateral rectus causes abduction of the eyeballs.

There are two types of squint

1. Paralytic
2. Nonparalytic

Paralytic squint results from the inability of the ocular muscles to move the eye because of neurologic deficit or muscular dysfunction.

The dysfunctional muscle can be identified by watching as the patient attempts to move the eyes to each of the cardinal positions of gaze.

This type of squint may be caused by

- Tumour
- Infection
- Injury to the brain or the eye

Nonparalytic squint is a defect in the position of the two eyes in relation to each other. This condition is inherited. The person cannot use the two eyes together but has to fix with one or the other. The eye that looks straight at a given time is the fixing eye.

This may be

- **Alternating squint** – Patient uses one eye and then the other
- **Monocular squint** – It affects only one eye

Visual acuity diminishes with diminished use of an eye and suppression amblyopia may develop.

Nonparalytic strabismus and suppression amblyopia are treated most successfully in early childhood.

Pulsating eyeball

A communication between the internal carotid artery (ICA) and the cavernous sinus (**carotid cavernous aneurysm**) leads to pulsating and bulging eye ball.

Ptosis

The paresis or paralysis of the muscles of the upper eyelid cause drooping of the eyelid thereby reducing the size of palpebral aperture. The muscles affected are orbital and palpebral parts of **orbicularis oculi**.

It is an abnormal condition involving one or both upper eyelids in which the eyelid droops because of a congenital or acquired weakness of the levator palpabrae superioris muscle or paralysis of III CN.

Partial ptosis may be caused by a disorder of the sympathetic portion of the autonomic nervous system.

In **Horner's syndrome**, pseudoptosis is observed because of sympathetic dennervation of levator palpabrae superioris. Involvement of oculomotor nerve (III CN) leads to ptosis accompanied by various degrees of squint. This is because III CN supplies levator palpabrae superioris (LPS) and as well as superior rectus (SR), medial rectus (MR), inferior rectus (IR) and inferior oblique (IO).

The condition can be treated surgically by shortening the levator palpabrae superioris muscle.

Lesions of different nucleus components of III CN

A. Lesions of Edinger Westphal nucleus will manifest as

- Dilatation of pupil - constrictor pupillae is affected
- Accommodation reflex is lost - ciliaris is affected

B. Lesions of Motor nucleus

- Eye ball is abducted (LR) and depressed (SO)
- All muscles are paralyzed except LR and SO
- Ptosis - LPS is also affected
- Exophthalmos – Paralyzed muscles slacken and their bulk pushes eye ball forwards
- No Diplopia Since the ptosis of the lid covers the affected eye

Lesion of Trochlear Nerve

The person cannot look down and laterally on the affected side. To compensate for this, the person bends the neck to the sound side. There will be diplopia

Argyl Robertson's Pupil

This is characterized by a pupil that constricts on accommodation but not in response to light. It is most often seen with miosis and in advanced neurosyphilis.

Cavernous Sinus

These are paired, irregularly shaped, bilateral venous channels situated on either side of the body of sphenoid bone in the middle cranial fossa. These are formed by the splitting of endosteal and meningeal dura mater.

It is one of the five anterior inferior venous sinuses that drain blood from the dura mater into the internal jugular vein. Like the other anterior inferior sinuses, the cavernous sinus has no valves.

Structures passing through the sinus

- Oculomotor nerve III CN
- Trochlear nerve IV CN
- Abducent nerve VI CN
- Ophthalmic division of trigeminal nerve
- Maxillary divisions of the trigeminal nerve
- Internal carotid artery

Cavernous sinus receives

- Superior and the inferior ophthalmic veins
- Some cerebral veins
- Sphenoparietal sinus

It is connected to the cavernous sinus of the opposite side by the anterior and posterior intercavernous sinuses thus completing circular sinus.

The cavernous sinus drains into inferior petrosal sinus.

Cavernous Sinus Thrombosis

This is generally secondary to infections near the eye or nose.

This is characterized by

- Orbital edema
- Venous congestion of the eye
- Palsy of III, IV and VI cranial nerves - supply extraocular muscles, resulting in ophthalmoplegia.

The infection may spread to involve the cerebrospinal fluid and meninges.

Cavernous Sinus Syndrome

It is due to thrombosis of the cavernous sinus.

This is characterized by

- Oedema of the conjunctiva, upper eyelid and root of the nose
- Paralysis of the III, IV and VI cranial nerves.

Fracture of Orbital Floor

Fracture of the orbital floor may occur as a component of **zygomaticomaxillary complex** fracture, which usually causes

- Comminution (breaking into several pieces) of orbital floor
- Isolated fracture
- Orbital blowout fracture, caused by a rapid increase in intraorbital pressure

The force producing a blowout fracture is usually delivered by a blunt object (e.g., a fist or a ball) directed at the eyeball and lid.

The sudden increase in pressure fractures the bony orbit at areas of weakness, namely

- Orbital floor
- Medial wall

In comminution of the orbital floor, the fibrous septa of the periorbital tissue become tethered to the bony edges of the fracture and pulled or displaced with the fragments.

In some cases, orbital soft tissue may protrude into the maxillary sinus, causing it to appear clouded in inferior oblique view (**Waters' sinus view**) radiograph.

Most common presenting ocular problems from orbital floor injury

- Diplopia - double vision
- Depression of the eyeball

Fracture Base of Skull

Increased intracranial pressure causes descent of brain stem (**Coning**).This puts strain on the two bends that the abducent nerve has in its course. These pull may severe the nerve and result in paralysis of lateral rectus (LR) manifesting as medial squint.

Horner's Syndrome

A syndrome is a set of symptoms and signs peculiar to a particular disease.

In Horner's syndrome, a set of symptoms are observed due to involvement of sympathetic innervation to the eyeball and face.

This is usually seen after cervical sympathectomy performed for improving blood flow to the distal parts of upper limbs (**Reynard's disease**).

These symptoms are also seen in **klumpke's paralysis** where the lower trunk of brachial plexus is affected.

Sympathetic innervation for the smooth muscles of blood vessels, sweat glands and arrector pilorum muscle of the upper limb is carried in the brachial plexus and thereafter via the blood vessels to the effector organ.

Symptoms of Horner's syndrome

1. **Flushing of face** – dilatation of cutaneous blood vessels
2. **Anhidrosis** – loss of sweat glands secrections of face
3. **Pseudoptosis** – drooping of upper eyelid because of paresis of smooth muscle component of levator palpabrae superioris (LPS)
4. **Enophthalmos** –sinking of eyeball in the orbit is known as enophthalmos. The inferior orbital fissure is bridged by a smooth muscle – **Muller's** muscle which is supplied by sympathetic fibers. Thus the paresis / paralysis of this muscle cause the eyeball to sink in the orbit. It is termed as an optical illusion due to narrowing of the palpable fissure.
5. **Miosis** – constriction of the pupil is known as miosis. It is due to interruption in the nerve supply to the dilator pupillae muscle.

Horner's syndrome is unavoidable after **cervico-thoracic ganglionectomy** as all preganglionic sympathetic fibers to the head region course upwards through the part of the sympathetic chain that is excised.

All the symptoms observed in Horner's syndrome are unilateral.

Oculocephalic Reflex

By this reflex the integrity of brainstem function is tested.

When the patient's head is quickly moved to one side and then to the other, the eyes normally lag behind the head movement and then slowly assume the midline position. Failure of the eyes to either lag or revert back to the midline position indicates a lesion at the level of brainstem on the ipsilateral side.

Ocular Myopathy

It is slowly progressive weakness of ocular muscles which is characterized by decreased mobility of the eye and drooping of the upper lid. The condition may be unilateral or bilateral.

This may be caused by

- Damage to the oculomotor nerve
- Intracranial tumor
- Neuromuscular disease

51

Ear

Ear has three components
- External ear
- Middle ear
- Internal ear

EXTERNAL EAR

It has two parts

Pinna or auricle

External acoustic meatus

The external acoustic meatus acts as a tubular resonator. Therefore, the vibrations of sound at the eardrum (tympanic membrane) have a considerably higher intensity of pressure than at the external ear.

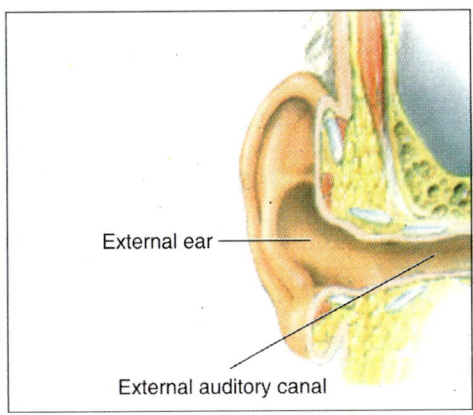

External ear

External auditory canal

Fig. 51.1: External Ear

At the eardrum, airborne pressure changes of sound waves are transformed into mechanical vibrations.

External acoustic meatus is approximately one inch long. Its lateral one third is cartilaginous and medial two third is osseous. It shows two bends: **lateral bend** is at the junction of cartilaginous and ·osseous part and the **medial bend** is five mm from lateral wall of middle ear (**tympanic membrane**).

To examine the tympanic membrane, the pinna is pulled upwards and backwards. This straightens the lateral bend of the auditory canal. Ceruminous glands line the walls of the canal. External acoustic meatus is supplied by following nerves:
- Great auricular nerve
- Auriculotemporal nerve
- **Arnold's** nerve (X CN)

In a newborn, there is no osseous part since the tympanic plate is in the form of an incomplete ring. In infants, external acoustic meatus is very short and narrow.

MIDDLE EAR

The eardrum and ossicles transfer airborne sound waves to the fluid-filled inner ear. The middle ear compensates for the change in density of the conducting medium (from air to water) by amplifying the sound via two relationships:

- Size difference between the handle of the malleus and the long limb of the incus
- Relative difference in the areas of the large eardrum and the small oval window.

Middle ear is a six walled cavity placed in petrous part of temporal bone. Its **lateral wall** separates it from external ear. **Medial wall** is related to internal ear. **Anterior wall** is connected to the pharynx through the auditory tube. Posteriorly it opens into mastoid antrum that leads into mastoid air cells. **Roof** is formed by tegmen tympani that separates it from the meninges covering the temporal bone. **Floor** has internal carotid artery anteriorly placed and bulb of internal jugular vein placed posteriorly. The roof and floor are cartilaginous in the early part of life. Hence meningitis, thrombosis of IJV and infections of middle ear (**otitis media**) are not uncommon in children.

Dimensions of middle ear

- Height and length: 15mm
- Roof and floor are 6 mm and 4 mm respectively
- In the middle it is only 2 mm wide.

It contains

1. Tympanic ossicles (**Malleus, Incus, Stapes**)
2. Ligaments and muscles attached to the ossicles
3. Chorda tympani and tympanic plexus

The **epitympanic recess** is above the level of tympanic membrane. It contains greater part of incus and upper half of malleus.

Features of ear ossicles

- Their size remain constant
- They show presence of marrow cavity
- They help in conduction of sound

Malleus

It is 8 mm long. It has following features

- Head – lies in the epi-tympanic recess
- Neck
- Lateral process
- Handle
- Anterior process – gives attachment to anterior ligament of malleus which is continuous with sphenomandibular ligament

Incus

Its body is large and lies in epi-tympanic recess.

It gives posteriorly a short crus and inferiorly continuous as long crus.

Its bent end is called lenticular process.

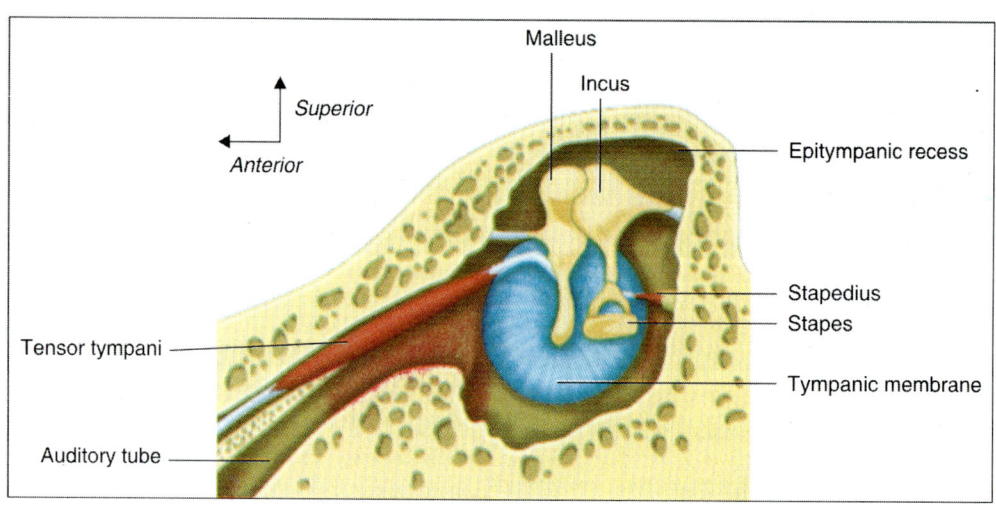

Fig. 51.2: Middle Ear

Stapes

It has head, neck, crus (limbs) and a footplate. Stapedius muscle is attached on the posterior surface of neck.

Joints between the ossicles

1. **Malleus & incus** – Saddle joint
2. **Incus & stapes** – Ball and socket joint
3. **Fenestra vestibuli & foot plate of stapes** – Syndesmosis

Muscles acting on ear ossicles

Tensor tympani - Runs in the groove in the anterior and medial wall. It tenses the tympanic membrane by pulling it medially.

Stapedius - It pulls the stapes laterally thus deepens the sound

INTERNAL EAR

The spiral organ (of **Corti**) is composed of supporting cells, which are interspersed with hair cells (**sensory end organs**).

The hair cells are arranged segmentally in rows of inner and outer hair cells. The free surface of each hair cell is covered with clumps of hair. The ends of the hairs are embedded in the tectorial membrane, overhanging the hair cells.

The wave of perilymph through the scala induces movement in the basilar membrane. This membrane is wider and thinner at the apex of the cochlea and narrower and thicker at the base. Vibrations of the basilar membrane cause a pull on the hair cells attached to the tectorial membrane.

This action transforms mechanical energy into electric impulses. This stimulates the fibers of the cochlear nerve of the vestibulocochlear nerve (VIII CN) to produce the action potentials. This action potential is responsible for transmission of nerve impulses to the brain.

- Hair cells transmitting specific frequencies are arranged together.
- Those transmits the higher tones are situated at the base of the cochlea
- Those transmits lower tones are placed near the apex

Each hair cell is supplied by at least one nerve fibre. A single neuron supplies ten outer hair cells while each inner hair cell is supplied by twenty neurons. 95% of cochlear neurons innervate the inner hair cells.

This overlap of nerve connections is important for functional flexibility and allows compensation for damage to single hair cells or certain neurons.

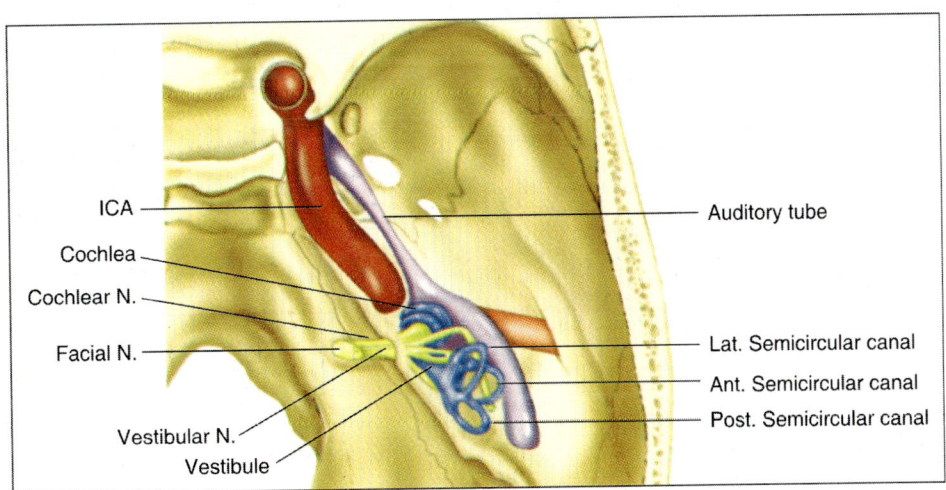

Fig. 51.3: Internal Ear

The cochlear nerve consists of 35,000 neurons. The nerve cell bodies are located in the cochlear (spiral) ganglion situated in the spiral canal of the modiolus (**Rosenthal's canal**).

TYMPANIC MEMBRANE

It is pearl grey in appearance. It is one cm in diameter with 50 degree angle with external acoustic meatus with a concavity towards lateral side – **umbo**. Its periphery is attached to a bony sulcus except in the upper part.

Handle and lateral process of malleus are embedded within it.

The mallear folds extend from lateral process to the tympanic sulcus. Pars flaccida (**Shrapnel's membrane**) is enclosed by the mallear folds. The remaining part of tympanic membrane is **Pars tensa**. The tympanic membrane has outer cuticular layer, middle fibrous layer and inner patchy ciliated layer. It has a rich nerve supply.

On the external side it is supplied by
- Auriculotemporal nerve
- Arnold's nerve

On the medial side it is supplied by
- Tympanic branch of glossopharyngeal nerve (**Jacobson's nerve**)
- Chorda tympani

PHARYNGO-TYMPANIC TUBE (AUDITORY TUBE/EUSTACHIAN TUBE)

It is trumpet shaped which is about 1.5 inch long. It extends from the anterior wall of tympanic cavity. It is directed forwards, downwards and medially to open on the lateral wall of nasopharynx. It has osseous and cartilaginous parts.

Osseous part is about half inch long. It is present in temporal bone. It is lateral to carotid canal and posteromedial to upper part of temporo-mandibular joint (TM joint).

Cartilaginous part is one inch long. It is paced in the groove between greater wing of sphenoid and petrous part of temporal bone. The tensor palati arises from its anterolateral surface. The posteromedial surface gives attachment to levator palati.

Its pharyngeal opening presents **tubal elevation,** which is caused by origin of salpingo-pharyngeus muscle.

Function

During deglutition, the tube in opened by the muscles attached to it. This equalizes the pressure between the nasopharynx and the tympanic cavity. At its pharyngeal orifice, lymphoid tissue is present (**pharyngeal tonsil**). The tube is supplied by tympanic plexus, and branches from sphenopalatine ganglion (**pterygo-palatine ganglion**).

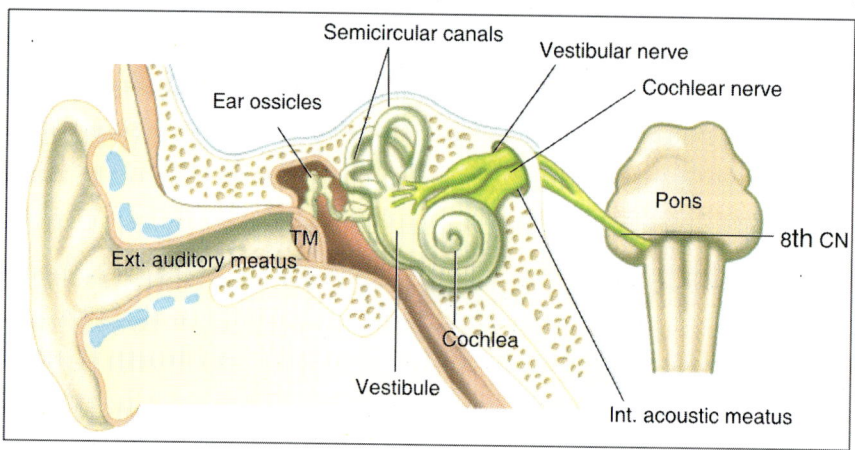

Fig. 51.4: Vestibulocochlear Nerve

CLINICAL CONSIDERATIONS

Tympanic Reflex

It is the reflection of a beam of shining light on the tympanic membrane. In the normal ear a bright, wedge-shaped reflection is seen with its apex is at the end of the malleus and its base is at the anterior inferior margin of the tympanic membrane. In the diseases of middle ear or tympanic membrane this shape is distorted.

Syringing

The wax like secretion in the ear gets hardened to block the external acoustic meatus thus causing hearing impairment. To remove this hardened wax, lukewarm water is injected slowly into external auditory meatus (EAM).

Precautions

- Water should not be hot
- Water should not be injected forcibly

This is to avoid stimulation of Vagus nerve, which may cause **vaso-vagal attack.**

Myringotomy (Tympanotomy)

This is making an opening in the tympanic membrane. This is carried out to drain the collected pus in the middle ear. The incision is given in the postero-inferior quadrant of tympanic membrane. This is seen behind the antero-inferior quadrant that appears as a cone of light when examine under illumination.

Otitis Externa

It is the infection of the external ear canal or the auricle of the external ear.

Causes

- Allergy
- Infection by bacteria, fungi and viruses
- Trauma

Otitis externa is more prevalent during hot, humid weather.

Prevention - to reduce maceration of the skin and to avoid trauma

Otitis Media

It is the infection of the middle ear a commonly seen in children. It may be

- Acute otitis media
- Chronic otitis media
- Allergic otitis media

Otitis media is often preceded by an upper respiratory tract infection.

The causative organisms enter middle ear through the eustachian tube. The small diameter and horizontal orientation of the tube in infants predisposes them to infection.

Obstruction of the eustachian tube and accumulation of exudate increases pressure within the middle ear. This forces infection to spread into the mastoid bone or causing the rupture of the tympanic membrane.

Symptoms of acute otitis media

- Sense of fullness in the ear
- Diminished hearing
- Pain and fever

Usually only one ear is affected. Squamous epithelium may grow in the middle ear through a rupture in the tympanic membrane. This leads to development of a **cholesteatoma** and deafness may result if repeated infections cause the opening to persist. The otitis media may spread to the meninges causing meningitis.

Management includes analgesics, nasal decongestants, needle aspiration of secretions and myringotomy.

Chronic otitis media may result in delayed speech development.

Tympanoplasty

This is the surgical operative procedure on the tympanic membrane or ear ossicles of the middle ear to restore or improve hearing in patients with conductive deafness.

This may be used in

- Perforation of tympanic membrane
- Otosclerosis
- Dislocation or necrosis of ear ossicles

Myringoplasty

This is the surgical repair of perforations of the tympanic membrane with a tissue graft. This is performed to correct hearing loss.

Under local or general anesthesia, the openings in the tympanic membrane are enlarged and the grafting material is sutured over the openings.

Deafness

This is characterized by partial or complete loss of hearing. To assess deafness the ears are examined for

1. Discharge
2. Crusts formation
3. Accumulation of wax
4. Structural abnormality of the ear
5. Deafness may be
   - Conductive or sensory
   - Temporary or permanent
   - Congenital or acquired

Management

- Removal of impacted wax from the external auditory meatus
- Hearing aids
- Amplification of sound
- Speech therapy

Conductive deafness

In this deafness sound is inadequately conducted through the external or middle ear to the sensorineural apparatus of the inner ear. Sensitivity to sound is diminished, but interpretation of the sound is not changed.

Sensorineural hearing loss

In this deafness sound is conducted normally through the external and middle ear. There is a defect in the inner ear or auditory nerve resulting in hearing loss. Sound discrimination may or may not be affected. Amplification of the sound with a hearing aid helps in these cases.

Mastoiditis

It is an infection of mastoid bone. This usually results from an extension of a middle ear infection. This is characterized by

- Earache
- Fever
- Headache and malaise

The swelling of the mastoid process displaces the pinna anteriorly and inferiorly. Children are affected most. Residual hearing loss may be seen following the infection.

Mastoidectomy

It is the surgical excision of a part of the mastoid temporal bone. This is performed.

- Chronic suppuartive otitis media (CSOM)
- Mastoiditis

The entry is made through the ear canal or from behind the ear.

Simple mastoidectomy - infected bone cells are removed and the tympanic membrane is incised to drain the middle ear.

Radical mastoidectomy - tympanic membrane and most of the middle ear structures are removed. The stapes is left intact so that a hearing aid may be used.

Modified radical mastoidectomy - tympanic membrane and the middle ear structures are saved. The patient will have better hearing compared to radical mastoidectomy.

Stapedectomy

This consists of removal of the stapes of the middle ear and insertion of a graft and prosthesis. This is performed to restore hearing in the treatment of otosclerosis.

The fixed stapes is replaced so that vibrations again transmit sound waves through the oval window to the fluid of the inner ear.

Complications

- Infection of the ear (outer, middle, or inner)
- Displacement or rejection of the graft

- Leaking of perilymph around the prosthesis into the middle ear

Otosclerosis (Otospongiosis)

It is a hereditary condition of unknown etiology in which irregular ossification in the bony labyrinth of the inner ear occurs. This causes tinnitus and then deafness. Females are affected twice.

Stapedectomy is done to restore hearing.

Tympanogram

It is a graphic representation of the acoustic impedance and air pressure of the middle ear and mobility of the tympanic membrane.

In the normal middle ear the air pressure is the same as the atmospheric pressure which is shown by a peak in the middle of the tympanogram. Distinctive tympanograms are observed in

- Otitis media
- Otosclerosis
- Perforation of tympanic membrane

Deafness

This may be due to abnormal ossification between the base of stapes and margins of fenestra cochleae (**otosclerosis**).

Hyperacusis

Thos may results due to paralysis of stapedius.

52

Eye

EYE

It is situated in the anterior part of the orbit. This organ of special sense. It is almost spherical (about one inch in diameter).

FASCIA BULBI (Tenon's capsule)

It is a thin membrane which envelops the eyeball from the optic nerve to the ciliary region and allows the eyeball to move freely. It has a smooth inner surface which is pierced by vessels and nerves. It fuses with the sheath of the optic nerve and with the sclera. The lower part of the membrane thickens into the suspensory ligament (**checks ligaments**). These are attached to the zygomatic arch and the lacrimal bone.

STRUCTURE OF EYE BALL

Three coats enclose concentrically
A. **Outer** or fibrous coat is composed of
   - Sclera
   - Cornea
B. **Middle** or vascular coat comprises
   - Choroid
   - Ciliary body
   - Iris
C. **Inner** or nervous coat consists of
   - Retina

The three coats enclose refracting media. From anterior to posterior these are
1. Cornea
2. Aqueous humour
3. Lens
4 Vitreous body

CORNEA

It is the convex and transparent layer. It is about half an inch wide. Anterior chamber separates it from the iris. It has no blood supply. It is nourished by lymph and has a rich nerve supply. Its junction with sclera is termed as **limbus**.

SCLERA

It is the visible white part of the eye covered with conjunctiva. It is made up of dense fibrous tissue. It receives arteries and nerves while **sinus venosus sclerae** communicates with scleral veins and anterior chamber. It provides attachments to tendons of recti and obliqui. It is pierces by numerous nerves and vessels.

CHOROID

It lines the sclera and separates it from retina. It consists of pigmented tissue containing nerve

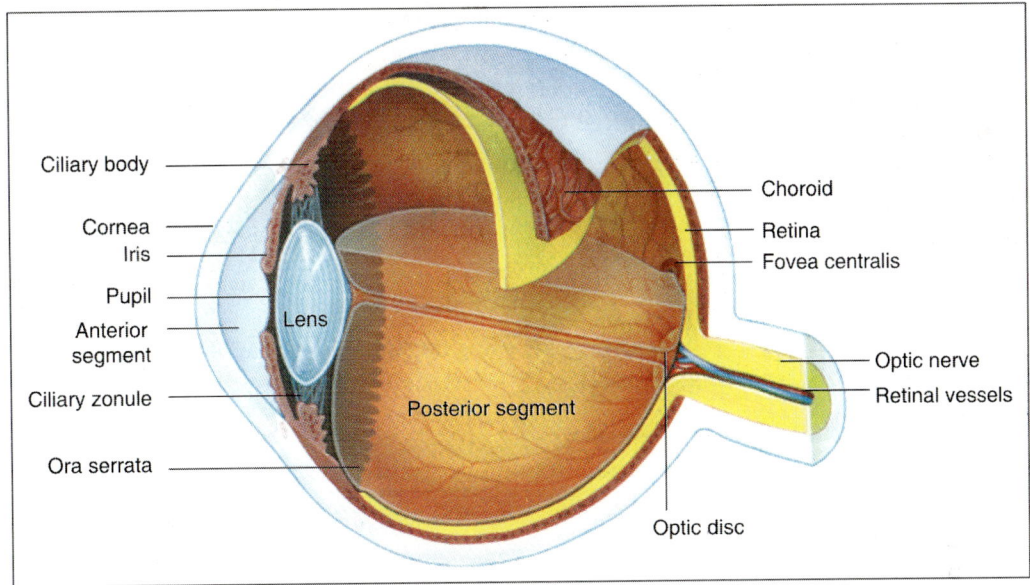

Fig. 52.1: Eye ball in section

plexuses, network of capillaries, arteries and superficial veins.

CILIARY BODY

It connects choroid with iris. It is made up of ciliary processes (internally) and ciliary muscle (externally)

Ciliary processes are similar to choroid in structure. They appear as radially arranged folds. These are about seventy in number that lie behind the periphery of iris. They form a flat ring with free and rounded central ends.

CILIARY MUSCLE

It is a muscular ring placed deep to anterior part of sclera. It is made up of radial and circular fibers. The ciliary muscle is brought into action during accommodation e.g. it slackens suspensory ligament of lens thus making it move convex as is required for near vision.

IRIS

It is placed behind the cornea and in front of lens. It is a circular, colored and contractile curtain. Its central aperture is pupil whose margins rest on lens while its peripheral margin is continuous with ciliary body. It is made up of smooth muscle – **sphincter pupillae** and **dilator pupillae**.

RETINA

It has two components

Pigmented layer (external layer) – This is attached to choroid and is continuous over ciliary body to iris.
Retina proper (internal layer) –This is in contact with vitreous. Ora serrata divides it into

- Posterior optic part
- Anterior ciliary part

Ora serrata is a wavy border behind the ciliary body. Posterior to this, retina contains nervous elements while anterior to this there is thin layer of columnar cells over ciliary body to iris.

Macula lutea – A small yellowish spot. The posterior pole of eyeball on retina. It presents **fovea centralis**.

Optic disc – Here optic nerve fibers converge to leave the eyeball. It is one mm below and three mm medial to the posterior pole. Its circumference is raised while its center is depressed. It is called **optic cup**. The disc is the blind spot of the eye as it lacks nervous elements.

LENS

It is transparent and circular measuring about ten mm in diameter. It is four mm thick. It is biconvex which lies on vitreous anteriorly and placed behind the iris and pupil. At rest it is more flattened. Looking at a near object, the ciliary muscle pulls the choroid and ciliary processes causing slackening of suspensory ligament. This makes the lens more convex.

ANTERIOR CHAMBER OF EYE BALL

It is the space between cornea anteriorly and iris and central part of lens posteriorly

POSTERIOR CHAMBER OF EYE BALL

It is placed behind the iris and suspensory ligament and adjoining part of the lens posteriorly. Two chambers communicate through the pupil and are filled with a clear fluid termed **aqueous humour**.

VITREOUS HUMOUR (Corpus vitreum, Vitreous body)

It is transparent and jelly like substance that fills posterior 4/5 of eyeball. It is enclosed in a transparent membrane (**hyaloid membrane**). It consists of
- Liquid aqueous humour
- Loose vitreous fibrous stroma

Some indications of the hyaloid canal may persist in the vitreous humor. This is not penetrated by any

blood vessels and is nourished at its periphery by vessels of the retina and the ciliary processes. The vitreous humor is concave anteriorly to accommodate the lens and is closely applied to the retina around the wall of the eyeball.

CLINICAL CONSIDERATIONS

Cataract

It is an abnormal progressive condition of the lens of the eye which is characterized by loss of transparency. This results in a gray-white opacity within the lens. The tendency to develop cataracts is inherited.

Most cataracts are caused by degenerative changes in the lens after fifty years of age. Trauma (puncture wound) may result in cataract formation. **Congenital cataracts** are usually hereditary but may be caused by viral infection during the first trimester of gestation.

Senile cataracts are uncomplicated cataracts of old age. Sight is lost if cataracts are not treated.

Management

These are treated with excision of the lens and implantation of interocular lens (IOL).

Retinal Detachment

It is the separation of the retina from the choroid. It usually results from a hole in the retina that allows the vitreous humor to leak between the choroid and the retina. In the majority of cases retinal detachment is the result of internal changes in the vitreous chamber associated with aging or with inflammation of the interior of the eye.

Retinal detachment develops slowly. The retina does not contain sensory nerves that relay the sensation of pain thus the condition is painless.

Detachment usually begins at the thin peripheral edge of the retina and extends gradually beneath the thicker and more central areas. The condition does not resolve itself. Blindness resulting from retinal detachment is irreversible.

Corneal Grafting (Keratoplasty)

It is the surgical procedure of transplantation of corneal tissue from one human eye to another person. It is performed to improve vision in

- Corneal scarring
- Distortion
- Perforation.

Glaucoma

This is an abnormal condition of elevated intraocular pressure because of obstruction of the outflow of aqueous humor.

Glaucoma may be

Acute (narrow-angle) glaucoma occurs if the pupil with a narrow angle between the iris and cornea dilates markedly. This causes folded iris to block the exit of aqueous humor from the anterior chamber.

Chronic (open-angle or **wide-angle) glaucoma** is more common and often bilateral. It is genetically determined and develops slowly. The obstruction is in the canal of Schlemm.

Acute glaucoma presents with extreme ocular pain, blurred vision, red eye and dilated pupil. Untreated cases results in complete and permanent blindness within two to five days.

Chronic glaucoma presents gradual loss of peripheral vision over a period of years. This may present with headaches, blurred vision and dull pain in the eye.

Cupping of the optic discs is noted in ophthalmoscopic examination.

Corneal Reflex

It is a protective mechanism for the eye in which the eyelids close when the cornea is touched. The reflex is mediated by the ophthalmic division of the 5th cranial nerve (sensory) and 7th cranial nerve (motor).

This reflex may be used as a test of integrity of those nerves.

Conjuctival Reflex

It is a protective mechanism for the eye in which the eyelids close whenever the conjunctiva is touched.

Conjunctivitis

It is the inflammation of the conjunctiva. This may be caused by

- Bacterial or viral infection
- Allergy
- Environmental factors

Clinical features

- Red eyes with a thick discharge
- Sticky eyelids in the morning
- Inflammation without pain

Uveitis

It is the inflammation of the uveal tract including the iris, ciliary body, and choroid.

Causes

- Allergy
- Infection
- Trauma
- Collagen disease

It is characterized by

- Irregularly shaped pupil
- Inflammation around the cornea
- Pus in the anterior chamber
- Opaque deposits on the cornea
- Pain and lacrimation

Major complication – development of glaucoma.

Vitreous Degeneration

It is a form of hyaline degeneration. This results in the formation of glassy material in the connective tissue of blood vessels and other tissues.

Chorioretinitis

It is an inflammatory condition of the choroid and retina of the eye. It usually results from parasitic or bacterial infection.

Clinical features

- Blurred vision
- Photophobia
- Distorted images

Section-IV
Neuroanatomy

CONTENTS

53. **Meanings and Blood Vessels**   299-312

54. **Medula Oblongata**   313-315

55. **Pons**   316-318

56. **Cerebellum**   319-322

57. **Midbrain**   323-324

58. **Cerebrum**   325-332

59. **Thalamus and Hypothalamus**   333-335

60. **Limbic System**   336-337

61. **Spinal Cord**   338-345

62. **Autonomic Nervous System**   346-350

Meanings and Blood Vessels

MENINGES

DURA MATER

It is the outer tough and fibrous covering of brain dura mater. It has two layers

Endosteal layer is the outer layer, which is firmly adherent to internal aspect of cranium all around. Part of this dura extends as a sheath along with cranial nerves emerging from various foramina.

Meningeal layer is the inner and relatively thin layer, which covers brain. Beyond foramen magnum it continues as spinal dura mater.

Within the cranium, at places, the meningeal layer duplicates to form partitions:

- Falx cerebri
- Falx cerebelli
- Tentorium cerebelli
- Diaphragma sallae

The intracranial dural venous sinuses are formed as:

- By the separation between the two layers of dura (**superior sagittal sinus**)
- By the reduplication of meningeal dura (**inferior sagittal sinus**)

SUBARACHNOID CISTERNS

Deep to meningeal dura mater the arachnoid mater is placed which unsheathes the brain and spinal cord. The subarachnoid space is filled with cerebrospinal fluid (**CSF**). It acts as a shock absorber. At places the subarachnoid space is enlarged in dimensions to form sub-arachnoid cisterns. These cisterns have been named as per their locations e.g. **Cisterna interpeduncularis, Cerebello- medullary cistern, cisterna pontis** etc.

Cerebello medullary cistern - It is formed by the arachnoid mater bridging the interval between medulla oblongata and the under surface of cerebellum. Below it continues as subarachnoid space of spinal cord.

Cisterna Pontis - It is present on the ventral aspect of pons containing basilar artery.

Cisterna Interpeduncularis - At the base of the brain is the interpeduncular fossa. It contains circle of Willis and roots of oculomotor nerves.

Cisterna Ambiens - A dilated space all around midbrain is termed as cisterna ambiens.

Among the meninges, only dura mater is sensitive to pain. Thus the sensory nerves innervate it.

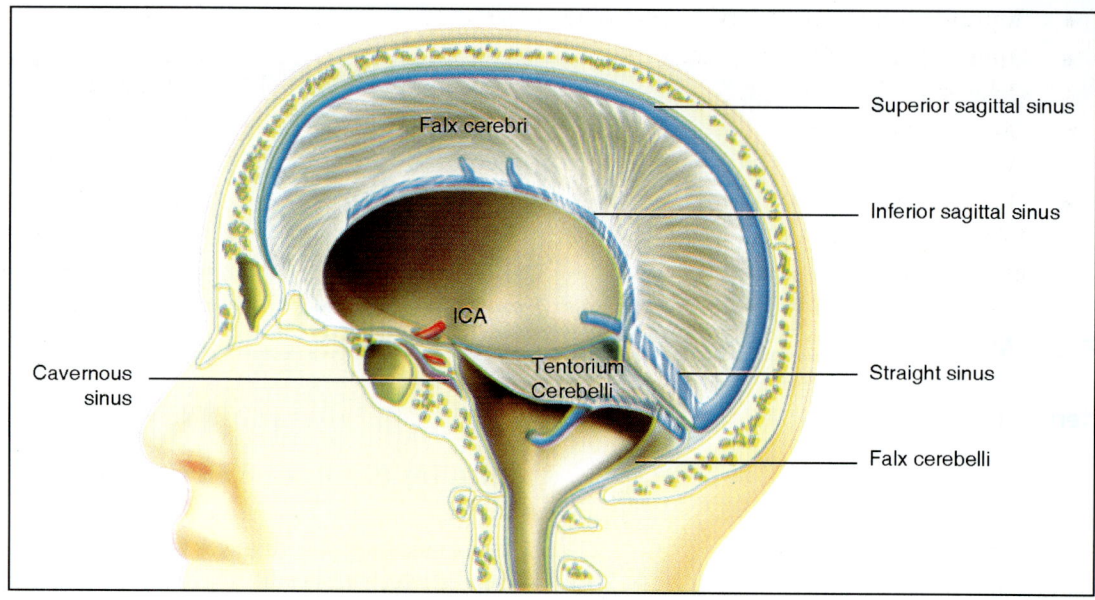

Fig. 53.1: Meninges and Dural Venous Sinuses

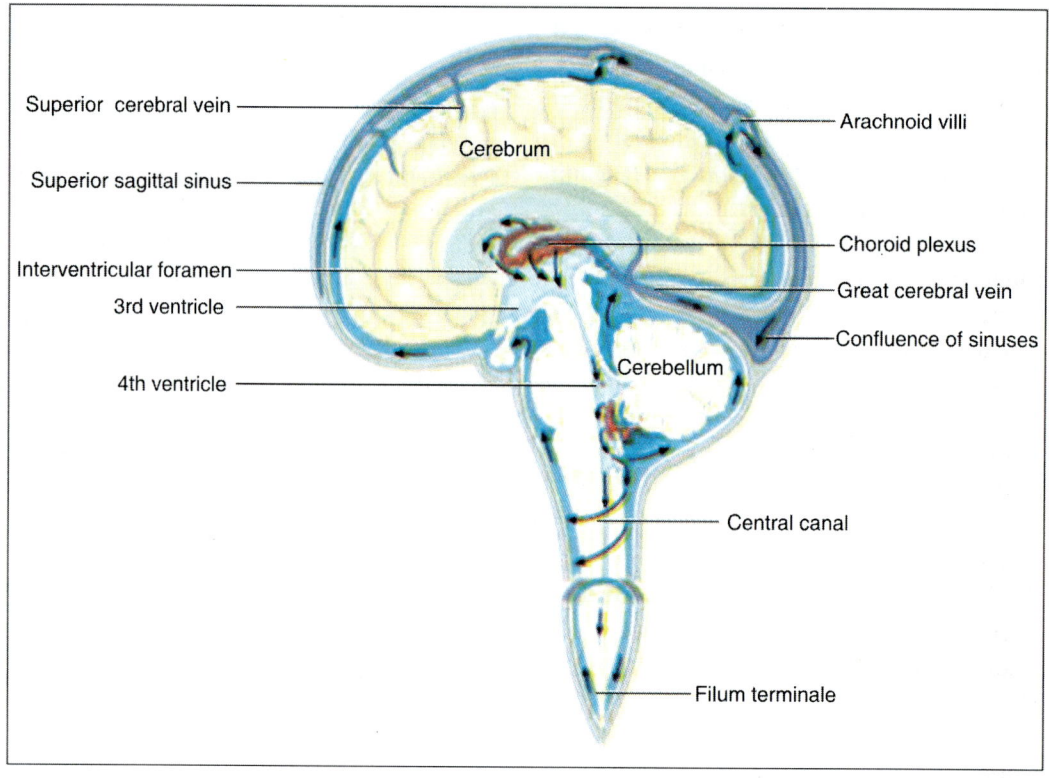

Fig. 53.2: CSF & its circulation

- **Supratentorial part** – Nervous spinosum
- **Dura of anterior cranial fossa** – Ophthalmic division (V-1)
- **Dura of middle cranial fossa** –Maxillary (V-2) and Mandibular (V-3)
- **Dura of posterior cranial fossa** – Recurrent branch of X and XII cranial nerves.

ARTERIAL SUPPLY OF MENINGES

Arterial supply of dura mater

It is mainly supplied by middle meningeal and accessory meningeal arteries (branches of first part of maxillary artery).

Arachnoid and pia mater

These are collectively termed as leptomeninges. **Pia mater** is closely applied to the surface of the brain / spinal cord. The double-layered fold of pia mater encloses a tuft of capillaries termed as **choroid plexus**. This plexus invaginates into the ventricular cavities of brain – cerebrospinal fluid formation. In the vertebral canal lateral extensions of the pia mater – **ligamentum denticulation** – attach the spinal cord laterally to the vertebral canal by piercing the arachnoid mater. They are 21 pairs, triangular in shape and present serrated appearance. They anchor the spinal cord to the vertebral canal. **Arachnoid mater** is the middle layer of meninges covering the brain and spinal cord. A thin film of fluid separates it from dura mater. The subarachnoid space is a potential space containing CSF. The CSF is absorbed into superior sagittal sinus through arachnoid granulations / villi.

Lateral lacunae are the extension of subarachnoid space through the meningeal dura to enter superior sagittal sinus. Here CSF and venous blood are separated by squamous epithelium. This is the site where from CSF is absorbed into circulation.

BLOOD SUPPLY OF BRAIN

The brain is supplied by branches of ICA and vertebral artery, which join to form **circle of WILLIS** at the base of brain (carotido-vertebral system).

The circle of WIILLIS is more polygonal than circular. It is placed in inter-peduncular cistern. Following arteries forms it:

- Posterior cerebral artery (terminal branch of Basilar artery)
- Middle and anterior cerebral arteries (branches of CIA)

Anterior and posterior communicating arteries complete the circle. This anastomotic channel is meant to equalize the flow of blood. About 60% of circles display anomalies. The circle gives off:

Cortical branches,

Central branches (ganglionic – striate branches)

Cortical branches

These supply the grey matter. These large branches form a superficial plexus, which issue smaller terminal branches. These branches enter the brain substance at right angles and run for variable distances. Short branches arborize in the cortex while the longer branches supply the deeply placed medullary substance.

The anastomosis between the cortical branches is rarely sufficient to prevent brain damage in case of occlusion. Most of the occlusions occur before these vessels enter the substance of brain. In a vascular injury **internal capsule**, **basal ganglia** and a part of cerebral cortex, which lie between the distributions of two primary arteries, are the sites most severely involved.

Central branches

They arise from circle of Willis and proximal portions of three cerebral arteries. To supply **diencephalon**, **corpus striatum** and **internal**

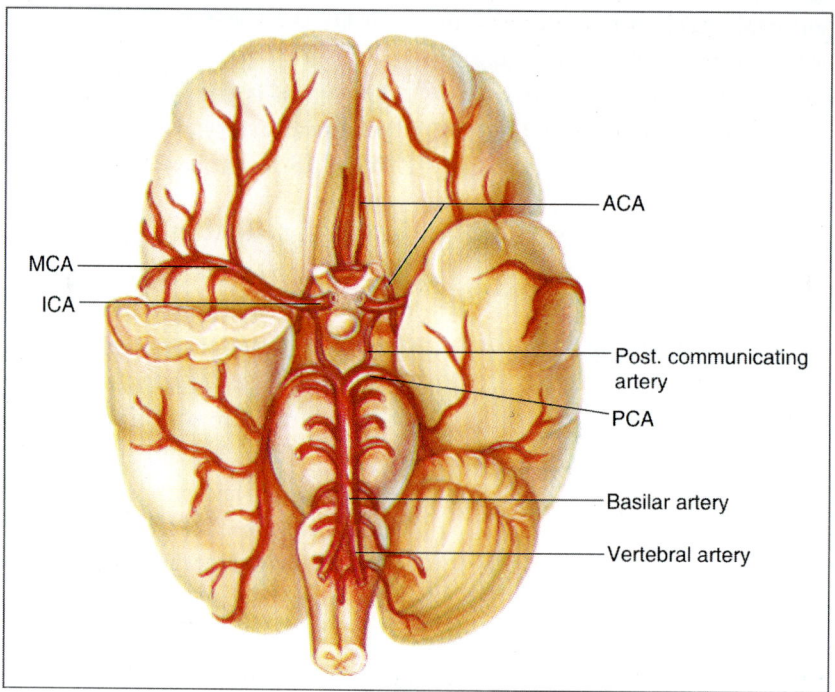

Fig. 53.3: Blood supply of Brain

capsule there branches dip perpendicularly in the brain substance. These arteries are not end arteries but the precapillary anastomosis is insufficient to maintain adequate circulation if a major vessel is occluded suddenly. The lesion leads to infarction / softening in the area deprived of an adequate blood supply.

The striate arteries constitute:

Group A – Which arise form inside of
- Circle of Willis
- Anteromedial (AM)
- Posteromedial (PM)

Group B – Which arise form the constituting branches of circle of Willis
- Anterolateral (AL)
- Posterolateral (PL)

CRANIAL AND INTRACRANIAL VEINS

DIPLOIC VEINS

These valves-less venous channels are present in the diploë of some cranial bones. These are large with dilatations at irregular intervals. These are absent at birth and begin to develop with the diploë at about two years.

These communicate with
- Meningeal veins
- Dural venous sinuses
- Veins of pericranium

Regular channels include
- **Frontal diploic vein** – Passes through the supraorbital foramen and joins the supraorbital vein

- **Anterior temporal (parietal) diploic vein** - Pierces the greater wing of the sphenoid to end in the sphenoparietal sinus
- **Posterior temporal (parietal) diploic vein** - Descends to the parietal mastoid angle to join the transverse sinus through a foramen at the angle or mastoid foramen
- **Occipital diploic vein** (largest) - Opens into occipital veins or the transverse sinus near the confluence of sinuses

Numerous small diploic veins emerge near the superior sagittal sinus to end in its venous lacunae.

MENINGEAL VEINS

Meningeal veins begin from plexiform vessels in the dura mater and drain into efferent vessels which are connected with lacunae of the superior sagittal sinus and with other sinuses.

VEINS OF BRAIN

Features

- Veins of the brain have no valves
- Their thin walls are devoid of muscular tissue
- They pierce the arachnoid mater and meningeal layer of dura mater
- They open into dural venous sinuses

These comprise

- Cerebral veins
- Cerebellar veins
- Veins of the brainstem

The cerebral veins (external and internal) drain the surfaces and the interior of the hemispheres.

EXTERNAL CEREBRAL VEINS

These veins form three groups

- Superior
- Middle
- Inferior

Superior cerebral veins

These are about eight to twelve in each cerebral hemisphere.

They drain superolateral and medial surfaces.

As these ascend towards the superomedial border, they receive small veins from the medial surface and open into the superior sagittal sinus.

Anterior veins open at right angles.

Posterior veins are directed obliquely forwards against the flow of blood in the sinus. This resists the collapse of thin-walled cerebral veins which might result from a rise of intracranial pressure.

Superficial middle cerebral vein

It begins on the superolateral surface. It follows the posterior ramus and stem of the lateral sulcus to end in the cavernous sinus.

Superior anastomotic vein runs postero-superiorly between the middle cerebral vein and the superior sagittal sinus which connects the superior sagittal and cavernous sinuses.

Inferior anastomotic vein runs over the temporal lobe which connects the middle cerebral vein to the transverse sinus.

Inferior cerebral veins

Veins on the frontal orbital surface join the superior cerebral veins and drain into the superior sagittal sinus

Veins on the temporal lobe anastomose with basal and middle cerebral veins and drain into the cavernous, superior petrosal and transverse sinuses.

BASAL VEIN

It begins at the anterior perforated substance by the union of:

- **Anterior cerebral vein**
- **Deep middle cerebral vein** - runs in the lateral cerebral sulcus
- **Striate veins -** emerge from the anterior perforated substance

The basal vein passes backwards around the cerebral peduncle to join the great cerebral vein. It receives tributaries from

- Interpeduncular fossa
- Inferior horn of the lateral ventricle
- Parahippocampal gyrus
- Midbrain

INTERNAL CEREBRAL VEIN

It is formed near the interventricular foramen by the union of thalamostriate and choroid veins. It drains the deep parts of cerebral hemisphere.

Thalamostriate vein

It runs anteriorly between the caudate nucleus and thalamus. It receives veins from thalamus and caudate nucleus.

Behind the anterior column of the fornix it joins with the choroid vein to form the internal cerebral vein.

Choroid vein

It runs along the whole choroid plexus. It receives veins from

- Hippocampus
- Fornix
- Corpus callosum

Great cerebral vein

It is formed by the union of the two internal cerebral veins. It curves upwards around the splenium to open into the anterior end of the straight sinus. It receives basal veins.

CEREBELLAR VEINS

These veins run over the cerebellar surface. These comprise superior and inferior sets.

Superior cerebellar veins

These run anteromedially across the superior vermis to open in the straight sinus or great cerebral vein

while others run laterally to terminate in the transverse and superior petrosal sinuses.

Inferior cerebellar veins

These run backwards on the inferior vermis to enter the straight or sigmoid sinus while the laterally running vessels open in the inferior petrosal and occipital sinuses.

VEINS OF BRAINSTEM

These form a superficial venous plexus placed deep to the arteries.

Veins of midbrain reach the great cerebral or basal vein.

Veins of pons form a lateral vein on each side which enter the petrosal sinuses, transverse sinus or cerebellar veins.

Veins of inferior medulla communicate with spinal veins and drain into the adjacent venous sinuses or along radicular veins. The veins following the last four cranial nerves terminate in the inferior petrosal or occipital sinus.

Anterior and posterior median medullary veins run along the anterior medial fissure and posterior median sulcus. These veins are continuous with the spinal veins in corresponding positions.

DURAL VENOUS SINUSES

These venous channels drain blood from the brain and cranial bones.

Features

- Placed between two layers of dura mater
- Lined by endothelium
- Do not have valves
- Their wall is devoid of muscular tissue

They are divided into

- **Posterosuperior group**
- **Antero-inferior group**

POSTEROSUPERIOR GROUP OF VENOUS SINUSES

It comprises

- Superior sagittal sinus
- Inferior sagittal sinus
- Straight sinus
- Transverse sinus
- Petrosquamous sinus
- Sigmoid sinus
- Occipital sinus

Superior sagittal sinus

It runs in the attached, convex margin of the falx cerebri. It begins near crista galli. It receives a vein from the nasal cavity when the foramen caecum is patent. The initial tributaries are cortical veins from the frontal lobes. The sinus runs backwards. It grooves the inner surface of the frontal bone, the adjacent margins of the parietal bones and the squamous occipital bone. Near the internal occipital protuberance it deviates (usually to the right) and continues as the transverse sinus. It is triangular in cross-section which gradually enlarges backwards.

Its interior shows the openings of superior cerebral veins, projections of arachnoid granulations and many fibrous bands across its inferior angle.

It also communicates by small orifices with irregular venous lacunae which are situated in the dura mater near the sinus. These lacunae are usually three on each side:

- Frontal (small)
- Parietal (large)
- Occipital (intermediate)

In old age the lacunae become confluent as one elongated lacuna on each side and numerous arachnoid granulations project into them.

Superior sagittal sinus receives

- Superior cerebral veins
- Veins from the pericranium

The lacunae drain the diploic and meningeal veins.

Confluence of sinuses

It is the dilated posterior end of the superior sagittal sinus, situated to one side (usually right) of the internal occipital protuberance, where it turns to become transverse sinus. It is also connected with the occipital and opposite transverse sinus.

Clinical relevance

Connections between the superior sagittal sinus and veins of the nose, scalp and diploë explain the spread of infective thrombosis in these parts.

Inferior sagittal sinus

It is located in the posterior two-thirds of the free margin of the falx cerebri. It increases in size gradually towards the posterior end. It terminates in the straight sinus. It receives veins from the falx cerebri and the medial surfaces of cerebrum.

Straight sinus

It is placed at the junction of the falx cerebri with the tentorium cerebelli. It is triangular in cross-section. It runs postero-inferiorly and may communicate terminally at the confluence of sinuses. Its tributaries include

- Superior cerebellar veins
- Great cerebral vein

Transverse sinuses

These begin at the internal occipital protuberance. One (right) is continuous with the superior sagittal sinus while the other with the straight sinus. Each sinus curves anterolaterally to the posterolateral part of the petrous temporal bone and it turns downwards as sigmoid sinus. It is placed in the attached margin of the tentorium cerebelli.

The sinus is triangular in section and the one (right) which drains the superior sagittal sinus is larger. The sinus is joined by the superior petrosal sinus where it continues as sigmoid sinus.

It receives

- Inferior cerebral vein
- Inferior cerebellar veins
- Diploic veins
- Inferior anastomotic veins

Petrosquamous sinus

It runs backwards in a groove which is seen along the junction of the squamous and petrous parts of the temporal bone. It opens posteriorly into the transverse sinus.

Anteriorly it is connected with the retromandibular vein through a postglenoid or squamous foramen. The sinus may be absent.

Sigmoid sinuses

These are continuations of the transverse sinuses beyond the tentorium cerebelli. The sinus curves inferomedially in a groove on the mastoid temporal bone. It crosses the jugular process of occipital bone and beyond the jugular foramen it continues as IJV.

It is connected with pericranial veins via mastoid and condylar emissary veins.

Occipital sinus

This smallest sinus lies in the attached margin of the falx cerebelli. It commences near the foramen magnum.

It is connected to the internal vertebral plexuses and terminates in the confluence of sinuses.

ANTERO-INFERIOR GROUP OF VENOUS SINUSES

This includes

- Cavernous sinus
- Intercavernous sinuses
- Inferior petrosal sinus
- Sphenoparietal sinus
- Superior petrosal sinus
- Basilar sinuses
- Middle meningeal veins

Cavernous sinuses

These are placed by the sides of the body of the sphenoid bone.

The sinus extends from the superior orbital fissure to the apex of the petrous temporal bone.

Measurements – Length: two cm and width: one cm

The internal carotid artery accompanied with sympathetic plexus passes forwards through the sinus along the abducent nerve which is placed inferolateral to the artery.

Structures in the lateral wall

- Oculomotor nerve
- Trochlear nerve
- Ophthalmic division of V CN
- Maxillary divisions of V CN

Sphenoidal air sinus and hypophysis cerebri are placed medial to it

Cavum trigeminale is near the inferoposterior part of its lateral wall which encloses trigeminal ganglion.

Tributaries

1. Superior ophthalmic vein
2. Branch from the inferior ophthalmic vein
3. Superficial middle cerebral vein
4. Inferior cerebral veins
5. Sphenoparietal sinus
6. Central vein of retina
7. Frontal tributary of the middle meningeal vein (sometimes)

It drains into

- Transverse sinus via the superior petrosal sinus
- Internal jugular via the inferior petrosal sinus
- Pterygoid plexus by veins passing through emissary sphenoidal foramen, foramen ovale and foramen lacerum
- Facial vein via the superior ophthalmic vein

Two sinuses are interconnected by anterior and posterior intercavernous sinuses and the basilar plexus.

All connections are valve-less. Thus the blood can flow in either direction.

Propulsion of blood in the sinus is due to

- Pulsation of the internal carotid artery
- Gravity - position of the head

Clinical relevance

An arteriovenous communication may occur between the cavernous sinus and internal carotid artery. This causes a pulsating orbital swelling. Ligation of the internal or common carotid artery may be required.

Suppuration in the upper nasal cavities and paranasal sinuses may lead to septic thrombosis of the cavernous sinuses.

Ophthalmic veins

These are superior and inferior. These are valve-less which connects the facial and intracranial veins.

Superior ophthalmic vein is formed posteromedial to the upper lid from two tributaries which are connected anteriorly with the facial and supraorbital veins. It runs with the ophthalmic artery and passes through the superior orbital fissure to terminate in the cavernous sinus.

Inferior ophthalmic vein is formed near the anterior part of the orbital floor and medial wall. It receives veins from the inferior rectus, inferior oblique, lacrimal sac and eyelids. It runs backwards above the inferior rectus and may join the superior ophthalmic vein. It terminates in the cavernous sinus. It is connected to the pterygoid venous plexus by small rami passing through the inferior orbital fissure.

Central vein of retina

This vein first traverses the optic nerve. Then it leaves the nerve to have a long course in the subarachnoid space. It terminates in the cavernous sinus or the superior ophthalmic vein.

Sphenoparietal sinuses

These are placed below the periosteum of the lesser wings of the sphenoid near their posterior edges. Each sinus receives small veins from the adjacent dura mater and sometimes the frontal ramus of the middle meningeal vein. It curves medially and opens into the anterior part of the cavernous sinus.

Intercavernous sinuses

These two sinuses (anterior and posterior) interconnect the cavernous sinuses in the anterior and posterior attached borders of the diaphragma sellae. These along with two cavernous sinuses constitute **circular sinus**.

Superior petrosal sinuses

These are paired, small and narrow sinuses which drain the cavernous sinuses to the transverse sinuses. Each leaves the posterosuperior part of the cavernous sinus and runs posterolaterally in the attached margin of the tentorium cerebelli. It crosses above the trigeminal nerve to a groove on the superior border of the petrous temporal bone. It ends by joining transverse sinus.

It receives

- Cerebellar veins
- Inferior cerebral vein
- Tympanic veins

It is connected to the inferior petrosal sinus and basilar plexus.

Inferior petrosal sinuses

These drain the cavernous sinuses to the internal jugular veins. Each sinus begins postero-inferiorly at its cavernous sinus and runs backwards in a groove between the petrous temporal and basilar occipital bones. It traverses the anterior part of the jugular foramen to ends in the superior bulb of IJV.

It receives

- Labyrinthine veins
- Vestibular aqueduct
- Tributaries from the medulla, pons and inferior cerebellar surface

Relations of structures in the jugular foramen

These are as follows

- **Inferior petrosal sinus** is anteromedial with a meningeal branch of the ascending pharyngeal artery, and the sinus descends obliquely backwards
- **Sigmoid sinus** is situated at the lateral and posterior part of the foramen with a meningeal branch of the occipital artery
- **Between the sinuses** are in succession, posterolaterally: IX, X and XI cranial nerves

Basilar venous plexus

It consists of interconnecting channels between layers of dura mater on the clivus.

It interconnects the inferior petrosal sinuses and joins with the internal vertebral venous plexus. It is also connected with the cavernous and superior petrosal sinuses at its anterior end.

Middle meningeal veins (sinuses)

These communicate above with the superior sagittal sinus through its venous lacunae. Below these converge and unite as frontal and parietal trunks, which run in the grooves on the inner surfaces of parietal bone accompanied by arteries. The veins are closer to bone and sometimes occupy separate grooves.

Termination is variable.

Parietal trunk may traverse the foramen spinosum to the pterygoid venous plexus

Frontal trunk may also reach pterygoid venous plexus via the foramen ovale or may terminate in the sphenoparietal or cavernous sinus.

SURFACE ANATOMY

Superior sagittal sinus runs from the glabella to the inion.

Transverse sinus begins at the inion and runs laterally, with slight upward convexity to the base of the mastoid process.

Sigmoid sinus starts from the base of mastoid process and passes downwards just anterior to the posterior mastoid border to a point about one cm above its tip.

EMISSARY VEINS

These are the connections between the dural venous sinuses and extracranial veins. Some are constant while others may be absent at times.

- **Mastoid emissary vein** in the mastoid foramen joins the sigmoid sinus with the posterior auricular or occipital vein.
- **Parietal emissary vein** traverses the parietal foramen to connect the superior sagittal sinus with the veins of the scalp.
- **Venous plexus of the hypoglossal canal** connects the sigmoid sinus to the internal jugular vein.
- **Posterior condylar emissary vein** connects the sigmoid sinus with the veins in the suboccipital triangle via the condylar canal.
- **Venous plexus of foramen ovale** joins the cavernous sinus to the pterygoid plexus via the foramen ovale.
- **Small veins** traverse the foramen lacerum and connect the cavernous sinus with the pharyngeal veins and pterygoid plexus.
- **Vein in the emissary sphenoidal foramen** (of Vesalius) connects the cavernous sinus with pterygoid venous plexus
- **Internal carotid venous plexus** which passes through the carotid canal connects the cavernous sinus to IJV.
- **Petrosquamous sinus** connects the transverse sinus with the EJV
- **Vein may traverse the foramen caecum** (patent in 1%) which connect nasal veins with the superior sagittal sinus.
- **Occipital emissary vein** connects the confluence of sinuses with the occipital vein.

- **Occipital sinus** is connected with veins around the foramen magnum (**marginal sinuses**) and thus with the vertebral venous plexuses - alternative venous drainage when the jugular vein is blocked
- **Ophthalmic veins** are potentially emissary because they connect intracranial to extracranial veins.

These connections are significant in the spread of infection from extracranial foci to venous sinuses.

CIRCULATIONS OF CSF

The CSF is a colorless, acellular fluid. The CSF is secreted by the choroid plexus placed in lateral, 3rd and fourth ventricles of the brain. The secretion flows from the lateral ventricle into the third ventricle through **inter-ventricular foramina of Monroe**. The third ventricle communicates with the fourth ventricle through cerebral aqueduct. It has no choroid plexus. The fourth ventricle communicates with subarachnoid space (cerebello-medullary cistern) through three foramina (median – foramen of **Megendie** and lateral – foramina of **Luschka**). It is absorbed into superior sagittal sinus through sub-arachnoid villi / granulations.

The central canal of spinal cord is continuous superiorly with fourth ventricle while inferiorly it presents a dilated blind sac – **terminal ventricle**. The composition of CSF is clinically relevant. It has mononuclear cells (less than 5/units). Red blood cells are seen only in subarachnoid haemorrhage, trauma or ruptured aneurysm. Glucose levels differ in viral and bacterial meningitis. Total proteins increases in bacterial meningitis.

The normal CSF pressure in lateral recumbent position ranges from 100 to 180 mm of mater. The pressure increases in brain tumor and meningitis. Among the various functions, it can be ascribed to

- Support to the CNS
- Protection against concessive injury

- Transportation of hormones
- Removal of metabolic waste products

CLINICAL CONSIDERATIONS

Queckenstedt's Test

The CSF is absorbed in the superior sagittal sinus. Raising the pressure in the superior sagittal sinus by compressing the internal jugular veins (IJVs) or the liver will affect the absorption of SCF. The secretion of CSF is a continuous process and if increasing the intracranial pressure slows its absorption down, the rate of flow of CSF (drops/min) through the lumbar puncture needle would increase. Any block in the CSF circulation above the lumbar puncture needle would not change rate of CSF through the lumbar puncture (LP) needle.

Direction of blood flow in veins

Superficial cerebral veins drain the superolateral surface of cerebral hemisphere. The superior veins open into superior sagittal sinus against the flow of blood in superior sagittal sinus. Thus any venous stasis/venous collapse is prevented by blood rushing from superior sagittal sinus into these veins.

The general direction of flow of blood in these veins is towards neighboring venous sinuses.

Hydrocephalus

This clinical condition is characterized by dilatation of cerebral ventricles resulting from blockage of CSF circulation. Thus there is an excessive accumulation of CSF in the cerebral ventricles or subarachnoid space.

The condition dilates the ventricles of the brain and causes a separation of the bones of the calvaria in infants.

The Cerebrospinal fluid (CSF) is produced by the choroid plexuses located in the ventricles. The CSF produced in the ventricles reaches the subarachnoid space through the median foramen of Megendie and the lateral foramen of Luschka. These foramina are located in the roof of the fourth ventricle .The Choroid plexuses are made of vascularized double layers of pia matter (tela choroidea) covered by a layer of ependyma. Excessive CSF could be a result of excess production, obstruction of its flow or impaired absorption into the dural venous sinuses.

Internal hydrocephalus is an accumulation of fluid in the ventricles. A block in the median aperture of the fourth ventricle results in the thin wall of the ventricle herniating out through the foramen magnum into the superior part of the vertebral canal.

External hydrocephalus is an accumulation of fluid in the subarachnoid space due to a block in the subarachnoid space. The common sites of block are

- Where the brain stem passes through the tentorium cerebelli and
- Where the medulla passes the foramen magnum.

Blockage of the CSF circulation results in the dilatation of the ventricles superior to the point of obstruction. The enlarging ventricles now compress the substance of the brain between the ventricles and the bones of the skull. In infants, this results in an expansion of the skull as the suture lines and the fontanelles are still open.

1. **Non-communicating hydrocephalus** – Due to obstruction within the ventricles Example: Congenital stenosis of aqueduct
2. **Communicating hydrocephalus** – Due to blockage within the subarachnoid space Example: Adhesions after meningitis
3. **Normal pressure hydrocephalus** – Due to non-absorption of CSF from the arachnoid villi. It may be seen secondary to post traumatic haemorrhage. Its clinical features include a triad of dementia, ataxia and urinary incontinence.

Lumbar Puncture

In many neurological conditions, examination of CSF is imperative to diagnose. For this CSF is drawn by carrying out lumbar puncture. The procedure can be conducted by placing the patient either in left lateral or sitting position. The vertebral column is flexed so as to increase the gap between the adjacent vertebral spines. Under aseptic conditions, the lumbar puncture needle is pushed in the midline to enter subarachnoid space. It is carried out at the lower border of L-3 vertebra. This is to avoid injury to the caudal end of spinal cord, which normally ends at the lower of L-1 vertebra. The procedure is strictly contraindicated where there is raised intracranial pressure suggested by clinical findings and fundus examination. The lumbar puncture has diagnostic and therapeutic usage.

Intracerebral Haemorrhage

Bleeding within the substance of the brain is usually a result of rupture of one of the lenticulostriate branches of the middle cerebral artery. The lenticulostriate arteries supply vital areas of

- Internal capsule
- Lentiform nucleus
- Caudate nucleus

One of the lateral lenticulostriate branches of the middle cerebral artery is especially prone to rupture and is called as the Charcot's artery of cerebral haemorrhage. Rupture of this vessel produces a paralytic stroke because of the interruption of motor pathways from the motor cortex to the brain stem and the spinal cord.

These arteries have a small lumen, thin wall and are numerous in number. Hence any sudden rise in blood pressure can cause rupture of one of these vessels. The haemorrhage may cause compression of motor pathways leading to paralytic stroke.

Subarachnoid Haemorrhage

Bleeding which accumulates in the space between the arachnoid and pia mater is called as subarachnoid haemorrhage. The subarachnoid space contains the cerebrospinal fluid. It also contains all the major blood vessels, which supply blood to the brain.

The blood vessels supplying the CNS have to run for some distance of their course in the subarachnoid space. As this space is a potential space, blood may accumulate in this space. The causes of bleeding are many, most common being rupture of an aneurysm. Fracture of skull also leads to subarachnoid haemorrhage. The haemorrhage is characterized by symptoms of meningeal irritation. These include severe headache, stiff neck and loss of consciousness. This can be diagnosed by performing a lumbar puncture.

A subarachnoid haemorrhage is usually the result of a rupture of an arterial aneurysm. Blood in the subarachnoid space causes meningeal irritation, which produces

- Headache
- Stiffness of the neck
- Loss of consciousness

Subdural Haemorrhage

Bleeding which accumulates in the space between the dura and arachnoid is termed as subdural haemorrhage. The subdural space normally contains a thin film of fluid.

This haemorrhage is especially common in the elderly in whom some shrinkage of the brain is usually present. This type of haemorrhage is usually a result of trauma, which violently moves the brain within the skull resulting in rupture of the cerebral veins draining into the superior sagittal sinus.

It is more common than extradural hemorrhage. The bleeding is venous in nature.

Clinically there are signs of cerebral compressions, presence of blood in CSF and absence of lucid internal (time internal between the infliction of injury and appearance of signs of cerebral compression).

Extradural Haemorrhage

It is due to blow to the head. The bleeding is between meningeal and endosteal layer of dura mater. Here, the meningeal vessels (middle meningeal artery and its anterior division) are torned. There is loss of consciousness followed by lucid internal and thereafter drowsiness and coma.

The **features include** a brief period of concussion immediately after the injury after which there is a lucid interval in which the patient is apparently normal. This is followed by period of drowsiness and coma. The accumulation of blood in the extradural space causes cerebral compression. A large supratentorial extradural hematoma can push the cerebral tonsils through the foramen magnum, which results in compression of the medulla. This can cause fatal effects due to involvement of the vital cardio respiratory centres in the medulla.

Extradural Hematoma

It is slow and localized accumulation of blood at sites where endosteal dura is firmly attached to skullcap. With the increase in the bleeding the size of hematoma increases causing compression of brain. Supra-tentorial extradural hematoma causes raised supra-tentorial pressure. This may result in herniation of cerebellar tonsils through foramen magnum causing compression of medulla that can prove fatal.

Features:
- Sensory loss along the distribution of affected spinal nerves
- Lower motor neuron paralysis
- Bladder and bowel involvement is late.

Conus Medullaris Syndrome

The terminal part of spinal cord is termed **conus medullaris**. Here there is involvement of S-2, S-3 and S-4 spinal segments. Its essential features are:
- Bladder and bowel involvement is early
- Loss of sensations along the distribution of S-2, S-3 and S-4 spinal nerves result in a **saddle shaped anesthesia**.

Direction of blood flow in cerebral veins

Superficial cerebral veins drain the superolateral surface of cerebral hemisphere. The superior veins open into superior sagittal sinus against the flow of blood in superior sagittal sinus. Thus any venous stasis/venous collapse is prevented by blood rushing from superior sagittal sinus into these veins.

The general direction of flow of blood in these veins is towards neighbouring venous sinuses.

Fractures of the skull

Fractures of the skull are common in the adults but less so in case of infants and children. The skull of an adult can be likened to an eggshell. It has some resilience of its own and beyond which it fragments. A severe localized blow will produce a local indentation often accompanied by splintering of bone. Blows to the vault of skull often produce linear fractures, which radiate out through thin areas of bone. The petrous parts of the temporal bones and the occipital crests strongly reinforce the base of the skull and tend to deflect linear fractures.

The skull of an infant can be likened to a table tennis ball in that a localized blow produces a depression without splintering. This common type of circumscribed lesion is referred to as a "**pond fracture**".

Fractures of Anterior Cranial Fossa

The cribriform plate of ethmoid may be damaged resulting in tearing of the overlying meninges and underlying mucoperiosteum. The patient will have bleeding from the nose (epistaxis) and leakage of cerebrospinal fluid into the nose (cerebrospinal rhinorrhoea). Fractures involving the orbital plate of the frontal bone will result in haemorrhage beneath the conjunctive and into the orbital cavity causing exophthalmos. The frontal air sinus may also be involved with haemorrhage into the nose.

Fractures of Middle Cranial Fossa

These are very common since this is the weakest part of the skull. Anatomically this weakness is due to the presence of numerous foramina and canals in this region. The cavities of the middle ear and the sphenoidal sinuses are particularly liable to damage. The leakage of CSF and blood from the external auditory meatus is common. The VII and VIII cranial nerves can get damaged as they pass through the internal auditory meatus. The III, IV and VI cranial nerves may get damaged if the lateral wall of the cavernous sinus is torn. Blood and CSF may leak into the sphenoidal air sinuses and then into the nose.

Fractures of the Posterior Cranial Fossa

Blood may escape into the nape of the neck deep to the postvertebral muscles. Some days later, it tracks between the muscles and appears in the posterior triangle, close to mastoid process. The mucous membrane of the roof of the nasopharynx may be torn and blood could accumulate there. In fractures involving the jugular foramen, the IX, X and XI cranial nerves could get damaged. The strong bony walls of the hypoglossal canal usually protect the hypoglossal nerve from injuries.

Ventriculoatirial Shunt

It is a surgical drainage procedure done to relieve increased pressure and thus helping in lessening the damage to the brain.

54

Medula Oblongata

It is the caudal part of hindbrain. The medulla beyond the foramen magnum continues as spinal cord. Hence, proximal to foramen magnum, its features should resemble that of spinal cord.

Gross features

It is pyriform in shape and extends superiorly to become continuous with pons.

It has anterior median fissure presenting:

- Foramen caecum in the cranial part
- Decussation of pyramidal fibers in lower part

Anterolateral sulcus – It has exit of **Hypoglossal nerve** and superiorly **Abducent nerve** at the function of pons.

Pyramid – Elevation between anterior median fissure and anterolateral sulcus. Superiorly it is continuous with basilar part of pons and inferiorly with anterior funiculus of spinal cord. It contains corticospinal fibers.

Posteromedian septum – corresponds to posteromedian septum of spinal cord.

Posterolateral sulcus – Has the attachments of rootlets of X, XI and cranial part of XI cranial nerves.

This sulcus corresponds with similar sulcus on spinal cord that has the attachments of dorsal roots of spinal cord.

Olive – An elevation placed between anterolateral and posterolateral sulci. This is caused by underlying inferior olivary nucleus. Inferiorly, olive is continuous with lateral funiculus of spinal cord.

Posterior region: Placed between postero-lateral and posteromedial sulci. It has two components:

- Gracile and cuneate fasciculi
- **Gracile** and **Cuneate nuclei** with accessory cuneate nucleus placed laterally.

The diverging upper posterior region encloses part of fourth ventricle and connects the medulla with the cerebellum by inferior cerebellar peduncle.

Central canal: It is continuous inferiorly with that of spinal cord while superiorly it enlarges into fourth ventricle.

Inferior cerebellar peduncle

The cerebellum is connected to brain stain by three sets of peduncles

- **Medulla** – inferior cerebellar peduncle
- **Pons** – middle cerebellar peduncle

- **Midbrain** – superior cerebellar peduncle

The inferior cerebellar peduncle has afferents and efferents concerned which are concerned with unconscious proprioception.

CLINICAL CONSIDERATIONS

Damage to Medulla

In hanging and automobile accidents (whip-lash injury) the medulla is damaged. Here the odontoid process comes out of median atlanto-axial joint and compresses the medulla from posterior aspect. This may cause damage to the vital centers in the medulla (**respiratory and cardiovascular**)

Motor Neuron Lesions

The motor impulses upon reaching the skeletal muscle involve two neurons.

Upper motor neuron (UMN) Betz cells situated in the motor cortex

The axons of UMN reach / synapse with:
- Cranial nerve nuclei
- Anterior horn cells of spinal cord

To reach these cells, the UMN runs in:
- Corona radiata (cerebral hemisphere)
- Internal capsule (between thalamus and corpus striatum)
- Crus cerebri (midbrain)
- Spread out corticospinal fibers (basilar part of pons)
- Pyramid (medulla)
- Lateral corticospinal and anterior corticospinal tracts (spinal cord)

Lower motor neuron (LMN) starts from
- Cranial nerve nuclei
- Anterior horn cells of spinal cord

Any lesion (traumatic, inflammatory, vascular, degenerative or neoplastic) can affect any where in this two neuronal motor pathway.

Features of UMN Lesion

- Paresis of muscles as the lower motor neuron is still functioning
- Muscles become spastic due to hyperactive lower motor neuron as they have no cortical control
- Exaggerated tendon reflexes (**deep reflexes**): This is due to hyperactive LMN – superficial reflex is present
- Muscle twitching – due to unopposed action of LMN
- Affected muscles do not show wasting or loss of tone since UMN do not innervate the muscles directly.

Features of LMN Lesion

LMN include involvement of either nuclei (**nuclear lesions**) or nerve fibers arising from them (**infra-nuclear lesions**). Examples are Poliomyelitis and Bell's palsy (Facial nerve palsy).
- Flaccid paralysis of affected muscles
- Wasting of muscles. These features result as there is no impulse reaching the affected muscle.
- Absence of tendon reflexes (deep reflex)
- Absence of muscle twitching

Babniski's Sign

It is a clinical sign to evaluate UMN lesion. The sign is marked by:
- Dorsiflexion of great toe
- Fanning of other toes

This is elicited by scratching the skin along the lateral border of sole.

Anatomical basis: Sensory stimulation of skin of sole causes plantar flexion of the toes by the corticospinal tracts. It these tracts are damaged, the other descending tracts take over causing dorsiflexion of great toe and fanning of other toes. This is thought to be flexor withdrawal reflex kept under check by the corticospinal tract. Hence, in UMN lesion Babniski's sign is positive and in LMN lesion it is absent.

Myelination of corticospinal tract starts in neonates and is completed by the age of two years. Thus Babniski's sign is normally seen in children up to two years of age.

Medial Medullary Syndrome

Occlusion of anterior spinal artery leads to set of features due to infarction of a portion of medulla oblongata involving:

- **Pyramid** – Contralateral LMN paralysis
- **XII CN** – Ipsilateral paralysis of muscles of tongue
- **Medial lemniscus** – Contralateral loss of proprioception

Lateral Medullary Syndrome (of Wallenberg)

Here posterior inferior cerebellar artery is affected. It involves:

- **Lateral spinothalamic tract–** Contralateral loss of pain and temperature below the neck
- **Spinal nucleus of Trigeminal and its tract** - Ipsilateral loss of pain and temperature of the face.
- **Nucleus Ambiguous–** Ipsilateral paralysis of muscles of larynx, pharynx and soft palate
- **Posterior spinocerebellar tract** – Ipsilateral ataxia
- **Vestibular nuclei** – Giddiness
- **Descending sympathetic pathway** – Horner's syndrome

55

Pons

It is part of brainstem continuous superiorly with midbrain and inferiorly with medulla. Externally it presents a midline groove on the ventral aspect for basilar artery, which runs in **cisterna pontis**. Laterally, middle cerebellar peduncle (**MCP**) connects basilar part of pons with cerebellum. Posteriorly it forms part of floor of fourth ventricle. Internally, its components are:

- **Anterior** – Basilar part
- **Posterior** – Tegmentum, which is a true continuation of medulla.

At the pontomedullary junction anteriorly, from medial to lateral, following cranial nerves are attached:

- Abducent (VI CN)
- Motor root of facial (VII CN)
- Sensory root of facial (nervous intermedius)
- Vestibulocochlear (VIII CN)

Anterolaterally, at the junction of middle cerebellar peduncle and basilar part of pons is the attachment of motor and sensory roots of Trigeminal nerve (V CN).

PATH OF FACIAL NERVE FIBERS

The motor nucleus of facial nerve corresponds to the branchial efferent column. By **neurobiotaxis**

(migration of neuron towards the source of stimulus) the neurons of VII CN nucleus shift towards the sensory inputs of the face -- main sensory nucleus trigeminal nerve. Thus the fibers of facial nerve arising as axons from the neurons placed in the motor nucleus; take a route, which winds around the motor nucleus of VI CN to descend anterolaterally to emerge at the ponto-medullary junction as the motor root of facial nerve. These winding fibers of facial nerve around VI cranial nerve nucleus cause an elevation termed **facial colliculus** in the middle part of floor of fourth ventricle.

CLINICAL CONSIDERATIONS

Pontine Haemorrhage

The pontine lesions are predominantly due to pontine hemorrhage. The clinical picture varies, as there is involvement of different nuclei and fiber bundle.

MEDIAL INFERIOR PONTINE SYNDROME

The resultant deficits are due to following affected structures

- **Corticospinal tract** – Contralateral spastic hemi paresis
- **Medial lemniscus** – Contralateral loss of touch from trunk and extremities

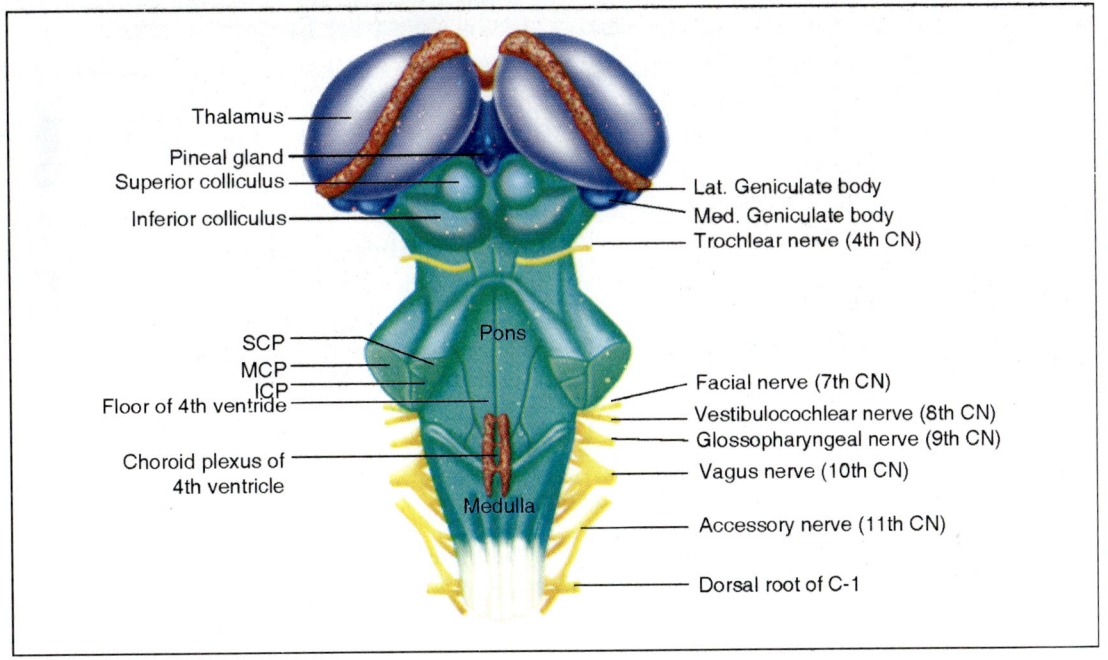

Thalamus

Pineal gland

Superior colliculus

Inferior colliculus

Lat. Geniculate body

Med. Geniculate body

Trochlear nerve (4th CN)

SCP

MCP

ICP

Floor of 4th ventricle

Pons

Facial nerve (7th CN)

Vestibulocochlear nerve (8th CN)

Glossopharyngeal nerve (9th CN)

Choroid plexus of
4th ventricle

Vagus nerve (10th CN)

Medulla

Accessory nerve (11th CN)

Dorsal root of C-1

Fig. 55.1: Brain stem: Dorsal view

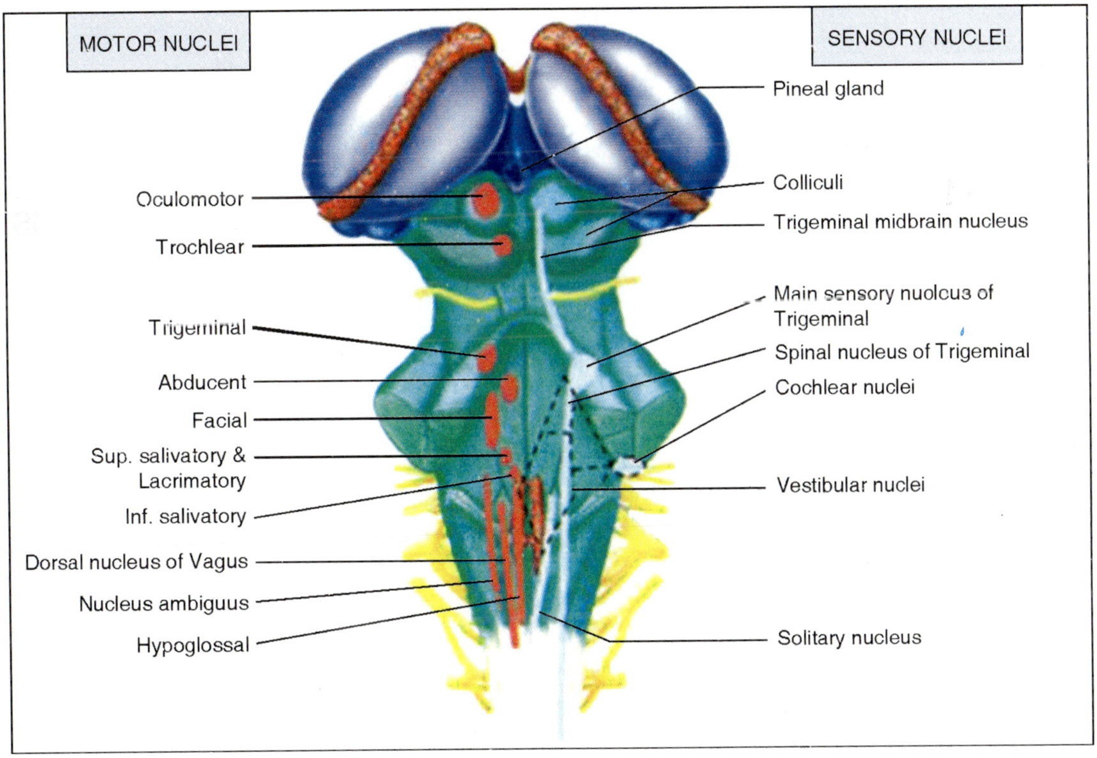

MOTOR NUCLEI

SENSORY NUCLEI

Pineal gland

Oculomotor

Colliculi

Trigeminal midbrain nucleus

Trochlear

Main sensory nuclcus of
Trigeminal

Trigeminal

Spinal nucleus of Trigeminal

Abducent

Cochlear nuclei

Facial

Sup. salivatory &
Lacrimatory

Inf. salivatory

Vestibular nuclei

Dorsal nucleus of Vagus

Nucleus ambiguus

Hypoglossal

Solitary nucleus

Fig. 55.2: Brain stem: Nuclei

- **Abducent nerve roots** – Ipsilateral lateral rectus paralysis

Lateral Inferior Pontine Syndrome

Here, anterior inferior cerebellar artery is involved. The affected structures and the resultant deficits are:

- **Facial nucleus** – Ipsilateral facial nerve paralysis
- **Cochlear nuclei** – Unilateral central deafness
- **Vestibular nuclei** – Nystagmus, nausea, vomiting and vertigo
- **Spinal nucleus of trigeminal and its tract** – Ipsilateral facial hemi-anesthesia - pain and temperature only
- **MCP and ICP** – Ipsilateral limb and gait ataxia
- **Spinal lemniscus** – Contralateral loss of pain and temperature from the trunk and extremities.

Medial Longitudinal Fasciculus Syndrome

This is also called inter-nuclear ophthalmoplegia. This lesion may occur in multiple sclerosis. Here there is involvement of ipsilateral medial rectus. Sub-nucleus of III CN and contralateral abducent nerve fibers passing through medial longitudinal fasciculus (**MLF**). It causes:

- Medial rectus palsy
- Nystagmus

Facial Colliculus Syndrome

Besides vascular accidents, this may results from pontine gliomas.

Lesion of facial nerve fibres causes
- Ipsilateral facial paralysis
- Ipsilateral loss of corneal reflex

Lesion of Abducent nucleus causes
- Lateral rectus paralysis
- Convergent squint

Cerebello Pontine Angle

It is the junction of medulla, pons and cerebellum. The VII and VIII cranial nerves are placed here. The cistern (dilated subarachnoid space) here is infamous for brain tumors including a cyst.

The tumors are: **Schwamnoma**, **Arachnoid cyst**, **Meningioma**, **Ependymoma**.

The clinical features include:

- Progressive deafness – damage to VIII CN
- Ipsilateral facial paralysis and loss of taste sensations from anterior two third of tongue - damage to VII CN
- Ipsilateral cerebellar ataxia – due to compression of neo- cerebellum.

Millard Gubler Syndrome

The lesion is in the lower part of the pons. It involves corticospinal fibers, VI CN and VII CN. It presents following features:

Contralateral hemiplegia – corticospinal fibers
Ipsilateral medial squint – VI CN
Ipsilateral facial paralysis – VII CN

56

Cerebellum

Cerebellum is the largest part of hindbrain placed in the posterior cranial fossa under tentorium cerebelli. Its morphology includes **floculonodular lobe** separated from **corpus cerebelli** by posterolateral fissure. Its median strip is called **vermis**. There are various transversely running sulci, which divide cerebellar hemispheres and the vermal cortex into smaller lobules. Prominent among them are anterior and posterior lobes divided by **primary fissure**. Developmentally, the cerebellum has three components:

- **Archicerebellum** – Oldest and includes floculonodular lobe
- **Paliocerebellum** – Relatively newer acquisition developmentally having anterior lobe with pyramid and uvula.
- **Neocerebellum** – Recent addition and includes posterior lobe and remaining part of vermal cortex.
- Situated in the posterior cranial fossa
- Weighs about 150 grams
- lies under the cover of tentorium cerebelli
- Connected to the brain stem with the help of three pairs of peduncles - cerebellar peduncles
- Superior peduncle connects it to midbrain
- Middle peduncle connects it to pons
- Inferior connects it to the medulla

The cerebellum is essentially a motor part of the brain.

It is **responsible for**

- Maintenance of equilibrium
- Muscle tone
- Muscle co-ordination

Parts, surfaces and lobes

The cerebellum has a superior surface and an inferior surface. **Vermis** is the midline structure on both the surfaces. The vermis blends imperceptibly into the superior surface but it is separated from the inferior surface by a deep notch called as **vallecula**.

The surface of cerebellum shows numerous, horizontally running leaf like folds called as folia. Adjacent folia are separated by clefts called as fissures. Some of these fissures are so deep that they divide the cerebellum into lobes.

The **fissura prima** is on the superior surface and divides the cerebellum into an anterior lobe and a posterior lobe (also called as middle lobe).

The **horizontal fissure** is situated at the junction of the superior and inferior surfaces at the posterior aspect of the cerebellum. This fissure is present in the posterior (or middle lobe).

The **postero-lateral fissure** is present on the

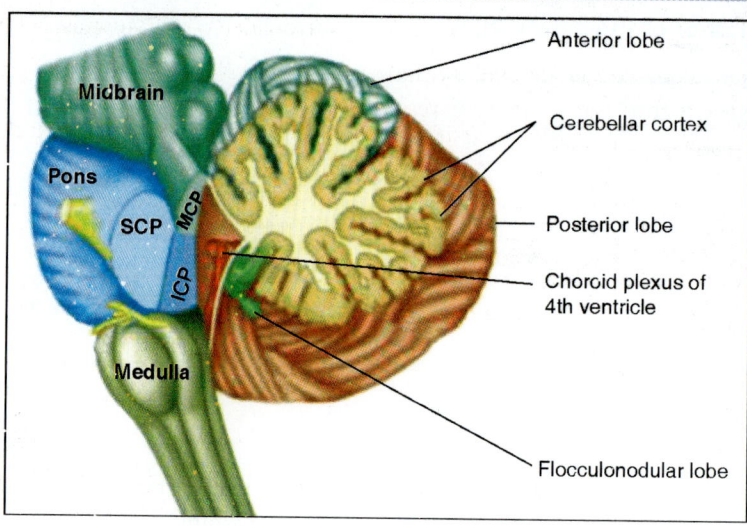

Fig. 56.1: Cerebellum

inferior surface and demarcates the posterior lobe (middle lobe) from the **floculonodular lobe**. Despite its name, fissura prima is not the first fissure to appear developmentally, it is the postero-lateral fissure, which develops first.

Subdivisions of vermis from anterior to posterior

- Lingula
- Central lobule
- Culmen
- Declive
- Folium
- Tuber
- Pyramid
- Uvula
- Nodule

The cerebral hemispheres also have subdivisions, which are grossly related to the vermal subdivisions. The ala is related to central lobule, anterior quadrate lobule to culmen, posterior quadrate lobule to declive, superior semilunar lobule to folium, inferior semilunar lobule to tuber, biventral lobule to pyramid, tonsil to uvula and flocculus to nodule.

From the point of view of its connections, the cerebellar cortex may be divided into a vermal part, a paravermal part and lateral parts. The cerebellar

cortex may also be classified as vestibulocerebellum, spinocerebellum and corticocerebellum.

Phylogenitically the cerebellum can be divided as

- Archicerebellum
- Paleocerebellum
- Neocerebellum

Archicerebellum corresponds to the lingual and the floculonodular lobe.

Paleocerebellum corresponds to the central lobule, culmen, pyramid and uvula.

Neocerebellum corresponds to declive, folium and tuber.

The phylogenetic evolution of this type of structural arrangement in the cerebellum may be explained as follows. The earliest forms of life evolved in water and balance of the body in the medium of water was essential. Such life forms developed lateral line sense organs, which were connected to vestibulo-cerebellum. As life forms moved from water to land, balance of the body with the help of limbs became essential and thus the spinocerebellum came into being. At the highest forms of evolution, fine motor co-ordination was essential to perform various skilled activities and thus the corticocerebellum came into being.

Grey and white matter of the cerebellum

Like the cerebral hemispheres, the cerebellum has an outer layer of grey matter and an inner core of white matter.

Layers of cerebellar cortex

- **Outer molecular layer** – Contains the dendrites of Punkinje cells, which synapse, with processes of stellate cells and basket cells present in this layer.
- **Punkinje cell layer** – Lies between molecular and granule cell layer. These cells constitute the first order neuron of the efferent pathway from the cerebellum. These cells are arranged in a single row and are the largest cells of cerebellum.
- **Granule cells layer** – Overlies the white matter. This inner layer contains granule cells, Golgi cells and mossy fibers.

The white matter contains afferent and efferent fibers. Embedded in the white matter are the cerebellar nuclei, which include from medial to lateral:

- Vestibular nuclei
- Fastigeal nucleus
- Nucleus interpositus (Globose and Emboliformis)
- Dentate nucleus

Deep within the inner core of white matter are certain aggregates of grey matter, which are referred to as the cerebellar nuclei.

- **Nucleus Fastigius** is the nucleus of the vestibulocerebellum
- **Globose and Emboliform nuclei** (together called as nucleus interpositus in primates) belong to spinocerebellum
- **Dentate nucleus** belongs to the corticocerebellum

A sagittal section through the cerebellum shows a tree like branching pattern of the white matter surrounded on its outer aspect by a thin core of grey matter. This branching pattern is referred to as **arbour vitae cerebelli**.

Three pairs of cerebellar peduncles connect the cerebellum to brain stem.

Middle cerebellar peduncle contains only afferent fibers (corticoponto- cerebellar).

Pattern of connections

The following is a broad generalization to the pattern of connections

- Most afferent fibres to the cerebellum first reach the cerebellar cortex where they relay. Subsequent fibres run from the cortex to the various cerebellar nuclei.
- Efferent fibres from the cortex run back, either through the cerebellar cortex or directly via the cerebellar peduncles into the spinal cord and finally reach their destinations.

Types of afferent fibres

Afferent fibres to the cerebellum are either **Mossy fibres** or **Climbing fibres**. Olivocerebellar fibres are climbing fibres.

All other afferent fibres are Mossy fibres.

Climbing fibres end in relation to the dendrites of Punkinje cells. The dendrites of adjacent Punkinje cells are connected by the axons of granule cells. Axons of Punkinje cells reach the cerebellar nuclei.

Mossy fibres end in relation to synaptic glomeruli formed by dendrites of granule cells. Impulses from the granule cells are taken by their axons to reach the dendrites of Punkinje cells. Axons of Punkinje cells finally convey the impulses to cerebellar nuclei.

Final efferent impulses from the cerebellar cortex to the cerebellar nuclei are carried by the axons of Punkinje cells.

Primary functions of cerebellum

- Maintenance of posture and balance (**Archicerebellum**)

- Maintenance of muscle tone (**Paliocerebellum**)
- Coordination of voluntary motor activity (**Neocerebellum**)

CEREBELLAR PATHWAYS

The afferent impulses reach the Punkinje cell through the **internuncial neuron**.

The efferent impulses start as first order neuron in the axon of Punkinje cells. These synapse with cerebellar nuclei where from second order neuron arises. These may enter inferior cerebellar peduncle or superior cerebellar peduncle.

CLINICAL CONSIDERATIONS

Cerebellar Dysfunctions

It include a triad
- Hypotonia
- Disequilibrium
- Dyssynergia

Hypotonia: Loss of resistance during passive movement of the limb.

Disequilibrium: This is reflected as loss of balance manifested in gait.

Asynergia/Dyssyringia: Loss of coordinated muscle activity. It includes:
- Nystagmus
- Intention tremors
- Failure to check movements. Over reaching target, past painting.
  Example: Rapid supination and pronation (**dysmetria**)
- Inability to perform repeated movements

Cerebellar Syndromes

Anterior Vermis Syndrome

This results from atrophy of caudal vermis caused by alcohol abuse. It is reflected as ataxic gait with trunk and leg dystaxia.

Posterior Vermis Syndrome

Floculonodular lobe is affected. It causes truncal dystaxia

Hemispheric Syndrome

Here, only one cerebellar hemisphere is involved. It leads to ipsilateral cerebellar signs as well as dystaxia of gait.

Cerebellar Tumours

70% of brain tumors are found in posterior cranial fossa in children. in adults, 70% of brain tumors are found in the supra-tentorial compartment. These tumors in the order of frequency are:
- Astrocytoma
- Medulloblastoma
- Ependymoma

Chorea

It means dancing. Here involuntary movements of the extremities especially hands and feet are present. These fine movements are random and disorganized. Progressive dementia is also a feature. It is associated with single gene defect of chromosome 4 (autosomal dominant).

Athetosis

It means variable. The lesion in putamen causes severance of cortical connections. Here involuntary movements are repetitive, slow and twisting in nature. Finger and toes are move commonly affected.

Ballismus

It means violent and flinging. Here the lesion is vascular and affects the subthalamic nucleus. The patient presents with sudden and out of control irregular movement of one limb (**monoballismus**) or both upper and lower limbs (**hemiballismus**)

57

Midbrain

Developmentally midbrain is a part of mesencephalon. It connects forebrain with hindbrain thus termed as mid brain. Externally, on the ventral aspect it presents crus cerebri with **interpeduncular fossa** in between. Posteriorly a cruciate sulcus separates a pair of superior colliculi from a pain of inferior colliculi. The components of midbrain are:

CEREBRAL PEDUNCLE

These include crus cerebri, substantia nigra and tegmentum. From anterior to posterior side the posterior part is called tectum. The mid brain contains cerebral aqueduct with central grey matter around it. The crus cerebri has **corticofugal fibers** emerging from the cerebral cortex to the cranial nerve nuclei, cerebellum and spinal cord. The tegmentum has various ascending tracts. It also has the nuclei of different cranial nerves. The tectum is concerned with:

- Auditory pathway
- Visual pathway

Lateral to the crus cerebri, are lateral and medial geniculate bodies (**Metathalamus**)
Superior brachium connects lateral geniculate body (**MGB**) with inferior colliculus. The subarachnoid space all around the midbrain is termed as **cisterna ambiens**. The sub arachnoid space between the medial parts of cerebral peduncle, the subarachnoid cistern is termed as **cisterna interpeduncularis**. On the ventral surface, III CN emerges on either side in the **interpeduncular fossa** while the IV CN emerges from posterior aspect below inferior colliculus. Fourth cranial nerve is the slenderest nerve and only nerve which emerges from the dorsal aspect of brain stem.

CLINICAL CONSIDERATIONS

Crossed Paralysis

The lesion is at basal mid brain. There is involvement of III CN and part of cerebral peduncle. The clinical picture includes:

- III CN palsy on the side of lesion
- Contralateral hemi paresis

This is because the lesion is above pyramidal decussation

Weber's Syndrome (Medial Midbrain Syndrome)

The deficits are caused by the following structures those are affected.

- **Ipsilateral oculomotor paralysis** manifesting as abduction and depression, ptosis and dilatation of pupil – all these features are because of complete involvement of oculomotor nerve roots.

- **Contralateral spastic hemi-paresis** due to corticospinal tracts involvement.
- **Contralateral weakness of**
  Lower part of face (VII CN)
  Tongue (XII CN)
  Palate (X CN)

Benedikt's Syndrome (Paramedian midbrain syndrome)

The clinical features result because of the involvement of following structures:

- **Complete ipsilateral oculomotor paralysis** causing abduction and depression because of sparing of lateral rectus (VI CN) and superior oblique muscle (IV CN). There is also ptosis and dilatation of ipsilateral pupil. All these are manifestations of involvement of oculomotor nerve roots.
- **Contralateral cerebellar dystaxia with intention tremors**. This is because of involvement of superior cerebellar peduncle (**Dentalo- thalamic fibers**)
- **Contralateral loss of tactile sensatory** from extremities and trunk – because of medial lemniscus involvement.

Perinaud's Syndrome (Dorsal midbrain syndrome)

The clinical features appear as the following structures are affected

Absence of convergence – Medial rectus paralysis
Paralysis of upwards and downwards movement – Both oblique paralysis
Pupillary disturbance – Edinger Westphal nucleus involvement
Non communicating hydrocephalus – Compression of cerebral aqueduct
Thus, the syndrome is due to involvement of:

- Superior colliculus
- Pretectal area
- Cerebral aqueduct

58

Cerebrum

CEREBRAL HEMISPHERES

Each cerebral hemisphere shows four lobes
- Frontal lobe
- Parietal lobe
- Temporal lobe
- Occipital lobe.

The frontal lobe lies in front of the central sulcus and above the posterior ramus of the lateral sulcus.

The temporal lobe lies below the posterior ramus of the lateral sulcus.

The occipital lobe is located posterior to an imaginary line drawn between the parieto-occipital sulcus and the preoccipital notch.

The parietal lobe is sandwiched between the frontal and occipital lobes

Landmarks used to demarcate the different lobes on the supero lateral surface are:
- Central sulcus
- A line joining parieto-occipital sulcus to the pre-occipital notch
- Posterior ramus of lateral sulcus and its extension joining this line

Thus the lobes are
- **Frontal lobe** – In front of central sulcus
- **Occipital lobe** – Behind the line b

- **Temporal lobe** – Below the posterior ramus of lateral sulcus
- **Parietal lobe** – Above the posterior ramus of lateral sulcus.

Broad functional demarcation
- Frontal lobe is associated with motor activity
- Parietal lobe is predominantly sensory, receiving somesthetic inputs
- Temporal lobe is for auditory function
- Occipital lobe is for vision

SURFACES

Each cerebral hemisphere consists of
- Superolateral surface
- Inferior surface
- Medial surface

The surfaces are bounded by the Superomedial, inferomedial and inferolateral boundaries.

Superolateral surface

The frontal lobe shows the following sulci and gyri:
- In front of the central sulcus is the precentral sulcus with the precentral gyrus in between.

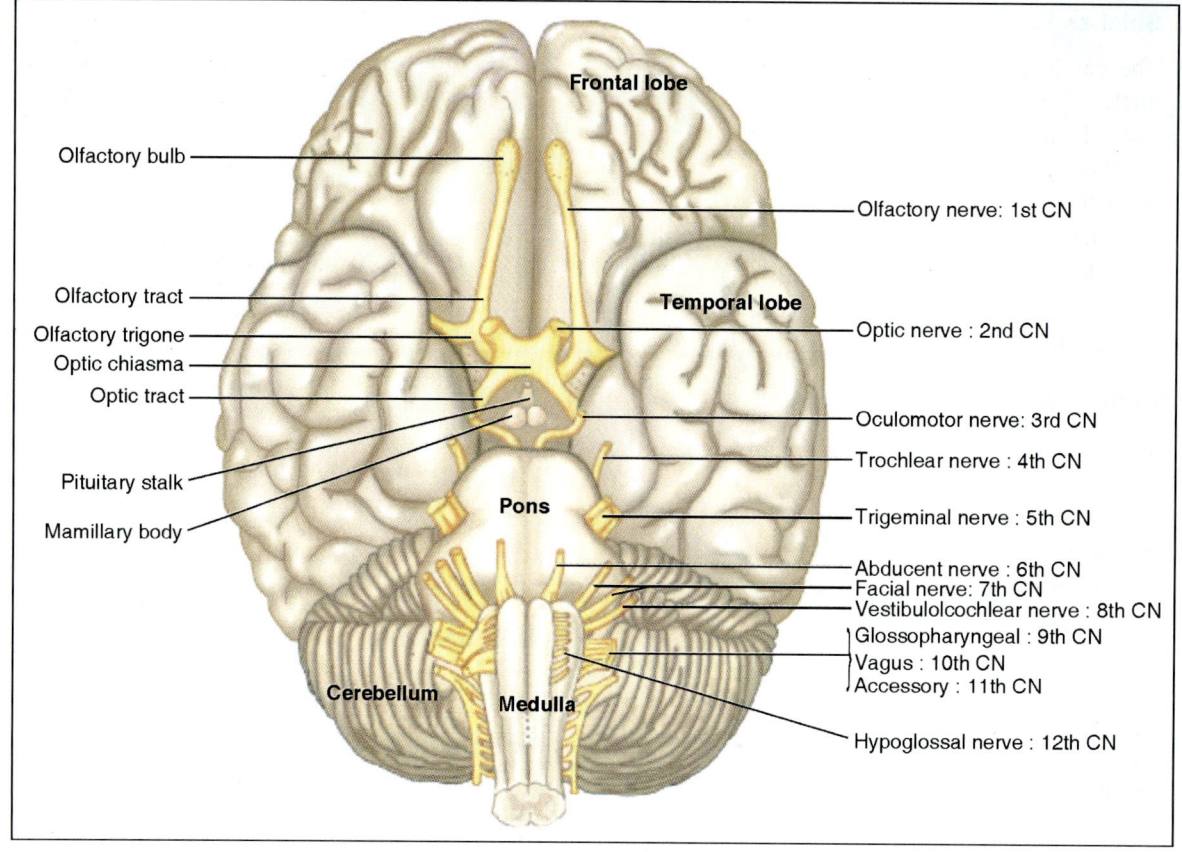

Fig. 58.1: Brain: Ventral aspect

- In the anterior part of the frontal lobe are two horizontally running sulci, the superior and inferior frontal sulci. These divide the frontal lobe into superior, middle and inferior frontal gyri.
- The stem of the lateral sulcus ramifies into three parts in the lower part of frontal lobe. The three branches are anterior ramus, ascending ramus and a posterior ramus. These rami divide the frontal cortex into pars orbitalis, pars triangularis and pars opercularis.

Parietal lobe shows the following sulci and gyri:
- The post central gyrus is present between the central sulcus and post-central sulcus.

- The intra parietal sulcus is a horizontally running sulcus which divides the parietal lobe into superior and inferior parietal lobule.
- The posterior end of the posterior ramus of the lateral sulcus extends into the parietal lobe and forms the supramarginal gyrus.

Temporal lobe shows
- Superior and inferior temporal sulci with the corresponding superior, middle and inferior temporal gyri

Occipital lobe shows
- Lunate sulcus
- Transverse occipital sulcus
- Inferior occipital sulcus

Sulci and gyri

The cerebral hemispheres have covering of grey matter – cerebral cortex, comprising of six layers of cells. To accommodate larger number of cells the cerebral cortex undergoes folding resulting in formations of **sulci** and **gyri**.

The sulci can be classified as

Those which reach to the ventricles

- Complete – Calcarine sulcus
- Incomplete

Primary and secondary sulci

These are associated with the development of cerebral hemisphere

Limiting sulcus - Central sulcus: Limits functionally different areas

Operculated sulcus - Lunate sulcus: two lips of the sulcus have functionally different areas, while in the depth another functional area.

Axial sulcus - Post Calcarine sulcus. The two lips of the sulcus have same functional area. Since this sulcus develops in the line of development of cerebrum it is termed as axial sulcus.

Secondary sulci result from relative growth of cerebrum. Example – Lateral sulcus. Here, insular cortex develops at a slower rate compared to temporal and parietal lobes. Other example is **parieto-occipital sulcus**.

The temporal, parietal and occipital fibers converge to reach the splenium and in the process they form a number of axial sulci which fuse to form a single sulcus **parieto-occipital sulcus**.

FUNCTIONAL AREAS

On the basis of cytoarchitecture, **Broadmann** classified different regions of cerebral hemisphere. These areas are numerically designated and are not in a chronological order. This study was based on associating clinical features with findings in autopsy. The superolateral and the medial surfaces of the cerebral hemispheres have specific areas responsible for specific functions. These areas are assigned random numbers and are referred to as **Brodmann's areas**.

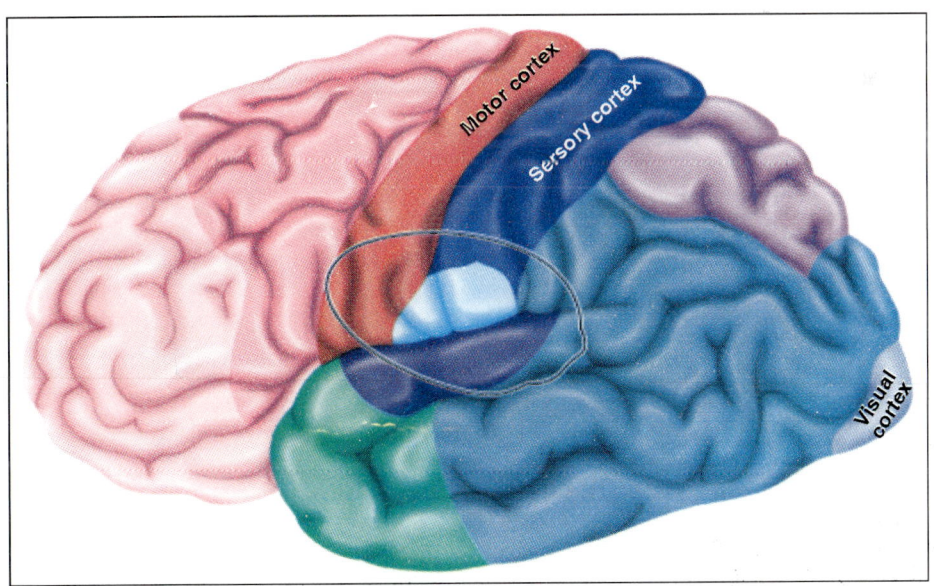

Fig. 58.2: Cerebrum: Superolateral surface

FRONTAL CORTEX

Area 4: Covering the **precentral gyrus** is concerned with initiation of organized movements of the contralateral side of the body. Here it is the movement, not the muscles that are represented. The **motor homunculus** represents the entire body. This representation is not in the morphological sequence of the body as well as the area ascribed for a particular set of movement does not correspond with the size of the body. **Example:** Lips and thumb have a greater representation compared to trunk and neck. Area 4 is predominantly motor which also contains sensory neurons (hence abbreviated as **Ms-1**). Para central lobule is abbreviated as **Ms-2** on the same line. Since the numbers of corticospinal fibres in the pyramid are more than number of Betz cells in motor cortex, it is presumed that remaining motor neurons should be distributed elsewhere – sensory areas.

Main motor area (area 4)

- Located in the precentral gyrus

- Controls gross voluntary movements of the opposite side of the body
- Area of cortex representing a part of the body is not proportional to the size of the body part but to the intricacy of movements in the region
- Body is represented as a motor homunculus with the face erect and the rest of the body inverted
- Knees lie at the superomedial border
- Legs and feet are represented on the medial surface of the paracentral lobule

Area 6: It lies in front of area 4. It is concerned with skilled acts – a sequence of movements performed for a proper length of time and in an order. **Example:** driving a motor cycle. These movements get registered permanently on these neurons.

Premotor area (area 6)

- Area is located anterior to the precentral gyrus
- Responsible for skilled motor activity

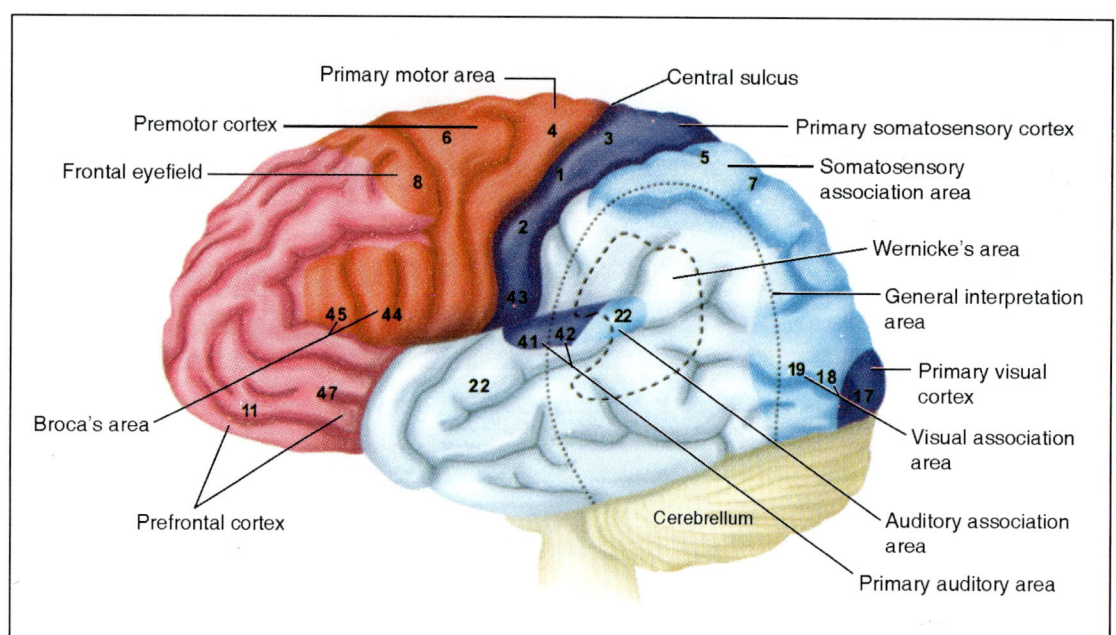

Fig. 58.3: Functional areas on superolateral surface

- A skill is a motor act, which is learnt over a period of time. It involves co-ordination of a series of gross motor acts
- Lesion in this area causes **apraxia** – loss of skilled motor movements.

Area 44 and 45: Broca's area of motor speech. This is concerned with movements of lips, tongue, jaw and larynx leading to articulated speech. It lies in line with area 6 in between anterior and ascending rami of lateral sulcus.

Motor speech area (areas 45, 44)

- Area lies in the lowest part of the inferior frontal gyrus in relation to the pars triangularis and pars opercularis
- Lesions in this area on the dominant side (usually the left side in right handed individuals) cause **motor aphasia - inability** to speak with comprehension of heard speech being left intact

Frontal eyefields (Area 8) – Is concerned with the conjugate movements of the eyeball. It is connected to the occipital cortex by long association fibers. This is placed in the middle frontal gyrus in front of area 6.

- Located in the posterior parts of the middle frontal gyrus
- Area is connected to the visual cortex
- Mediates conjugate deviation of eyes to opposite side
- Stimulation of this area with electrodes causes deviation of eyes to the opposite side

Prefrontal cortex The remaining part of frontal lobe is termed as prefrontal cortex. These include **area 9, 10, 11 and 12**. Earlier since on the basis of studies after injury and diseases to this part of brain were not projected as gross subjective deformities. Hence it was felt that this area has no effect on the body. But on the basis of connections with other parts of CNS this area is no longer termed as silent area.

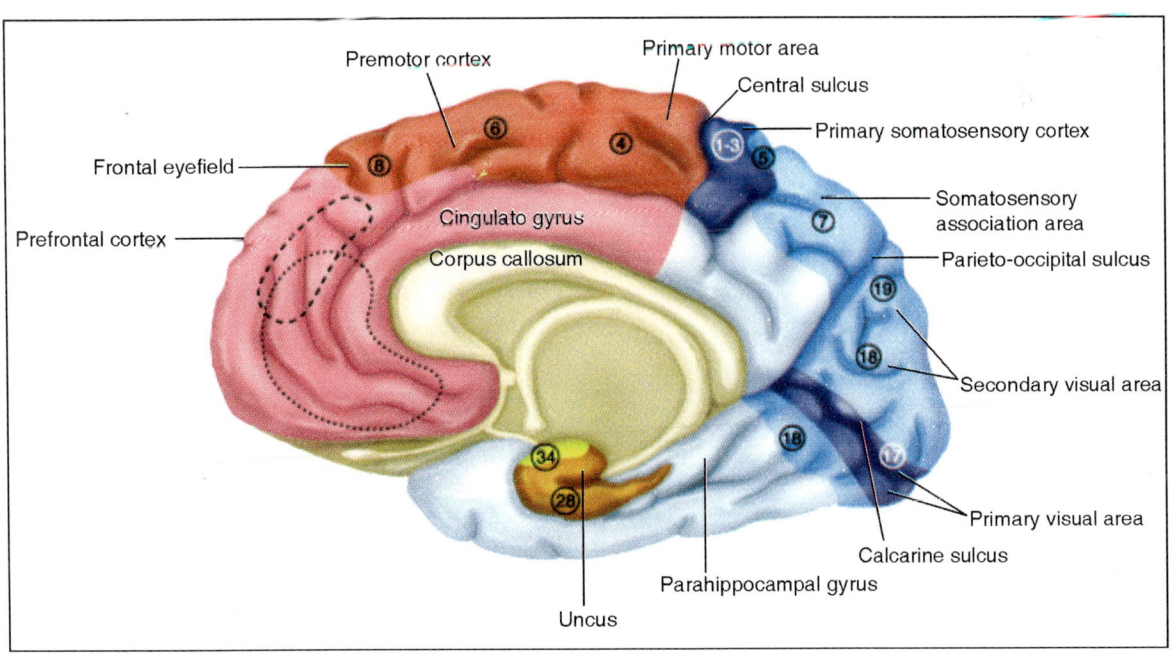

Fig. 58.4: Functional areas on Medial Surface

It is concerned with attention, mental concentration and personality of an individual. **Frontal lobotomy** – This area is often ablated to relieve the patient of excruciating pain. Example: Carcinoma of urinary bladder.

Prefrontal areas (areas 9, 10, 11, 12)

- Part of the frontal lobe excluding the motor and premotor areas
- Includes the parts of frontal gyri anterior to the premotor area, the orbital gyri, most of the medial frontal gyrus and the anterior parts of gyrus cinguli
- Have numerous connections with thalamus, corpus striatum, limbic system, hypothalamus, reticular formation, cranial nerve nuclei and pontine nuclei
- Concerned with the personality of an individual and governs mood, behaviour, emotions and ability to predict consequences of actions.

PARIETAL CORTEX

The **sensory homunculus** in the post central gyrus receives somesthetic sensations. It is represented as **Sm-1.** In the upper lip of posterior ramus of lateral sulcus is **Sm-2**. Area 3 receives sensory impulses while area 1 and 2 interpret these impulses on the basis of past experience.

Area 5 and 7 are in superior parietal lobule and are associated areas.

In inferior parietal lobule **area 39 and 40** are placed. They are concerned with sensory speech area of **Wernicke**. This is in association with **area 22** (*Auditory psychic*) of superior temporal gyrus. **Stereognosis:** ability to recognize an object with eyes closed is associated with this area because of its proximity to other sensory areas like visual, auditory and somesthetic. Sensory speech is a form of expression that includes writing, reading and listening

OCCIPITAL CORTEX

Area 17, 18 and 19

Area 17 is also called striate cortex as well marked **stria of Gennari** can be seen in a section passing through post-calcarine sulcus. These are outer **band of Bellarger** (layer number 4 of cerebral cortex). This area receives the visual impulses in the form of shape, size, colour, illumination and transparency.

- Area 18 and 19 are visual psychic area.
- Area 18 is peristriate
- Area 19 is parastriate

There interpret the visual impulses on the basis of past experience.

TEMPORAL CORTEX

Area 41 and 42 are placed in the depth of superior temporal gyrus.

It receives sound, its intensity and direction. **Area 22** is placed in the posterior part of superior temporal gyrus. It interprets the sound on the basis of past experience.

FUNCTIONAL AREAS ON MEDIAL SURFACE

Area 23, 24, 31 and 32 are concerned with visceral activity.

FUNCTIONAL AREAS ON INFERIOR SURFACE

Area 13 is placed on the postorbital gyrus. This is concerned with parasympathetic activity.

BLOOD SUPPLY OF CEREBRUM

Superolateral surface

- **ACA** supplies a strip of one-inch cerebral cortex up to parieto- occipital sulcus from the frontal pole.

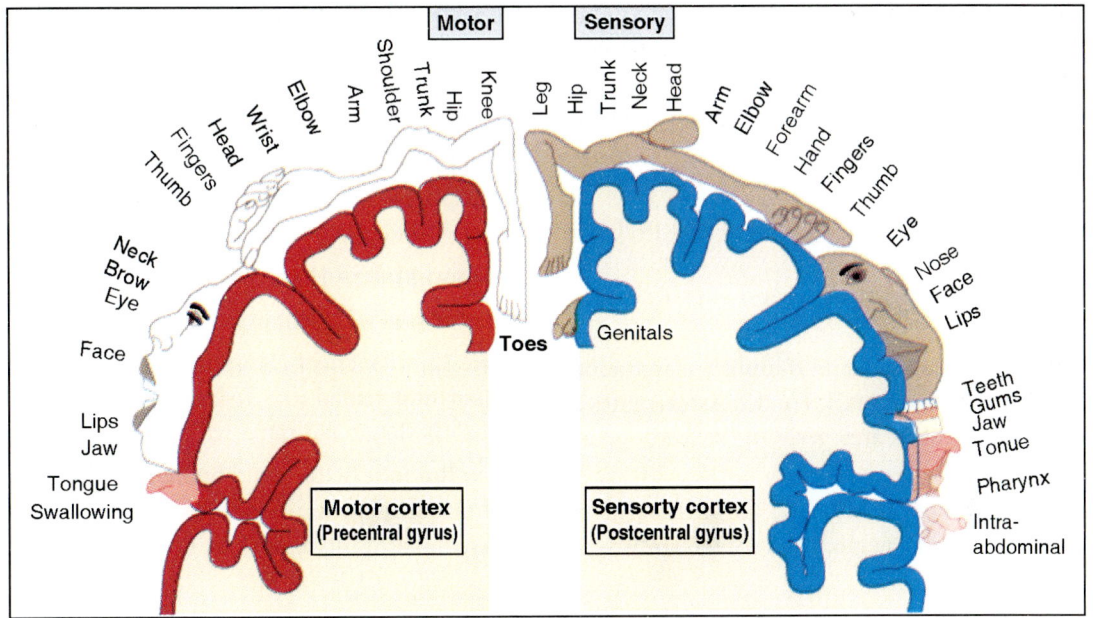

Fig. 58.5: Motor & Sensory Homenculus

- **PCA** supplies part of cerebral cortex below parieto-occipital sulcus and it includes occipital lobe and inferior temporal gyrus.
- **MCA** supplies remaining parts of frontal, temporal and parietal lobes. Thus it is the major artery of superolateral surface.

Medial surface

- **ACA** supplies frontal and part of parietal lobe including corpus callosum
- **PCA** supplies occipital lobe and adjoining part of parietal lobe as well as part of temporal lobe excluding temporal pole
- **MCA** supplies temporal pole

Inferior surface

- **ACA** supplies medial part of orbital surface of frontal lobe
- **PCA** supplies posterior three fourth of tentorial surface

- **MCA** supplies lateral part of orbital surface and anterior one fourth of tentorial surface including temporal pole.

CLINICAL CONSIDERATIONS

Lesions of Functional Areas

The cause of lesions could be traumatic, inflammatory, vascular, degenerative or neoplastic. In the vascular lesions since the areas supplied by a particular branch is extensive, the clinical picture is variegated.

Motor cortex (Area 4) – Causes contralateral spastic paresis (UMN)

Area 6 – coordinated movements are not possible but individual movement may be performed – **apraxia**.

Area 44 and 45 – In a right handed person, it is placed in left hemisphere. Lesions result in **Broca's aphasia** – verbal expression is affected. Here, the patient understands spoken and written language but cannot articulate his speech or write normally. This condition is usually associated with contralateral weakness of face and arm.

Area 8 - Lesions leads to ipsilateral deviation of the eye.

Prefrontal cortex – Lesion results in lack in concentration, judgment, orientation and problem solving ability. Other lesions may manifest as inappropriate behavior, and sphincteric incontinence.

Parietal lobe – contralateral diminished sensation results due to lesion of area 3, 1 and 2. **Astereognosis** may also result as this area gives the sensory inputs to area 39 and 40.

Superior parietal lobule – Lesion results in contralateral sensory neglect and **astereognosis**.

Inferior parietal lobule of dominant hemisphere. Here the damage causes deficits, which include confusion between right and left, **dyslexia**, **dysgraphia** and **dyscalculia**.

Inferior parietal lobule of non-dominant – hemisphere – Lesion leads to loss of topographic memory and contralateral sensory neglect.

Temporal lobe - Here lesions may affect:

Area 41 and 42 – Slight loss of hearing

Area 22 – Wirnecke's aphasia in which patient cannot understand any form of language but the speech is fluent and rapid without much sense.

Occipital lobe – Cortical blindness due to bilateral lesion while in unilateral lesions, contralateral hemianopia results in lesions involving area 17.

Thalamus and Hypothalamus

The diencephalon is the principal sensory relay station between the nuclei in the brain stem and cerebral cortex. It is concerned with sensory and motor functions. **Components of diencephalon**

- Epithalamus
- Thalamus
- Hypothalamus
- Sub thalamus
- Metathalamus

Epithalamus consists of:
- Pineal gland
- Habenular nuclei
- Stria medullaris thalami

Metathalamus comprise of geniculate bodies
- Medial geniculate body (MGB)
- Lateral geniculate (LGB)

THALAMUS

It is a relay station, which send it afferents to cerebral cortex and receive afferents from:
- All sensory impulses except olfaction
- From cerebellum through superior cerebellar peduncle
- From basal ganglia
- From cerebral cortex

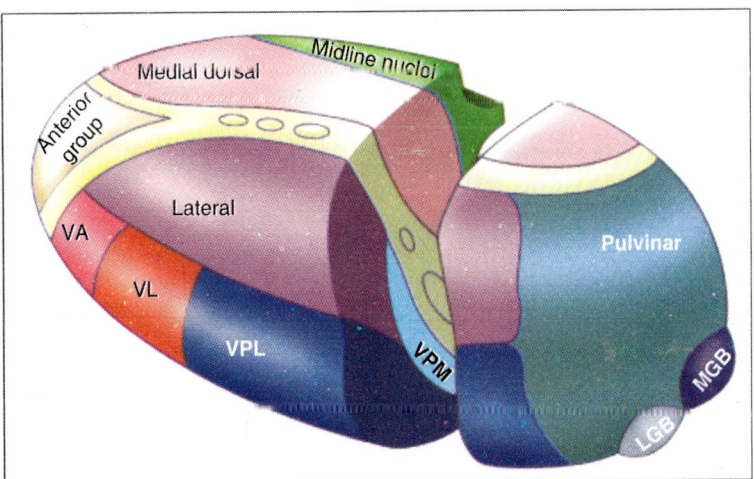

Fig. 59.1: Thalamus & its Nuclei

- From hypothalamus and Subthalamus
- From reticular formation in brain stem

Superiorly, the choroid fissure separates it from fornix. Inferiorly, sulcus limitans (**Hypothalamic sulcus**) demarcates it from hypothalamus. Anteriorly, interventricular foramen demarcates its anterior end. The posterior end termed **pulvinar**, lies at level with superior colliculus. Medial surface forms the lateral wall of third ventricle and is covered by ependyma. Laterally, internal capsule separates it from caudate nucleus and lentiform nucleus. Third ventricle is placed between the two thalami. Inter-thalamic adhesion is seen in anterior part of its medial surface.

Y shaped inter-medullary lamina into divides thalamus:

- Anterior group of nuclei
- Medial group of nuclei
- Lateral group of nuclei
- Posterior group of nuclei
- Midline nuclei

HYPOTHALAMUS

It is a component of diencephalon, governing:

- Autonomic system
- Endocrine system
- Limbic system

Thus it helps to maintain homeostasis. It has a number of nuclei with specific functions ascribed to them.

Major hypothalamic nuclei and their associated functions are as under:

- **Medial preoptic nucleus** – Regulates release of gonadotropic hormones
- **Supra chiasmatic nucleus** – Regulates circadian rhythms as it is connected with nature
- **Anterior nucleus** – Regulates temperature. It stimulates parasympathetic nervous system
- **Par-ventricular nucleus** – Functions and connections:

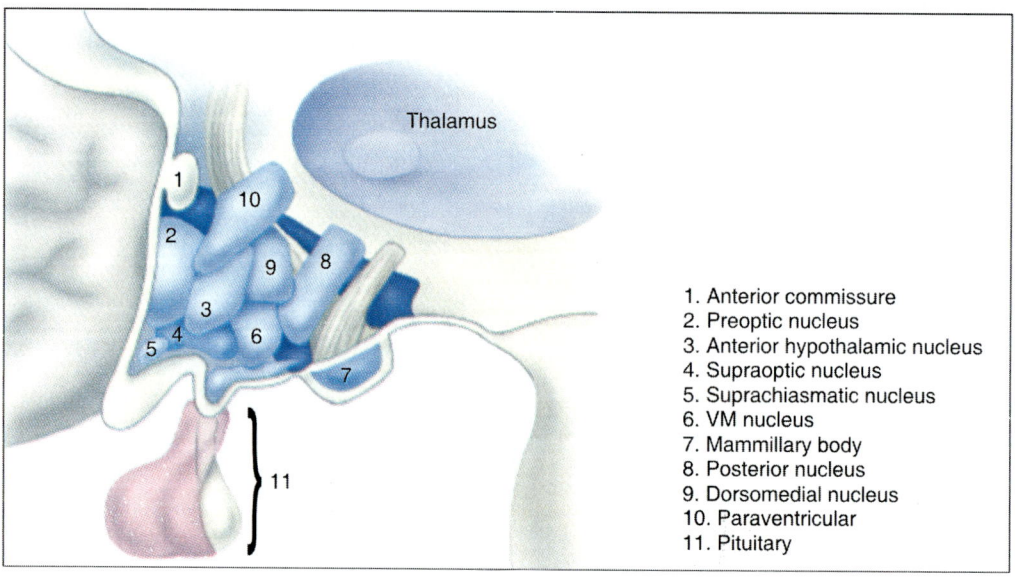

1. Anterior commissure
2. Preoptic nucleus
3. Anterior hypothalamic nucleus
4. Supraoptic nucleus
5. Suprachiasmatic nucleus
6. VM nucleus
7. Mammillary body
8. Posterior nucleus
9. Dorsomedial nucleus
10. Paraventricular
11. Pituitary

Fig. 59.2: Hypothalamus & its Nuclei

Production of hormones – ADH, Oxytocin

Connected to neurohypophysis by supra-opticohypophyseal tract

Regulates water balance

Diabetes insipidus results due to malfunction of this nucleus

Supraoptic nucleus – Oxytocin and ADH are synthesized

Venteromedial nucleus – Considered as the satiety centre.

Infundibular nucleus – It produces dopamine.

CLINICAL CONSIDERATIONS

Hypothalamic lesions can account for:

- Diabetes insipidus
- Disturbance of temperature regulations
- Adiposity
- Drowsiness

The lesions are primarily because of pressure caused by tumours such as **Craniopharyngeoma** and **pituitary adenoma**

Thalamic Syndrome

Thrombosis of arteries supplying the thalamus causes infarction leading to thalamic syndrome. This is characterized by:

- **Hemianesthesia** – Contralateral, followed by hyperesthesia / excrucicating pain due to thalamic rebound
- **Abnormal voluntary movements**, intention tremors, chorea, athetosis and ataxia.

The other symptomatology would vary with the extent of the lesion. Thus there may be loss of stereognosis and memory.

60

Limbic System

RHINENCEPHALON

Developmentally it is a component of **prosence-phalon.** It differs from rest of the tract system by the following:

- It has five neurons as against two to four neurons of other fiber system
- Impulses start in the cortex, go to the thalamus and to the cortex

RHINENCEPHALON HAS TWO COMPONENTS

1. **NOSE BRAIN OR TRUE RHINENCE-PHALON** –It is concerned with olfaction. Fiber tract projects olfactory sensation to the cortex. It has regressed in human. Its components are:
   - Olfactory nerve
   - Olfactory tract
   - Olfactory bulb
   - Lateral olfactory stria ending in **piriform lobe** which includes:
     - Lateral orbital gyrus
     - Anterior part of parahippocampal gyrus
     - Uncus
     - Amygdaloid body

2. **LIMBIC SYSTEM**

   The cortical center and the fiber tract are arranged in a circular (limbus) manner. The limbic system has **telencephalic areas** (hypothalamus and tegmental nuclei), which govern somatic and visceral activities. The limbic system is not primarily concerned with olfaction but the olfactory sensations have some relation with **somatomotor** and **visceromotor** function. It has cortical areas and multi synaptic pathways.

Functions of limbic system

Assigning specific functions to limbic system is difficult since its different components are related to other structures also. Experimentally on stimulation of different cortical centers of the limbic system, some specific responses are achieved. Examples are:

Amygdaloid body
   - Basolateral part – behavior
   - Cortico-medial part – somato motor and visceromotor responses

Hippocampal formation – concerned with memory
Reticular nuclei – concerned with alertness
Hypothalamic connections with pituitary - endocrinal influences

Papez circuit – Interconnection of limbic structures with hypothalamus and thalamus provide an anatomical pathway for emotional responses.

This has been experimentally supported.

- Marked behavior changes – Agnosia, loss of fear, heightened sexual behavior result

after bitemporal lobectomy in monkey – **Kliiver Bucy syndrome.**

- Similar behavioral disturbances are seen in cat after removal of amygdaloid body and adjacent cortex.

61

Spinal Cord

Spinal cord is the continuation of medulla oblongata. It begins at the foramen magnum or upper border of atlas (first cervical vertebra) and ends at the lower border of first lumbar vertebra or upper border of second lumbar vertebra. It may extend as high as T-12 or as low as L-3. It is however, elevated by the flexion of the vertebral column. It is about 45 cm in length.

Extent

- **Foetus:** S-2 vertebra
- **Newborn:** L-3 vertebra
- **Adult:** L-1 vertebra

The spinal cord is placed within the vertebral canal. The diameter of spinal cord is small as compared to the diameter of vertebral canal. This space is filled with **three meningeal coverings** that surround the spinal cord. These are Dura, Arachnoid and Pia mater. The pia mater closely invests the cord and is reflected onto it along the blood vessels that supplying it. The three meninges are separated from each other by subdural and subarachnoid spaces. A thick layer of epidural fat containing venous plexus surrounds dura mater.

The lower tapering end of the cord is known as **conus medullaris**. From the apex of conus

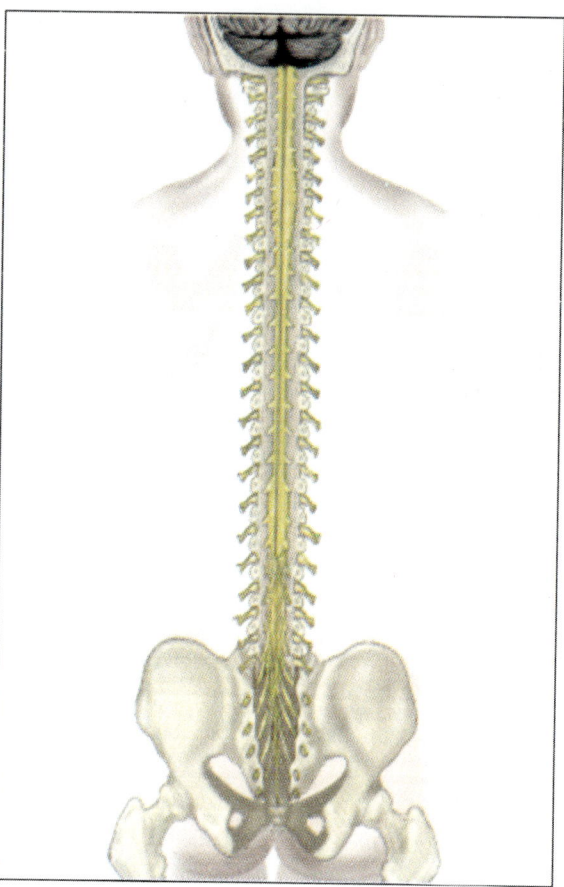

Fig. 61.1: Spinal Cord

medullaris, a fine connective tissue filament descends to the dorsal surface of first coccygeal vertebral – **filum terminale (pia-glial process)**.

Filum terminale is about 20 cm in length. It is divided into two parts:

Filum terminale internum

It is the cranial part (15 cm). Dura and arachnoid mater surround it. It extends till lower border of S-2.

Filum terminale externum

It is the caudal part (5 cm). It descends to first coccygeal segment.

The filum terminale is mainly made up of
- Fibrous tissue continuous with pia
- Few strands of nerve fibers (**rudiments of coccygeal 2, 3**)

The lumbar and spinal nerves, which surround filum terminale and conus medullaris, constitute **cauda equina**.

The central canal of spinal cord is also continued into the filum terminale for 5 to 6 cms. This fusiform dilatation in the conus medullaris is known as **terminal ventricle**.

Spinal cord enlargements

The diameter of spinal cord is not uniform. It shows two swellings:

- **Cervical enlargement** – Corresponds to the portion of spinal cord from where brachial plexus arises (**C-3 to T-2**)
- **Lumbar enlargement** – Corresponds to the portion from where lumbar plexus arises (**L-1 to S-3**).

These enlargements are not present during early embryonic life and appear subsequent to the development of limbs.

Segmentation of spinal cord

A spinal segment is the region of attachment of one pair of spinal nerves. There are 31 segments in the spinal cord.

Cervical
- $C3 \rightarrow C3$
- $C6 \rightarrow C6 + 1 = C\text{-}7$

Upper thoracic
- $T4 + 2 = T\text{-}6$
- $T9 + 2 = T\text{-}11$

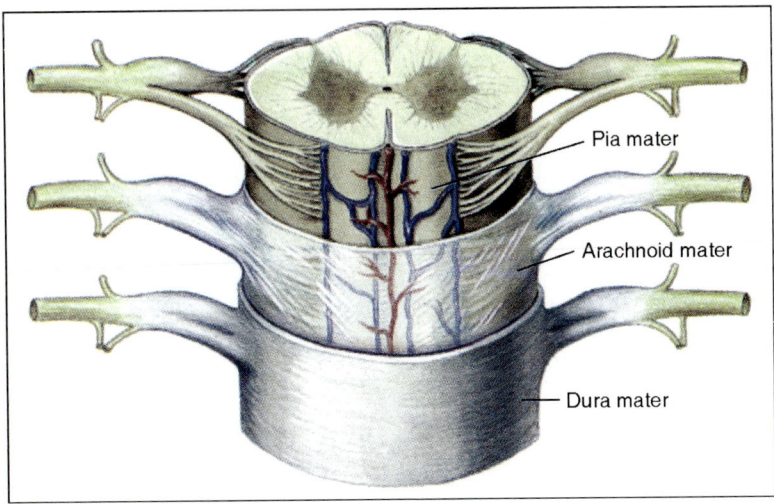

Fig. 61.2: Coverings of spinal cord

Lower thoracic

- T10 + 3 = L-1
- T11 + 4 = L-3
- T12 + 6 = S-1

Lumbar L-1

- Sacral and coccygeal

Fissures and sulci

Several longitudinal fissures are seen upon the surface of spinal cord.

Anterior median fissure: Present in the middle of the ventral surface. It extends into the cord to a depth of 1/3 of its anteroposterior diameter. It contains a fold of pia mater.

Posterior median sulcus: Present in the middle of dorsal surface. These divide the cord into two lateral halves.

Anterolateral sulcus: Corresponds to attachments of ventral nerve roots on either side

Posterolateral sulcus: Corresponds to attachments of dorsal nerve roots on either side

These six furrows extend throughout the length of the spinal cord. In the cervical region, an additional longitudinal groove may be seen on the dorsal surface between posterior median and posterolateral sulcus termed **posterior intermediate sulcus**.

Internal structure

On cross section, the spinal cord is seen to have an **H shaped** centrally placed grey matter surrounded by white matter. The central grey matter is called **substantia grisea**. The two halves of grey matter are connected across the midline by an anterior and posterior grey commissure in front and behind the central canal respectively. Each half of grey matter presents dorsal and ventral projections called posterior and anterior grey columns.

The posterior column is long and narrow reaching up to posterolateral sulcus. It does not reach the surface. From the lateral aspect in the thoracic region (**T-2 to L-1**) opposite grey commissure, projects a triangular mass known as **lateral column**

Grey matter consists of

- Multipolar nerve cells
- Nerve fibers
- Neuroglia
- Blood vessels

White matter consists of

- Long nerve fibers (myelinated)
- Neuroglia

STRUCTURE OF SPINAL CORD AT DIFFERENT LEVELS

Features	Cervical	Thoracic	Lumbar	Sacral
Posterior horn	Slender	Slender	Bulbous	Bulbous
Lateral horn	Absent	Present	Absent	Absent
Anterior horn	Broad	Slender	Bulbous	Bulbous
Central canal	In front of midpoint	In front	At midpoint	Behind midpoint

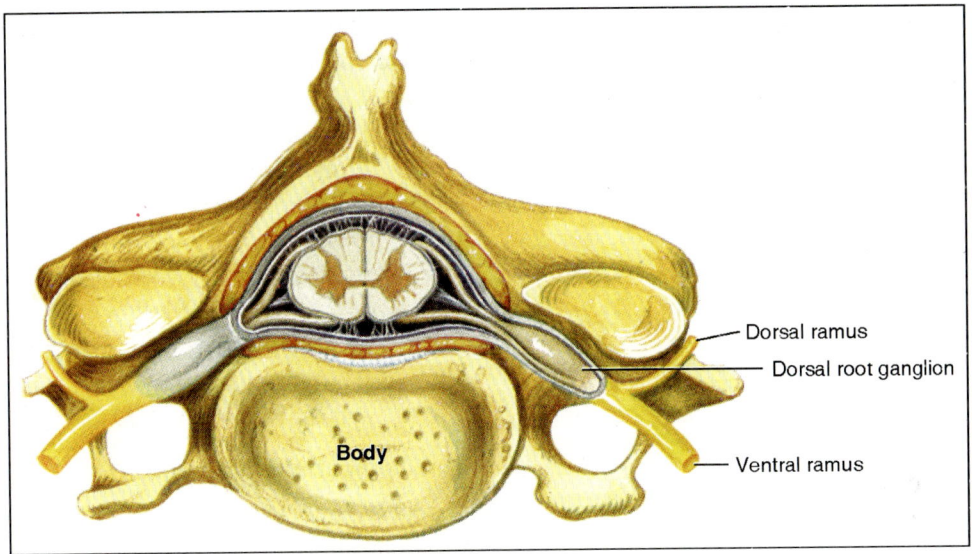

Dorsal ramus

Dorsal root ganglion

Body

Ventral ramus

Fig. 61.3: Spinal Nerve

BLOOD SUPPLY OF SPINAL CORD

Arterial supply

- Spinal branches of vertebral arteries
- Spinal branches of deep cervical artery
- Spinal branches of intercostal – Arteries **of Adamkiewicz (T1-T11)**
- Spinal branches of lumbar arteries
- Anterior spinal artery – branch of vertebral artery
- Posterior spinal arteries – branches of vertebral artery
  Spinal branches are:
  - Anterior redicular branch
  - Posterior redicular branch

Anterior redicular supplies anterior funiculus, anterior grey column, and base of posterior horn till nucleus dorsalis, much of lateral funiculus.

Anterior spinal artery supplies anterior two third of cross sectional area of the cord.

Posterior spinal arteries supply posterior area of funiculus and posterior grey column. It supplies posterior 1/3 of cross sectional area of the cord.

Venous drainage

Six veins

- One along anterior spinal artery
- One along posterior median septum
- Four on both sides along with nerve roots.

These veins form long tortuous channels, which communicate with veins of the cerebellum and dural venous sinuses.

CLINICAL CONSIDERATIONS

Involvement of spinal cord in injury and diseases

- Traumatic causes
- Affection of dorsal root
- Affection of ventral root
- Semi-section of spinal cord (**Brown Sequard syndrome**)
- Complete and incomplete transection of spinal cord

Vascular causes

- Cerebral haemorrhage (**Charcot's artery**)

- **Wallenberg syndrome** (posterior inferior cerebellar artery)
- Thrombosis of anterior spinal artery

Infectious causes

- Poliomyelitis

Degenerative diseases

- Syringomyelia
- Amyotrophic lateral sclerosis
- Subacute combined degeneration of spinal cod

Neoplastic

Tumour in:

- Interpeduncular space
- Lesion in mesencephalic tegmentum
- Pontine syndrome

Wallarian Degeneration

- When a nerve fiber is cut degenerative changes are termed as Wallarian degeneration.
- Degenerative changes in the cells termed **chromatolysis.**
- If the spinal cord is cut, there would be degenerative changes above and below the level of cut.

Dorsal Rhizotomies

Features

- Ipsilateral loss of proprioceptive sensations at the level of section
- Ipsilateral loss of pain, temperature and touch at the level of section
- Movements of particular group of muscles corresponding with the level of same nerve supply would be affected as the afferent impulses are severed (**spinal reflex arc is affected**)

Affection of Ventral Roots

Ventral roots include

- LMN
- Preganglionic sympathetic fibers (**Thoraco lumbar region**)
- Preganglionic para sympathetic (**sacral region**)

The clinical features would include LMN type of paralysis at the level of lesion and:

- **Horner's syndrome** if T-1 is involved
- Bladder disturbances if sacral para-sympathetic is involved

Involvement of Mixed Nerve

It would be a composite picture of sensory and motor involvement.

Hemi-section of Spinal Cord

Sensory loss

- **Posterior column** – Proprioception below the level of same side
- **Anterior and lateral spinothalamic** – Pain, temperature and touch are lost below the level of opposite side
- **Crossing fibers of spino thalamic** – Loss of pain, temperature and touch of both sides only at the level of lesion

Motor loss

- **Lateral corticospinal tract** - UMN paresis (**ipsilateral**) below the level of lesion
- **Anterior corticospinal** (**contralateral**) - At and below the level
- **Anterior horn cells** - LMN paralysis (**ipsilateral**) at the level
- **Lateral horn** - Vasomotor paralysis at the level

Complete Transection of Spinal Cord

This may result from

- Missile wounds

- Fracture -dislocation
- Ischaemic necrosis due to redicular arteries involvement
- Neoplasms

Features

All ascending tracts - Loss of all sensations below the level including the level of transection.

All descending tract - Loss of all voluntary movements below the level (**UMN**) and at the level (**LMN** type of paralysis)

Descending autonomic fibers

- Bladder and bowel dysfunctions
- Conus medullaris syndrome
- Permanent paralysis of external sphincter
- Faecal incontinence
- Bladder distention
- Impotency
- Saddle anesthesia
- Motor and sensory function in lower extremity remains affected

Fasciculi proprii (intraspinal reflex arc)

- Above the level: loss of reflexes in several cord segments
- Below the level: until six weeks "**spinal shock**" is observed

All somatic and visceral reflex activities including muscle tone abolished for variable period. Once restored there will be:

- Enhanced deep reflexes
- Loss of superficial reflexes
- Hypertonia
- Spasm of extensors and flexors

Incomplete Transection of Spinal Cord

- Some of the sensory and descending tracts escape injury
- Sensory deficit may not correspond to the level of motor loss
- Vasomotor and visceral disturbances are less pronounced

- **Irritative sensory phenomenon** ranging from pain, paraesthesia to hyperesthesia is observed.

Inflammatory Lesions – Anterior Poliomyelitis

Anterior horn cells are partially or completely affected leading to **flaccid paralysis**.

In bulbar poliomyelitis, vital functions are also affected along with spastic (**UMN**) paralysis.

DEGENERATIVE CONDITIONS

Syringomyelia

This is characterized by **degeneration of ependymal cells** of central canal, which may expand all around leading to involvement of

- **Crossing fibers of spinothalamic tract**
  - Bilateral loss of pain and temperature within the segment of lesion
  - No changes seen above and below the lesion
- **Anterior horn cells**
  - Ipsilateral lower motor neuron paralysis at the level of lesion
- **Preganglionic sympathetic fibers**
  Ipsilateral Horner's syndrome

Amyotrophic Lateral Sclerosis

It is a progressive degenerative disease of the spinal cord of unknown etiology. It selectively **affects corticospinal tract** and **anterior horn cells**. There is no involvement of lateral spinothalamic tract, which is placed adjacent to corticospinal tract.

Clinical features include

- **Corticospinal tract** - UMN paralysis below the level of lesion
- **Anterior horn cells** – LMN paralysis at the level of lesion
- **Descending autonomic fibers** – Disturbance of rectum and bladder

Seen due to **deficiency of vitamin B12**

Clinical Features include

- **Posterior column involvement** – Loss of proprioceptive impulses below the level of the same side
- **Lateral corticospinal tract** – UMN paralysis below the level of same side.
- **Spinocerebellar tract** – Ipsilateral ataxia causing tottering, stiff gait.
- **Visceral fibers** - Visceral disturbances

LESIONS OF THE SPINAL CORD

Divided into five neuroanatomic syndromes

- Anterior cord
- Central cord
- Brown-Sequard
- Conus medullaris
- Cauda equina

Most commonly result from occlusion of the anterior spinal artery.

- Loss of motor function
- Loss of pain and temperature sensation below the level of lesion
- Relative preservation of vibration and position sense

The anterior two thirds of the spinal cord is supplied by the anterior spinal artery. Thus this syndrome has been correlated anatomically with damage to the **corticospinal** and **lateral spinothalamic tracts** with relative sparing of the posterior columns.

Central Cord Syndrome

Usually follows an acute cervical injury and is characterized by:

- Greater weakness in the arms than the legs
- Almost constant sacral sensory sparing

Patients with cervical spondylosis/stenosis are predisposed to central cord injuries.

The proposed mechanism of injury suggests that the spinal cord is pinched between a dorsally displaced vertebral body and a buckled ligamentum flavum during hyperextension.

The underlying pathology consist of

- Contusion
- Haemorrhage, and/or
- Necrosis of the central cervical gray matter

Both the corticospinal and spinothalamic tracts in man are laminated such that the most rostral projections are most medial. The central damage in the cervical cord would injure the cervical laminations most severely and spare the sacral laminations, resulting in the characteristic pattern of deficit.

Brown-Sequard Syndrome

It is due to a purely unilateral transverse lesion above midlumbar spinal cord levels.

Most common trauma associated with this syndrome is a fall on the back from a considerable height. Stab wounds may also be responsible.

Clinical features

- Loss of proprioception and motor control ipsilateral to the lesion reflects damage to the corticospinal tract and posterior columns on the side of the lesion
- Contralateral loss of sensitivity to pin and temperature is due to damage to the crossing spinothalamic tracts

Conus Medullaris Syndrome

Damage to the sacral spinal segments alone produces a pure conus medullaris syndrome resulting in

- Areflexic bladder
- Faecal incontinence
- Saddle anesthesia

It may result in a variable degree of flaccid paralysis in the legs with accompanying multimodal sensory loss.

Lesions that occur **higher in the sacral cord** may effectively isolate the distal-most cord and thus these injuries exhibit preservation of bowel, bladder and genital reflexes.

It is caused by injuries **below the level of the sacral segments**.

Damage to lumbosacral nerve roots results in

- Flaccid paralysis of the bowel, bladder and legs
- Loss of all sensory input

The cauda equina is more resistant to trauma than the spinal cord and shows a greater propensity for recovery.

It is composed of peripheral nerve roots rather than central nervous system tissue may account for its resistance to injury. Nerve roots are ensheathed by a substrate that includes fibrous tissue. This covering renders them more resistant to trauma than the spinal cord.

The peripheral axons are myelinated by **Schwann cells** rather than the oligodendrocytes found in the spinal white matter is a major factor that accounts for the unique ability of peripheral nerves to regenerate following trauma. Following injury to the cauda equina, Schwann cells provide a substrate for axonal elongation. This sets the stage for restitution of the peripheral nerves and neurological recovery.

62

Autonomic Nervous System

The motor part of ANS is concerned with innervations of cardiac and smooth muscles and glands. It differs from somatic system in that the pathway from nerve cells in the CNS to the target organ is interrupted in a ganglion. The preganglionic cell bodies are always within the CNS.

Autonomic system is divided into

- Sympathetic component
- Parasympathetic component

These systems present ganglia which are the sites of synapses of neurons. These are preganglionic fibers and postganglionic fibers. The cell bodies of postganglionic fibers lie in the ganglion.

In sympathetic system they are in lateral horn cells of all thoracic and upper two lumber spinal segments (Thoracolumbar outflow). The post ganglionic cell bodies are situated in the ganglia in PNS.

In parasympathetic system the ganglia are either in sympathetic trunk or within the walls of the viscera. In the case of certain system in head and neck structures, four ganglia are situated a little away from the structures innervated. This system controls involuntary activities of the body – gut motility. It consists of

- Preganglionic fibers
- Ganglia for relay
- Postganglionic fibers

SYMPATHETIC NERVOUS SYSTEM

The **Sympathetic trunk** extends from base of skull to the coccyx. Theoretically there is one ganglion for each spinal nerve but there occurs fusion; thus:

Cervical region presents

- Superior cervical ganglion (fusion of C-1 to C-4)
- Middle cervical ganglion (fusion of C-5 and C-6)
- Inferior cervical ganglion (fusion of C-7 to T-1)

Thoracic region - 11
Lumbar region – 4
Sacral region – 4

- Each sympathetic trunk ganglia has a visceral branch called splanchnic nerve in thoracic lumbar and sacral region and cardiac branch in cervical region. Cardiac branches descend to the cardiac plexus which is supplemented by fibers from upper thoracic ganglia.
- From lower thoracic ganglia splanchnic nerves pierce diaphragm to reach the coeliac plexus.

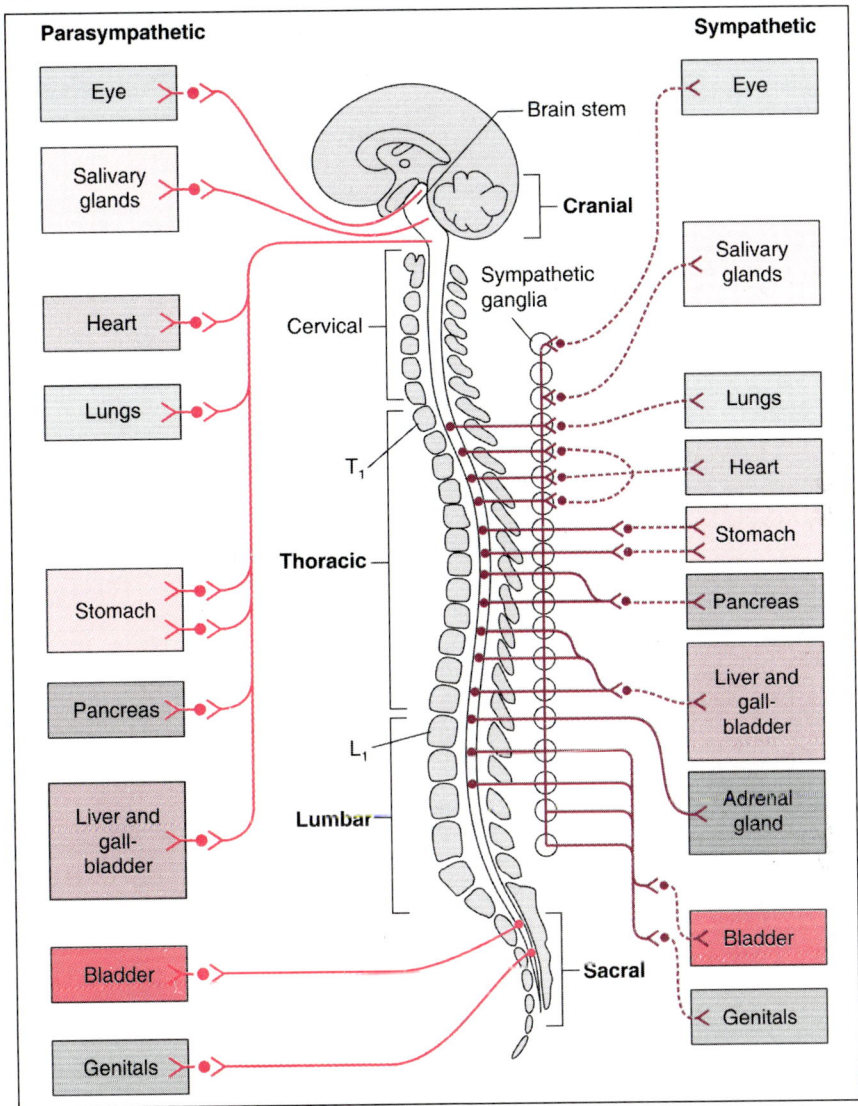

Fig. 62.1: Autonomic Nervous System

- Upper lumber splanchnic nerves reach superior hypogastric plexus and this divides to enter the right and left inferior hypogastric plexuses. They are joined by sacral splanchnic nerves. These plexuses are joined by parasympathetic nerves.

- Preganglionic fibers – cell – bodies in lateral horn (intermediate horn) of spinal cord from T-1 to L-2 or L-3 to form **thoracolumbar outflow.**

- Ganglia from two chains - one on either side of vertebral column called sympathetic chain / trunk.

- Preganglionic fibers are short while post ganglionic fibers are long

- Post ganglionic fibers pass through spinal nerves.

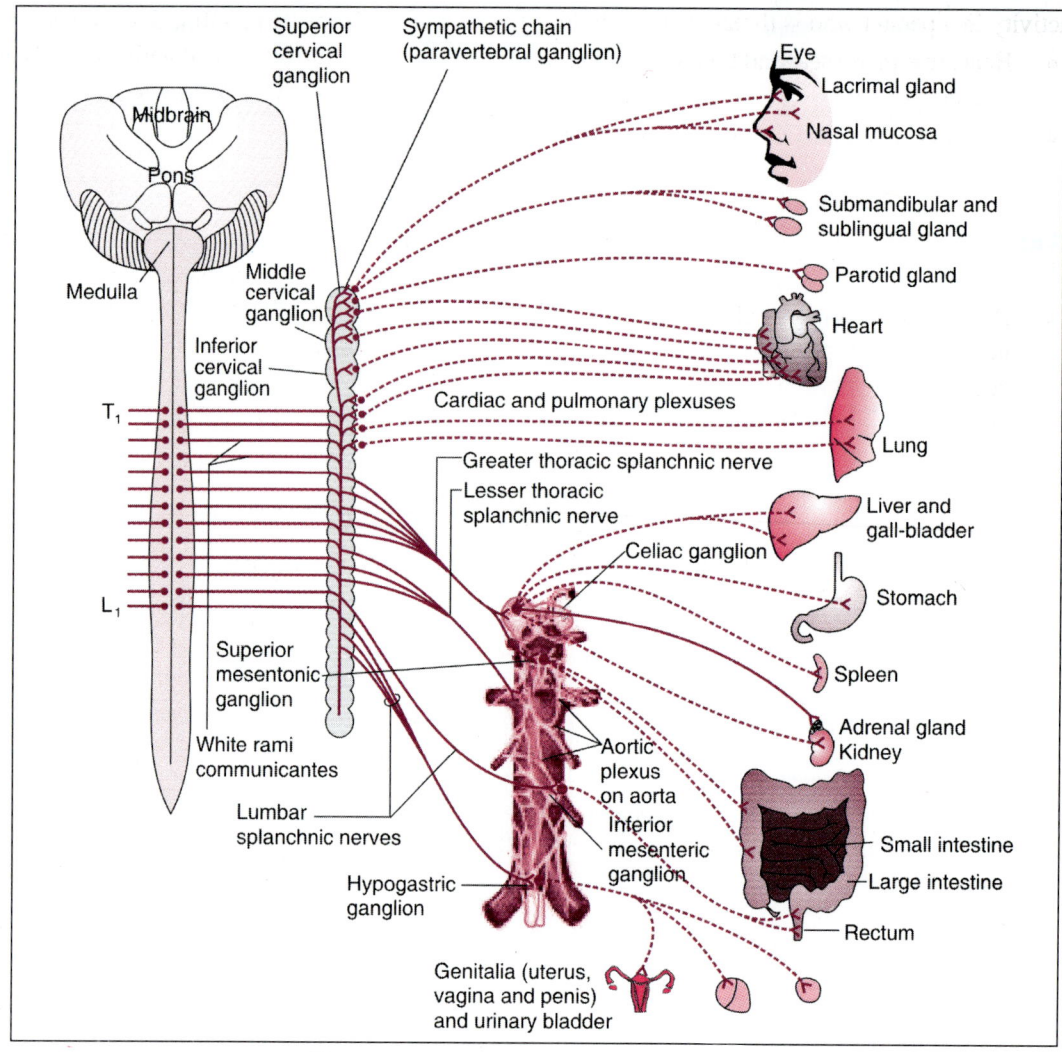

Fig. 62.2: Sympathetic Nervous System

- Supply blood vessels, sweat glands and arrector pilorum muscle of skin. Some preganglionic fibers form **splanchnic nerves** which synapse on distant ganglia called collateral ganglia or terminal ganglia and supply the viscera.

- Sympathetic fibers use adrenaline and noradrenaline as their neurotransmitters (**adrenergic**) except postganglionic fibers supplying sweat glands and blood vessels of skeletal muscle (**cholinergic**)

- Symptoms system is responsible for fight, flight, fright reactions – work during stress.

- The sympathetic division is the "**fight-or-flight**" system

- Involves **E** activities – exercise, excitement, emergency and embarrassment

- Promotes adjustments during exercise – blood flow to organs is reduced, flow to muscles is increased

Its activity in a person who is threatened would be:

- Heart rate increases, and breathing is rapid and deep
- The skin is cold and sweaty, and the pupils dilate

PARASYMPATHETIC NERVOUS SYSTEM

- Preganglionic fibers – cell bodies in cranial nerve nuclei or in lateral horn of spinal cord from S-2, 3, 4 segments to form **craniosacral out flow.**

- Nuclei of IIIrd, VIIth, IXth and Xth cranial nerves are associated with parasympathetic ganglia. These are **Ciliary, Pterygopalatine, Otic** and **Submandibular** ganglia.

- The pre-ganglionic fibers of cranial origin of these ganglia have their cell bodies in:
  Edinger Westphal nucleus (**III CN**)
  Superior salivatory nucleus (**VII CN**)
  Lacrimatory nucleus (**VII CN**)
  Inferior salivatory nucleus (**IX CN**)
  Dorsal nucleus of Vagus (**X CN**)

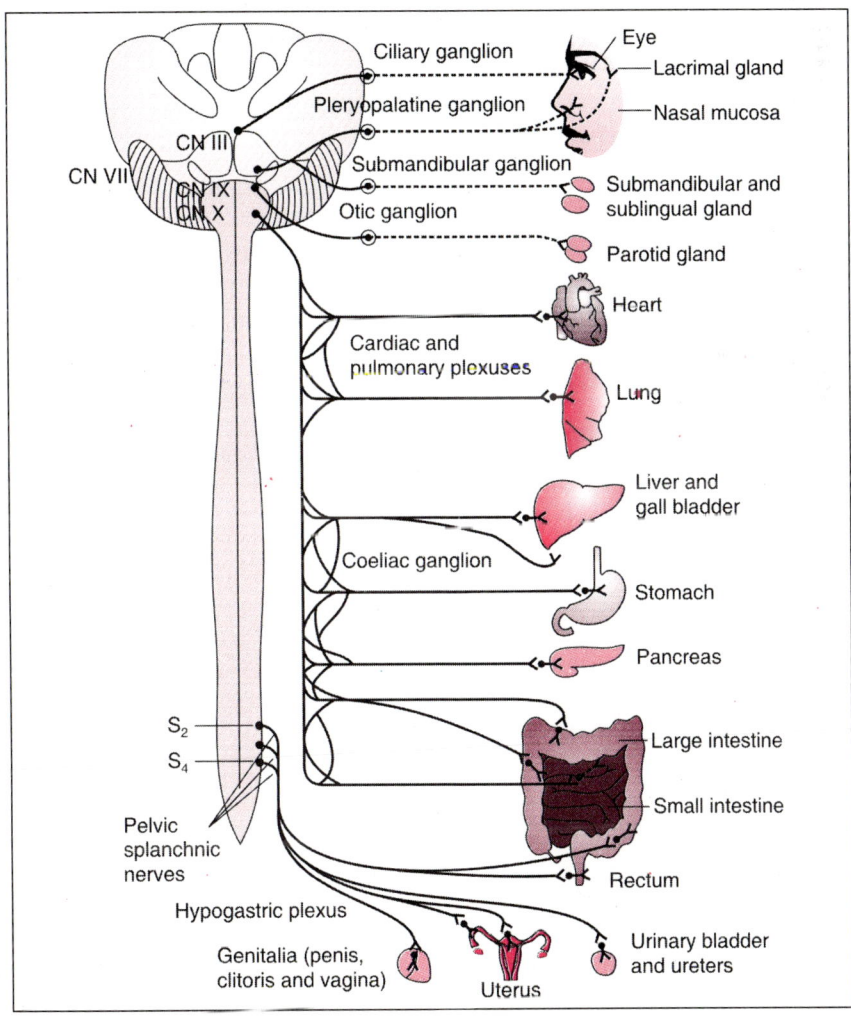

Fig. 62.3: Parasympathetic Nervous System

- Postganglionic cells lie in
  Ciliary ganglion
  Pterygopalatine ganglion
  Otic ganglion
  Submandibular ganglion
- The pre-ganglionic fibers of sacral origin arise from **S-2, 3 and 4** constituting **pelvic splanchnic nerves**. These join the inferior hypogastric plexuses. From here they supply the pelvic viscera and hindgut.
- These parasympathetic ganglia lie nearer to the viscera or gland they supply.
- Preganglionic fibers are long and postganglionic fibers are short.
- Parasympathetic fibers use acetylcholine as their neurotransmitter (**cholinergic**)
- All the smooth muscles in the body except those of blood vessels and all the glands except sweat glands are supplied by parasympathetic nervous system.
- Parasympathetic system is responsible for anabolic (building up) activities – digestion, absorption, conservation of energy, and facilitates acts of micturition, defecation and sexual function.

Role of Parasympathetic activity

Concerned with keeping body energy use low

Involves the **D** activities – digestion, defecation, and diuresis

Its activity in a person who relaxes after a meal would be:

- Blood pressure, heart rate, and respiratory rates are low
- Gastrointestinal tract activity is high
- The skin is warm and the pupils are constricted

CONTROL OF ANS

- The hypothalamus is the main integration center of ANS activity.
- Subconscious cerebral input via limbic lobe connections influences hypothalamic function.
- Other controls come from the cerebral cortex, the reticular formation, and the spinal cord.

Section-V
Histology

CONTENTS

63. **Epithelium**   353-359

64. **Connective Tissue**   360-364

65. **Cartilage**   365-366

66. **Bone**   367-368

67. **Muscle**   369-370

68. **Blood Vessels**   371-373

69. **Nervous Tissue**   374-377

70. **Salivary Glands**   378-381

71. **Lymphoid Tissue**   382-386

72. **Integumentary System**   387-389

73. **Lip, Tooth and Tongue**   390-392

74. **Gastrointestinal Tract**   393-395

75. **Respiratory System**   396-398

76. **Endocrine Glands**   399-404

63

Epithelium

EPITHELIUM CHARACTERISTICS

- Consists almost entirely of cells
- Covers body surfaces and forms glands
- Has free and basal surface
- Specialized cell contacts
- Avascular
- Undergoes mitosis

FUNCTIONS OF EPITHELIAL TISSUE

- Protecting underlying structures
- Acting as barriers
- Permitting the passage of substances
- Secreting substances
- Absorbing substances

CLASSIFICATION OF EPITHELIUM

Simple
- Squamous
- Cuboidal
- Columnar

Stratified
- Squamous
- Cuboidal
- Columnar

Pseudostratified
- Columnar

Transitional
- Cuboidal to columnar when not stretched
- Squamouslike when stretched

SIMPLE EPITHELIUM

It consists of only a single layer. According to the shape of the cells it is classified into
- Simple squamous
- Simple cuboidal
- Simple columnar

1. Simple squamous epithelium

It consists of single layer of very thin cells. Nuclei bulge on the membrane. The cytoplasm is very.

E.g. Endothelium of blood vessels, mesothelium of serous cavities

2. Simple cuboidal epithelium

The height and breadth of the cell is same. Rounded nucleus is placed centrally.

E.g. Small collecting tubules of kidney medulla, lining of thyroid follicle

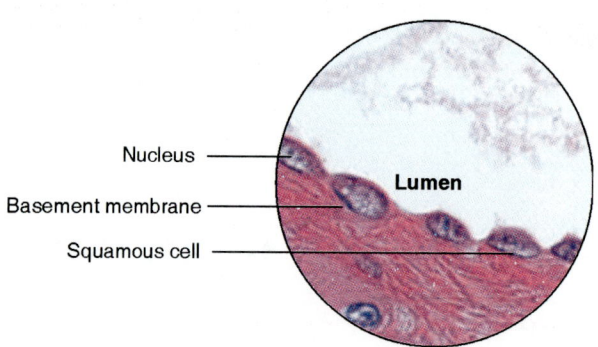

Nucleus
Basement membrane
Squamous cell
Lumen

Fig. 63.1: Simple Squamous Epithelium

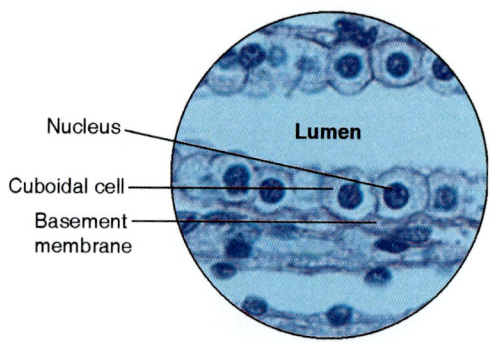

Nucleus
Cuboidal cell
Basement membrane
Lumen

Fig. 63.2: Simple Cuboidal Epithelium

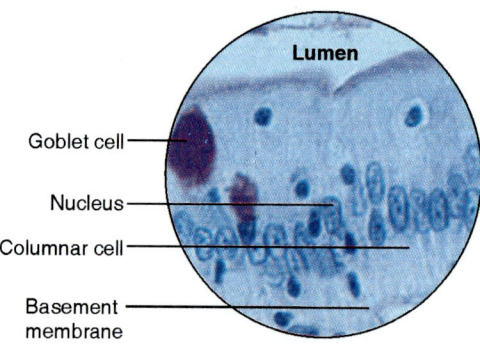

Lumen
Goblet cell
Nucleus
Columnar cell
Basement membrane

Fig. 63.3: Simple Columnar Epithelium

3. Simple columnar epithelium

Cells are tall. Nucleus is basal which may be oval or elongated.

Variants of simple columnar

– **Simple columnar nonciliated** - provides protection along wet surfaces. The cytoplasm is light eosinophilic.

E.g. Lining epithelium of gastrointestinal tract

– **Simple columnar ciliated** - cells are provided with cilia which help in the movement of mucous along the membrane.

E.g. Fallopian tube

– **Simple columnar with goblet cells** - Goblet cells are mucous secreting cells which are present in between the columnar lining cells. These are bowl-like shapes. Mucous is washed during H&E staining so they appear vacuolated or empty.

E.g. Large intestine

– **Simple columnar with microvilli** - Apical surface of the cells are provided with microvilli - striated border or brush border. It increases the absorptive surface area.

E.g. small intestine

STRATIFIED EPITHELIUM

They have more than two layers of cells and are mainly protective in function. These are:

1. Stratified squamous

It consists of five to six layers of cells. The superficial cells are squamous. It may be:

2. Stratified squamous nonkeratinised

The deepest layer consists of a single row of columnar cells. The intermediate layers show polyhedral cells but the surface cells are squamous. Keratin layer is absent on the surface.

E.g. Oesophagus, vagina, cornea

3. Stratified squamous keratinised

Here the superficial cells are dead and non-nucleated. They appear as eosinophilic fibrillar strands - nonliving layer of keratin.

E.g. Skin

4. Stratified cuboidal

It consists of many layers of epithelial cells where

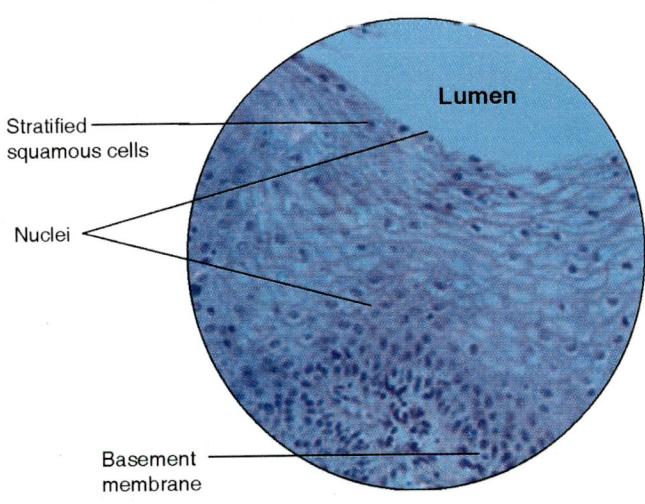

Fig. 63.4: Stratified Squamous Epithelium

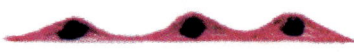

Simple squamous epithelium

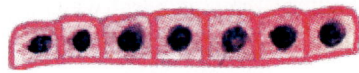

Cuboidal epithelium

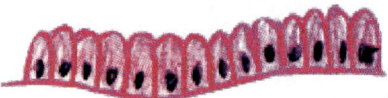

Columnar epithelium

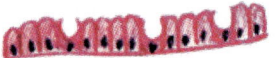

Goblet cells

Ciliated columnar epithelium

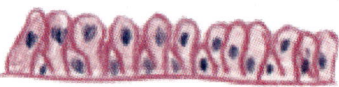

Pseudostratified epithelium

Pseudostratified epithelium with cilia

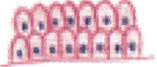

Stratified columnar

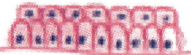

Stratified Cuboidal

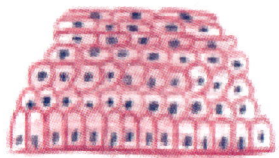

**Stratified Squamous
(Non-Keratinised)**

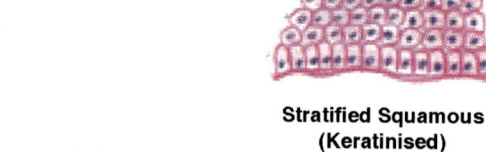

**Stratified Squamous
(Keratinised)**

**Urothelium
(Tranistional Epithelium)**

Fig. 63.5: EPITHELIAL TISSUE

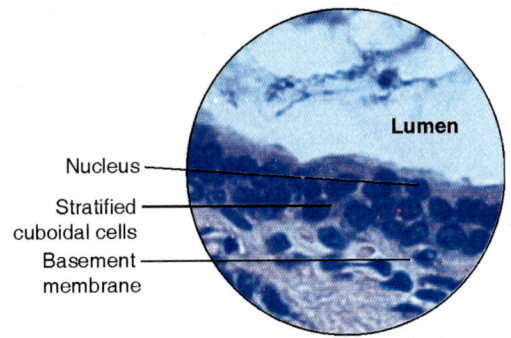

Fig. 63.6: Stratified Cuboidal Epithelium

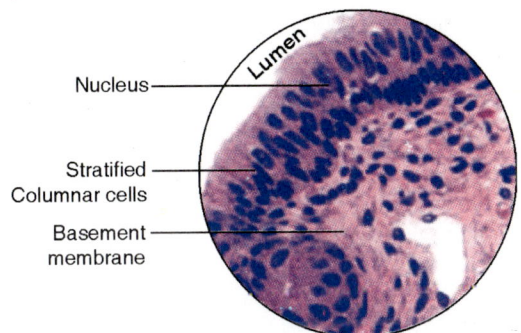

Fig. 63.7: Stratified Columnar Epithelium: Nonkeratinized

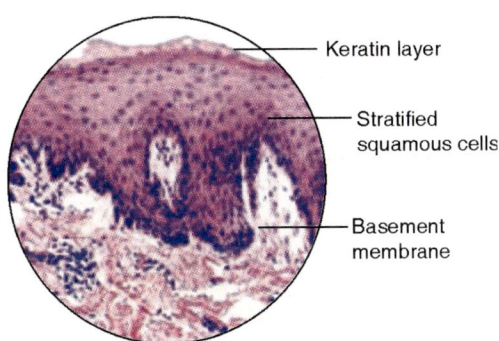

Fig. 63.8: Stratified Columnar Epithelium: Keratinized

deeper layers consist of polyhedral while superficial layer is cuboidal in shape.

E.g. Duct of sweat gland,

5. Stratified columnar ciliated

Here superficial cells are columnar shaped. It is present at the transitional zone between different types of epithelium.

E.g. Large ducts of exocrine glands

TRANSITIONAL EPITHELIUM

It is stratified epithelium. It consists of five to six layers. The basal cells are columnar. The intermediate cells are pear shaped while the surface cells are umbrella shaped. Most of the layers show similar cells with rounded nuclei.

E.g. Urinary bladder

When stretched

Transitional epithelium can be stretched (full bladder) without superficial cells pulling apart from one another; they become broader thinner cells. When stretched it is similar to stratified squamous nonkeratinised epithelium.

When relaxed

In relaxed state, the more superficial cells are rounded in appearance. The surface cells are commonly multinucleated.

PSEUDOSTRATIFIED EPITHELIUM

It is a simple epithelium where cells are of different height and their nuclei are placed at different level so that it gives a false appearance of two layers. It is of following types:

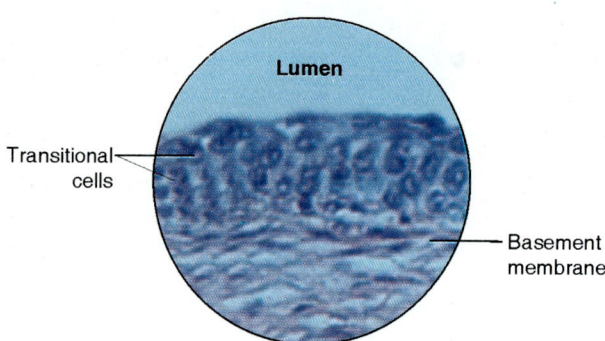

Fig. 63.9: Transitional Epithelium

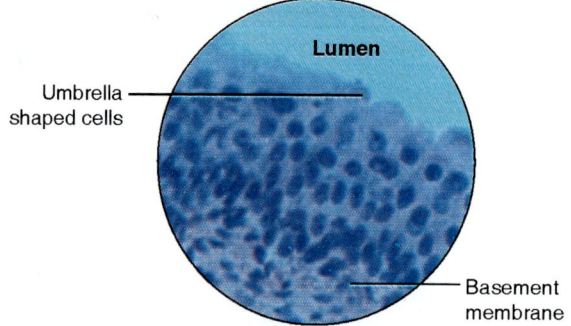

Fig. 63.10: Epithelium Relaxed

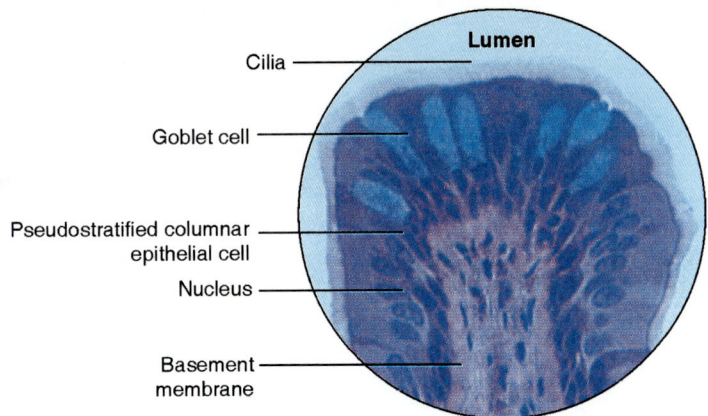

Cilia

Goblet cell

Pseudostratified columnar
epithelial cell

Nucleus

Basement
membrane

Lumen

Fig. 63.11: Pseudosrtatified columnar epithelium

1. Pseudostratified columnar nonciliated

All cells rest on the basement membrane. Many cells reach the luminal surface; some cells do not. Thus it appears as stratified as the cut surface shows nuclei at two different levels. More deeply placed cells are short basal cells while superficial cells are columnar with goblet cells.

2. Pseudostratified columnar ciliated

Here the cells reaching the surface are of two types; one having cilia and others are goblet cells (secrete mucous). This mucous forms a film on the luminal surface and the cilia moves the mucous - **respiratory epithelium**. The basal cells not reaching the surface act as stem cells for the taller cells when they are lost from the membrane. Cilia arise from basal bodies located just beneath the surface membrane of the columnar cells.

E.g. Trachea

3. Pseudostratified columnar with stereocilia

Here columnar cells reaching the lumen show long stereocilia which are nonmotile. These are long and branching microvilli. These columnar cells are absorptive cells.

E.g. Duct of epididymis

64

Connective Tissue

FEATURES OF CONNECTIVE TISSUE

- Abundant
- Consists of cell separated by extracellular matrix
- Diverse
- Performs variety of important functions

Functions of Connective Tissue

1. Enclosing and separating as capsules around organs
2. Connecting tissues to one another as tendons and ligaments
3. Supporting and moving as bones
4. Storing as fat
5. Cushioning and insulating as fat
6. Transporting as blood
7. Protecting as cells of the immune system

TYPES

- Loose & dense connective tissue
- Adipose tissue,
- Blood
- Cartilage
- Bone

Histologically it is divided into

- Cells
- Non-cellular component

Non-cellular component is subdivided into

- Nonfibrous component
- Fibrous component

CONNECTIVE TISSUE CELLS

1. Specialized cells produce the extracellular matrix

Suffixes

- **blasts:** create the matrix
- **cytes:** maintain the matrix
- **clasts:** break the matrix down for remodeling

2. Adipose or fat cells
3. Mast cells that contain heparin and histamine
4. White blood cells that respond to injury or infection
5. Macrophages that phagocytize or provide protection
6. Stem cells

These are divided into

- Fixed cells
- Wandering cells

Fibroblast

They are fusiform or spindle shaped with branching processes. Nucleus has prominent nucleolus and chromatin is euchromatic type. They are present in all types of connective tissue.

Fibrocyte

Fibroblast surrounded with the intercellular substance produced by it - loses its ability to divide & synthesize - **fibrocyte**. These are elongated pink cells with rod shaped nucleus and small cytoplasm. Nucleus is heterochromatic. They are seen in all types of connective tissue.

Adipose cell

These are oval or spherical in shape containing a large globule of fat surrounded by thin rim of cytoplasm. Since fat is dissolved during staining; appear empty spaces - characteristic signet ring appearance. These are present in superficial fascia in large amount.

Macrophage

These are phagocytic in nature. Its shape varies (**pleomorphic**) with the content. The cytoplasm is granular vacuolated and basophilic. Ingested particles are present in the vacuole - **unstained**. The nucleus is small & rounded. These are most numerous in loose connective tissue.

Mast cell

These are large, round or oval cells having metachromatic granules. Nucleus is small. These require **Alcian blue** staining.

E.g. In serous cavities and loose areolar tissue

Plasma cell

These are oval or round having basophilic cytoplasm in which **Russell bodies** may be seen. Nucleus is eccentric and chromatin is cart-wheel in appearance. These are derived from B- lymphocytes and produce antibodies.

Other cells
- Blood cells
- Marrow cells
- Bone cells
- Cartilage cells

EXTRACELLULAR MATRIX

Components
Protein fibers
- Collagen which is most common protein in body
- Reticular fill spaces between tissues and organs
- Elastic returns to its original shape after distension or compression

Ground substance
- Shapeless background

CATEGORIES OF CONNECTIVE TISSUE

Embryonic or mesenchyme
Adult
- Loose
- Dense
- Connective tissue with special properties
- Cartilage
- Bone
- Blood

LOOSE CONNECTIVE TISSUE

- Also known as areolar tissue
- Loose packing material of most organs and tissues
- Attaches skin to underlying tissues
- Contains collagen, reticular, elastic fibers and variety of cells

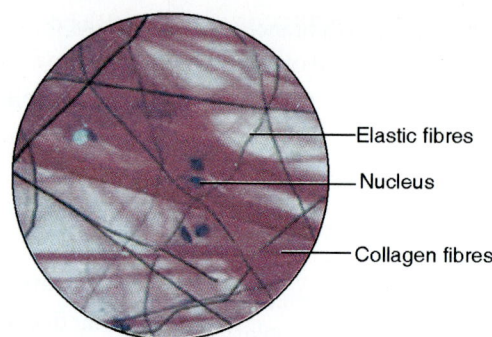

Fig. 64.1: Loose Connective Tissue

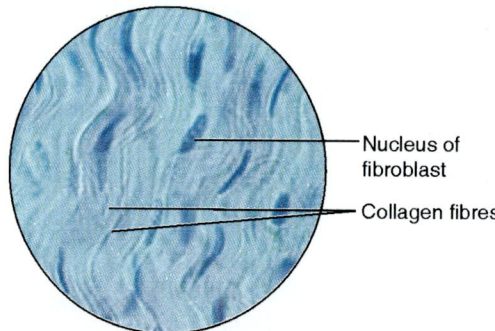

Fig. 64.2: Dense regular Connective Tissue

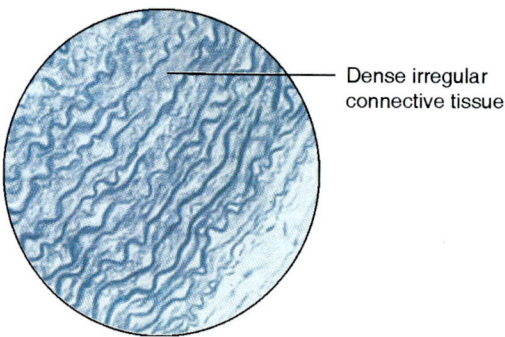

Fig. 64.3: Dense Irregular Connective Tissue

DENSE CONNECTIVE TISSUE

Dense regular
Have abundant collagen fibers
- Tendons: Connect muscles to bones
- Ligaments: Connect bones to bones

Dense regular elastic
- Ligaments in vocal folds

Dense irregular
- Scars

Dense irregular collagenous
- Forms most of skin dermis

Dense irregular elastic
- In walls of elastic arteries

CONNECTIVE TISSUE WITH SPECIAL PROPERTIES

Adipose tissue
Consists of adipocytes

Types

Yellow (white)
Most abundant, white at birth and yellows with age

Brown
Found only in specific areas of body as axillae, neck and near kidneys

Reticular tissue
Forms framework of lymphatic tissue
Characterized by network of fibers and cells

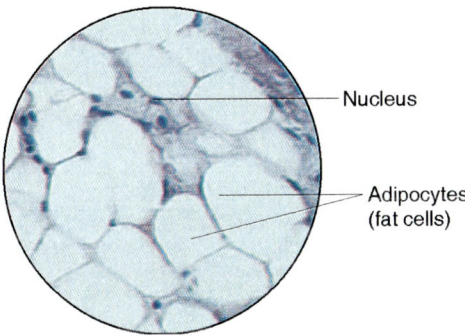

— Nucleus

— Adipocytes (fat cells)

Fig. 64.4: Adipose Tissue

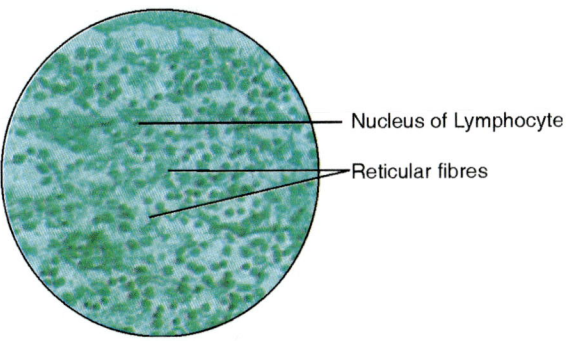

— Nucleus of Lymphocyte

— Reticular fibres

Fig. 64.5: Reticular Tissue

FIBRES

There are three types of connective tissue fibres which are synthesized by the connective tissue cells (fibroblast).

Collagen fibres

These are wide and wavy fibres which are eosinophilic. Each collagen fibre is made up of fibrils. Unfixed fibres are white so they are also known as white fibres. Under microscope they appear in bundles and some bundles appear wavy.

E.g. Tendon, aponeurosis

Elastic fibres

These show branching and can be stretched by tensile force and on being released they return to their original length. Because of their different refractive index unstained fibres appear darker and yellow. They branch and anastomose freely and run singly.

E.g. Ligamentum nuchae

Reticular fibres

These are very fine, branched and arranged in delicate network. These are not stained so cannot be identified under H & E; seen in **silver stain**. They are present in basement membrane, glands, etc.

LOOSE AREOLAR TISSUE

Here most of the constituents of the connective tissue i.e. cells, fibrous and nonfibrous parts are seen.

Collagen fibre bundles are wavy, thick and eosinophilic. Elastic fibres are single branched and may be straight or wavy when cut. Adipose cells can be seen with vacuolated cytoplasm. Most of the nuclei in this tissue are of fibroblast and fibrocytes. These cells are flat, branching cells with oval nuclei. Plasma cells, lymphocytes and eosinophils can also be identified.

E.g. Superficial fascia

ADIPOSE TISSUE

Fat cells are special type of cell. Mature fat cells do not divide in adult. Fat lobules are separated by connective tissue septa. About 50% cells of adipose tissue are not fat cells but cells of stroma. Under microscope fat cell appears as a **signet ring** only if the section passes through the nucleus. Fat is unstained so the cell appears as empty or vacuolated. White fat is abundant in man but brown fat is less.

TENDON

It is a dense regular connective tissue having great tensile strength. In longitudinal section it shows compact parallel bundles of collagen fibres with rows of fibroblast (**tendon cells**) in the loose connective tissue. In the transverse section collagen bundles are seen covered by interfascicular connective tissue.

65

Cartilage

CARTILAGE

Composed of chondrocytes located in spaces called lacunae.

Next to bone firmest structure in body

Types

- Hyaline
- Fibrocartilage
- Elastic

HYALINE CARTILAGE

It is mainly seen in

- Respiratory system
- Joints

It is also seen in

- Articular costal
- Cellular cartilage

The matrix is glistening, smooth and glassy in appearance. It is covered by **perichondrium**. It consists of

- Outer fibrous layer
- Inner cellular layer

It is avascular.

E.g. Trachea, laryngeal cartilages

Features

The fibrous layer shows dense regularly arranged connective fibres with flattened fibroblast and fibrocytes. Cellular layer has chondrogenic cells- **chondrocytes** and **chondroblast**. The chondroblast secretes matrix and can divide. Cells are present in lacunae. The matrix consists of collagen fibres and nonfibrous amorphous substance. The refractive index of collagen is same as that of matrix so they are not seen separately.

A chondroblast secretes the matrix around itself and forms lacuna. When it divides then two or more daughter cells are seen in the lacuna (**primary lacuna**). These daughter cells continue to secrete the matrix around them so that the primary lacuna is divided into two or four small secondary lacunae. This group of cells in the lacunae is called as a **cell nest**.

Articular cartilage

Here the perichondrium is absent. It is seen as epiphyseal cartilage at the ends of long bones on the free joint surface. Superficial cells are more scattered and lie parallel to the surface. In the next zone mitotic figures can be seen in deeper parallel cell layers. In the deeper column cells are large and

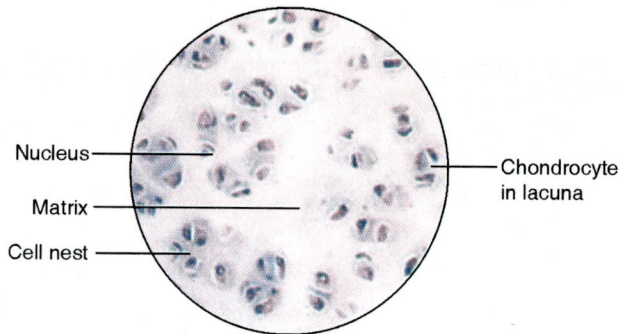

Fig. 65.1: Hyaline Cartilage

secrete matrix while the deepest zone is calcified. Articular cartilage is extremely smooth.

Costal cartilage

It has perichondrium where cellular layer may not be seen after full development. Chondrocytes are large cells with eosinophilic cytoplasm and prominent nucleus. Cells are seen in groups around the periphery.

WHITE FIBROCARTILAGE

Perichondrium is absent in the fibrocartilage It shows dense white fibrous tissue (pink in H&E) with fibroblasts and small groups of chondrocytes. The chondrocytes are ovoid, surrounded by concentrically striated matrix, and lie in rows or layers. Between the rows there are bundles of collagen fibres.

E.g. Intervertebral disc

ELASTIC CARTILAGE

Perichondrium is present and shows both layers (fibrous & cellular). Elastic cartilage is firm and elastic. Chondrocytes produce collagen and elastic fibres as well as intercellular substance. The ground substance contains branching and anastomosing elastic fibres. Chondrocytes are larger and are present singly or in small groups. Elastic fibres are better seen in **orcein stain.**

E.g. Epiglottis, Pinna of external ear

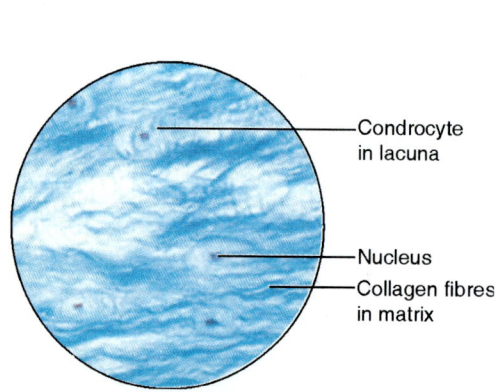

Fig. 65.2: Fibrocartilage

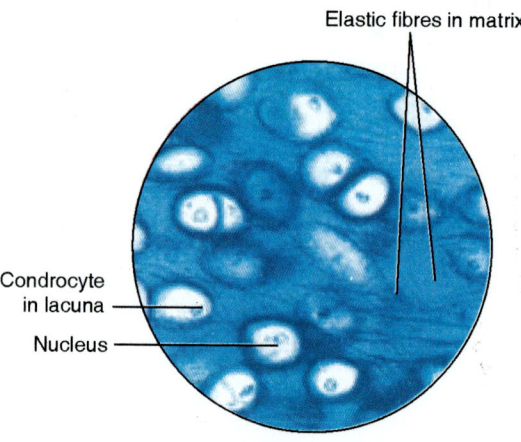

Fig. 65.3: Elastic Cartilage

66

Bone

It consists of cells and matrix. The matrix consists of collagen and amorphous component and cells placed in lacunae. The matrix is rich in inorganic salts. It is vascular and grows by **appositional growth**.

Bone is covered by periosteum.

It consists of

- Outer fibrous layer
- Inner cellular layer

Bone cells are

- Osteoblast
- Osteocytes
- Osteoclast

The bone matrix is made up of organic and inorganic elements.

Organic element - collagen dense bundles embedded in an amorphous ground substance composed of hyaluronic acid and protein polysaccharides.

Inorganic matrix - calcium phosphates, carbonate, fluoride and magnesium chloride.

Dried compact bone T.S

As this is a dry tissue, periosteum and cells are not seen but lacunae and canaliculi are easily seen. A number of **Haversian systems** or **Osteon**s are seen with central Haversian canal surrounded by concentrically arranged laminae. Between the lamellae are oval spaces called as **lacunae** and fine channels radiating from each lacunae **canaliculi**. Between the Haversian systems the space is filled

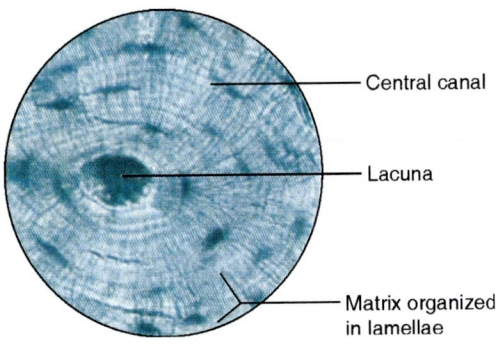

Fig. 66.1: Compact Bone

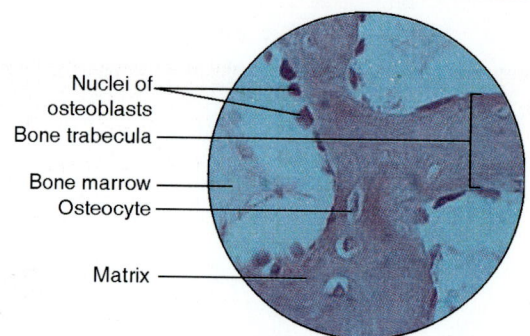

Nuclei of osteoblasts
Bone trabecula
Bone marrow
Osteocyte
Matrix

Fig. 66.2: Cancellous Bone

by irregularly arranged interstitial lamellae containing lacunae and canaliculi.

Ground compact bone L.S

Haversian canals are seen in long axis and they are interconnected by transverse or oblique channels known as **Volkmann's canals** which communicate with the medullary cavity. Haversian and Volkmann's canals in living contain blood vessels nerves and lymphatics. At the outer periphery of the compact bone the lamellae run parallel with the surfaces- **outer circumferential lamellae**. The **inner circumferential lamellae** are parallel with the inner surface. They are covered with periosteum and endosteum respectively. Histologically periosteum and endosteum is same.

BONE CEILS

Osteogenic cell in periosteum

They are present in the osteogenic layer of periosteum. They divide and redivide to form other varieties of bone cells.

Osteoblast

They are present where bone deposition is going on. Osteoblast shows many cell cytoplasmic processes and basophilic cytoplasm. Nucleus is round and eccentric. They do not divide and synthesize & secrete matrix. These appear as round or polygonal cells. The nucleus is located away from the cell surface where bone deposition is going on.

Osteocyte

These are mature osteoblasts (after completing their role in bone formation). These are present in lacunae with processes in canaliculi. These cells are imprisoned in the intercellular matrix.

Osteoclast

These are bone resorption cells; mainly present at site where bone resorption is going on (**endosteal surface**). These are **multinucleated giant cells** with eosinophilic cytoplasm and vacuoles.

67

Muscle

These are of three types
- Striated, skeletal or voluntary
- Nonstriated, smooth or involuntary
- Cardiac muscle

SKELETAL MUSCLE

The muscle is covered by connective tissue sheath - **epimysium**. Fibrous partitions extending into the muscle to surround bundles of muscle fibres- **perimysium**. From it a delicate sheet of connective tissue covering each muscle fibre - **endomysium**. All three coverings transmit blood vessels, nerves and lymphatics to the muscles.

Muscle fibres are large cylindrical and are multinucleated which are ovoid and elongated with long axis parallel to the muscle fibre. They lie just beneath the sarcolemma. Cytoplasm is acidophilic and cross striations are not always clearly seen under low power. In addition to the myofibrils the cytoplasm contains numerous mitochondria and substantial amount of glycogen.

The cytoplasm contains numerous longitudinal fibrils – **myofibrils.** Striations are alternate dark and light bands- **A and I bands** respectively. **Isotropic** - refracts light evenly in all direction while **anisotropic-** reflects light unequally in different planes. These striations are better seen in

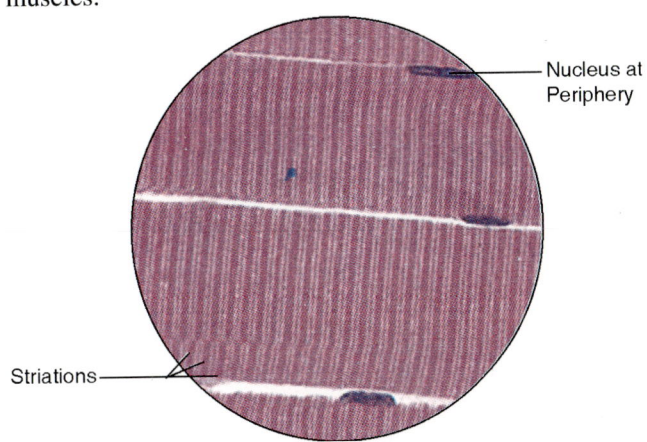

Nucleus at Periphery

Striations

Fig. 67.1: Skeletal Muscle

369

polarized light. I band shows **Z lines** in the centre and A band shows **H zone** in the middle. The centre of the light H zone shows a dark **M band.**

SMOOTH MUSCLE

Smooth muscle fibre is a single cell with single central nucleus. Layers of smooth muscles are commonly subdivided into bundles of fibres. Muscle fibres are elongated and tapered at the ends. The nucleus lies in the widest part of the fibre i.e. in the middle. The cytoplasm is eosinophilic and uniform. Relaxed smooth muscle is **spindle shaped** while contracted muscle is **ellipsoid shaped** and the cell membrane and cytoplasm bulge out. They lack striations because filaments overlap each other in no definite pattern and **Z lines** are absent. -

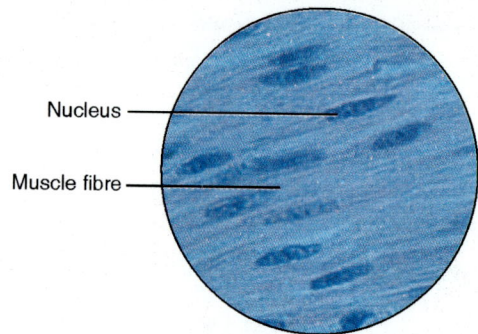

Nucleus

Muscle fibre

Fig. 67.2: Smooth Muscle

CARDIAC MUSCLE

It is striated but involuntary in nature. The structure of the sarcomere is same seen in the skeletal muscle.

Muscle fibres are branch and anastomose to form a network or **syncytium.** Each muscle cell has single central nucleus. The myofibrils are relatively few so that the striations are not as distinct as in skeletal muscles. Cytoplasm of the cardiac fibre is eosinophilic.

The junctions between adjacent muscle cells are seen as dark staining transverse lines running across the fibres - **intercalated discs.** These discs lie **opposite I band** of the striations.

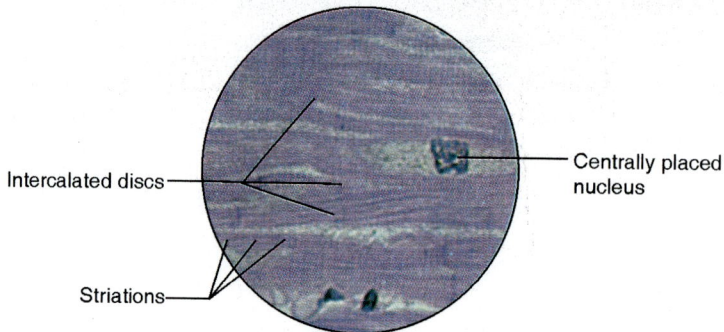

Intercalated discs

Centrally placed nucleus

Striations

Fig. 67.3: Cardiac Muscle

68

Blood Vessels

Histologically blood vessels show three basic layers:

- Tunica intima
- Tunica media
- Tunica adventitia

In artery media is thicker than other two coats, while in vein adventitia is thicker than the other two coats.

Depending upon the amount of elastic fibres or smooth muscles, arteries are either elastic or muscular.

ELASTIC ARTERY

Elastic artery shows **thick tunica intima**, one fifth of total thickness of the wall. It shows incomplete laminae of elastic fibres embedded along with cells in an amorphous intercellular substance. The luminal surface is lined by the simple squamous endothelium. Internal elastic lamina is difficult to identify. The **tunica media** is mainly formed by concentrically arranged elastic fibres with smooth muscle cells. The media is limited externally by external elastic lamina. **Tunica adventitia** shows thin irregularly arranged connective tissue containing both collagen and elastic fibres and vasa vasorum.

E.g. Aorta, pulmonary artery.

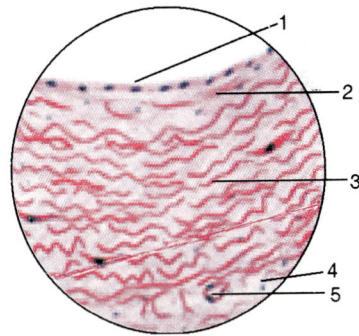

1. Endothelium 2. Subendothelium layor
3. Tumica media with elestic fibres
4. Tunica adventitia 5. Vasa vasorum

Fig. 68.1: Elastic Artery

MUSCULAR ARTERY

Tunica intima shows simple squamous epithelium (**endothelium**) with a small amount of subendothelial connective tissue. Internal elastic lamina is seen at the junction of tunica intima and media. Generally it is in contracted condition giving a wavy appearance to the intima and identified as pink line. **Tunica media** showsspirallyarrangedsmoothmusclecellswithelastic fibres. External elastic lamina is at the junction of the media and adventitia. **Tunica adventitia** is two third the thickness of media and shows collagen and elastic fibres. Vasa vasorum and lymphatics are also seen.

E.g. Axillary, femoral artery.

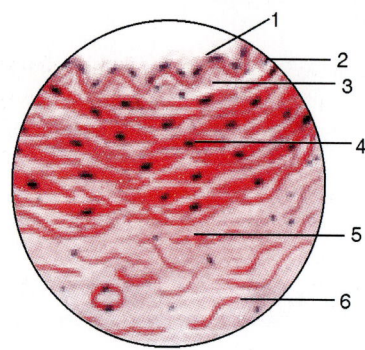

1. Endothelium 2. Subendothelium layer
3. Internal elastic lamina
4. Tunica media with smooth muscle
5. Exteral elastic lamina
6. Tunica adventitia

Fig. 68.2: Muscular Artery

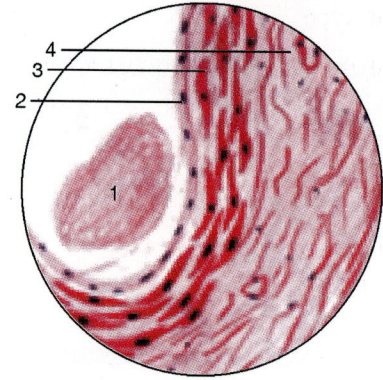

1. Blood in lumen
2. Endothelium
3. Tunica media
4. Tunica adventitia

Fig. 68.3: Vein

ARTERIOLE

Arterioles - These are smaller branches of an artery with less than 100 micron diameter. The ratio of thickness of wall to the diameter of its lumen is **1:1.7 to 1:27**. **Tunica intima** shows simple squamous endothelial layer. Internal elastic lamina is present. **Tunica media** shows circularly arranged smooth muscle fibre and are limited on its outer surface by external elastic lamina. **Tunica adventitia** shows the mixture of collagen and elastic fibres. In smaller branches of arterioles internal elastic lamina is not seen, while only one or two, smooth muscle cells are seen in the media.

If the diameter is less than 50 micron then it is **terminal arteriole** while lateral branches of terminal arterioles are called **metaarterioles -** supply capillary bed.

Arterioles are best seen in spleen.

VEIN

Tunica intima shows simple squamous endothelial lining resting on poorly defined internal elastic lamina, which may be seen separated from the endothelium by scanty subendothelial collagenous connective tissue. **Tunica media** is thin and has circularly arranged smooth muscle fibres with more collagen and few elastic fibres. **Tunica adventitia** is the thickest coat which is made up of mainly collagen-fibres with the nuclei of fibroblast. Vasa vasorum are present in tunica adventitia.

Veins are well seen in the slides of liver and glands.

CAPILLARIES

These are of two types :

Continuous type: Simple squamous endothelial cells line the capillaries. Nucleus of these endothelial cells appears as a blue crescent partly bulging and encircling the lumen. Endothelial cells under EM shows many pinocytotic vesicles. Edges of endothelial cells are joined by tight junctions. Endothelial cells rest on the basement membrane, which also encircles the pericytes. These capillaries are for exchange of materials.

E.g. Capillaries in the muscle, lung

Fenestrated type

The wall of the capillaries has apertures in their endothelial lining. Some fenestrations are present within the endothelial cell cytoplasm. These are the cytoplasmic pores which pass through the entire thickness of the cell. Capillaries are meant for diffusion of substances.

E.g. Renal glomeruli, intestinal villi

Sinusoids

These are large thin-walled, irregular shaped. These are lined by endothelium. Lining simple squamous cells may show scattered reticuloendothelial cells. Sinusoids are supported by a thin layer of reticular fibres. Sinusoids are seen in liver, adrenal, pituitary etc. Sinusoids are of two types:

- Fenestrated type
- Discontinuous type

69

Nervous Tissue

Nervous tissue shows neurons and glial cells. Neuron is the structural and -functional unit of nervous system. It shows cell body and two types of processes, axon and dendrites. Glial cells are special type of connective tissue.

Axon - thin, long and single

Dendrites - thick short and one or more in number

TYPES OF NEURON

Depending upon the number of processes, the neurons are classified into four types:

Unipolar

These are relatively rare in nervous system. These have only one process. These are present in the **mesencephalic nucleus of Trigeminal nerve**.

Bipolar

Cells are spindle shaped having two poles. These have one axon and one dendrite extending from opposite surfaces of the cell body. They are present in **retina** and in the **spiral ganglion of vestibulocochlear nerve**.

Multipolar

They are most common type of neuron. These consist of a single axon and more than one dendrites. The shape of the cell varies with number of processes.

Pseudounipolar

In light microscope these neurons show a single process like but in high resolutions two processes are seen arising from one pole of the cells. These two processes later separate in a T-shaped manner. Out of the two processes one is axon and another is dendrite. These are seen in **spinal ganglia** and the **ganglia of the cranial nerves**.

CELL BODY (PERIKARYON)

It is acidophilic with some basophilic granules in it - **Nissl's** substance. They cannot divide. The soma may be 4 micron in diameter in small neurons to 130 micron in (**Betz cells**) pyramidal cortex. The nucleus is central in CNS while eccentric in PNS. The nucleolus is easily seen as the chromatin is vesicular type (**Owl's eye**). The Nissl's substance is the region of the cytoplasm rich in flattened cisternae of rough endoplasmic reticulum. The abundant free ribosomes and polysomes synthesize proteins.

NEUROGLIAL CELLS

In H & E stain neurons and neuroglia cannot be identified separately all the time. Neurons are supported by neuroglia in the nervous system.

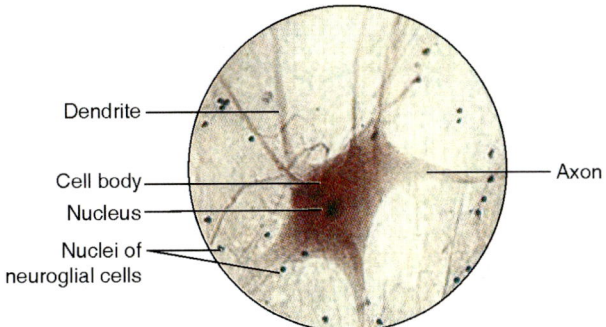

Fig. 69.1: Multipolar Neuron

Astrocyte (Fibrous)

This cell has many processes which extend out in star like fashion from its cell body. Processes are long and straight with very little or no branching. They are located in the white matter. They are seen well in **Cajal stain**.

Astrocyte (Protoplasmic)

They have branching cytoplasmic processes which extend from cell bodies. Their processes are shorter and branch extensively. Processes of both the types of astrocytes widen at the end and form an astrocyte foot along the capillaries-**blood brain barrier**. They play major role in the cohesion of Nervous system.

Oligodendroglial cell

These cells have tree like few processes. They are of three types **light larger**, **intermediate** and **dark small cells**. In adults, dark types are more common and they have less cytoplasm compared to light type. They are responsible for the **myelination in CNS**. Their processes wrap nerve fibres to form myelin. A single cell can wrap several nerve fibres.

Microglial cell

They are also called **brain macrophages**. They do not divide. These are smallest glial cells with flattened body and short processes and present in more number in grey matter. They are phagocytes derived from blood monocytes. They are stained by **silver carbonate method**.

Schwann cell

They are responsible for the **myelination of PNS**. They cover the internode region of a peripheral nerve fibre and form myelin of that internode region. Schwann cells are essential for the repair of the damaged peripheral nerves.

Ependymocyte

These line the lumen of all the cavities inside the CNS (ventricles, aqueduct and central canal). In the neural tube germinal cells after formation of nervous system remain as ependymal cells. According to the location they vary from squamous to columnar in shape. Their surfaces have numerous microvilli and cilia contributing to the flow of CSF. The nucleus is heterochromatic.

Tanycytes

These are ependymoglial cells, also called ependymal astrocytes. They have the function of transport of substances between the vascular system and ventricular system.

PERIPHERAL NERVES

Peripheral nervous system (PNS) consists of
- Ganglia
- Nerves

Ganglion - collection of neurons in the PNS
Nerves - bundles of axons (motor) or I and peripheral processes of sensory ganglia.

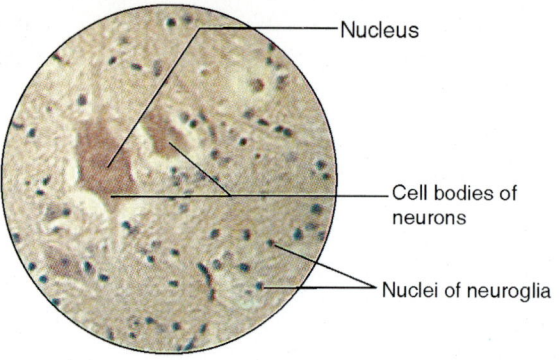

Nucleus

Cell bodies of neurons

Nuclei of neuroglia

Fig. 69.2: Neuroglia

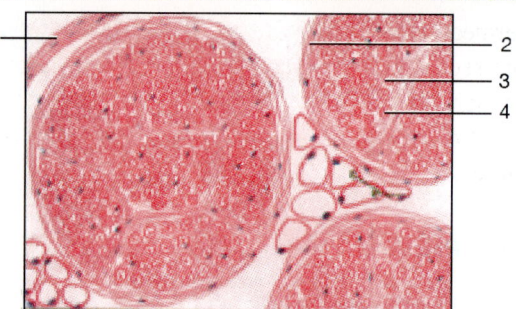

1. Epineurium 2. Perineurium 3. Endoneurium 4. Axon

Fig. 69.3: Nerve: T.S

The nerves are

- Motor (axons)
- Sensory (dendrite) r
- Mixed (both)

Ganglia are

- Sensory
- Sympathetic
- Parasympathetic

The sympathetic and parasympathetic are collectively known as autonomic and are motor in function.

PERIPHERAL NERVE (T.S)

They are covered by connective tissue, which is arranged in the form of tubular sheaths.

- **Epineurium** - covers the whole nerve.
- **Perineurium** - covers a fascicle of nerve fibres.
- **Endoneurium** – covers each nerve fibre (axon).

These sheaths carry blood vessels to the nerves. Nerve fibres cut transversely are covered by **Neurilemma** or **sheath of Schwann** cell cytoplasm. In myelinated fibres myelin covers axons.

At certain places the nucleus of Schwann cells and nuclei of fibroblast are seen in epineurium, perineurium and endoneurium.

PERIPHERAL NERVE (L.S)

Myelin dissolved away by dehydration and clearing agents. Myelin is seen in **osmic acid** staining. Longitudinal section of the peripheral nerve shows **streaky appearance** and the streaks run in a wavy manner. Many nuclei are seen in the bundle of fibres but the nuclei of Schwann, fibroblast or endothelial capillary cells cannot be differentiated. Perineurium and endoneurial connective tissue is seen with the blood vessels.

In high power it shows a central core formed by the axon - **axis cylinder**. **Axolemma** - plasma membrane surrounding the axon. The axon is surrounded by the myelin in myelinated nerve fibres. As myelin is washed during dehydration of the tissue, empty longitudinal space is seen in H&E stain along the axon.

The myelin is in the form of segments separated by short intervals. The segment of myelin is called **internode** and the gap in between the internode is termed **Node of Ranvier**. Myelin of each internode is formed by separate Schwann cell outside the myelin.

Cytoplasm with nucleus and surrounding cell membrane - **Neurilemma**.

In nonmyelinated nerve the neurilemma surrounds the axis cylinder directly (myelin absent). In the internodal myelin sheath little discontinuities termed clefts or incisures of **Schmidt-Lanterman** are seen. These are the places where the cytoplasm of Schwann cell was trapped during formation of myelin by rotation of the cells around the nerve fibres.

PERIPHERAL NERVOUS SYSTEM

Peripheral nervous system consists of ganglia and nerve fibres. Collection of neurons outside the central nervous system is ganglion. There are two types of ganglia:
Sensory and autonomic.

SPINAL (SENSORY GANGLION)

They are seen on the V and VII, IX and X cranial nerves and on the dorsal root of 'spinal nerves. They are the first order (afferent) sensory neurons. The cell body is large and rounded. They are pseudounipolar cells having peripheral process (**dendrite**) and central process (**axon**). Nucleus is central vesicular with a prominent nucleolus. There is capsule to each neuron formed by flattened cells called satellite cells. The cells are in groups separated by nerve fibres. The neurons show Nissl substance and sometimes **lipochrome pigment**. The satellite cells are with rounded or oval nuclei. There are many fibroblasts in the connective tissue. Part of the dorsal root (nerve fibres) may be seen entering and leaving the ganglion on either side. Endoneurium and perineurium of the root enters inside and ganglion as connective tissue while epineurium merges with the capsule of the ganglion.

SYMPATHETIC (AUTONOMIC GANGLION)

They are seen on the sympathetic chain and some migrated like coeliac ganglion. It consists of multipolar neurons (efferent). The cell body is smaller and irregular as many dendrites arise from the soma. The nucleus is eccentric and also has a prominent nucleolus. Satellite cells are seen but few in numbers. The neurons and nerve fibres are seen scattered. Neurons also show Nissl substance and sometimes two nucleoli and lipochrome.

The intercellular area shows fibroblast, supporting connective tissue, blood vessels, myelinated and unmyelinated fibres. The nerve fibres are preganglionic and postganglionic visceral efferents mainly. Outermost layer is connective tissue capsule.

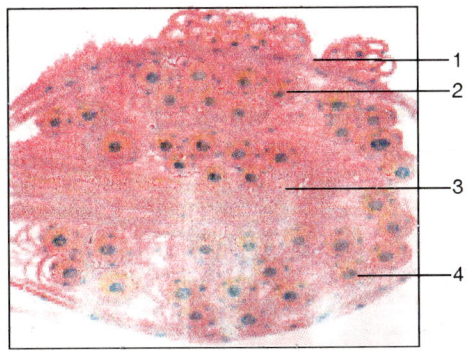

1. Epineurium 2. Ganglion cells in group
3. Nerve fibres 4. Central nucleus

Fig. 69.4: Spinal Ganglion

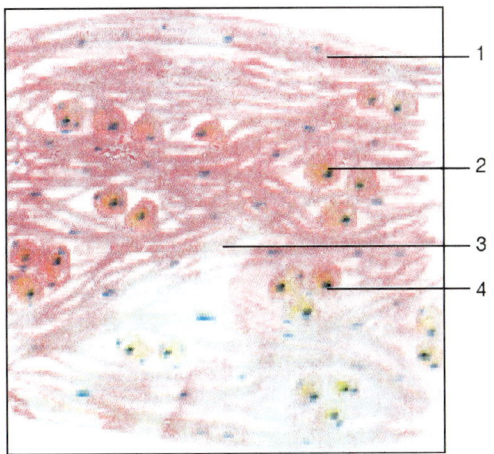

1. Connective tissue 2. Ganglion cell
3. Scattered nerve fibres 4. Eccentric nucleus

Fig. 69.5: Sympathetic Ganglion

70

Salivary Glands

There are three pairs of large salivary glands and many small scattered salivary glands. Saliva is a mixed secretion of salivary glands. Depending upon the type of the secretory unit salivary glands are either serous, mucous or mixed type.

SEROUS SALIVARY GLAND: PAROTID

The secretion is watery, and rich in digestive enzymes.

Under low power it shows capsule of collagenous connective tissue which covers the gland. The capsule sends septa inside the gland dividing the gland substance into many lobules. The connective tissue is divided into interlobular and intralobular. Interlobular connective tissue is easily seen in the form of septa containing blood vessels and ducts. Intralobular connective tissue is scanty and indistinct. It is present in the interalveolar areas. At places adipose tissue is present within the connective tissue and inside the lobules.

It is a **compound tubuloalveolar** or racemose gland. From the secretory alveoli excretory ducts arise. All excretory ducts finally open in the main parotid duct. Within each lobule are masses of serous alveoli, lined by pyramidal simple columnar cells. The lumen of the alveoli is not seen clearly. Nucleus is prominent and rounded. Serous alveoli show basal basophilia and apical eosinophilic cytoplasm. Intralobular ducts, blood vessels and adipose tissue are also seen within the lobule.

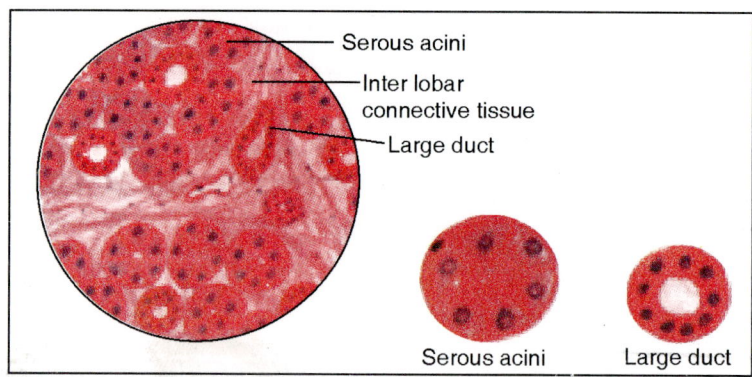

Serous acini

Inter lobar connective tissue

Large duct

Serous acini

Large duct

Fig. 70.1: Serious Salivary Gland

Serous alveolus

Under high power shows large triangular columnar cells resting on a basement membrane. Small lumen is present in the centre of each acinus. The cytoplasm of the basal aspect of the cell is basophilic as it is rich in rough endoplasmic reticulum. The apical cytoplasm contains eosinophilic **zymogen granules** which are membrane bound vesicles containing secretion. The nucleus of myoepithelial cell is seen around the alveolus.

DUCT SYSTEM

1. Intercalated duct

These are lined by cuboidal epithelium with prominent nuclei. Cells contain mitochondria, small rough endoplasmic reticulum, Golgi apparatus, lysosomes and secretory granules. It is involved in the addition of water and electrolytes to saliva. Lumen of the duct is small.

2. Striated duct

Here the cells show basal striations due to packed columns of elongated mitochondria. Between the columns the cytoplasm is divided in to basal processes by infolded basal plasmalemma. These cells are engaged in transport of K+ into the saliva and Na + from saliva, thus make saliva hypotonic. Luminal surface forms microvilli. Duct lining is simple cuboidal to columnar cells with central nuclei. Lumen of duct is distinctly seen.

3. Intralobular duct

All striated and intercalated ducts are intralobular ducts as they are seen only inside a lobule. Parotid can be differentiated from pancreas by large number of these ducts and prominent appearance. All these ducts are distinctly seen scattered within a lobule and surrounded by many secretory alveoli.

4. Interlobular duct

Interlobular duct is seen within the interlobular tissue along with blood vessels. They are cut in all planes. Lumen becomes progressively wider and the lining epithelium is simple columnar. As the duct becomes more and more wide it is lined by pseudostratified columnar nonciliated epithelium. Larger ducts are lined by stratified columnar epithelium.

MUCOUS SALIVARY GLAND

Because of the presence of serous demilunes, the mucous glands are not purely mucous in secretion.

Sublingual gland

It is predominantly mucous in nature. The connective tissue capsule sends septa which carries blood vessels, nerves and support the duct system. The gland is divided into lobules. Interlobular connective tissue is easily seen forming septa while intralobular connective tissue is scanty around the secretory units. Intralobular ducts are identified as these are surrounded by secretory units. Interlobular ducts are very prominent in the slide seen along with blood vessels within the interlobular connective tissue. The lining of the duct system is same as that in parotid gland.

Mucous secretory units are packed within a lobule. They are larger compared to serous alveoli and are lined by simple columnar cells resting on a basement membrane. Mucous cells are pale staining because mucous is washed during staining. The lumen is larger and easily seen. The nuclei are flat placed near the basement membrane.

Mucous alveolus with serous demilune

Columnar cells of a mucous alveolus rest on a basement membrane. Nucleus of each cell is flat with long axis parallel to the basement membrane. Nucleus is disk like and is squeezed up against the bases of the cells. Basal cytoplasm is less basophilic. Larger part of the cytoplasm is supranuclear containing membrane bound vesicles of mucous as in goblet cells. Mucous is a glycoprotein so does not

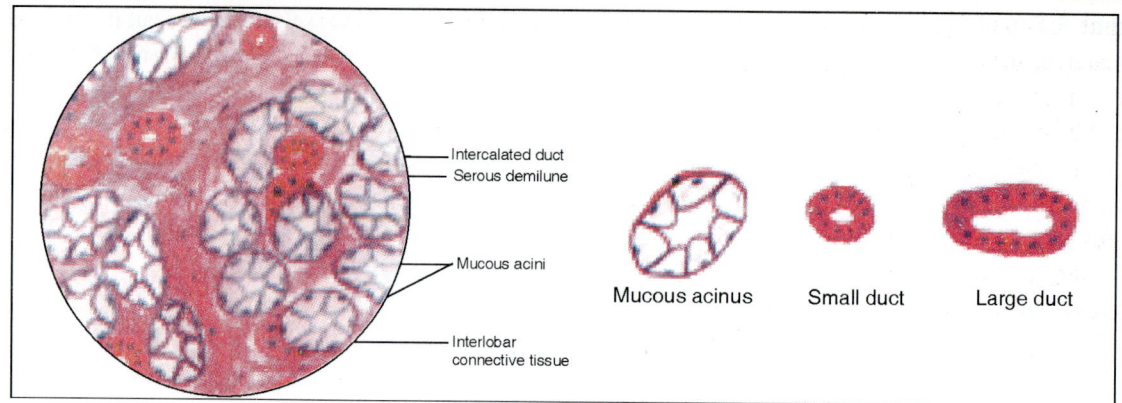

Fig. 70.2: Mucous Salivary Gland

stain with H & E and hence the cytoplasm is pale and vacuolated. These vacuoles are stained with PAS.

Demilune is half moon shaped cluster of serous secreting cells around a mucous secretory unit. Mucous alveolus is capped by crescent shaped group of serous cells. Nucleus and the cytoplasm of the serous cells are like that of other serous cells. Secretion of these cells reaches the lumen of the mucous alveolus to which they cap through tiny intercellular canals. Mucous secretory units are cradled in loose basket made up of cytoplasmic processes of myoepithelial cells lying between the bases of the secretory cells. Its basement membrane lies between the secretory unit and surrounding connective tissue. The nucleus of the myoepithelial cell is central. It shows many long cytoplasmic processes that extend to encircle the secretory units. These cells are epithelial in origin and are contractile. They help in expressing the secretion into the duct.

MIXED SALIVARY GLAND

A salivary gland showing both the serous and mucous secretory units is called mixed salivary gland submandibular gland. The gland is covered which by capsule send septa inside, dividing the gland into many lobules. The duct system is similar

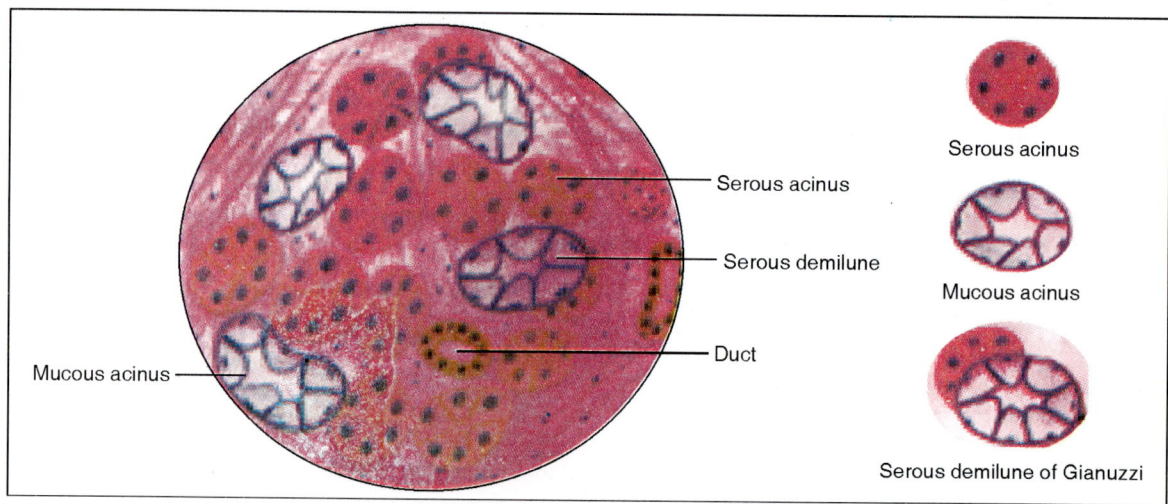

Fig. 70.3: Mixed Salivary Gland

to that of parotid salivary gland showing intercalated, striated and excretory ducts. These are seen under microscope as intralobular and interlobular ducts.

Inside a lobule many secretory alveoli are seen with some adipose tissue and ducts. Presence of mucous secretory units differentiates submandibular from parotid, while presence of many serous secretory units differentiates it from sublingual gland. Many mucous secretory units show serous demilune. **Serous alveolus** stains dark violet and small in size, with hardly any lumen, round basal nucleus, basal basophilia and apical eosinophilia. **Mucous alveolus** stains faint pink and large in size with a prominent lumen. Flat basal nucleus is situated very close to the cell membrane and cytoplasm is vacuolated. Myoepithelial cells and demilunes are also seen.

71

Lymphoid Tissue

LYMPH NODE

It is covered by connective tissue capsule containing adipose tissue. Capsule is thick at hilum; here it gives off trabeculae. Internal structure shows **cortex and medulla**.

Cortex is packed with lymphocytes. Lymph moves from cortex to medulla. Through the trabeculae blood vessels enter inside. Internal support is provided by reticular fibres formed by reticular cells. Cellular parenchyma exists as round cortical nodules in the cortex.

Islands of cellular parenchyma between the lymphatic sinuses - **medullary cords**. Efferent vessels empty the lymph in subcapsular sinus, which continues as subcortical sinuses between the pyramids and further continue as medullary sinuses between medullary cords.

Midcortical and deep cortical zones are called **Thymus dependant zone** of the lymph node. Subcapsular space contains **RE cells** and free cells like lymphocytes, macrophages and plasma cells. It is lined by endothelium while sinuses have discontinuous wall. Cortical primary nodules

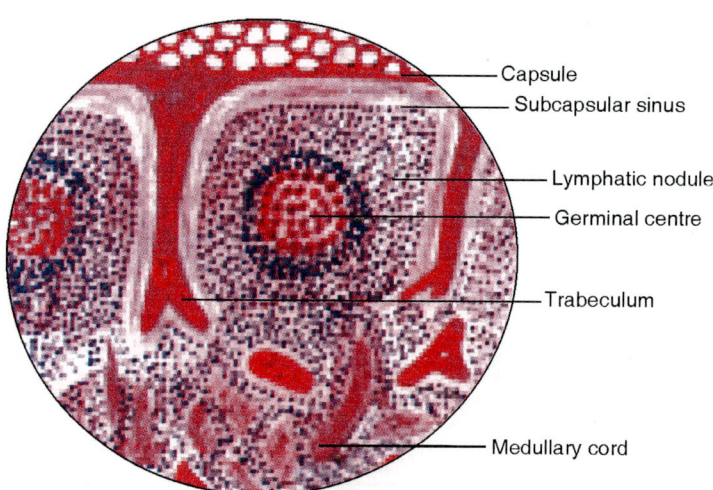

Capsule
Subcapsular sinus

Lymphatic nodule
Germinal centre

Trabeculum

Medullary cord

Fig. 71.1: Lymph Node

(follicles) are the areas of greater concentration of lymphocytes. The cytoplasm of these cells exists as a thin rim.

Lymphatic follicle (nodule) and Germinal centre

In the centre of the lymphatic nodule germinal centre may be seen. Lymphatic nodules are called **primary nodules** and germinal centre as **secondary nodule**. It develops after the exposure to an antigen. Lymphocytes become blast cells and multiply. It is a rounded mass of cells with basophilic cytoplasm. This is a light staining (faint violet) area within the dark basophilic primary nodule. It is a lymphopoietic centre. It contains large lymphocytes and plasma cells. Nuclei are larger and so appear as less concentrated and widely separated from each other, compared with surrounding zone of the primary centre.

Depending upon the packing density, cortex is subdivided into three zones. Germinal centre is seen in zone III.

CELLS

1. Small Lymphocyte

They are of two types **T and B lymphocytes**. They have round densely stained nucleus and relatively small amount of pale basophilic cytoplasm. T and B lymphocytes cannot be identified separately under microscope. Nucleus is heterochromatic and the, nucleoli are not seen. The cytoplasm is also not seen.

2. Large Lymphocyte

They make up about 3% lymphocytes in peripheral blood. They represent activated **B lymphocytes**. Cytoplasm is faint basophilic and chromatin condensed type; nucleoli are not seen. Cytoplasm can be seen in the form of a rim around the nucleus.

3. Lymphoblast

These have basophilic cytoplasm with rounded nucleus. Chromatin matter is euchromatic with two or more nucleoli. They are seen in the centre of the germinal centre.

4. Plasma cell

Cytoplasm is basophilic and nucleus is eccentric. The chromatin matter is distinctly "**cart wheel**" type. The cytoplasm may contain round acidophilic bodies known as **Russell bodies**. Activated B lymphocyte is converted into plasma cell and they secrete antibodies.

5. Macrophage

These are large cells which show eccentric nucleus and vacuolated cytoplasm due to dissolved lipid inclusions.

SPLEEN

Blood born antigen stimulates lymphocytes in spleen. There are no afferent lymphatics and efferents are confined to the connective tissue. Lymph is filtered in a lymph node while blood is filtered in the spleen.

Spleen

It is covered by connective tissue capsule containing smooth muscle fibres, collagen and elastic fibres. From hilum trabeculae extend inside and a few also extend from capsule. Its internal structure consists of **red and white pulp**. In routine H & E staining white pulp is dark violet mass and rest of the area is red pulp which appears pink. The basic framework of the pulp is a network of reticular fibres.

In white pulp lymphatic nodules are seen - site of lymphocyte production.

Red pulp contains large number of RBCs in its mesh. Trabeculae cut in multiple planes (histological feature) and these convey blood vessels and nerves.

Spleen (HP)

Arteries branch in the trabeculae and enter white pulp. **In white pulp** the arteries are covered by

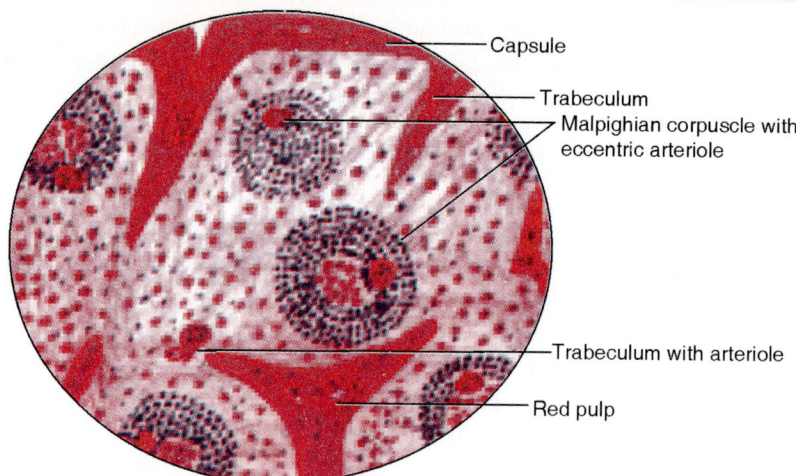

Fig. 71.2: Spleen

reticular sheaths which are infiltrated with lymphocytes. These are lymphatic nodules, which may show the **germinal centre**. White pulp is distributed along arteries that leave trabeculae. When a sheath is expanded to form the nodule, the artery gives off a branch to supply the nodule - **follicular artery**. A follicular artery leaves white pulp and enters the red pulp. Here it divides into two to six branches, which radiate in different directions - **penicillar arteries**. Each again divides in to two to three arterioles. Perivascular lymphatic sheaths of the arteries and arterioles are the thymus dependent zone of the spleen. The border between the red and white pulp is not sharp - **transitional zone**.

In red pulp there are sinusoids lined by long narrow endothelial cells showing slits. Red pulp between two sinusoids is like a cord so called **Billroth cords**. Red pulp contains RBCs, WBCs, plasma cells, macrophages and reticular cells. Basic cells of germinal centre are activated B cells. The rim that surrounds the centre is composed of T cells. From both positions plasma cells moves readily into the red pulp.

THYMUS

It shows **cortex** and **medulla** but no germinal centre. Presence of **Hassall's corpuscles** is the main identifying feature.

Thymus

It is covered by capsule, which sends incomplete septa and divides it into lobules. No lymphatics enter or drain in to the thymus. It gives off efferent vessels.

Cortex is concentrated with lymphocytes while **medulla** is pale and contains less lymphocyte. Outer cortex shows large lymphocytes and rapid mitosis which forms small lymphocytes, which are placed in the deeper zone of the cortex. Cortical nodules are absent so that the whole cortex is uniformly dark violet. The medulla of the adjacent lobules is continuous.

Thymus (HP)

Plasma cells may be seen in medulla. Thymus reticulum is formed by epithelial cells. Macrophages may be seen in

- Capsule

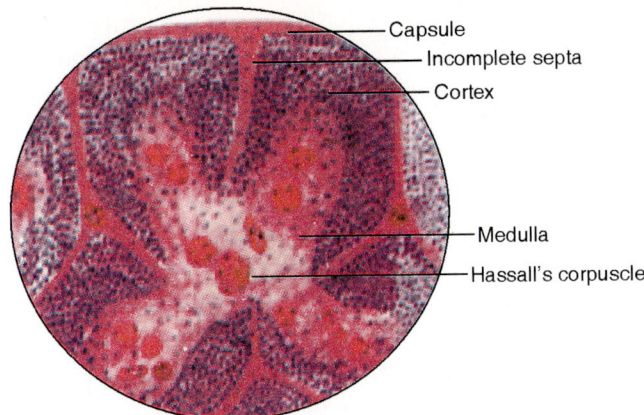

Fig. 71.3: Thymus

- Corticomedullary junction
- Medulla

Hassall's corpuscle

It is a pink staining hyaline mass around which there are concentrically arranged epithelial cells are seen. These are **keratinised epithelial cells**. Each Hassall's corpuscle has a central core formed by epithelial cells that have undergone degeneration. Hassall's' corpuscles increase in number and size as age advances.

Blood thymic barrier

Arterioles from **corticomedullary junction** ascend into cortex where they form anastomosing capillary arcades from which capillaries return to corticomedullary junction and drain into venules of medulla. A continuous epithelium surround the capillaries of the cortex. There is a space between capillary pericytes and epithelial membrane. Both the capillary endothelium and epithelial cells have separate basement membranes.

Component of barrier:
- Capillary endothelium
- Basement membrane
- Perivascular space
- Epithelial basement membrane
- Epithelial cell

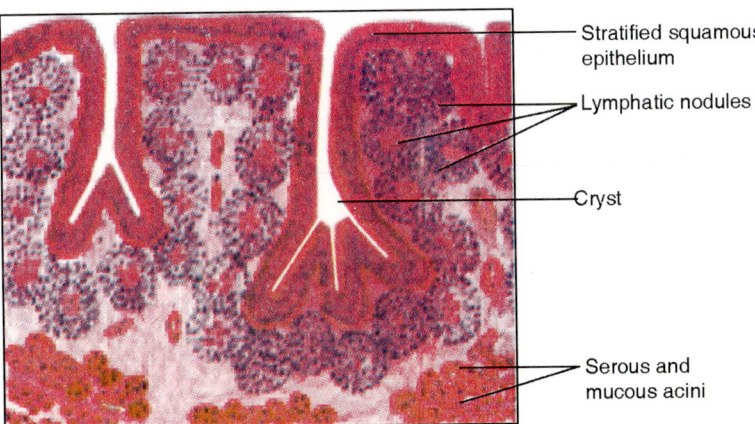

Fig. 71.4: Palantine Tonsil

PALATINE TONSIL

A lymphoid tissue covered by mucous membrane is termed as tonsil.

There are
- Lingual
- Pharyngeal
- Palatine

Palatine tonsil is covered by a capsule (fibroblastic connective tissue) which sends septa inside between the masses of lymphatic nodules. It forms wall of the crypts. Palatine tonsil is covered from oral side by stratified squamous nonkeratinised epithelium, which dips into the underlying lymphatic tissue to form ten to twenty pits (**primary crypts**). A primary pit may show many **secondary pits**. In the lamina propria lymphatic tissue lies below the epithelium and extends down along the sides of the crypts. In these lymphatic nodules there is loose lymphatic connective tissue with many plasma cells. In the lamina propria some mucous glands are seen and their ducts open on the surface.

Some lymphocytes infiltrate the epithelium and enter in the pharynx. These degenerating lymphocytes are termed **salivary corpuscles**.

72

Integumentary System

The integument consists of
- Skin
- Hair
- Nail
- Sweat gland
- Sebaceous gland

SKIN

Skin is the largest organ of the body which consists of two layers, firmly attached to each other.

Skin thickness varies from O.5mm to 4 mm. It rests on subcutaneous tissue.

It shows epidermis and dermis. **Epidermis** is stratified squamous keratinised. It is avascular and nourished by diffusion. Deepest cell layers proliferate and newer cells are pushed towards the surface. Here they die and are transformed into horny material - **keratin**. Dermis is made up of connective tissue which has dermal papillae extend which into epidermis fitting into epidermal papillae.

Outer layer of dermis is called **papillary layer** because it sends the papillae. Deeper layer of dermis is called **reticular layer**, which is made up of dense irregularly arranged connective tissue. Elastic fibres form network of very fine fibres in papillary layer while in reticular layer they form network of randomly arranged coarse fibres. The sweat and sebaceous glands, hair follicles with blood vessels are seen.

Skin under high power shows resting basal layer of columnar cells on a basement membrane- **stratum basale**. Here the nuclei are distinct and show mitosis. Next layer is **stratum spinosum** of polyhedral cells. Cells show many spine like processes. Third layer is **stratum granulosum** (two to four cells thick). They show keratohyaline granules in the cytoplasm which is basophilic in nature. Fourth layer is **stratum lucidum** which is thin, clear and homogenous line, consisting of eleidin substance - transformed keratohyaline. Outermost layer is **stratum corneum** (keratin). Here nuclei and cytoplasmic organelles disappear and keratohyaline granules fade away due to intracellular activity of lysosome derived enzymes. The granules are converted into a homogenous matrix. Keratin is tough fibrous protein highly resistant to chemical changes.

Apart from various skin appendages and fibres the dermis shows many fibroblasts, few macrophages and adipose cells.

- **Melanocytes** are derived from melanoblasts and they are situated in the basal layer of epidermis. They produce melanin.
- **Langerhans cells** show branching processes. They are macrophages in the epidermis.

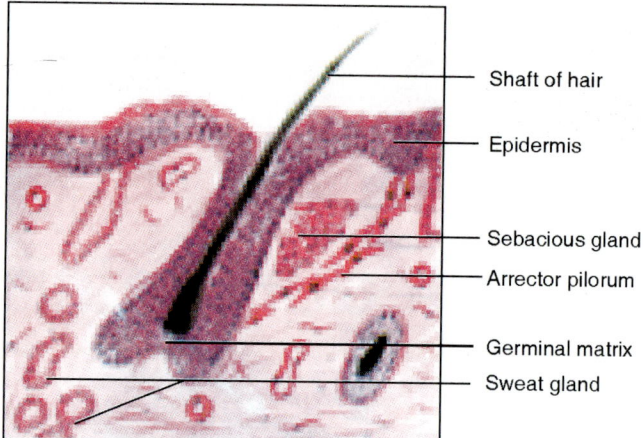

Fig. 72.1: Hairy skin

Shaft of hair
Epidermis
Sebacious gland
Arrector pilorum
Germinal matrix
Sweat gland

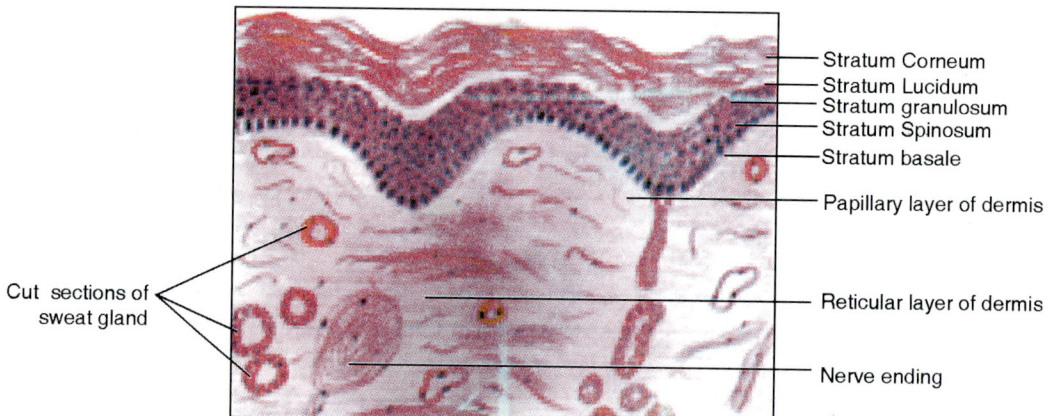

Fig. 72.2: Non-hairy skin

Stratum Corneum
Stratum Lucidum
Stratum granulosum
Stratum Spinosum
Stratum basale
Papillary layer of dermis
Reticular layer of dermis
Nerve ending

Cut sections of sweat gland

HAIR

Human skin is not very hairy. No hair follicles are formed after birth. Terminal hairs develop at puberty.

Hair follicle

Hair has shaft (visible part) and a root, which is embedded in the skin within the follicle.
Hair is composed of
- Central **medulla**
- Middle **cortex**
- Outermost **cuticle**

Epidermal downgrowth forms **hair follicle** and its terminal (deeper) expansion is the **hair bulb**. Invagination of the dermis in the concavity of the bulb is the **hair papilla**.

A hair follicle shows inner and outer coats. Inner coat is epithelial and outer coat is dermis of the skin. The inner coat shows inner root sheath and outer root sheath. Inner root sheath is made up of outer **Henle's layer**; middle **Huxley's layer** and outermost **cuticle** of inner root sheath. Outer root sheath is the continuation of stratum basale and stratum spinosum of the epidermis. Arrector pilorum is the smooth muscle which extends from the hair follicle to the dermis.

Melanocytes close to hair papilla produce melanin which is taken up by the cortex forming epithelial cells which are undergoing process of keratinization.

Layers studied under high magnification:

Medulla

It is made up of cornified cells forming two or three layers. Air spaces are present in between. Keratin of the medulla is soft.

Cortex

It shows many layers of cuboidal or cornified cells. Pigment granules are present in these cells. Keratin of cortex is hard.

Cuticle of hair

There are thin flat scales like single layer of cells with their free edges point upward. These free edges interrerlock with those of inner root sheath.

Henle's layer

It is formed by a single layer of cuboidal cells. It is the outermost layer. Nuclei are flattened.

Huxley's layer

It consists of a number of rows of elongated cells containing **tricohyaline granules**, which appear eosinophilic.

Cuticle of inner epithelial root sheath

This layer is similar to the cuticular layer of the cuticular layer of the hair. It lies against the cuticle of the hair and consists of flattened cornified cells.

Nail

A nail has

- Root
- Body
- Free edge

The nail root is covered by proximal nail fold and rests on the **germinal matrix** while body of the nail lies on the **sterile matrix**. Epidermis of the skin from the nail lies on the sterile matrix. Epidermis of the skin from the nail fold continues as germinal and then further as sterile matrix. The nail substance is formed by proliferation of cells in the germinal matrix which is thicker than sterile matrix. The stratum corneum lining the deep surface of the proximal nail fold extends for a short distance on to the surface of the nail termed **eponychium**. **Hyponychium** is present on the undersurface of the free distal edge of the nail.

Sebaceous gland

It is simple alveolar gland. These are seen on the side of the hair follicle towards which hair slants. Secretion is **holocrine** type. Basal cells resting on the basement membrane show mitosis. Newer cells are pushed in the inner layer towards the center of the gland. They synthesize **sebum** - fatty material that accumulates in the cytoplasm. As cells go away and away from nourishment they undergo necrosis releasing sebum.

The gland is seen between the hair follicle and arrector pilorum muscle like a bunch of grapes. Cells are polyhedral containing fat (vacuolated cytoplasm). The duct is lined by stratified squamous epithelium, which is continuous with the outer root sheath of the follicle. Duct of the sebaceous glands may usually open into the hair follicle but at places may open independent of hair

Sweat gland

These are of two types:

- Apocrine
- Merocrine

Sweat gland consists of a single long tube, lower end of which is highly coiled. The coiled part is called body of the gland and proximal uncoiled part is the duct. The duct follows a spiral course in the epidermis and opens on the surface as sweat pore.

Because of coiled nature single gland is cut at various levels so that clusters of secretory units are seen cut in various planes and above that duct is also seen. The secretory units are lined by simple cuboidal epithelium with a narrow lumen. Secretory cells are covered from outer side by myoepithelial cells. Their nuclei can be seen deep to the nuclei of secretory cells. The duct is lined by stratified cuboidal epithelium.

73

Lip, Tooth and Tongue

LIP

The slide shows two surfaces one covered by skin and opposite surface covered by mucous membrane. These two epithelial surfaces are continuous with each other at the transitional zone. Between the two epithelial coverings orbicularis oris muscle is present.

Epidermis of the skin contains hair follicles, sweat glands and sebaceous glands. Presence of stratified squamous keratinised epithelium helps to identify dermal connective tissue from lamina propria. Dermis shows number of well-developed and vascular dermal papillae. The skin of the red

margin of the lip shows absence of sweat and sebaceous glands or hair follicles. The mucous membrane is thicker stratified squamous non-keratinised type. Epithelium lies on a lamina propria. Papillae of lamina propria extend high into the epithelium of mucous membrane. Small clusters of mucous glands (labial glands) are embedded in the lamina propria which opens on the surface.

The surface of the lip consists of striated muscles cut transversely. The fascicles of the fibres are covered by fibroelastic connective tissue. At the edge of the lip neurovascular bundle is seen. At the transition zone near the border of the lip keratinised epithelium of the skin gradually changes to nonkeratinised epithelium.

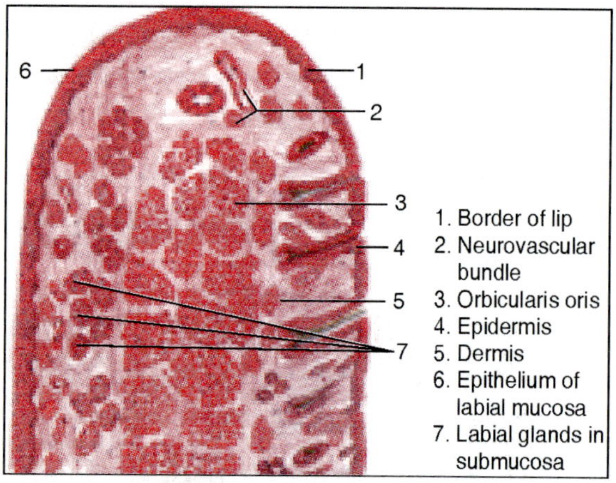

TOOTH

Tooth shows projected part called **crown** and the part within the gum and socket called as the **root**. Enamel is the hardest substance in the human body. The slide of tooth is unstained like ground bone as the tooth matrix is calcified.

Ground tooth

The central part shows a large cavity towards crown called **pulp cavity** and a narrow cavity towards the root called **root canal**. Both the cavities are

1. Border of lip
2. Neurovascular bundle
3. Orbicularis oris
4. Epidermis
5. Dermis
6. Epithelium of labial mucosa
7. Labial glands in submucosa

Fig. 73.1: Lip

continuous with each other and opens by a root pore through which vessels, nerves and connective tissue enters the canal. The cavity is surrounded from all sides by **dentin**. The dentin is covered from outside by **enamel** in the region of the crown and by **cementum** in the region of root. Dentin is made up of wavy parallel dentinal tubules. Enamel is composed of rods or prisms held together by a small amount of interprismatic cementing substance. Incremental growth lines or dark striae of **Retzius** represent variations in the rate of enamel deposition. Between the dark striae there are light striae or **band of Schreger**. These are seen due to refraction of light from enamel rods.

Decalcified tooth (LP)

A stained slide of decalcified developing tooth shows various types of cells. **Ameloblasts** are the enamel producing cells. These are columnar with apical surface towards the dentin and basement membrane to the opposite side. **Odontoblasts** are simple columnar cells lining the pulp or pulp cavity. Their apical surface is towards the enamel and basement membrane towards the pulp. In root part, the dentin is covered by **cementoblast** secrete cementum. Cementum is firmly adherent with the periosteum of the alveolar socket by strong periodontal ligament.

Enamel dentine junction

Dried tooth under microscope shows the enamel in the form of elongated rods while at the enamel dentine junction many enamel spindles are seen. These are extensions of dentinal matrix penetrating for a short distance into the enamel. There are groups of poorly calcified twisted enamel rods called **enamel tuft**. They extend from the dentinel enamel junction in to the enamel. Interglobular spaces are seen in the dentin filled with air and black colour. Dentinal canals are also seen in dentin. Interglobular spaces filled with incompletely calcified dentin are also called as interglobular dentin.

Dentine cementum junction

At the dentinal cementum junction **granular layer of Tomas** is seen. Dentin shows large irregular interglobular air filled black spaces.

Cementum shows lacunae and canaliculi, which were occupied by cementoblasts in living.

TONGUE

It is lined with stratified squamous epithelium on both the surfaces with a core of striated muscles in the centre cut in all directions.

Dorsal surface shows various papillae. The epithelium on the ventral surface is nonkeratinised. On the dorsal surface it varies from keratinised to nonkeratinised type. The epithelium is supported by the lamina propria of the connective tissue. The mucous membrane covering the dorsum of the tongue bears numerous projections called papillae. Each papilla consists of lining stratified squamous epithelium and a core of connective tissue of lamina propria.

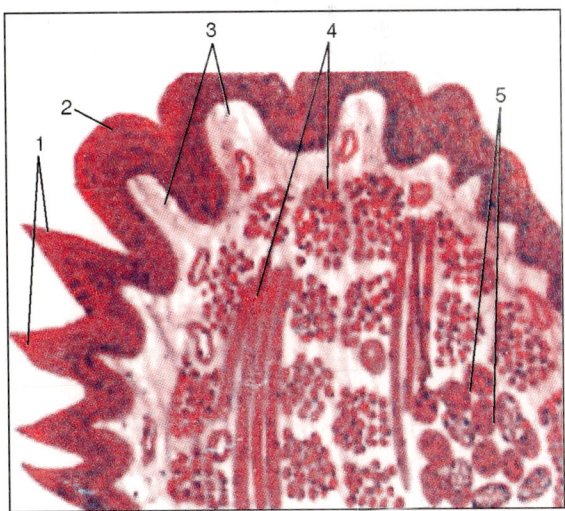

1. Filiform papillae 2. Stratified squamous non-keratinised epithelium 3. Lamina propria 4. Skeletal muscle 5. Mucous acini

Fig. 73.2: Anterior two third : Tongue

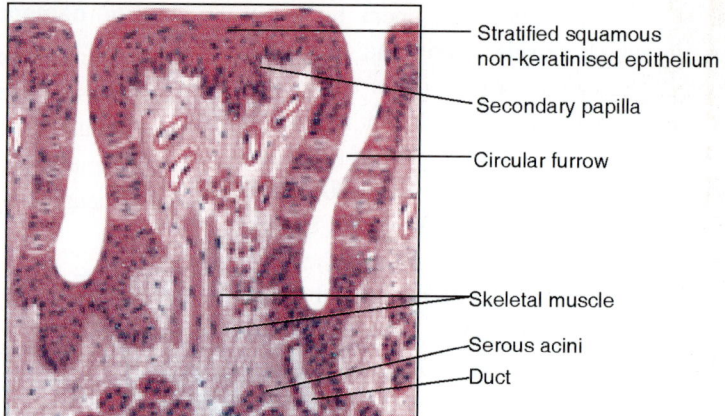

Fig. 73.3: Posterior one third tongue showing circumvallate papilla

Depending upon the shape, the papillae are:

- Filiform
- Fungiform
- Circumvallate

Taste buds are seen on the fungiform and circumvallate papillae.

Numerous mucous and serous secretory glands are present in the lamina propria. Their secretion dissolves the substance to be tasted and spreads it over the taste buds as well as washes away after it has been tasted.

Tongue papillae

They are present on the dorsal surface of the tongue. Following types of papillae can be seen: first two types in anterior 2/3rd and third type in the posterior 1/3rd of the tongue.

1. Filiform

They are tapered, thread like, composed of epithelium and lamina propria. There are oblique and transverse rows that run parallel to the sulcus terminalis. The core of primary papilla of the lamina propria shows secondary papillae.

2. Fungiform

They have narrower base, rounded top and less numerous than filiform. The shape is like little fungi. These are present more numerous at the tip of the tongue. They show a core of lamina propria with secondary papillae.

3. Circumvallate

They are located along 'V' shaped sulcus terminalis. These are about eight to twelve in number. Each papilla is surrounded by a trough that can be flushed out and cleared by the secretory activity of the underlying salivary glands. The papillae are narrow at the base than at the top. The papilla has a circumferential lateral wall that lies in the depth of the groove where taste buds are also present.

Taste bud

It is a barrel shaped structure protecting the gustatory receptors. There are three types of cells inside the bud. **Sustentacular cells** look like a segments of an orange, follow slightly curved course. They are arranged around a small central cavity, which communicates with the surface through the taste pore. **Receptor cells** synapse with nerve terminals. Membrane of basal cells possesses presynaptic densities and synaptic vesicles. Both these types of cells show microvilli on the apical surface. Third kind of cells is basal cells – stem cells. They proliferate and differentiate into two other types of cells. Taste bud is surrounded by epithelial cells which are modified also as sheath cells

74

Gastrointestinal Tract

Gastrointestinal tract (GIT) shows four basic layers, mucous membrane, submucosa, muscularis externa and serosa/adventitia. Mucous membrane shows epithelium, lamina propria and muscularis mucosa.

OESOPHAGUS

It shows four basic layers of the GIT. Its features include

- Stratified squamous epithelium
- Presence of submucosal glands

In animals that swallow rough material the epithelium is keratinised type.

First layer consists of mucosa, lamina propria and muscular is mucosa. The **mucous membrane** is stratified squamous epithelium. The epithelium rests on **lamina propria** (loose connective tissue). It carries blood vessels and lymphatics close to the epithelial surface. The third sub-layer of the mucous membrane is **muscularis mucosa**. It consists of smooth muscles (inner circular & outer longitudinal).

Second layer is the submucosa. It consists of loose connective tissue and larger vessels. An important feature of this layer is the presence of many mucous glands (submucosal glands).

Third layer is muscularis externa, which shows striated muscles in upper one third and nonstriated

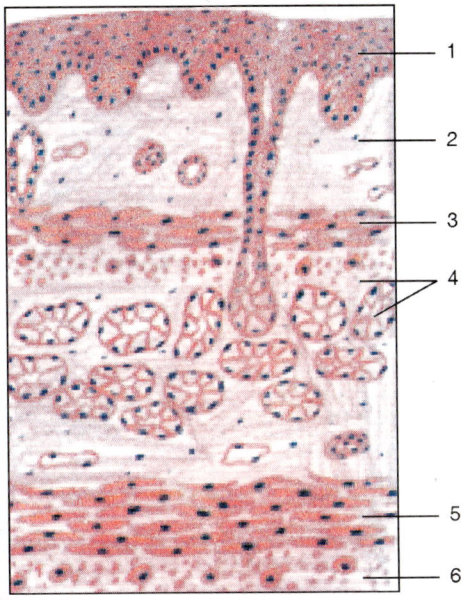

1. Stratified squamous non-keratinised epithelium
2. Lamina propria 3. Muscularis mucosa
4. Submucosa with mucous acini 5. Muscularis externa
6. Adventitia

Fig. 74.1: Oesophagus

in lower one third. However in the middle one third striated and nonstriated both are seen.

Fourth layer is adventitia.

The oesophagus is not covered by peritoneum so that it has adventitia and not serosa. Adventitia is made up of loose connective tissue.

393

Under high power basal cell layer of the epithelium rests on the basement membrane. They undergo continuous mitosis and the newer cells are pushed in the superficial (luminal) layers. Luminal cells desquamate in to the lumen. Except the basal cells other cells cannot divide but they appear basophilic due to accumulation of tonofilaments. The lamina propria contains collagenic, reticular and in some sites elastic fibres. Blood vessels and lymph capillaries are also seen. The papillae of connective tissue of lamina propria project in to the epithelial layer. At the upper and lower ends of the oesophagus mucous glands are seen in the lamina propria. The muscularis mucosa is poorly developed and may not be seen as a continuous layer. It is more distinct in lower part of oesophagus. In it both circular and longitudinal muscle fibres are seen. Submucosa shows at some places compound tubuloalveolar mucous glands, the ducts of which pass through the muscularis mucosa, lamina propria and epithelial layers to open in the lumen. Submucosa also shows small aggregation of lymphoid follicle especially near the cardiac end.

The mucous membrane of the oesophagus shows several longitudinal folds in the nondistended state. Abdominal part of oesophagus shows serosa. Submucosal glands are more common near the level of bifurcation of trachea. The circular muscle at the cardiac end of stomach acts as **physiological sphincter**.

PANCREAS

It is both exocrine and endocrine in function. Exocrine part is mostly like parotid or serous salivary glands. Endocrine part is in the form of small islands placed between the exocrine acini.

The gland is covered by thin capsule. The capsule sends septa inside the gland and divides the gland into lobules. From these septa connective tissue enters inside the lobule called intralobular tissue which is scanty and is seen in between the secretory units. Interlobular connective tissue contains interlobular ducts, blood vessels, nerves and lymphatics.

Inside the lobule the secretory units are arranged in groups resembling bunches of grapes. In a given section acini and ducts are cut in all planes. Secretory cells are pyramidal and cell boundaries are not always distinct while lumen is hardly seen.

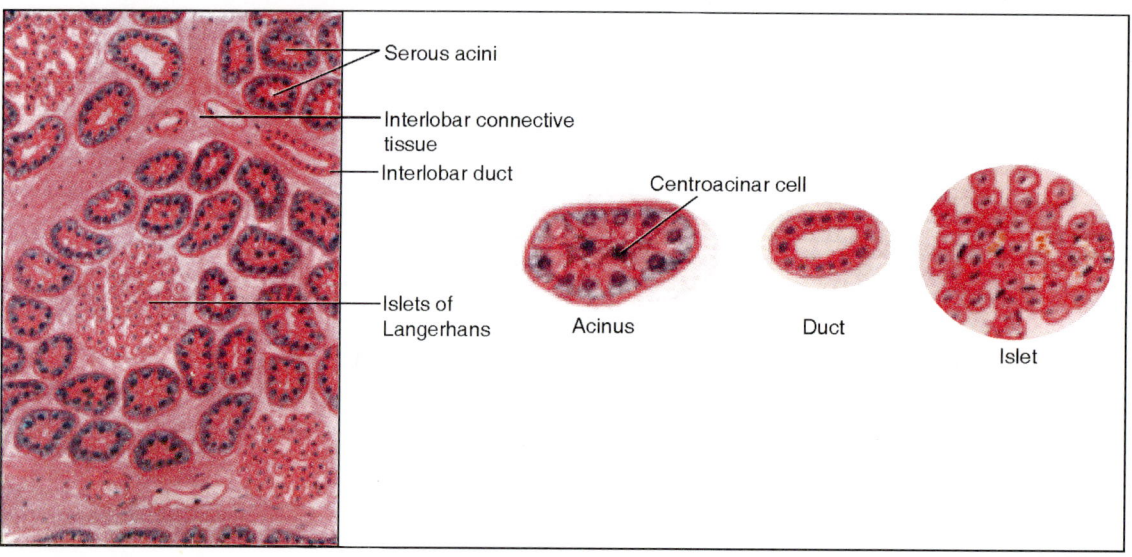

Fig. 74.2: Pancreas

Acini are packed together in a most irregular way with little intralobular loose connective tissue containing capillaries between them.

The main pancreatic duct (**Duct of Wirsung**) shows **Herring bone pattern**. Side branches are first interlobular ducts, which are formed by joining of many intralobular ducts. By relative paucity of intralobular ducts pancreas is distinguished from parotid.

Endocrine part of pancreas is seen as pale areas called **islets of Langerhans**. They are non-capsulated cords and irregular clumps of cells and capillaries.

Under high power each acinus has a central lumen that connects to a duct. Nucleus of secretory cell is near its broad base and infranuclear part of the cytoplasm is basophilic. The supranuclear part of the cytoplasm contains acidophilic zymogen granules and nucleoli are prominent. The nucleus of the **centroacinar cells** is seen in the central part of the acinus. The proximal duct cells are invaginated in to the lumen of the acinus. The duct cells thus begin in the centre (centroacinar cell) of an acinus. Thin basement membrane encloses the whole acinus.

Intercalated ducts are lined by simple squamous to simple cuboidal epithelium, intralobular ducts are lined by simple cuboidal to low columnar epithelium, while interlobular ducts are line by simple columnar epithelium. Interlobular ducts are surrounded by connective tissue with blood vessels.

A small amount of reticular tissue separates islets from acini. Internal support of islet is provided by reticular fibres associated with capillaries.

There are **10 to 30% alpha cells** and **60 to 80% beta cells** in the islets. Other types of cells -**D cells** are also present in the islets. Alpha cells contain water soluble and beta cells contain alcohol soluble granules in the cytoplasm. In H & E staining alpha and beta cells cannot be identified separately. Alpha cells are in the peripheral part and beta cells are placed in the central part of the islets. Special stains are **aldehyde fuchsin** (beta cells) and **acid fuchsin** (alpha cells).

75

Respiratory System

Special features of the respiratory system include

- Presence of large amount of elastic fibres
- Presence of cartilage

Presence of cartilage prevents the collapse of the wall of the conducting system as in sucking.

TRACHEA

Trachea (wind pipe) contains about 20 C-shaped cartilages. There is dense connective tissue between the adjacent cartilages. The trachea is lined by pseudostratified ciliated columnar epithelium with goblet cells. The epithelium also shows neuroendocrine cells, seen only after special staining. The epithelium rests on a basement membrane. Lamina propria contains high proportion of elastic fibres and occasional lymphatic nodule. Deeper part of the lamina propria shows a dense lamina of elastin. It contains secretory portion of many mucous glands with some serous secretory units. The duct pierces the elastic lamina and lamina propria and opens in the lumen. Sometimes glands are also seen in the lamina propria. Hyaline cartilage is deep to submucosa, covered by perichondrium. Trachealis is the smooth muscle bundle transversely arranged extending between the ends of 'C' shaped

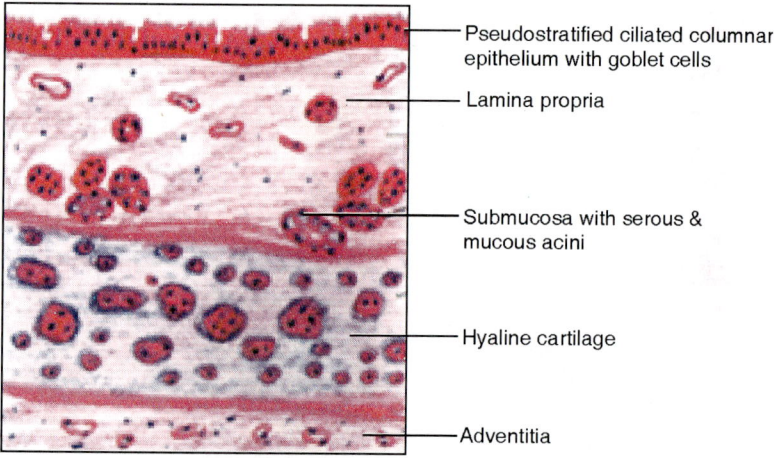

Pseudostratified ciliated columnar epithelium with goblet cells

Lamina propria

Submucosa with serous & mucous acini

Hyaline cartilage

Adventitia

Fig. 75.1: Trachea

396

cartilage on the posterior side. Tracheal glands are also present deep to the trachealis muscle. Outside the cartilage there is adventitia containing collagen fibres, adipose tissue and blood vessels.

LUNG

Lung is covered by pleura which shows surface simple squamous epithelium with small amount of subepithelial connective tissue.

Lung is divided into lobules which are separated by fibrous septa. Interlobular fibrous septa are incomplete. A lobule of a lung is aerated by a bronchiole and acinus is a unit supplied by terminal bronchiole.

The section shows many empty spaces some communicating with each other. The wall of these spaces is thin and pink in staining. Bronchioles are seen cut in various planes. Respiratory bronchioles open into the alveolar duct, which further continues in to alveolar sacs and alveoli. These spaces exist in a elastic sponge like arrangement of capillary beds. The alveolar ducts are long and branching. They communicate with round spaces termed as alveolar sacs. Spur like partitions project inward

from the periphery of alveolar saccule. These partitions divide the peripheral zone of each saccule into a series of alveoli which open into the central part of the saccule. There are three million alveoli and total surface area is 70 to 80 square meters.

Overexpansion of the alveolar wall is prevented by the internal support of the elastic fibres. Respiratory epithelium in the lung is lined by simple squamous cells. Single line seen in the slide is made up of alveolar walls of adjacent alveoli, capillaries and connective tissue in between.

Air-blood barrier in lung

The bottom of the alveoli has a small opening called **alveolar pore** which permits passage of air from one alveolus to another. Capillary network is present in the interalveolar septum. **Lambert channels** are the communications from the wall of the preterminal bronchioles and provide passage for air into alveolar sac belonging to the same or neighbouring units. Alveolar pores and Lambert channels play an important role during obstruction.

Simple squamous epithelium is lined by **pneumocyte I and II**. First type of cells are squamous, more numerous and through their

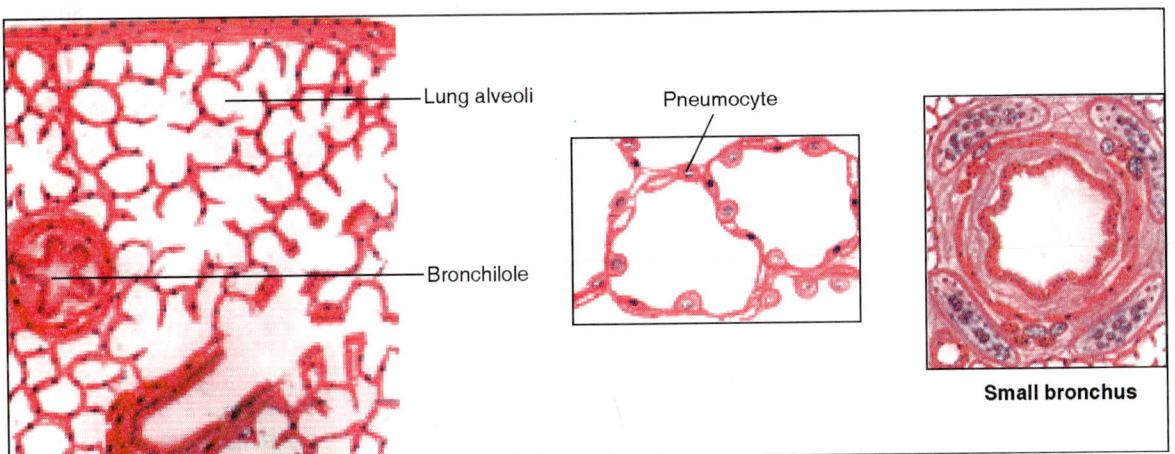

Lung alveoli

Bronchilole

Pneumocyte

Small bronchus

Fig. 75.2: Lung

thickness the exchange between air and blood occurs. Pneumocyte II are interspersed among the type-1 cells and are less numerous. They are larger cells and secrete chiefly **Dipalmitoyl phosphatidylcholine**. This secretion spreads as a thin film over the entire surface of the squamous epithelium – surfactant.

Blood air barrier is formed by the alveolar pneumocytes, basement membrane of alveolar epithelium, basement membrane of capillary endothelium and capillary endothelial connective tissue. At some places interalveolar connective tissue forms the part of the barrier between two basement membranes. If both basement membranes are very close and fuse together then the common membrane is called alveolocapillary basement membrane.

76

Endocrine Glands

The endocrine or ductless glands are devoid of ducts and the secretions are poured directly into the blood through the capillaries and numerous sinusoids. They have rich blood supply. Each gland secretes specific hormone/s with distinct functions. The principal endocrine glands are

- Hypophysis cerebri
- Thyroid gland
- Parathyroid gland
- Suprarenal gland
- Pineal gland
- Parts of pancreas, testis and ovary

THYROID GLAND

Thyroid gland is responsible for maintaining the basal metabolic rate of the body by means of **thyroxine** and **tri-iodothyronine** secreted by the follicular cells. Another smaller number of cells called the **parafollicular cells** lower the calcium in the blood by **thyrocalcitonin**.

Thyroid gland is covered by the false capsule derived from pretracheal fascia. The true capsule is comprised of collagen fibres. This capsule sends connective tissue septae into the gland to form lobes and lobules. These septae provide support

the abundant fenestrated capillaries present in the gland. The structural and functional unit of thyroid gland is a follicle. Each follicle is an oval or round space lined by single layer of epithelial cells. The epithelial cells vary in size according to activity of the gland. The epithelium is cuboidal in normal functioning status, columnar in hyperactive stage and low cuboidal in resting phase. Different areas of gland show variance in height of cells.

The epithelial cells rest on a basal lamina. The connective tissue is sporse around capillaries as thyroid hormones are absorbed both by blood and lymph capillaries. The lumen of the follicles contains colloid which represents the stored product of the secretory activity of the gland and takes up acidophilic stain. Its main constituent is thyroglobin and iodothyroglobulin.

In addition to the follicular cells, another smaller population of cells are seen. These are lighter in colour, bigger in size and are present amongst the follicular epithelium situated between the basement chorine and the epithelial cells between the follicles. These cells are termed as **parafollicular or 'C' cells**. These secrete hormone called thyrocalcitonin or calcitonin responsible for lowering blood calcium level.

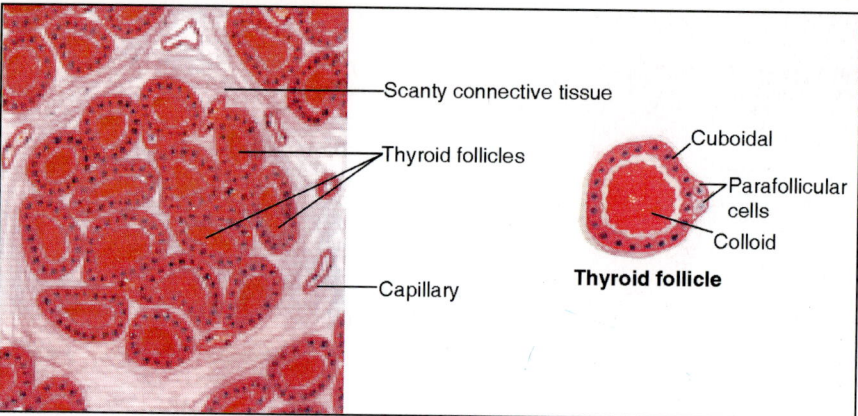

Fig. 76.1: Thyroid gland

Synthesis and release of thyroid hormones:

- Iodide circulating in blood is selectively taken up by the follicular cells.

- Iodine is liberated from iodide by peroxidase which enters the lumen of follicle.

- Follicular cells synthesize protein molecules from amino acids especially tyrosine. Carbohydrate is added to this protein molecule forming thyroglobulin which is also pushed into the lumen of the follicle.

- Iodine already present in the lumen combines with the tyrosine radicle of thyroglobulin to form mono and di-iodotyrosine which further combine to generate tri-iodothyronine and tetra-iodothyronine (thyroxine). All this occurs in the lumen.

- According to the requirements of the body, iodothyroglobulin is taken by the follicular cells from the lumen of the follicle. It is acted upon by enzymes present in these cells and tri and tetra iodothyronine are released from the basal /aspects of follicular cells. Tri-iodothyronine is quick and short lasting in action, whereas thyroxine is slower and long lasting in its effects on the various tissues of the body.

PARATHYROID GLAND

These are two pairs of small, yellow brown bodies intimately connected with the posterior aspect of the thyroid gland. These glands are separated from the thyroid by a thin connective tissue capsule. The capsular connective tissue extends into the parathyroid gland. Along these trabeculae that larger branches of blood vessels, nerves and lymphatics enter and leave.

The reticular tissue forms framework of the parathyroid gland. The parenchyma consists of **principal cells** and **oxyphilic cells**.

Principal cells or chief cells are arranged in sheets with numerous sinusoids and capillaries traversing them. The principal cells are polygonal or round with a centrally placed vesicular nucleus and a pale staining acidophilic cytoplasm. These cells show granules with special stains.

Oxyphilic cells are few in number; occur singly or in small groups. These are larger than principal cells. They have darkly staining nuclei and strongly acidophilic cytoplasm. Oxyphilic cells increase with age.

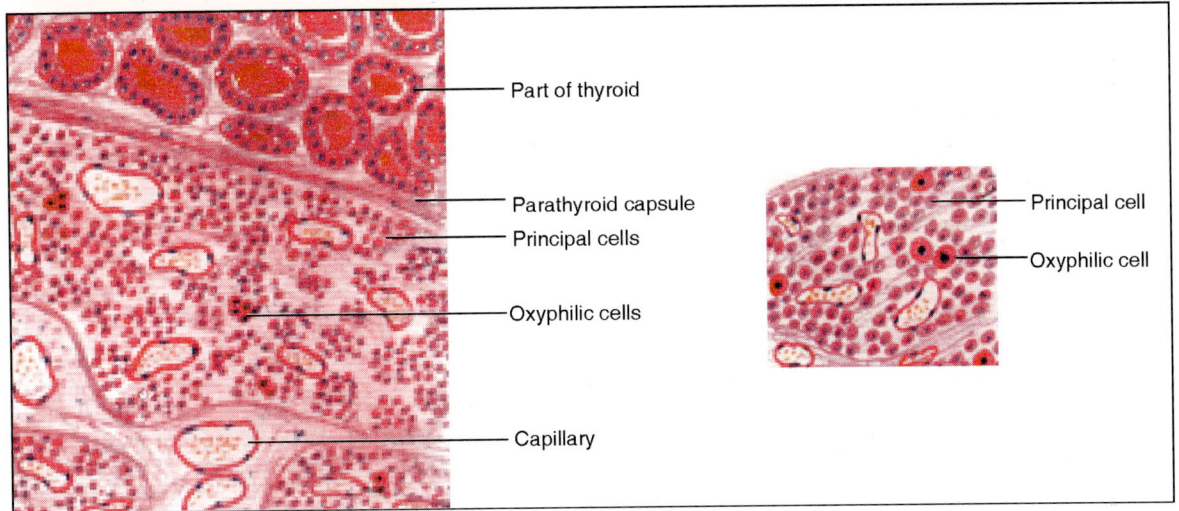

Fig. 76.2: Parathyroid gland

The principal or chief cells secrete parathormone responsible for maintaining the blood calcium level. In cases of hyper activity of parathyroid gland, blood calcium level is elevated by withdrawing it from the bones, thereby causing osteoporosis. Increased calcium level also favours tendency for renal stone formation.

SUPRARENAL GLAND

The paired suprarenal or adrenal glands are roughly triangular or semilunar flattened glands situated at the upper pole of each kidney. It is surrounded by a thick capsule in which are branches of main vessels, nerves and lymphatics are placed. The septa penetrate the capsule into the interior carrying blood vessels along them.

Each gland is comprised of outer yellow **cortex** surrounding the inner dark brown **medulla**.

Cortex develops from the coelomic epithelium (mesoderm) whereas medulla originates from neural crest cells (ectoderm). Cells of medulla are comparable to sympathetic ganglion cells as it is supplied by preganglionic sympathetic fibres.

Blood Supply: Supra renal is supplied by superior, middle and inferior suprarenal arteries. These form a plexus in its capsule. Cortical capillaries supply cells of the cortex before reaching the sinusoids of medulla. The medullary vessels pass through the cortex to reach the medulla. Thus

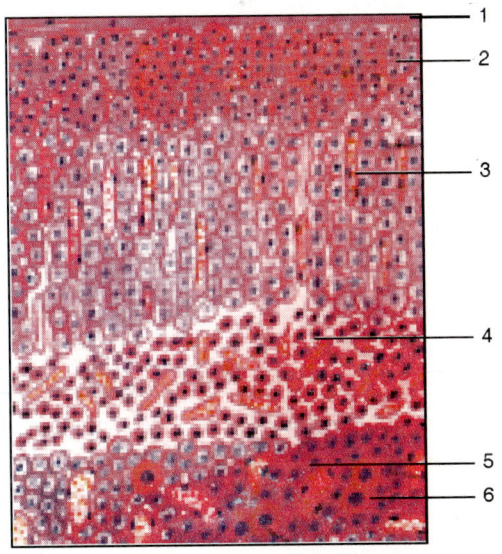

1. Capsule 2. Zona glomerulosa 3. Zona fasciculata
4. Zona reticularis 5. Medulla 6. Sympathetic ganglion

Fig. 76.3: Suprarenal gland

the sinusoids of medulla receive blood both from cortex and medulla.

Cortex

The cortex shows three zones, outermost is the **zona glomerulosa**, a thick middle layer is the **zona fasciculata**, and moderately thick inner layer is the **zona reticularis** which is continuous with the medulla. The transition from one zone to the other is gradual and is not well demarcated.

1. The zona glomerulosa consists of closely packed groups and arches of columnar cells. The nuclei are spherical and stain deeply. The cytoplasm shows vacuoles. Sinusoids are seen in between the groups of cells. The cells of the zona glomerulosa secrete **mineralocorticoids**.

2. In zona fasciculata the cells are arranged in vertical columns, with large vacuoles in their cytoplasm. These cells are also called spongiocytes. The cytoplasm is slightly basophilic and nuclei are central. The sinusoids follow a vertical course in this zone. The cells of the zona fasciculata secrete **glucocorticoids**.

3. In zona reticularis, the regular parallel arrangement of cords is replaced by an anastomosing network. The cytoplasm of cells contains fewer lipid droplets and is less vacuolated. Some of the cells contain yellow pigment. The intervening capillaries are irregularly arranged. These cells secrete **sex hormones**.

Another view about the functions of the cortex is that zona glomer-ulosa is the cell producing zone; zona fasciculata the hormone-producing zone and the zona reticularis the graveyard of the cells.

Medulla

Medulla is composed of chromaffin cells or pheochromocytes. These are arranged in irregular rounded groups or short cords isolated by fine septa.

These are surrounded by blood capillaries and venules. The cytoplasm of the cells is basophilic. When the tissue is fixed in solution containing potassium bichromate, these cells are filled with fine brown granules **chromaffin reaction**. These granules are precursors of the hormone epinephrine (adrenalin) and norepinephrine (noradrenalin). Norepinephrine producing cells are relatively more densely granulated. Between these cells autonomic ganglion cells are interposed which are seen singly or in groups of two to four. The ganglion cells are large with big vesicular nuclei and nucleoli.

HYPOPHYSIS CEREBRI

It lies in the cranial cavity. It is attached to the base of the brain by the stalk or infundibulum. The hypophysis has two main regions:

Neurohypophysis - develops as a process growing downwards from the floor of the diencephalon

Adenohypophysis - originates in the embryo as a dorsal outpouching from the roof of the mouth. The neurohypophysis is also known as the posterior lobe. There are three sub divisions of the adenohypophysis

- Pars distalis or anterior lobe
- Pars intermedia
- Pars tuberalis

Pars distalis

It forms the largest sub-division of the hypophysis cerebri. It is composed of glandular cells arranged in irregular cords or clumps. These are related to the extensive system of thin walled capillaries and sinusoids. The glandular cells are

Chromophobes (50 percent of the total cell population)

Chromophils (50 percent of the cell population)

These are of two types:

- Acidophils or alpha cells
- Basophils or beta cells

Chromophobes

These are small cells, with homogeneous light staining cytoplasm. Nuclei are pale and lie in the centre of the cells. The cells are arranged in groups or clumps. These cells give rise to chromophils.

Chromophils

These cells are larger than the chromophobes and contain granules in their cytoplasm. These cells are usually present at the periphery of the clump. Chromophils consist of alpha or acidophilic cells and beta or basophilic cells. Acidophilic cells can be further distinguished by differential histochemical stains into type A acidophil and type B acidophil.

- Type A acidophil secretes Somatotropin (STH) or growth hormone.
- Type B acidophil secretes lactoge-nic hormone (LTH).

Basophils can be differentiated into Beta basophils, responsible for the secretion of thyrotropic hormone (TSH)

Delta basophils -elaborate gonadotropins (FSH, LH and ICSH).

Pars intermedia

The pars distalis is separated from the neurohypophysis by a cleft lined on the juxtaneural side by a multilayered epithelium of basophilic cells comprising the pars intermedia. The cells here are low columnar in shape and are basophilic in their staining properties. The cells are arranged in the form of vesicles which are lined by low columnar cells and contain colloid in their cytoplasm. The hormone secreted by the pars **intermedia is the melanocyte stimulating hormone (MSH)**. It is also thought to be responsible for the secretion of adreno-corticotrophic hormone.

Pars Nervosa

It consists of terminal portions of axons of extrinsic secretory neurons (supraoptic and paraventricular nuclei) whose cell bodies are located in the hypothalamus and modified neuroglial cells called the pituicytes. These cells are highly variable in size, shape and have cytoplasmic processes. In the neurohypophysis spherical masses that stain deeply with chrome-alum haematoxylin stain and are called Herring bodies. These are local accumulations of

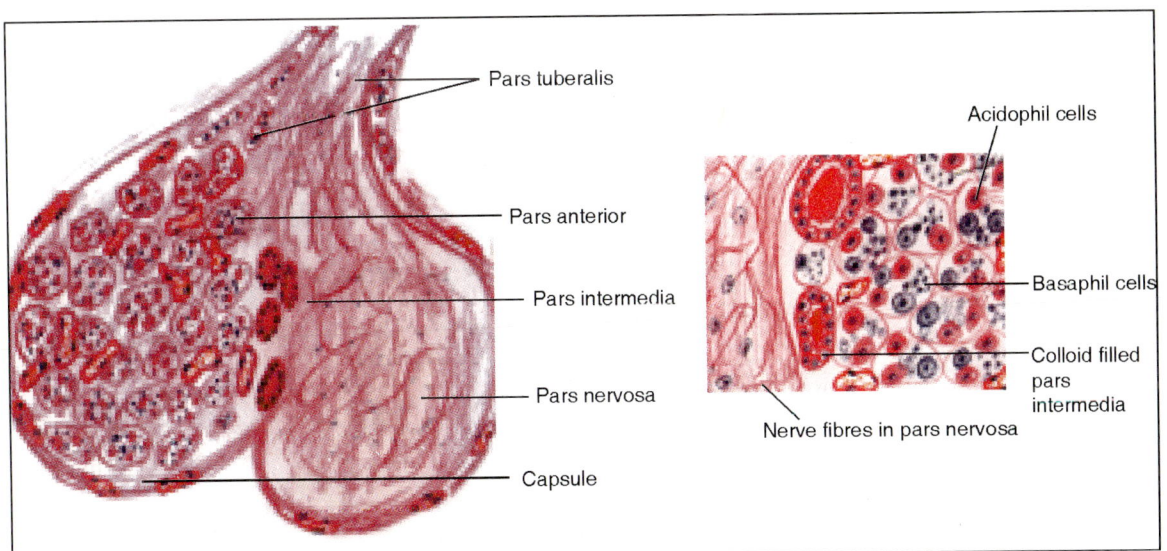

Fig. 76.4: Pituitary gland

neurosecretory material in the axoplasm of the hypothalamo-hypophyseal tract which is discharged into the sinusoids. Hormones secreted by pars nervosa are **oxytocin, antidiuretic hormone (ADH)** and **vasopressin**.

Blood supply of Hypophysis

It is related to the secretory activity of the gland Two inferior hypophyseal arteries from cavernous part of internal carotid (ICA) supply the posterior lobe and to a lesser extent anterior lobe of the gland Many superior hypophyseal arteries arise from internal carotid and posterior communicating branch of circle of Willis supply median eminence of hypothalamus and base of pituitary. The blood from these regions is collected by long and short portal veins which open into a second set of sinusoidal capillaries in the anterior lobe of hypophysis. The veins from here drain into cavernous sinus. This type of circulation is called **hypothalamo-hypophyseal portal circulation**.

Section-VI
Embryology

CONTENTS

77. **General Aspects**   407-415

78. **Gametogenesis : Conversion of Germ Cells into Male and Female Gametes**   416-432

79. **Developments of Systems**   433-464

80. **Glossary : Germ Layer Derivatives**   465-466

81. **Critical Periods of Human Development**   467-473

82. **Correlated Human Development**   474-487

General Aspects

Study of the origin and development of single individual – Developmental anatomy.

Prenatal period

- Embryonic period – First 8 weeks
- Foetal period – Remaining 30 weeks

Human Body is made up of millions of cells.

All these cells are derived from fertilized ovum.

The diverse cell population is achieved by two processes

- **Cell division** – increase the cellular population
- **Cell differentiation** – different tissues are derived.

CELL DIVISION

Human body cells can be put broadly in two types

- **Germ cells** (Oogonia and Spermatozoa)
- **Somatic cells** (Various tissues of body ; bone muscle)

The Chromosome composition of these cells is 2n i.e. 46 Chromosomes.

Chromosomes are

- **Autosomes** - 22 pairs or 44
- **Sex chromosome** - 2 (In **female: XX** and **male: XY** hence also termed hetrosomes)

Autosomes are arranged in pairs that are similar in morphology (homologous chromosome)

The cellular population can be classified on the basis of rate of cell division as

Renewing: Cells are rapidly dividing in tissues where wear and tear occurred eg. Epithelia

Expanding: Cells divide as and when required e.g. uterine mucosa, healing of wound

Static: Cells never divide eg. Neurons, neural retina, muscle

Cell division is controlled by two factors

- **Stimulating** e.g. – Somatotrophic hormones carcinogens
- **Inhibiting** e.g. Chalones – decline in the concentration allows cell division

MITOSIS

- Occurs in all cells including germ cells
- Proliferation of cellular population in an orderly manner
- No change in number of chromosome

Phases

- **Prophase** – Very short
- **Metaphase** – Chromosomes get arranged in "Single file" on equatorial zone)

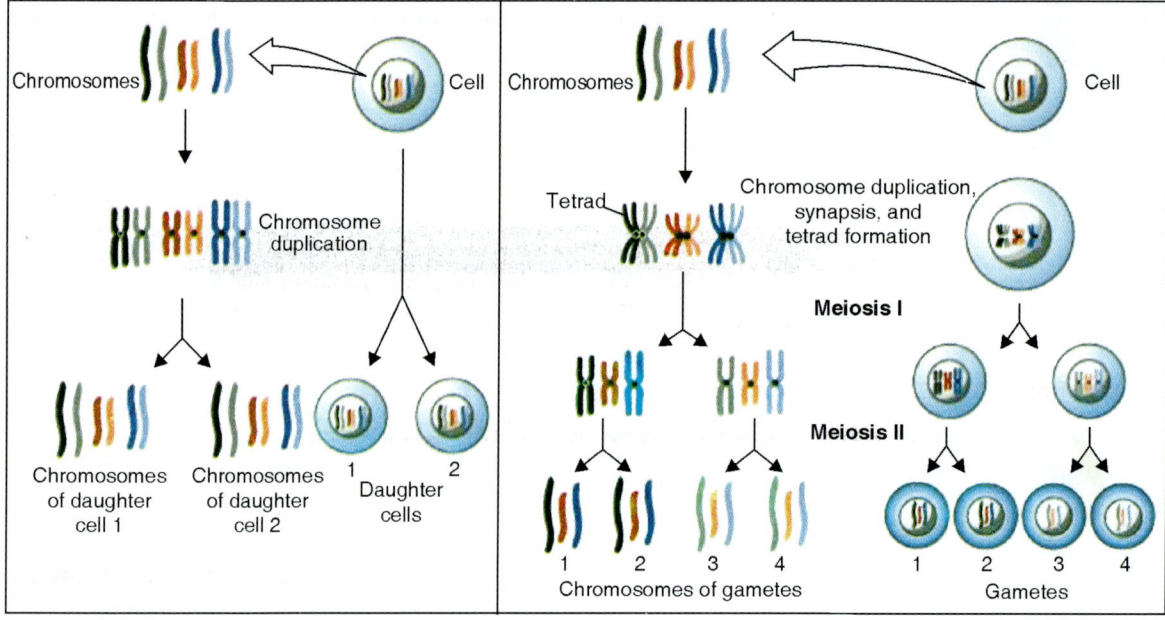

Fig. 77.1

- **Anaphase** – Longitudinal division of chromosomes
- **Telephase** – Two daughter cells

Each cell has 2 n (Diploid number of chromosomes)

MEIOSIS

Occurs only in germ cells

- Number of chromosomes is reduced to half (n) (hence also called reduction division).
- To prepare for eventual fertilization so that resultant zygote would have 46 chromosomes.

Changes take place in the nucleus as well as cytoplasm – Ovum enlarges in size while sperm loses cytoplasm and acquires a tail.

- **Prophase:** It is extended with following stages
- **Leptotene** – Chromosomes become visible as beaded strands.
- **Zygotene** – Pairing of homologous chromosomes "Bivalents"
- **Pachytene** – Chromatids are replicated "Tetrad".
- **Diplotene** – Chromosomes strands break and recombine with strands on the homologous Chromosomes "Chiasma "(crossing over)
- **Diakinesis** – Centromere separate

GAMETOGENESIS

Formation of germ cell i.e. Oocyte / Sperm.

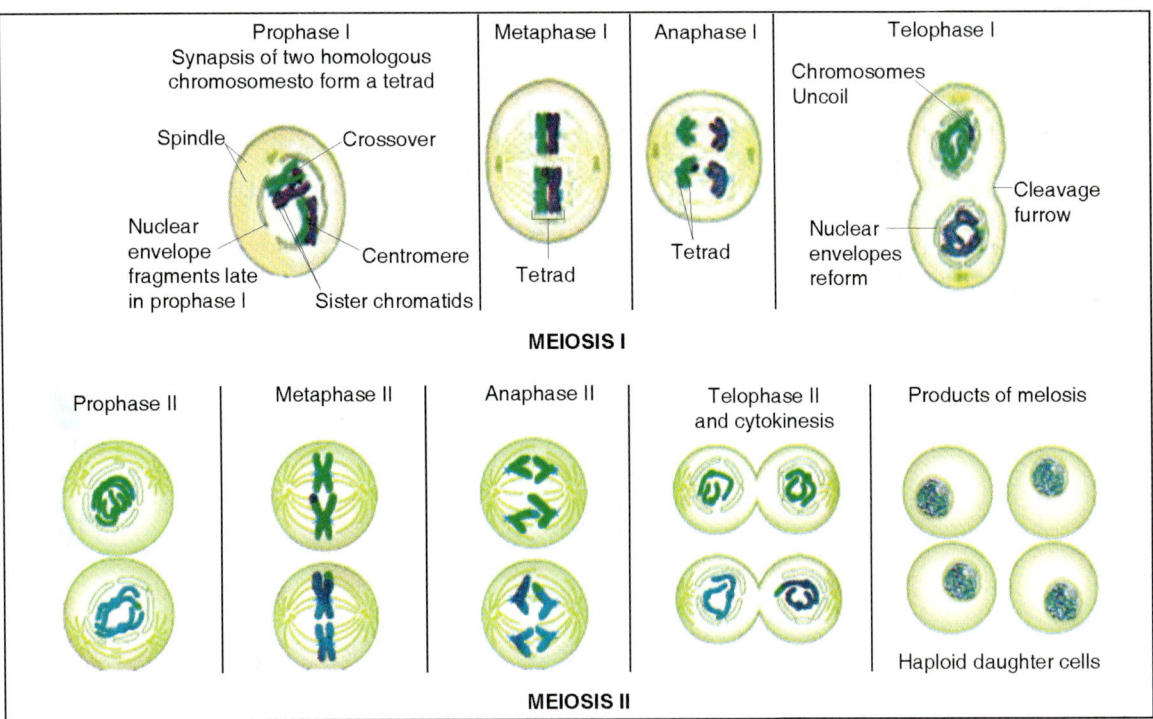

Fig. 77.2

OOGENESIS

Formation of ovum

3rd Week:

- PGC appear in the wall of yolk sac.

5th Week:

- Migrate and settle in the gonadal ridge.

3rd Month:

- Primordial germ cells divide and give rise to oogonia (2n)

7th Month:

- All primordial germ cells are converted into oogonia.
- Oogonia differentiate into primary oocyte (2n)
- All primary oocyte enter first meiotic division
- All primary oocyte are in the diptotene stage (chaisma formation, "crossing over") of prophase

At Birth:

- 40,000 to 3,00,000 primary oocytes are seen in cortex of the ovary as primary follicle (primary oocytes are surrounded by flattened / cubical cells)

After puberty:

- Under the influence of hormones, every month a group of primordial follicle enter the race for maturity – leading to formation of
  - Growing follicle
  - Larger follicle with follicular cavity
  - Mature follicle (**Graafian follicle**)

Features of Graafian follicle

- Big antrum filled with follicular fluid
- Theca cells (**Interna** - vascular, **Externa** - fibrous) surround the follicle
- Graffian follicle reaches the surface of ovary

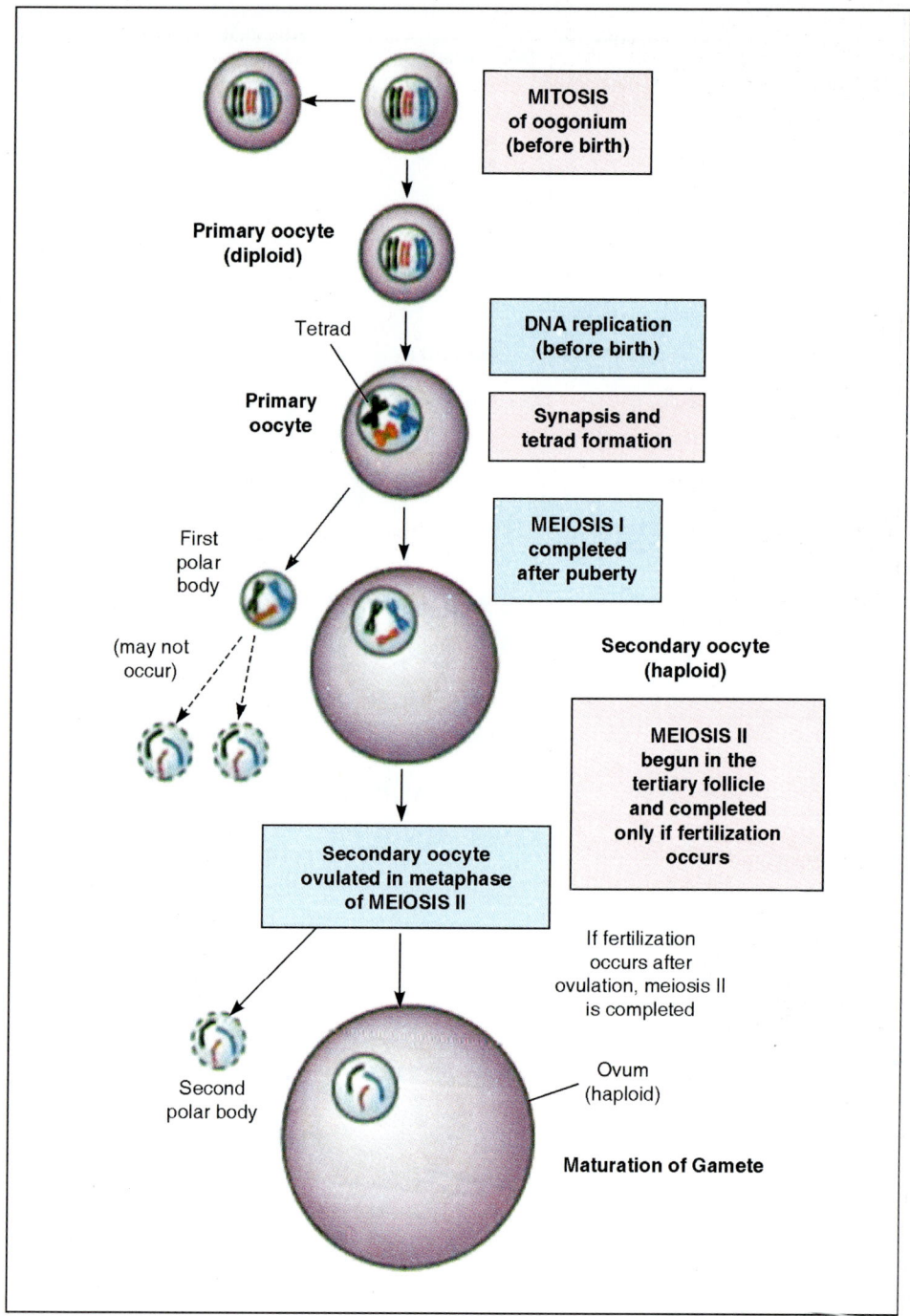

Fig. 77.3: Oogenesis

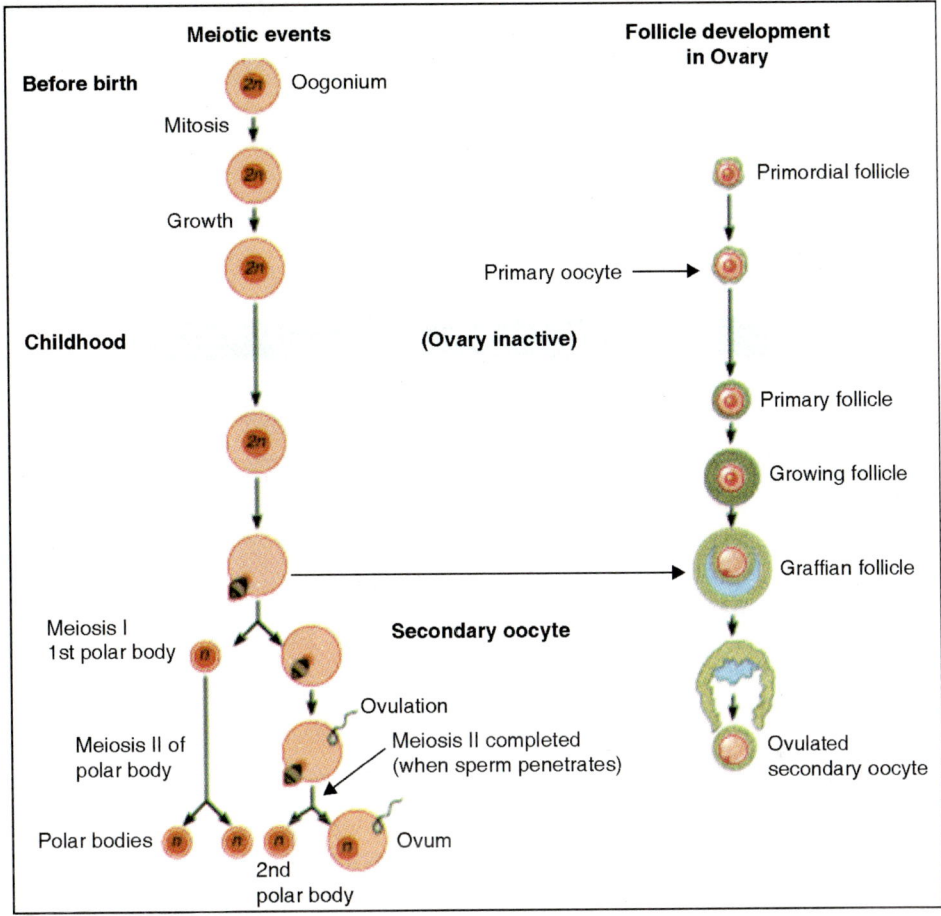

Fig. 77.4: Oogenesis

Primary oocyte completes 1st meiotic division to form secondary oocyte (n) and 1st polar body.

Secondary oocyte has following features

- Surrounded by zona pellucida
- Cummulus oophorus" are follicular cells surrounding zona pellucida towards follicular cavity
- 1st Polar body (n) is within the zona pellucida

Ovulation

- Graffian follicle stretches the surface epithelium of ovary. The resultant ischaemia and increasing pressure of follicular fluid causes rupture of Graffian follicle
- Secondary oocyte with follicular cells (**corona radiata**) liberated in the peritoneal cavity
- Secondary oocyte is taken up by the Fallopian tube
- On fertilization it completes 2nd meiotic division to from mature oocyte (n) and 2nd polar body

If fertilization does not take place the secondary oocyte undergoes degeneration and is extruded per vaginum along with the menstrual fluid.

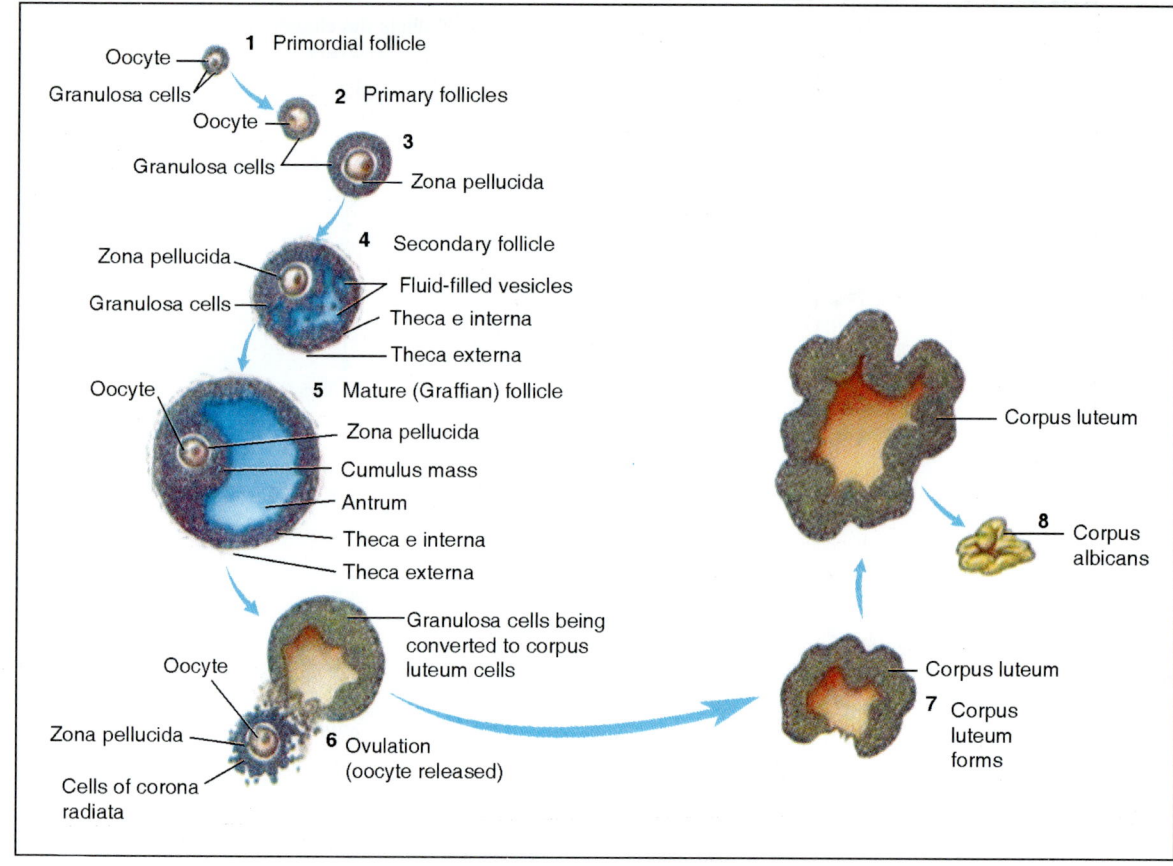

Fig. 77.5: Maturation of follicle & oocyte

Formation of sperm is achieved by two processes

- **Spermatogenesis -** till the formation of spermatids
- **Spermiogenesis** -metamorphosis of spermatid into sperm

SPERMATOGENESIS

3rd week of intrauterine life – Primordial germ cells appear in dorsal wall of yolk sac.

5th week of intrauterine life – Primordial germ cells settle in gonadal ridge and form solid sex cords with cells of gonadal ridge.

Before puberty – Sex cords acquire lumen and form seminiferous tubules.

Each seminiferous tubule is multilayered having from periphery towards the human the following cells

- Spermatogonia
- Primary spermatocyte
- Sertoli cells
- Secondary spermatocyte
- Spermatid
- Sperm

At puberty

- Primordial germ cells undergo mitosis to form Spermatogonia which divide to form Spermatogonia A

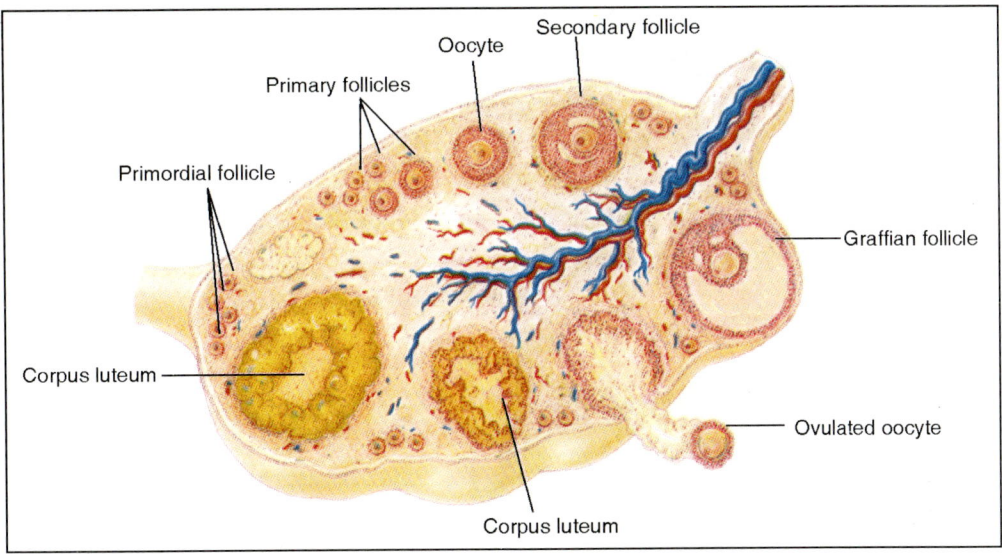

Fig. 77.6: Ovulation

- Spermatogonia B are derived from spermatogonia A
- Spermatogonia B undergoes mitotic division to form primary spermatocyte
- Primary spermatocyte undergoes 1st meiotic division to form two secondary spermatocyte with haploid (n) number of chromosome
- Each secondary spermatocyte undergoes second meiotic division (mitosis) to give two spermatids
- Thus from one spermatogonium (2n) four spermatids (n) are derived

SPERMIOGENESIS

- Metamorphosis of spermatid to sperm
- Nucleus gets elongated
- Condensation of Golgi material at one pole of nucleus (head cap) which is filled with acrosomic granules
- Centriole is placed at the other pole of nucleus which gives rise to axial filament / flagellum

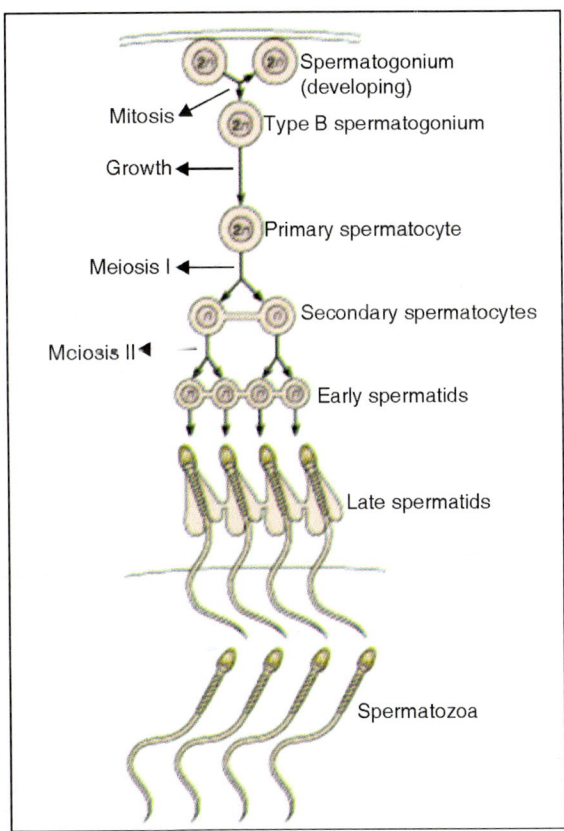

Fig. 77.7: Spermatogenesis

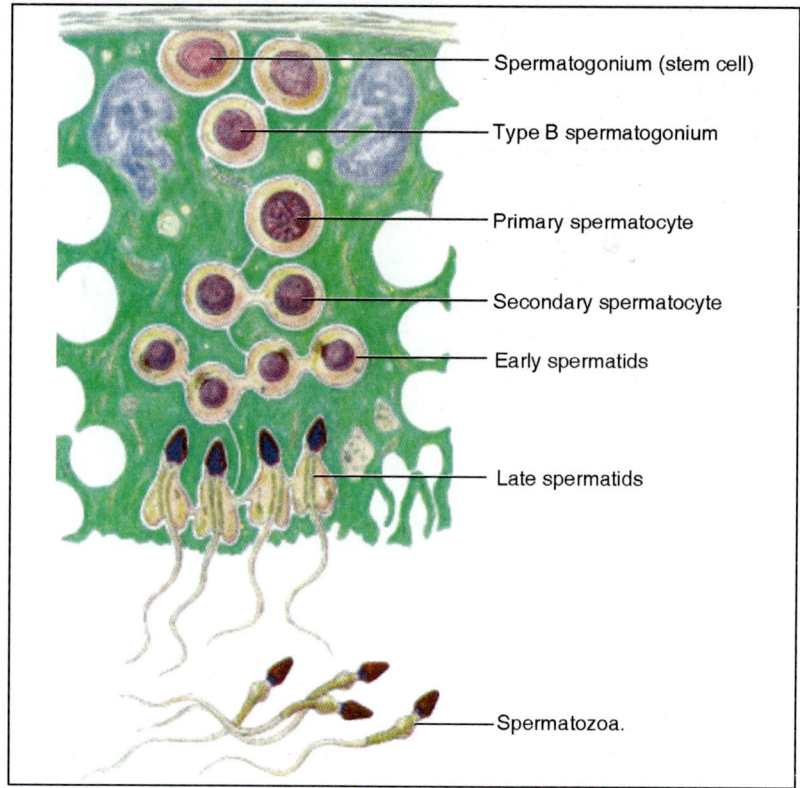

Spermatogonium (stem cell)

Type B spermatogonium

Primary spermatocyte

Secondary spermatocyte

Early spermatids

Late spermatids

Spermatozoa.

Fig. 77.8: Spermatogenesis

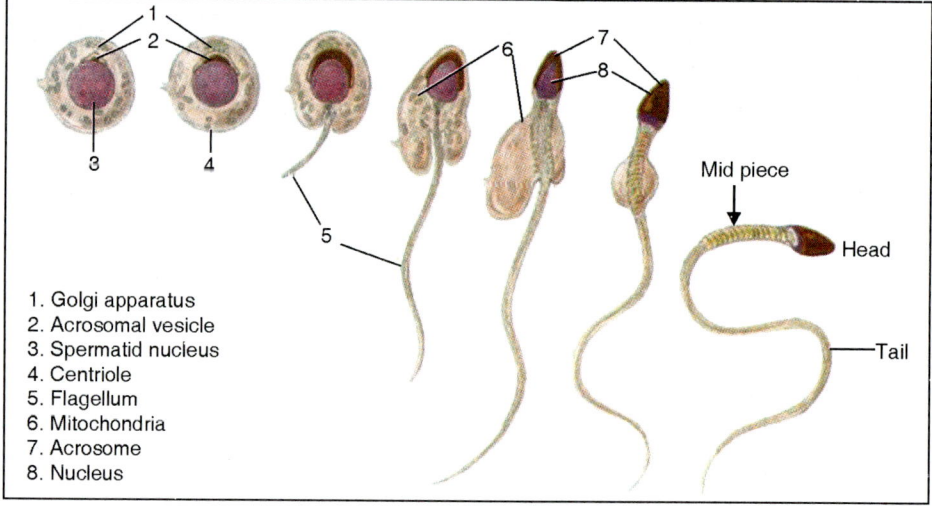

1. Golgi apparatus
2. Acrosomal vesicle
3. Spermatid nucleus
4. Centriole
5. Flagellum
6. Mitochondria
7. Acrosome
8. Nucleus

Mid piece

Head

Tail

Fig. 77.9: Spermatogenesis

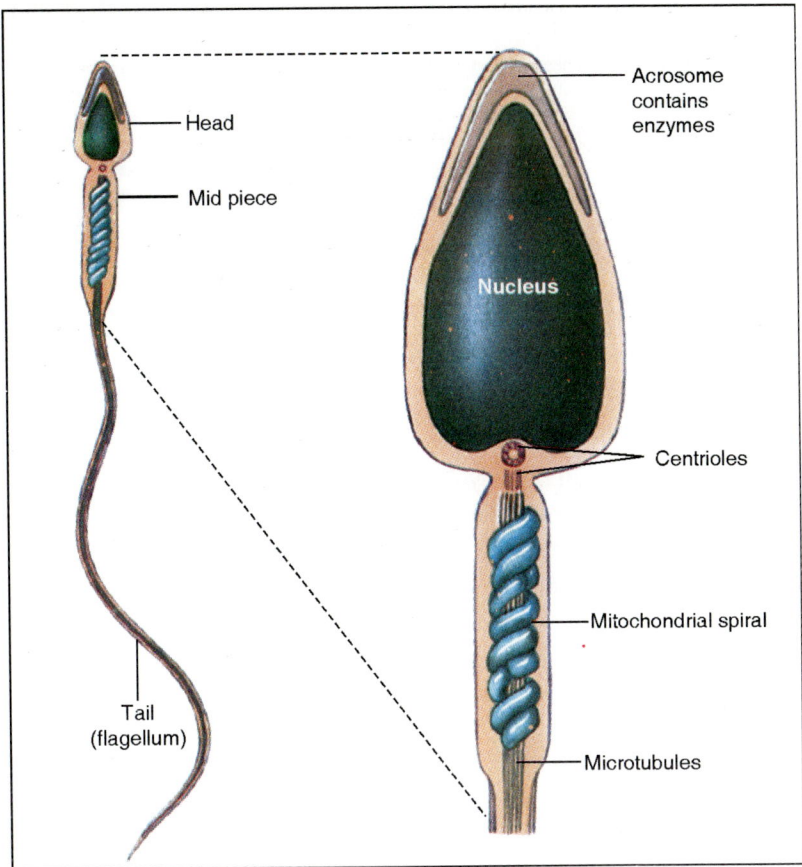

Fig. 77.10: Structure of Sperm

- Mitochondria get arranged spirally around proximal axial filament
- Residual cytoplasm is extruded
- Cytoplasm + axial filament = Tail

Metaphase
- Bivalents get arranged on spindle ("double file")

Anaphase
- Chromosomes are separate and move towards poles

- No division of centromere

Telophase
- Two daughter cells are formed with haploid (n) number of chromosomes

Meiosis II
- Simple mitosis
- Four cells
- Each with haploid (n) number of chromosomes
- Chromatids are genetically dissimilar

78 Gametogenesis : Conversion of Germ Cells into Male and Female Gametes

Primordial germ cells appear in the wall of the yolk sac during 4th week and migrate to the indifferent gonad and reach at the end of the 5th week.

In preparation for fertilization, both male and female germ cells undergo gametogenesis, which includes meiosis and cytodifferentiation.

During meiosis I homologous chromosomes pair and exchange genetic material.

During meiosis II cells fail to replicate DNA and each cell is thus provided with a haploid number of chromosomes and half the amount of DNA of a normal somatic cell.

Hence, mature male and female gametes have 22 + XY or 22 + XX chromosomes respectively.

Birth defects may arise due to abnormalities in

- Chromosome number
- Chromosome structure
- From single gene mutations

7 % of major birth defects are a result of chromosome abnormalities

8 % are due to gene mutations

Trisomies (**extra chromosome**) and monosomies (**loss of a chromosome**) arise during mitosis or meiosis.

During meiosis, homologous chromosomes normally pair and then separate. When this separation fails (**non-dysjunction**), one cell receives too many chromosomes and one receives too few.

The incidence of numerical aberrations increases with age of the mother (mothers aged 35 years or more).

Structural abnormalities of chromosomes include large deletions (cri-du-chat syndrome) and microdeletions.

Microdeletions involve contiguous genes which may result in

- **Angelman syndrome** (maternal deletion, chromosome 15q 11-15q 13)
- **Prader-Willi syndrome** (paternal deletion, 15q 11-15q 13)

These syndromes depend on whether the affected genetic material is inherited from the mother or the father.

Gene mutations may be

- Dominant (only one gene of an allelic pair is affected to produce an alteration)
- Recessive (both allelic gene pairs mutated)

In females - oogenesis begins before birth.

In males - spermatoge-nesis begins at puberty.

In females primordial germ cells form oogonia. After repeated mitotic divisions, some of these arrest in prophase of meiosis I to form primary oocytes. By 7th month, nearly all oogo-nia become atretic. Only primary oocytes remain surrounded by a layer of follicular cells which are derived from the surface epithelium of the ovary. Together they form primordial follicle.

At puberty everyday fifteen to twenty follicles begin to grow. As they ma-ture, they pass through three stages:

- Primary or preantral
- Secondary or antral (Graafian)
- Preovulatory

The primary oocyte re-mains in prophase of the first meiotic division until the secondary follicle is mature. At this point, a surge in luteinizing hormone (LH) stimulates pre-ovulatory growth - meiosis I is completed and a secondary oocyte and polar body are formed. Then, the secondary oocyte is arrested in metaphase of meiosis II approximately three hours before ovulation and this cell division will not be completed until fertilization.

In males primordial cells remain dormant until puberty. Only at puberty they differentiate into spermatogonia. These stem cells give rise to primary spermatocytes. These spermatocytes through two successive meiotic divisions produce four spermatids. Spermatids go through a series of changes (**spermiogenesis**) which include

- Formation of the acrosome
- Condensation of the nucleus
- Formation of neck, middle piece, and tail
- Shedding of most of the cytoplasm

The time required for a spermatogonium to become a mature spermatozoon is approximately 64 days.

FIRST WEEK OF DEVELOPMENT: OVULATION TO IMPLANTATION

During each ovarian cycle, a number of primary follicles begin to grow. Usually only one primary follicle reaches full maturity and only one oocyte is discharged at the time of ovulation. At ovulation, the oocyte is in metaphase of the second meiotic division and it is surrounded by the zona pellucida and some granulosa cells.

Before spermatozoa can fertilize the oocyte, these undergo

- **Capacitation** - A glycoprotein coat and seminal plasma proteins are removed from the spermatozoon head
- **Acrosome reaction** - Acrosin and trypsin-like substances are released to penetrate the zona pellucida

During fertilization the spermatozoon must penetrate

- Corona radiata
- Zona pellucida
- Cell membrane of oocyte

As soon as the spermatocyte has entered the oocyte

- Oocyte finishes its second meiotic division and forms the female pronucleus
- Zona pellucida becomes impenetrable to other spermatozoa
- Head of the sperm separates from the tail, swells and forms the male pronucleus

After both pronuclei have replicated their DNA, paternal and maternal chromosomes intermingle, split longitudinally and go through a mitotic division. This gives rise to the two-cell stage.

Results of fertilization

- Restoration of the diploid number of chromosomes
- Sex determination
- Initiation of cleavage

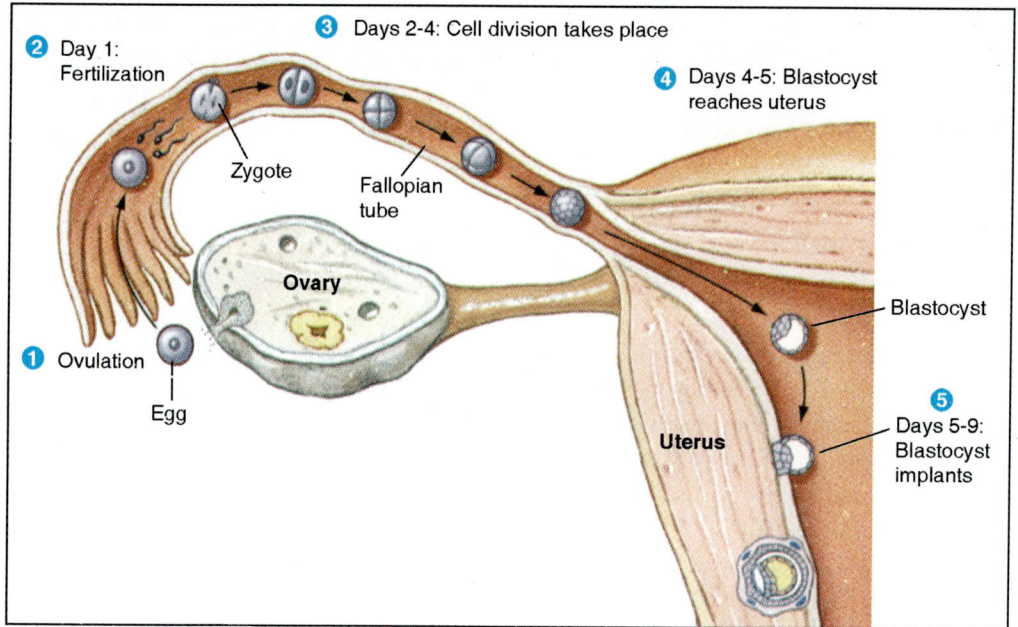

Fig. 78.1: Ovulation, Fertilization & Implantation

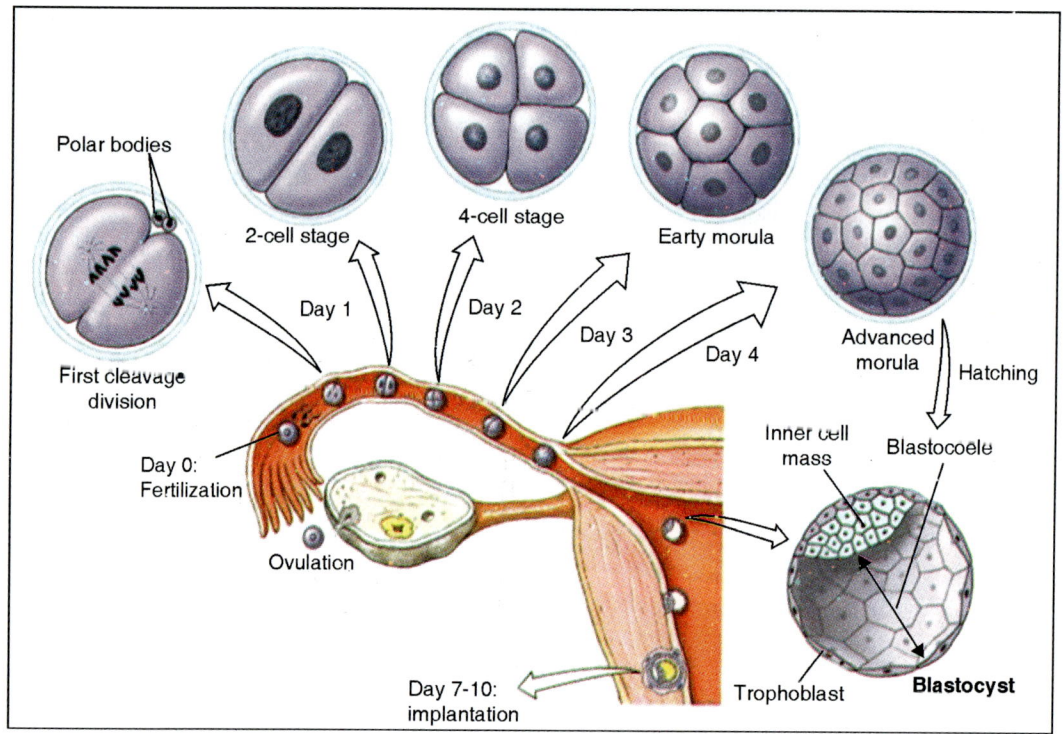

Fig. 78.2: Ovulation, Fertilization & Implantation

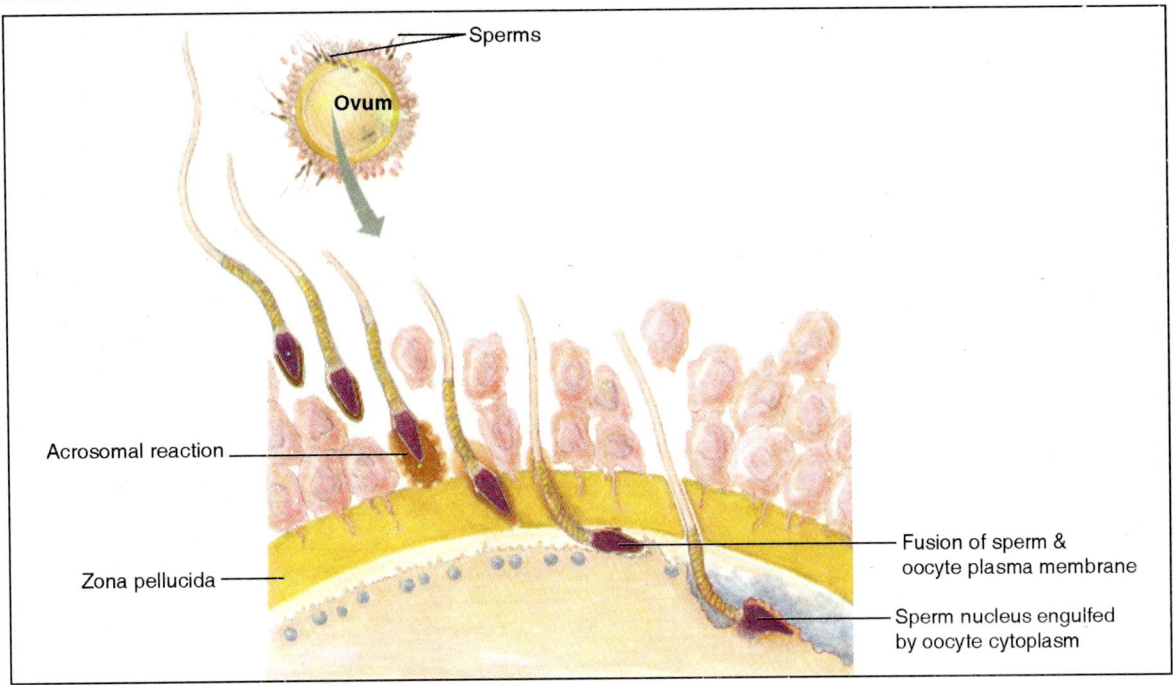

Fig. 78.3: Fertilization

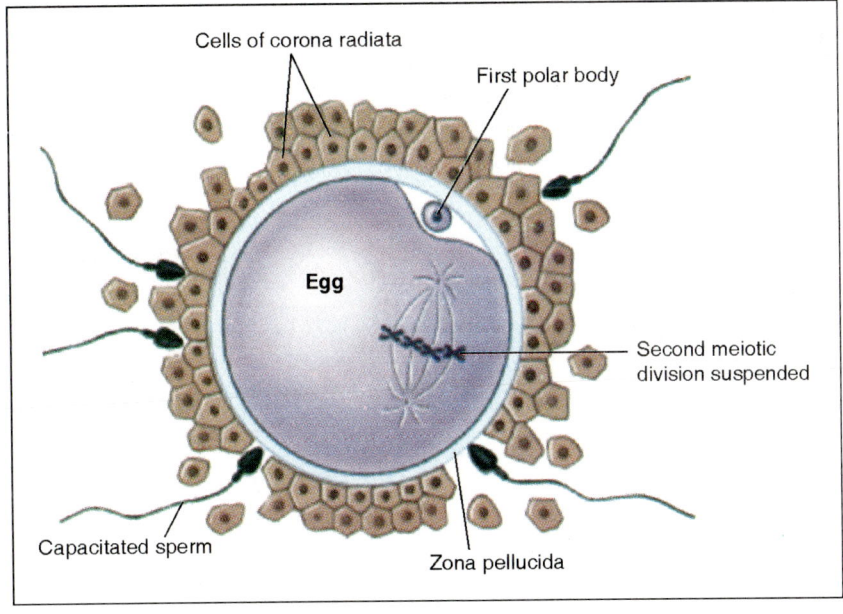

Fig. 78.4: Fertilization

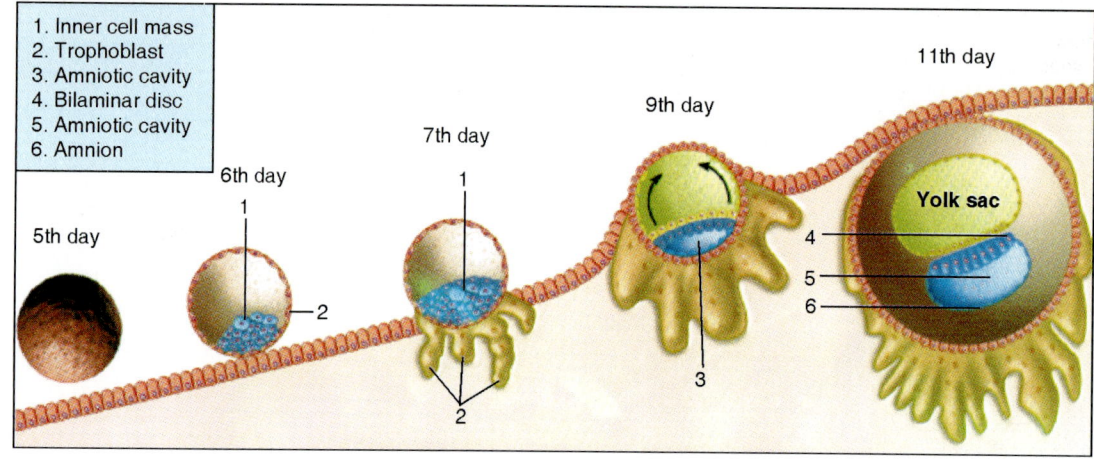

1. Inner cell mass
2. Trophoblast
3. Amniotic cavity
4. Bilaminar disc
5. Amniotic cavity
6. Amnion

5th day

6th day

7th day

9th day

11th day

Yolk sac

Fig. 78.5: Implantation

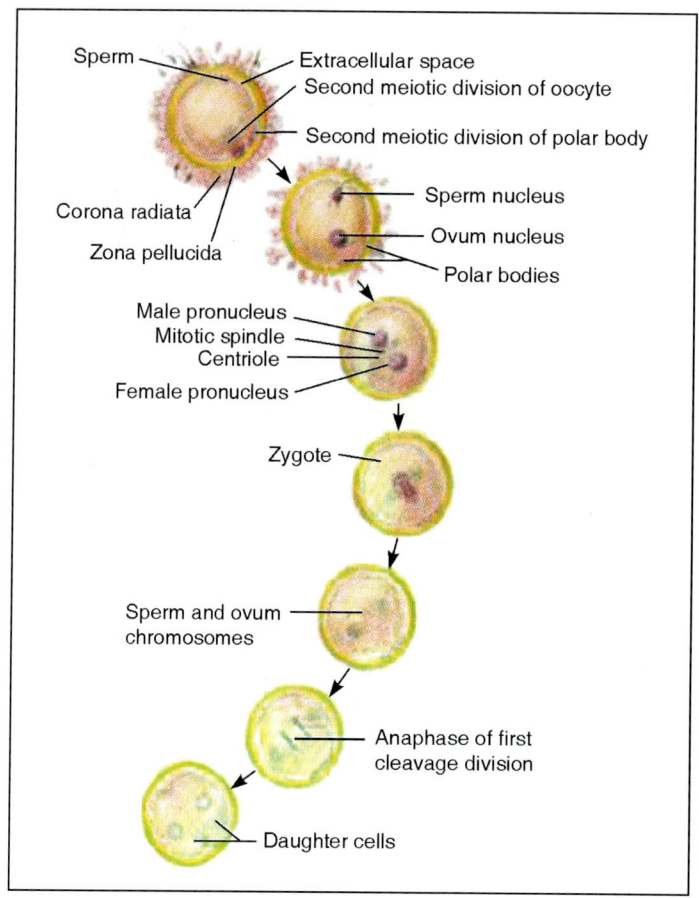

Sperm

Extracellular space
Second meiotic division of oocyte
Second meiotic division of polar body

Corona radiata

Zona pellucida

Sperm nucleus

Ovum nucleus

Polar bodies

Male pronucleus
Mitotic spindle
Centriole
Female pronucleus

Zygote

Sperm and ovum
chromosomes

Anaphase of first
cleavage division

Daughter cells

Fig. 78.6: Completion of Meiosis II & Fertilization

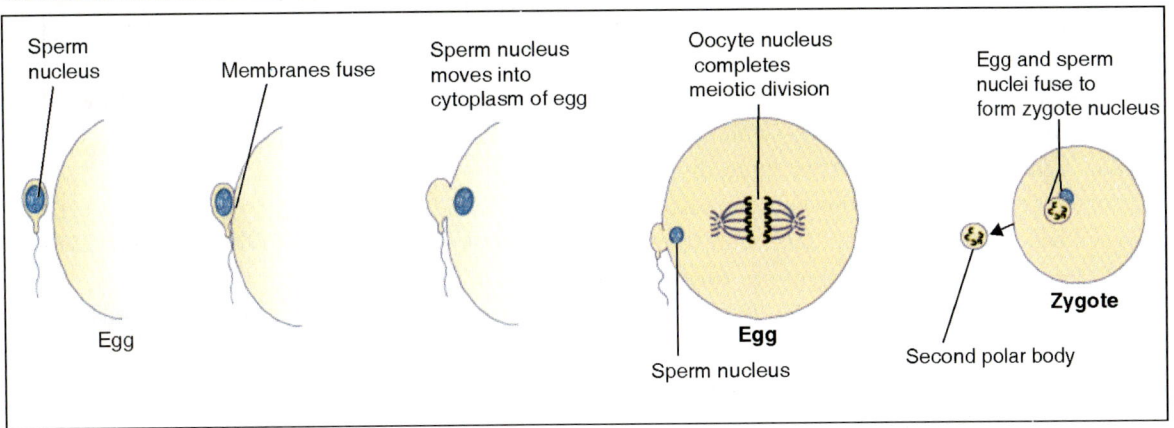

Fig. 78.7: Formation of Zygote

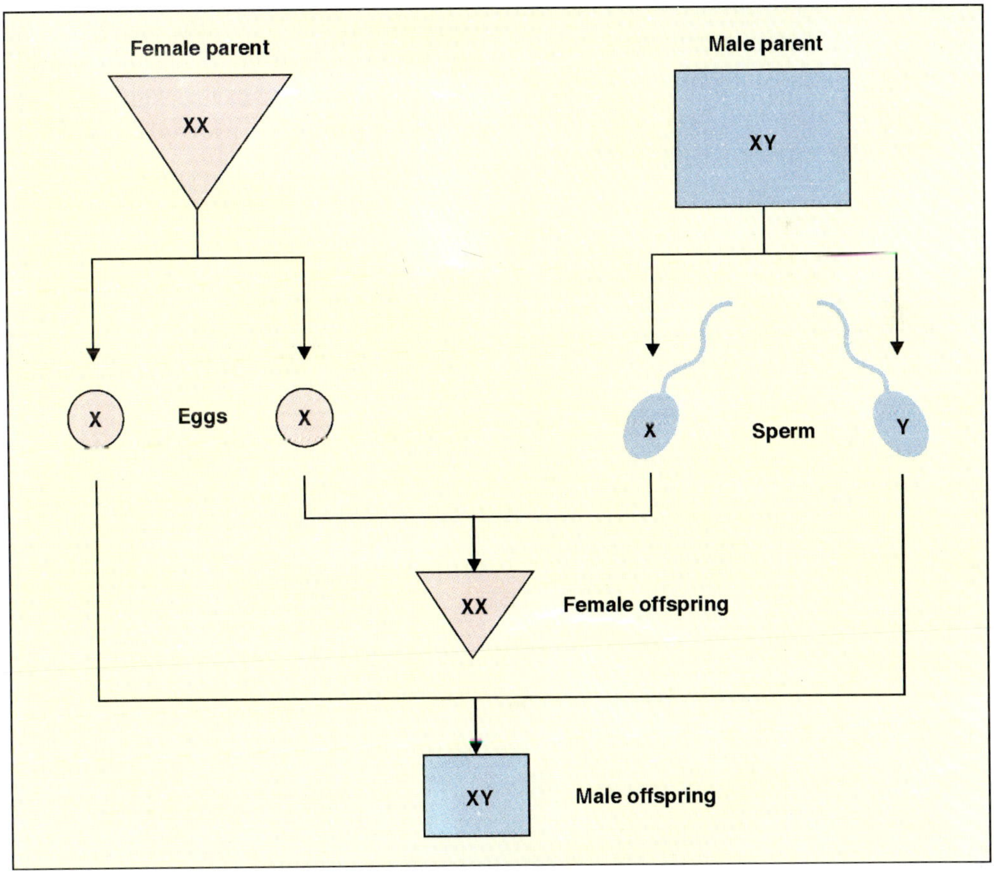

Fig. 78.8: Sex determination of Offspring

CLEAVAGE

It is a series of mitotic divisions that results in an increase in cells – **blastomeres** - which become smaller with each division. After three divisions, blastomeres undergo compaction to become a tightly grouped ball of cells with inner and outer layers.

Compacted blastomeres divide to form a 16-celled structure called **morula**. The morula enters the uterus on the 3rd or 4th day after fertilization. A cavity begins to appear in morula and the resultant structure is termed **blastocyst.**

Inner cell mass formed at the time of compaction develops into the embryo proper, is placed at one pole of the blastocyst.

Outer cell mass which surrounds the inner cells and the blastocyst cavity forms the trophoblast.

The uterus at the time of implantation is in the secretory phase. The blastocyst gets implanted in the endometrium along the anterior or posterior wall.

If fertilization does not occur, then the menstrual phase begins and the spongy and compact layers of endometrium are shed. The basal layer remains intact to regenerate the other layers during the next cycle.

SECOND WEEK OF DEVELOPMENT: FORMATION OF BILAMINAR GERM DISC

At the starting of the second week, the blastocyst is partially embedded in the stroma of endometrial. The trophoblast differentiates into

- Inner, actively proliferating layer - **cytotrophoblast**
- Outer layer – **syncytiotrophoblast** - erodes maternal tissues

By 9th day lacunae develop in the syncytiotrophoblast. Subsequently, maternal sinusoids are eroded by the syncytiotrophoblast and the maternal blood enters the lacunar network. By the end of 2nd week, a primitive **uteroplacental circulation** begins.

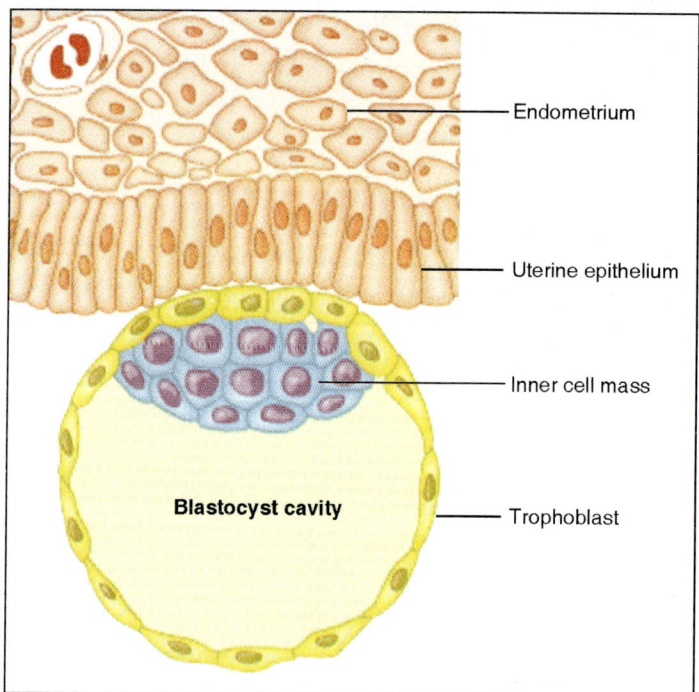

Endometrium

Uterine epithelium

Inner cell mass

Blastocyst cavity

Trophoblast

Fig. 78.9: Formation of Blastocyst

The cytotrophoblast forms cellular columns which penetrate into and are surrounded by the syncytium. These columns are termed **primary villi**. By the end of the second week the blastocyst is completely embedded.

The inner cell mass differentiates into

- Epiblast
- Hypoblast

Together these form a bilaminar disc.

Epiblast cells give rise to amnioblasts that line the amniotic cavity superior to the epiblast layer. Endoderm cells are continuous with the exocoelomic membrane and together they surround the primitive yolk sac.

By the end of the second week, extraembryonic mesoderm fills the space between the trophoblast and the amnion and exocoelomic membrane internally. Development of vacuoles in this tissue results in the formation of extraembryonic coelom (**chorionic cavity**).

Second week of development is known as the week of twos

- **Trophoblast** differentiates into two layers - cytotrophoblast and syncytiotro-phoblast

- **Embryoblast** forms two layers - epiblast and hypoblast

- **Extraembryonic mesoderm** splits into two layers – somatopleural layer and splanchnopleural layer

- **Two cavities** are formed – amniotic cavity and yolk sac

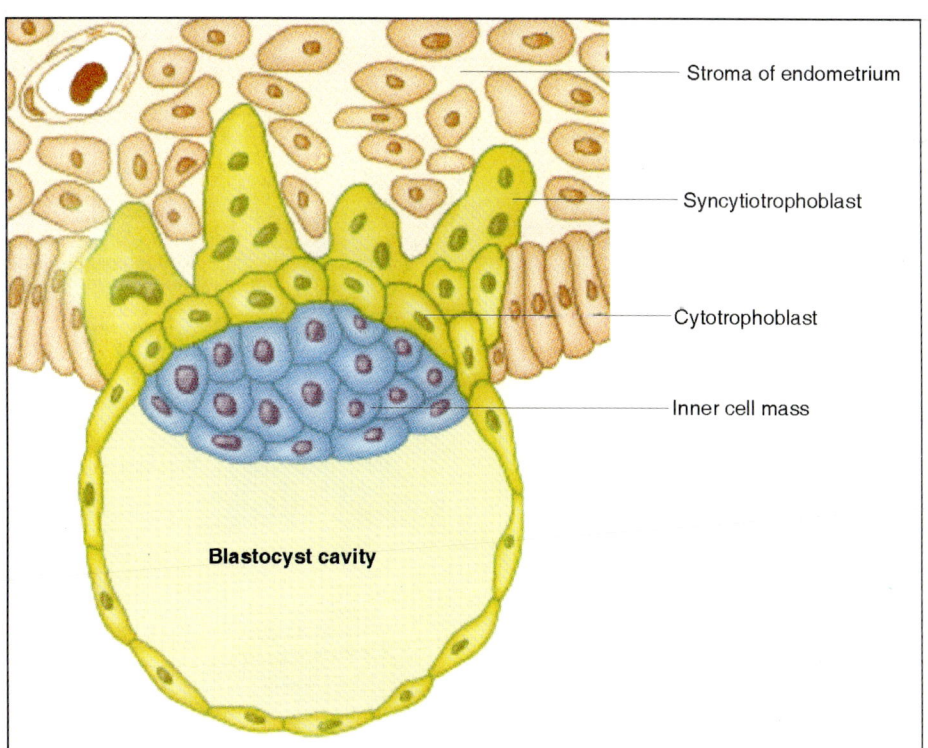

Stroma of endometrium

Syncytiotrophoblast

Cytotrophoblast

Inner cell mass

Blastocyst cavity

Fig. 78.10: Formation of Syncytiotrophoblast & Cytotrophoblast

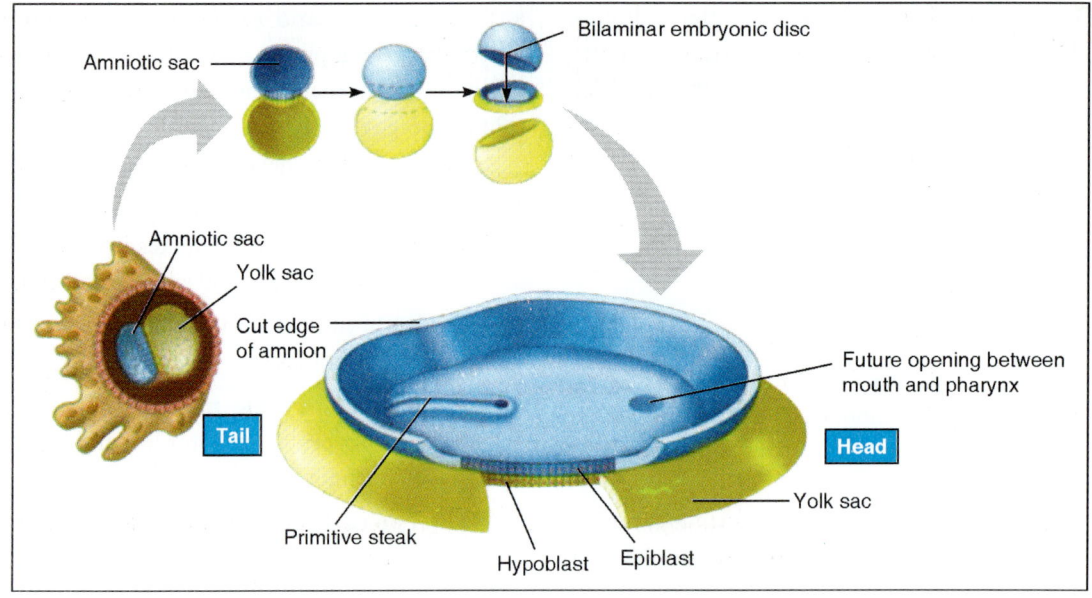

Fig. 78.11: Bilamminar embryonic disc: Lateral superior view

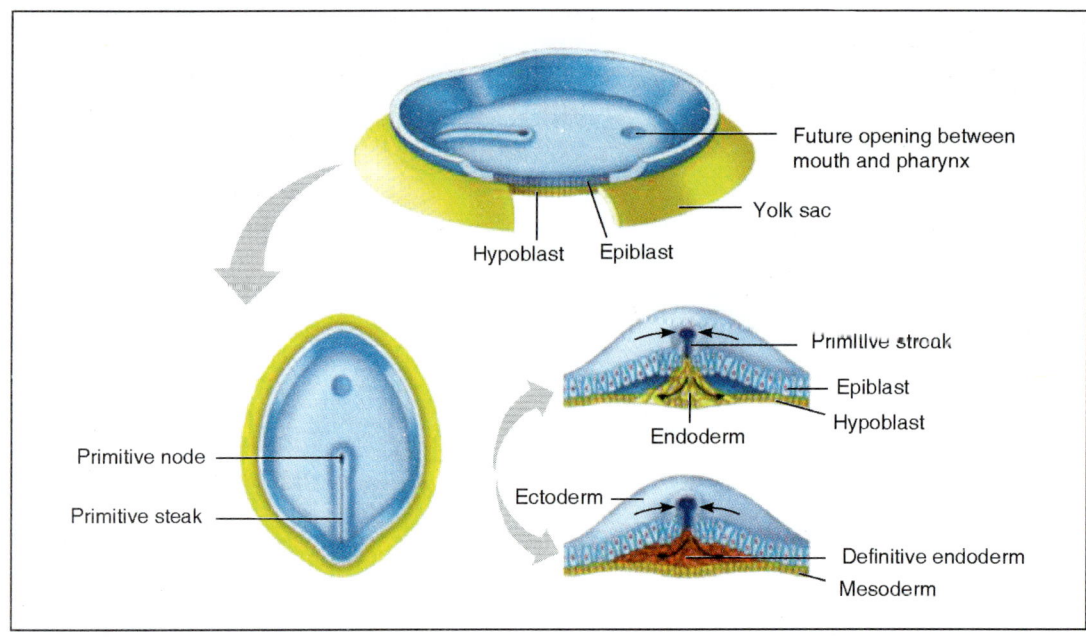

Fig. 78.12: Bilamminar embryonic disc: Superior view – Premitive streak

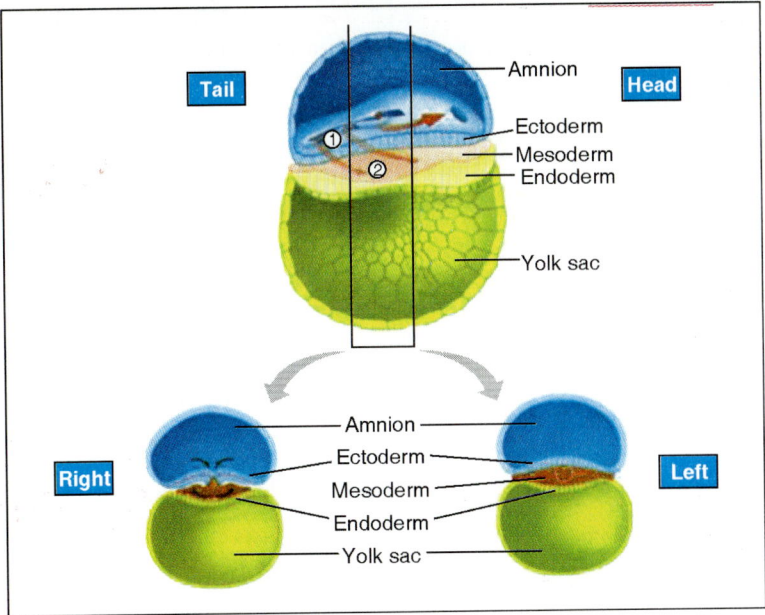

Fig. 78.13: Formation of mesoderm and notochord

Note

- Implantation occurs at the end of the first week
- Trophoblast cells invade the epithelium and underlying endometrial stroma with the help of proteolytic en-zymes
- Implantation may also occur outside the uterus (in the rectouter-ine pouch, in the uterine tube or in the ovary - **ectopic pregnancy**)

THIRD WEEK OF DEVELOPMENT: TRILAMINAR GERM DISC

The most characteristic event during third week is gastrulation. Gastrulation begins with the appearance of the primitive streak. Primitive streak at its cephalic end contains primitive node. In the region of the node and streak, epiblast cells move inward (invaginates) to form new cell layers - endoderm and mesoderm.

Thus epiblast gives rise to all three germ layers in the embryo.

Cells of the intraembryonic mesodermal germ layer migrate between the two other germ layers until they establish contact with the extraembryonic mesoderm covering the yolk sac and amnion.

Prenotochordal cells invaginates primitive pit, move forward until they reach prechordal plate. They intercalate in the endoderm as the notochordal plate. With further development, the plate is detached from the endoderm and a solid cord termed **notochord** is formed. It forms a midline axis which serves as the basis of the axial skeleton.

Cephalic and caudal ends of the embryo are established before the primitive streak is formed. Thus, cells in the hypoblast (endoderm) at the cephalic margin of the disc form the anterior visceral endoderm that expresses head-forming genes.

Epiblast cells moving through the node and streak are predetermined by their position to become specific types of mesoderm and endoderm.

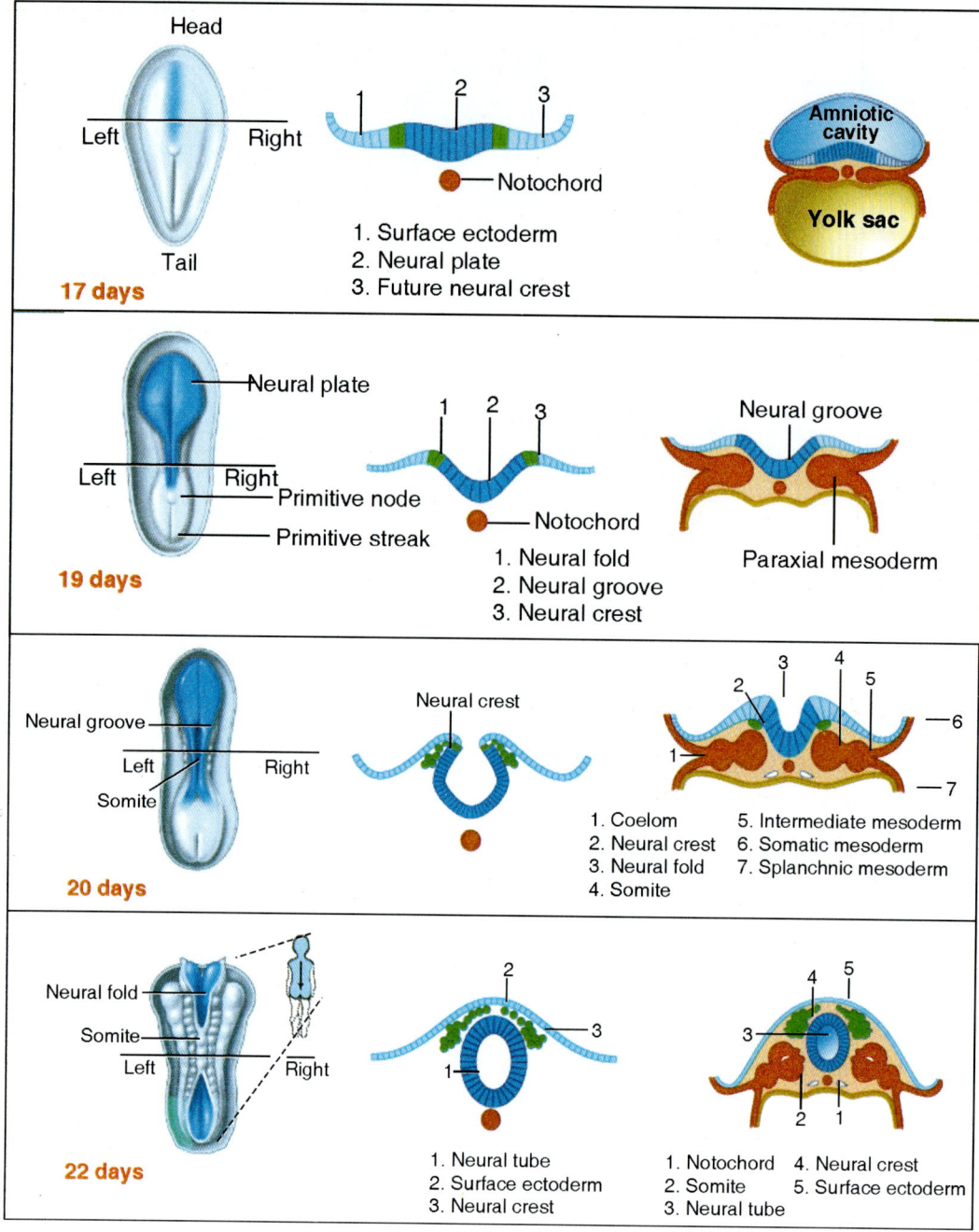

Fig. 78.14: Changes in the Embryo

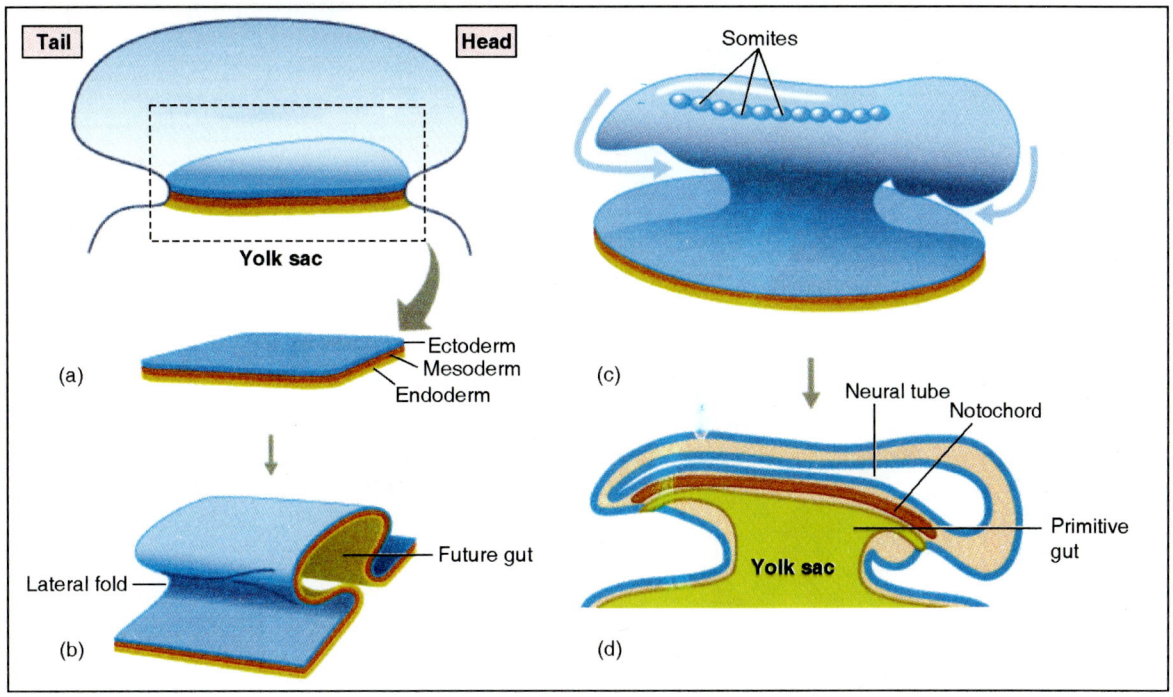

Fig. 78.15: 4th week of development

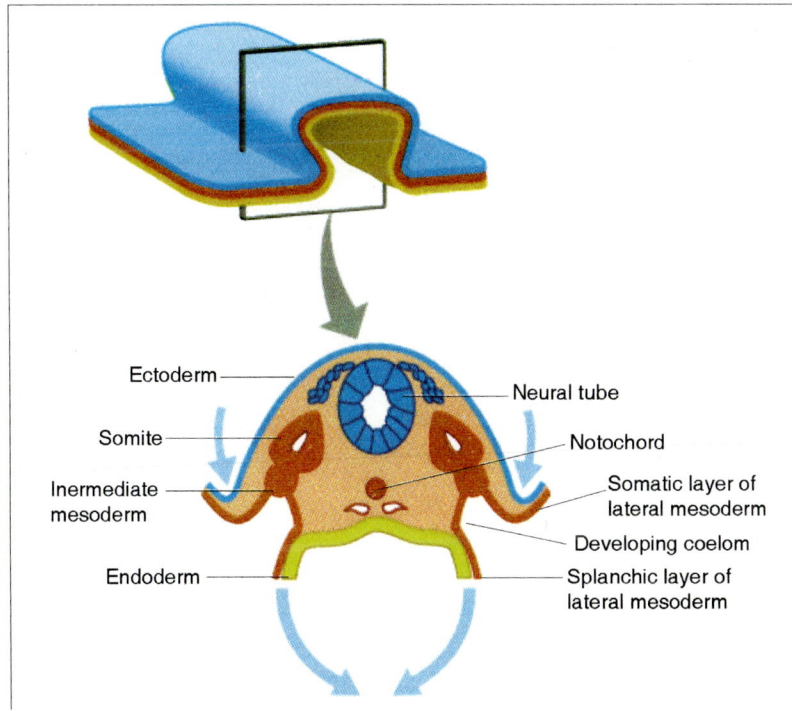

Fig. 78.16: Germ layers in 4th week

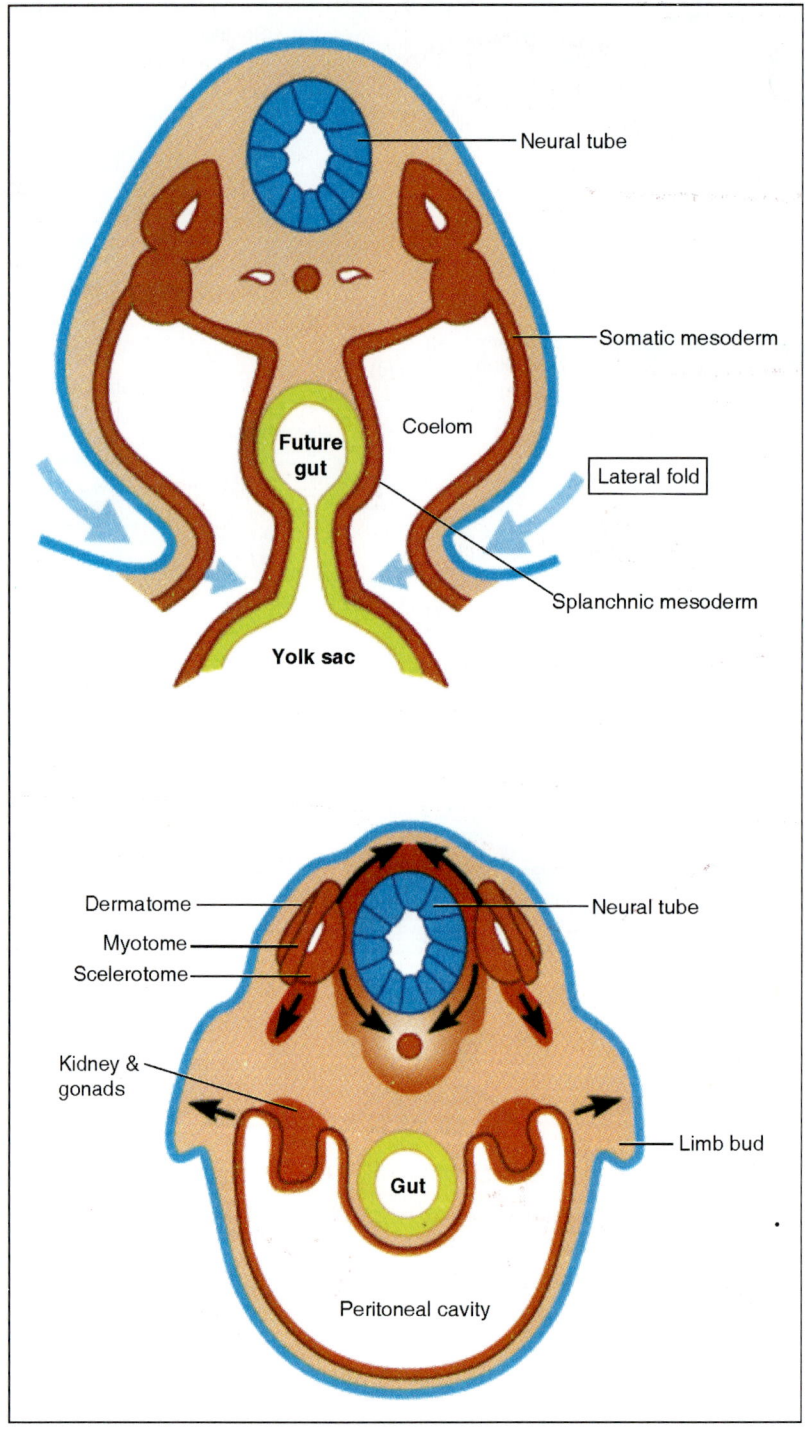

Fig. 78.17: Germ layers in 4th week

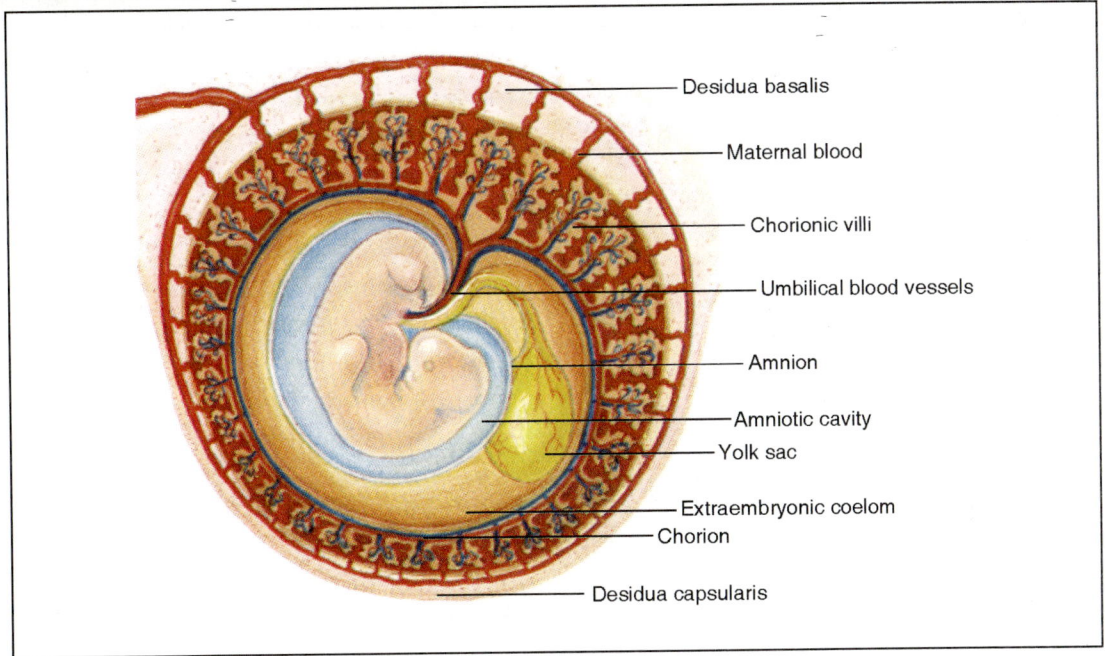

Fig. 78.18: Four week Embryo

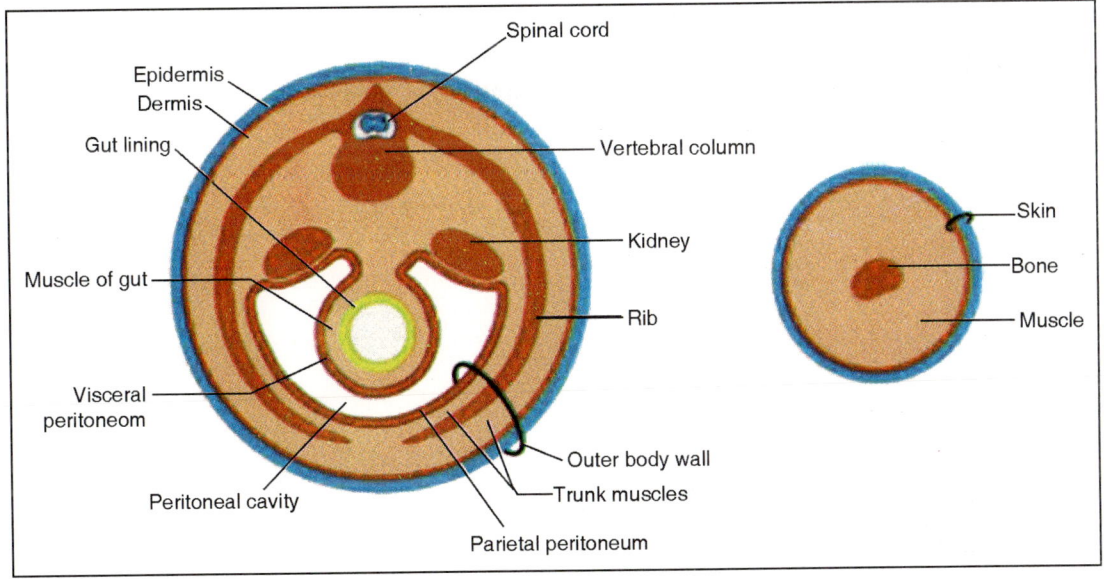

Fig. 78.19: Basic body plan

By the end of third week three basic germ layers (ectoderm, mesoderm and endoderm) are established in the head region. The process continues to produce these germ layers for more caudal areas of the embryo until the end of 4th week.

Tissue and organ differentiation starts which occur in a cephalocaudal direction as the gastrulation continues.

In the meantime, the trophoblast progresses rapidly. Primary villi obtain a mesenchymal core in which small capillaries arise. When these villous capillaries make contact with capillaries in the chorionic plate and connecting stalk, the villous system becomes ready to supply the embryo with its nutrients and oxygen.

EMBRYNIC PERIOD

The embryonic period extends from **3rd to 8th weeks** of development. During this period germ layers (ectoderm, mesoderm and endoderm) give rise to its own tissues and organ systems.

Ectodermal germ layer gives rise to the organs and structures that maintain contact with the outside world. These include:

- Central nervous system (CNS)
- Peripheral nervous system (PNS)
- Sensory epithelium of ear, nose and eye
- Skin including hair and nails
- Pituitary, mammary and sweat glands
- Enamel of the teeth

Mesodermal germ layer has

- Paraxial plate mesoderm
- Intermediate plate mesoderm
- Lateral plate mesoderm.

Paraxial mesoderm forms somitomeres. It gives rise to mesenchyme of the head and organizes into somites in occipital and caudal segments.

Somites give rise to

- Myotome (muscle)
- Sclerotome (cartilage and bone)
- Dermatome (subcutaneous tissue of the skin)

Signals for somite differentiation are derived from surrounding structures which include notochord, neural tube, and epidermis.

Mesoderm also gives rise to the vascular system which includes the heart, arteries, veins, lymph vessels, and blood and lymph cells.

It gives rise to the urogenital system: kidneys, gonads, and their ducts (not urinary bladder). Spleen and cortex of the suprarenal glands are also derived.

Endodermal germ layer forms.

Epithelial lining of:

- Gastrointestinal tract
- Respiratory tract
- Urinary bladder

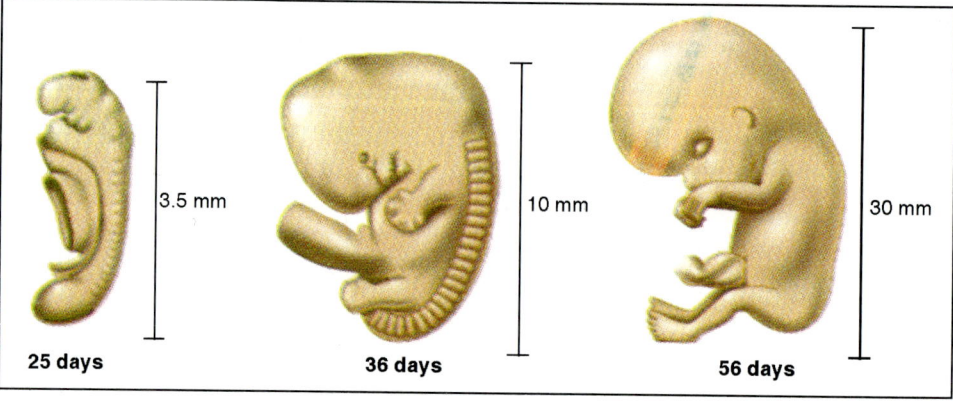

25 days   3.5 mm   36 days   10 mm   56 days   30 mm

Fig. 78.20

Forms the parenchyma of:

- Thyroid
- Parathyroids
- Liver
- Pancreas

Epithelial lining of:

- Tympanic cavity
- Auditory tube

As a result of formation of organ systems and rapid growth of the central nervous system, the initial flat embryonic disc begins to fold cephalocaudally. This establishes the head and tail folds. The disc also folds transversely (**lateral folds**), establishing the rounded body form. Connection with the yolk sac and placenta is maintained through the vitelline duct and umbilical cord respectively.

THIRD MONTH TO BIRTH: THE FOETUS AND PLACENTA

The foetal period extends from **9th week of gestation until birth**. This is characterized by rapid growth of the body and maturation of organ systems.

Growth in length is striking during 3rd to 5th months (approximately 5 cm per month), while increase in weight is most striking during the last two months of gestation (approximately *700* g per month).

There is relative slowdown in the growth of the head. In the 3rd month, it is about half of the crown rump length (CRL). By the 5th month the size of the head is about one-third of crown heel length (CHL) and at birth it is one-fourth of CHL.

During 5th month, foetal movements are recognized by the mother. The foetus is covered with fine, small hair.

A foetus born during 6th or the beginning of 7th month is difficulty to survive. This is mainly because the respiratory and central nervous systems have not differentiated sufficiently.

The length of pregnancy for a full-term foetus is considered to be 280 days or 40 weeks after onset

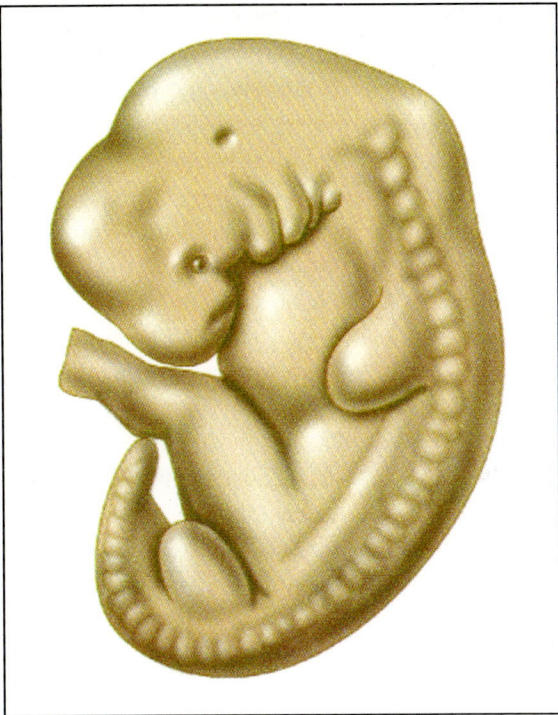

Fig. 78.21: 28 days Embryo

of the last menstruation or (more accurately) 266 days or 38 weeks after fertilization.

The placenta consists of two components

- **Foetal portion** – derived from the chorionic villous
- **Maternal portion** – derived from the decidua basalis

The space between the chorionic and decidual plates is filled with maternal blood. Villi grow into the maternal blood.

Foetal circulation is separated from the maternal circulation by:

- Syncytial membrane (derived from chorion)
- Endothelial cells from foetal capillaries

The human placenta is thus **hemochorial** in nature Intervillous spaces of the fully grown placenta contain approximately 150 ml of maternal blood, which is renewed three or four times per minute. The villous area varies from four to fourteen m2, thus facilitating exchanges between mother and the foetus.

Main functions of the placenta

1. Exchange of gases
2. Exchange of nutrients and electrolytes
3. Transmission of maternal antibodies – passive immunity to foetus
4. Production of hormones – progesterone, estradiol and estrogen (it also produces Hcg and somatomammotropin)
5. Detoxification of some drugs

The amnion is a large sac containing amniotic fluid in which the foetus is suspended by its umbilical cord. The fluid

- Absorbs jolts
- Allows for fetal movements
- Prevents adherence of the embryo to the surrounding tissues

The foetus swallows amniotic fluid, which is absorbed through its gut and cleared by the placenta. The foetus adds urine to the amniotic fluid which is mostly water.

An excessive amount of amniotic fluid (**hydramnios**) is associated with anencephaly and esophageal atresia while an insufficient amount (**oligohydramnios**) is related to renal agenesis.

The umbilical cord is surrounded by the amnion. It contains

- Two umbilical arteries
- One umbilical vein
- Wharton's jelly – serves as a protective cushion for the vessels

Foetal membranes in twins vary according to their origin and time of formation.

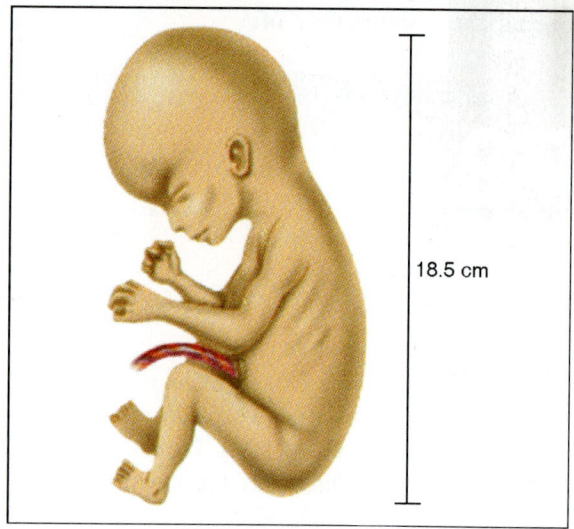

18.5 cm

20 week Foetus

Dizygotic twins (fraternal) have two amnions, two chorions and two placentas, which sometimes are fused.

Monozygotic twins usually have two amnions, one chorion and one placenta.

In conjoined twins where the foetuses are not entirely split from each other, there is one amnion, one chorion, and one placenta.

Signals initiating parturition (**birth**) are not clear. Preparation for labour usually begins between 34th and 38th weeks.

Labour consists of three stages

- Effacement and dilatation of the cervix
- Delivery of the foetus
- Delivery of the placenta and foetal membranes

79

Developments of Systems

SKELETAL SYSTEM

The skeletal system develops from mesenchyme - derived from the mesodermal germ layer and neural crest.

Some bones (flat bones of skull) undergo membranous ossification where mesenchyme cells are directly transformed into osteoblasts.

In most bones (long bones of limbs) the mesenchyme condenses and forms hyaline cartilage models of bones. The ossification centers appear in these cartilage models and the bone gradually ossifies by endochondral ossification.

Development of skull

Skull consists of

- Neurocranium
- Viscerocranium (face)

Neurocranium includes a membranous portion - forms the cranial vault and a cartilaginous portion (chondrocranium) - forms the base of the skull.

Neural crest cells form

- Face
- Most of the cranial vault
- Prechordal part of the chondrocranium (part rostral to notochord)

Paraxial mesoderm forms the remainder of the skull

Development of limbs

The limb buds appear along the body wall that appear in the 4th week.

Lateral plate mesoderm forms the bones and connective tissue whereas muscle cells migrate to the limbs from the somites.

Many of the genes that regulate limb growth and patterning have been defined.

Development of vertebral column and ribs

The vertebral column and ribs develop from the sclerotome compartments of the somites. Sternum is derived from mesoderm in the ventral body wall.

A definitive vertebra is formed by condensation of the caudal half of one sclerotome and fusion with the cranial half of the subjacent sclerotome.

Abnormalities of the skeletal system include:

- **Vertebral** - spina bifida
- **Cranial** - cranioschisis and cranio-synostosis
- **Facial** - cleft palate

Major malformations of the limbs are rare. Defects of the radius and digits are often associated with other abnormalities (syndromes).

DEVELOPMENT OF MUSCLES

Most muscles arise from the mesoderm.

Skeletal muscles are derived from paraxial mesoderm which include

- **Somites** - Forms muscles of the axial skeleton, body wall and limbs
- **Somitomeres** - Forms muscles of the head.

Progenitor cells for muscle tissues are derived from the dorsolateral and dorsomedial portions of the somites.

Cells in the dorsolateral portion migrate to form hypomeric muscle. The cells in the dorsomedial portion migrates ventral to the dermatome to form the myotome, and ultimately form epimeric musculature.

By 5th week muscle precursor cells divide into

- Small dorsal portion (**Epimere**) - innervated by dorsal primary ramus
- Larger ventral portion (**Hypomere**) - innervated by ventral primary ramus

Myoblasts from epimeres form extensor muscles of the vertebral column and the myoblasts of the hypomere form limb and body wall musculature.

Connective tissue is derived from

- Somites
- Somatic mesoderm
- Neural crest (head region)

This provides a template for the establishment of muscle patterns.

Most smooth muscles and cardiac muscle fibers are derived from splanchnic mesoderm. Smooth muscles of the pupil, mammary gland and sweat glands differentiate from ectoderm.

At the end of the third week, intercellular clefts appear in the mesoderm on each side of the midline. When these spaces fuse, the intraembryonic cavity (**body cavity**), bordered by a somatic mesoderm and a splanchnic mesoderm layer, is formed (Figs. 10.1 and 10.2). With cephalocaudal and lateral folding of the embryo, the intraembryonic cavity extends from the thoracic to the pelvic region. Somatic mesoderm will form the parietal layer of the serous membranes lining the outside of the peritoneal, pleural, and pericardial cavities. The splanchnic layer will form the visceral layer of the serous membranes covering the lungs, heart, and abdominal organs. These layers are continuous at the root of these organs in their cavities (as if a finger were stuck into a balloon, with the layer surrounding the finger being the splanchnic or visceral layer and the rest of the balloon, the somatic or parietal layer surrounding the body cavity). The serous membranes in the abdomen are called peritoneum.

DEVELOPMENT OF DIAPHRAGM

The diaphragm divides the body cavity into the thoracic and peritoneal cavities. It develops from four components

- Septum transversum (central tendon)
- Pleuroperitoneal membranes
- Dorsal mesentery of the esophagus
- Muscular components of the body wall

Congenital diaphragmatic hernias involve a defect of the pleuroperitoneal membrane. This defect on the left side occurs frequently.

The thoracic cavity is divided into the pericardial cavity and two pleural cavities for the lungs by the pleuropericardial membranes.

Two layers of peritoneum form mesenteries that suspend the gut tube from the posterior abdominal wall. These provide a pathway for vessels, nerves, and lymphatics to the organs. Initially, the gut tube from the caudal end of the foregut to the end of the hindgut is suspended from the dorsal body wall by dorsal mesentery. Ventral mesentery derived from the septum transversum is present only in the region of the lower part of the oesophagus, stomach and upper part of the duodenum.

CARDIOVASCULAR SYSTEM

The cardiovascular system (including heart, blood vessels, and blood cells) develops from the mesoderm.

The heart tube is initially paired (22nd day of development). Two tubes form a single, slightly bent heart tube which consists of an inner endocardial tube and a surrounding myocardial mantle.

During 4th to 7th weeks the heart is divided into a four-chambered structure.

Septum formation in the heart partly arises from development of endocardial cushion in the atrioventricular canal (atrioventricular cushions) and in the conotruncal region (conotruncal swellings). Because of the key location of cushion, many cardiac malformations are related to abnormal cushion morphogenesis.

Septum formation in the atrium

The septum primum is a sickle-shaped crest which descends from the roof of the atrium. It begins to divide the atrium in two but leaves a lumen - **ostium primum**, for communication between the two sides. Later the ostium primum is obliterated by the fusion of the septum primum with the endocardial cushions.

The ostium secundum is formed by cell death that creates an opening in the septum primum.

Finally, a septum secundum forms, but an interatrial opening - **oval foramen**, persists.

At birth, when pressure in the left atrium increases two septa press against each other and close the communication between the two.

Abnormalities in the atrial septum may vary from **total absence** to a small opening known as **probe patency** of the oval foramen.

Septum formation in the atrioventricular canal

Four endocardial cushions surround the atrioventricular canal. Fusion of the opposing superior and inferior cushions divides the orifice into right and left atrioventricular canals. Cushion then becomes fibrous and forms the mitral (**bicuspid**) valve on the left and the tricuspid valve on the right.

Defects include

- Persistence of the common atrioventricular canal
- Abnormal division of the canal

Septum formation in the ventricles

The interventricular septum consists of a thick muscular part and a thin membranous portion. The septum is formed by

- Inferior endocardial atrioventricular cushion
- Right conus swelling
- Left conus swelling

These three components may fail to fuse, resulting in an open interventricular foramen. Although this abnormality may be isolated, it is commonly combined with other defects.

Septum formation in the bulbus

The bulbus is divided

- Truncus (aorta and pulmonary trunk)
- Conus (outflow tract of the aorta and pulmonary trunk)
- Trabeculated portion of the right ventricle

The truncus region is divided by the spiral **aorticopulmonary septum** into the two main arteries.

The conus swellings divide the outflow tracts of the aortic and pulmonary channels and with tissue from the inferior endocardial cushion close the interventricular foramen.

Vascular abnormalities resulting from abnormal division of the conotruncal region include

- Transposition of the great vessels
- Pulmonary valvular atresia

The aortic arches lie in each of the five pharyngeal arches.

Four important derivatives of the original aortic arch system are

- Carotid arteries (**third arches**)

- Arch of the aorta (**left fourth aortic arch**)
- Pulmonary artery (**sixth aortic arch**) which is connected to the aorta through the ductus arteriosus in the foetal file
- Right subclavian artery formed by the right fourth aortic arch, distal portion of the right dorsal aorta and the seventh intersegmental artery

Most common vascular aortic arch abnormalities include

- Open ductus arteriosus
- Coarctation of the aorta
- Persistent right aortic arch
- Abnormal right subclavian artery

Vitelline arteries initially supply the yolk sac. Later these form the coeliac, superior mesenteric, and inferior mesenteric arteries, which supply the foregut, midgut and hindgut, respectively.

Umbilical arteries arise from the common iliac arteries. After birth the distal portions of these arteries are obliterated to form the medial umbilical ligaments, whereas the proximal portions persist as the internal iliac and vesicular arteries.

VENOUS SYSTEM

Three venous systems are

- **Vitelline system** - Develops into the portal system
- **Cardinal system** - Forms the caval system
- **Umbilical system** - Disappears after birth

Complicated caval system may results in

- Double inferior vena cava
- Double superior vena cava
- Left superior vena cava

CHANGES AT BIRTH

During prenatal life the placental circulation provides oxygen to the foetus but after birth the lungs take on gas exchange.

In the circulatory system the following changes take place at birth and in the first postnatal months

- Closure of ductus arteriosus
- Closure of oval foramen
- Obliteration of umbilical vein - ligamentum teres hepatis
- Obliteration of ductus venosus - ligamentum venosum
- Obliteration of umbilical arteries - medial umbilical ligaments

LYMPHATIC SYSTEM

It develops later than the cardiovascular system. It originates as five sacs

- Two jugular
- Two iliac
- One retroperitoneal
- One cisterna chyli

Numerous channels form to connect the sacs and provide drainage from other structures. **Thoracic duct** forms from

- Anastomosis of the right and left thoracic ducts
- Distal part of the right tho-racic duct
- Cranial part of the left thoracic duct

Right lymphatic duct develops from the cranial part of the right thoracic duct.

RESPIRATORY SYSTEM

- Respiratory system develops as an outgrowth of the ventral wall of the foregut.
- Epithelium of the larynx, trachea, bronchi and alveoli originates in the endoderm.
- Cartilaginous, muscular and connective tissue components arise in the mesoderm.

During 4th week of development, tracheoesophageal septum separates the trachea from the foregut, dividing the foregut into the lung bud anteriorly and the oesophagus posteriorly. The contact between them is through the larynx, which is formed by tissue of the 4th and 6th pharyngeal arches.

The lung bud develops into two main bronchi.

Right main bronchus forms three secondary bronchi and three lobes.

Left main bronchus forms two secondary bronchi and two lobes.

Faulty partitioning of the foregut by the tracheoesophageal septum causes

- Oesophageal atresias
- Tracheoesophageal fistulas

After a pseudoglandular (5th to 16th weeks) and canalicular (16th to 26th weeks) phase, cells of the cuboidal lined bronchioles change into thin, flat cells - **type I alveolar epithelial cells** which are intimately associated with blood and lymph capillaries.

In the 7th month, gaseous exchange between the blood and air in the primitive alveoli is possible. Before birth the lungs are filled with fluid with little protein, some mucus and surfactant - produced by **type II alveolar epithelial cells,** which form a phospholipid coat on the alveolar membranes.

At the commencement of respiration the lung fluid is resorbed except the surfactant coat, which prevents the collapse of the alveoli during expiration by reducing the surface tension at the air-blood capillary interface.

Absent or insufficient surfactant in the premature baby causes **respiratory distress syndrome** (RDS) because of collapse of the primitive alveoli (hyaline membrane disease)

Growth of the lungs after birth is primarily due to an increase in the number of respiratory bronchioles and alveoli and not to an increase in the size of the alveoli. New alveoli are formed during the first ten years of postnatal life.

Gross abnormalities of the lung and bronchial tree are rare which include

- Blind-ending trachea with absence of lungs
- Agenesis of one lung

Abnormal divisions of the bronchial tree are more common, some result in supernumerary lobules.

Ectopic lung lobes

These arise from the trachea or oesophagus. These lobes are formed from additional respiratory buds of the foregut that develop independently of the main respiratory system.

Clinically important

Congenital cysts of the lung - formed by dilation of terminal or larger bronchi. These cysts may be small and multiple which give the lung a honeycomb appearance on radiograph.

Cystic structures of the lung usually drain poorly and frequently cause chronic infections.

DIGESTIVE SYSTEM

- Epithelium and the parenchyma of its derivatives originate in the endoderm.
- Connective tissue, muscular components, and peritoneal components develop from the mesoderm.

Gut extends from the buccopharyngeal membrane to the cloacal membrane. It is divided into the

- Pharyngeal gut
- Foregut
- Midgut
- Hindgut

The pharyngeal gut gives rise to the pharynx and related glands.

Foregut gives rise to

- Oesophagus
- Trachea
- Lung buds
- Stomach
- Duodenum proximal to the entrance of the bile duct

Liver, pancreas and biliary apparatus develop as outgrowths of the endodermal epithelium of the upper part of the duodenum.

Since the upper part of the foregut is divided by a septum (**tracheoesophageal sep-tum**) into the oesophagus (posteriorly) and the trachea and lung buds (anteriorly), deviation of the septum may result in abnormal openings between the trachea and esophagus.

Epithelial liver cords and biliary system growing out into the septum transversum differentiate into parenchyma.

Hematopoietic cells, Kupffer cells and connective tissue cells originate in mesoderm.

Pancreas develops from a ventral bud and a dorsal bud that later fuse to form the definitive pancreas. Sometimes, the two parts surround the duodenum (**annular pancreas**) and cause constriction of the gut.

Midgut forms primary intestinal loop which forms

- Duodenum distal to the entrance of the bile duct
- Small intestine
- Large intestine up to the junction of the proximal two-thirds of the transverse colon with the distal third.

At its apex the primary loop remains temporarily in open connection with the yolk sac through the vitelline duct. During 6th week, the loop grows rapidly and it protrudes into the umbilical cord (**physiological herniation**).

- During the 10th week, it returns into the abdominal cavity. While these processes are occurring, the midgut loop rotates 2700 counterclockwise. Remnants of the vitelline duct, failure of the midgut to return to the abdominal cavity, malrotation, stenosis, and duplications of parts of the gut are common abnormalities.

Hindgut gives rise to

- Region from the distal third of the transverse colon to the upper part of the anal canal

Distal part of the anal canal develops from ectoderm.

Hindgut enters the posterior region of the cloaca (**future anorectal canal**) and the allantois enters the anterior region (**future urogenital sinus**).

Breakdown of the cloacal membrane covering this area provides communication to the exterior for the anus and urogenital sinus.

Abnormalities in the size of the posterior region of the cloaca shift the entrance of the anus anteriorly. This causes rectovaginal and rectourethral fistulas and atresias.

UROGENITAL SYSTEM

Urinary and genital systems develop from mesodermal tissue.

Three urinary systems develop in a temporal sequence from cranial to caudal segments:

Pronephros - forms in the cervical region. It is vestigial.

Mesonephros - forms in the thoracic and lumbar regions. It is large and characterized by

- Excretory units (**Nephrons**) and its own collecting duct
- Mesonephric or wolffian duct

In the human it may function briefly, but most of the system disappears. Ducts and tubules from the mesonephros form the channels for sperm from the testes to the urethra. In female, these ducts regress.

Metanephros (permanent kidney) develops from two sources.

It forms its own excretory tubules or nephrons like the other systems, but its collecting system originates from the ureteric bud - outgrowth of the mesonephric duct.

This bud gives rise to

- Ureter
- Renal pelvis
- Calyces
- Entire collecting system

Connection between the collecting and excretory tubule systems is essential for normal development.

Abnormalities

Early division of the ureteric bud may lead to bifid or supernumerary kidneys with ectopic ureters.

Abnormal posi-tions of the kidney (pelvic kidney) and horseshoe kidney

Genital system is consist of

- Gonads or primitive sex glands
- Genital ducts
- External genitalia

All three components go through an indifferent stage in which they may develop into either a male or a female.

When primordial germ cells fail to reach the indifferent gonad, the gonad remains indifferent or is absent.

The indifferent duct system and external genitalia develop under the influence of hormones. Testosterone produced by **Leydig cells** in the testes stimulates development of the mesonephric ducts (**vas deferens, epididymis**); while MIS produced by **Sertoli cells** in the testes causes regression of the paramesonephric ducts (**female duct system**).

Dihydrotestosterone stimulates development of

- External genitalia
- Pcnis
- Scrotum
- Prostate

Estrogens influence development of the female system

- Uterine tube
- Uterus
- Cervix
- Upper portion of the vagina

They also stimulate differentiation of

- External genitalia including the clitoris
- Labia majora and minora
- Lower portion of the vagina

Errors in the production or sensitivity to hormones of the testes lead to a predominance of female characteristics under the influence of the maternal and placental estrogens.

HEAD AND NECK

Pharyngeal (branchial) arches consist of bars of mesenchymal tissue, separated by pharyngeal pouches and clefts. These arches give the head and neck their typical appearance in the 4th week.

Each arch contains its own

- Artery
- Cranial nerve
- Muscle element
- Cartilage bar or skeletal element

Endoderm of the pharyngeal pouches gives rise to a number of endocrine glands and part of the middle ear.

In subsequent order the pouches give rise to

- Middle ear cavity and auditory tube (**Pouch 1**)
- Stroma of the palatine tonsil (**Pouch 2**)
- Inferior parathyroid glands and thymus (**Pouch 3**)
- Superior parathyroid glands and ultimobranchial body (**Pouches 4 and 5**)

Pharyngeal clefts give rise to only one structure

- External auditory meatus.

Thyroid gland develops from an epithelial proliferation in the floor of the tongue and descends to its final position in front of the tracheal rings in the course of development.

Maxillary and mandibular prominences and **frontonasal prominence** are the first prominences of the facial region.

Later, medial and lateral nasal prominences form around the nasal placodes on the frontonasal prominence.

These important structures determine (**fusion and specialized growth**) the size and integrity of the mandible, upper lip, palate and nose.

Formation of the upper lip

Occurs by fusion of the two maxillary prominences with the two medial nasal prominences.

Intermaxillary segment is formed by merging of the two medial nasal prominences in the midline. This segment is composed of

- Philtrum
- Upper jaw component - carries the four incisor teeth
- Palatal component - forms the triangular primary palate

Nose is derived from

- Frontonasal prominence - forms the bridge
- Medial nasal prominences - provide the crest and tip
- Lateral nasal prominences - form the alae

Fusion of the palatal shelves (formed from maxillary prominences) creates the hard (secondary) and soft palate.

Cleft deformities may result from partial or incomplete fusion of these mesenchymal tissues. This may be caused by hereditary factors and drugs (**diphenylhydantoin**).

Adult face is influenced by development of

- Paranasal sinuses (PNS)
- Nasal conchae
- Teeth

DEVELOPMENT OF TEETH

Teeth develop from epithelial-mesenchymal interactions between oral epithelium and neural crest derived mesenchyme.

Enamel is made by ameloblasts. It lies on a thick layer of dentin produced by odontoblasts - neural crest derivative.

Cementum is formed by cementoblasts - mesenchymal derivative found in the root of the tooth.

First teeth (**deciduous or milk teeth**) appear 6 to 24 months after birth.

Definitive or **permanent** teeth (supplant milk teeth) are formed during third month of development.

Tooth Abnormalities

Teeth may be abnormal in number, shape, and size. These may be

- Discolored by foreign substances - **Tetracycline**
- Deficient in enamel - caused by vitamin D deficiency (rickets)

Many factors affect tooth development which include:

- Genetic factors
- Environmental influences

THE EAR

Ear has three parts which have different origins, but function as one unit.

INTERNAL EAR

It develops from the otic vesicle, which in the 4th week of development detaches from surface ectoderm. This vesicle is divided into

- **Ventral component** - Forms saccule and cochlear duct
- **Dorsal component** - Forms utricle, semicircular canals, and endolymphatic duct

The epithelial structures are collectively known as the membranous labyrinth.

Except for the cochlear duct (forms **organ of Corti**), all structures derived from the membranous labyrinth are involved with equilibrium.

MIDDLE EAR

It consists of the tympanic cavity and auditory tube. It is lined with epithelium of endodermal origin and is derived from the first pharyngeal pouch.

Auditory tube extends between the tympanic cavity and nasopharynx.

Ear ossicles (transfer sound from the tympanic membrane to the oval window) are derived from the first (malleus and incus) and second (stapes) pharyngeal arches.

External auditory meatus develops from the first pharyngeal cleft. It is separated from the tympanic cavity by the tympanic membrane (**ear drum**).

Eardrum consists of

- Ectodermal epithelial lining
- Intermediate layer of mesenchyme
- Endodermal lining from the first pharyngeal pouch

Auricle develops from six mesenchymal hillocks along the first and second pharyngeal arches.

Defects in the auricle are often associated with other congenital malformations.

DEVELOPMENT OF EYE

The eyes begin to develop as a pair of outpocketings which become the optic vesicles on each side of the forebrain at the end of the 4th week of development.

The optic vesicles contact the surface ectoderm and induce lens formation. When the optic vesicle begins to invaginate to form the pigment and neural layers of the retina, the lens placode invaginates to form the lens vesicle.

Through a groove at the inferior aspect of the optic vesicle, choroid fissure, hyaloid artery (later central artery of retina) enters the eye.

Nerve fibers of the eye also occupy this groove to reach the optic areas of the brain.

Cornea is formed by

- Layer of surface ectoderm
- Stroma - continuous with the sclera
- Epithelial layer bordering the anterior chamber

SKIN

The skin and its associated structures (hair, nails and glands) are derived from surface ectoderm.

Melanocytes (give skin colour) are derived from **neural crest cells,** which migrate into the epidermis. The production of new cells occurs in the **germinative** layer.

After moving to the surface, cells are sloughed off in the horny layer (stratum corneum).

Dermis - deep layer of the skin; derived from lateral plate mesoderm and from dermatomes of the somites.

Hairs develop from down-growth of epidermal cells into the underlying dermis. By about 20 weeks, the foetus is covered by downy hair (**lanugo hair**). These hairs are shed at the time of birth.

Sebaceous glands, sweat glands and **mammary glands** develop from epidermal proliferations.

Polythelia - Supernumerary nipples

Polymastia - Supernummary breasts

CENTRAL NERVOUS SYSTEM

The CNS originates in the ectoderm and appears as the neural plate at the middle of the third week.

After the edges of the plate fold, the neural folds approach each other in the midline to fuse into the neural tube. The cranial end closes approximately at 25th day, and the caudal end closes at 27th day. The CNS then forms a tubular structure with a broad cephalic portion, the brain, and a long caudal portion, the spinal cord.

Failure of the neural tube to close results in defects such as **spina bifida** and **anencephaly,** defects that can be prevented by folic acid.

Spinal cord forms the caudal end of the CNS. It is characterized by

- **Basal plate -** Contains motor neurons
- **Alar plate -** For sensory neurons
- **Floor plate** and **roof plate -** Connecting plates between the two sides

Brain forms the cranial part of the CNS. It consists originally of three vesicles

- Rhombencephalon (**hindbrain**)

- Mesencephalon (**midbrain**)
- Prosencephalon (**forebrain**)

Rhombencephalon is divided into

- **Myelencephalon** - forms the medulla oblongata (this region has a basal plate for somatic and visceral efferent neurons and an alar plate for somatic and visceral afferent neurons)
- **Metencephalon** with its typical basal (effer-ent) and alar (afferent) plates. This brain vesicle is also characterized by formation of the **Cerebellum** - coordination center for posture and movement and the **Pons** - pathway for nerve fibers between the spinal cord and the cerebral and the cerebellar cortices.

The mesencephalon (midbrain) resembles the spinal cord with its basal efferent and alar afferent plates. The mesencephalon's alar plates form the anterior and posterior colliculi as relay stations for visual and auditory reflex centers, respectively.

The diencephalon (posterior portion of the forebrain) consists of a thin roof plate and a thick alar plate in which the thalamus and hypothalamus de-velop. It participates in formation of the pituitary gland, which also develops from Rathke's pouch.

Rathke's pouch forms

- Adenohypophysis
- Intermediate lobe
- Pars tuberalis

Di-encephalon forms the posterior lobe – **neurohypophysis** - contains neuroglia and receives nerve fibers from the hypothalamus.

The telencephalon (most rostral of the brain vesicles) consists of two lateral outpocketings, the cerebral hemispheres, and a median portion, the lamina terminalis. The lamina terminalis is used by the commis-sures as a connection pathway for fiber bundles between the right and left hemispheres.

The cerebral hemispheres, originally two small out-pocketings, expand and cover the lateral aspect of the diencephalon, mesencephalon, and metencephalon. Eventually, nuclear regions of the telencephalon come in close contact with those of the diencephalon.

Ventricular system

It contains cerebrospinal fluid and extends from the lu-men in the spinal cord to the 4th ventricle in the rhombencephalon, through the narrow duct in the mesencephalon, and to the third ventricle in the dien-cephalon. By the interventricular foramen (of **Monro**) the ventricular system extends from the third ventricle into the lateral ventricles of the cerebral hemispheres.

Cerebrospinal fluid is produced in the choroid plexus of the 3rd, 4th and lateral ventricles. Blockage of cerebrospinal fluid in the ventricular system or subarachnoid space may lead to **hydrocephalus**.

FORMATION OF NEURAL TUBE

Development of CNS begins in the 3rd week of intrauterine life

Neural plate:

- It is a pear shaped thickening of ectoderm.
- It overlies the notochord and paraxial mesoderm.
- It is cranial to primitive streak.

Neural folds:

- These appear due to folding of neural tube along longitudinal axis.

Neural groove:

- Longitudinal depression enclosed by the neural folds.

Neural tube:

- It is formed with the fusion of neural folds.
- It presents cranial and caudal neural pores.
- These neural pores get closed to form a tube by the 5th week.

DIFFERENTIATION OF NEURAL TUBE AND ITS DEVELOPMENTAL COMPONENTS

Neural tube differentiates into:
- Caudal cylindrical part (future spinal cord)
- Cranial bulbous part (future forebrain, midbrain and hindbrain)

The cranial part shows three dilatations from cranial to caudal. These are:
- Prosencephalon: Forebrain.
- Mesencephalon: Midbrain.
- Rhombencephalon: Hindbrain.

Due to the appearance of the cranial and caudal folds of the embryo, two flexures appear in the neural tube:
- Cranial – Between mesencephalon and rhombencephalon.
- Caudal – Between rhombencephalon and spinal cord.

Cranial part of neural tube differentiates as:

Prosencephalon shows:
- Two lateral dilatations – Telencephalon (future cerebral hemispheres)
- Median part – Diencephalon (future thalamus)

Mesencephalon does not modify. It forms midbrain.

Rhombencephalon shows:
- Cranial dilated part – Metencephalon (**future pons & cerebellum**)
- Caudal narrow part – Myelencephalon (**future medulla**)

Cavities of the neural tube show changes as:
- Spinal cord – remains unchanged – central canal.
- Rhombencephalon – dilates – 4th ventricle
- Mesencephalon – remains unchanged – cerebral aqueduct
- Prosencephalon :
  - Diencephalon – 3rd ventricle
  - Telencephalon – enlarges – lateral ventricle

HISTOGENESIS OF NEURAL TUBE

The neural tube presents three layers from within out:
- Ependyma
- Mantle
- Marginal

Ependymal layer: It is made up of two types of cells.
- Epithelial cells (Pseudostratified)
- Stem cells (Progenitor cells –show mitosis)

Mantle layer: It comprises neuroblasts derived from the stem cells. It constitutes the grey matter.

Marginal layer: It contains nerve fibers of the neuroblasts. It forms the white matter.

DEVELOPMENT OF SPINAL CORD

The mantle layer proliferates and shows a longitudinal sulcus- Sulcus limitans on lateral side. The sulcus limitans divides the mantle layer into:
- **Ventral part**: Basal laminae
- **Dorsal part**: Alar laminae.

Basal laminae grow ventrolaterally; hence they do not fuse. This leads to appearance of ventral fissure of the spinal cord. Basal lamina contains motor neurons.

Alar laminae grow medially; hence they fuse. It accounts for posterior median septum of spinal cord. Alar laminae contain sensory neurons.

Central canal reduces due to overgrowing basal and alar laminae.

GROWTH OF SPINAL CORD

During the intrauterine life the growth of the spinal cord and vertebral column are identical. Therefore the spinal nerves are transversely placed.

The vertebral column grows faster; hence spinal cord falls short of vertebral column.

At birth, tip of the spinal cord corresponds to lower border of L3 vertebra. Thus:

- Upper nerves – horizontally placed.
- Middle nerves – obliquely placed.
- Lower nerves – vertically placed.

CONGENITAL ANOMALIES OF SPINAL CORD

Rachischisis: Failure of fusion of neural folds can be complete or incomplete.

- Complete failure of fusion results in non-formation of neural tube. The embryo is non-viable, hence is aborted.
- Partial closure of neural tube leads to:
  - Anencephaly (cranial part is affected)
  - Myelocoele (caudal part is involved)

Failure of closure of vertebral arch is termed spina bifida. In such a condition there is no intrinsic defect in the spinal cord, but it may present as:

- **Spina bifida oculta**: Only a layer of skin covers the spinal cord and its meninges.
- **Meningocoele**: Here meninges protrude through the deficient vertebral arch.
- **Meningomyelocoele**: Spinal cord together with meninges is seen protruding through the deficient vertebral arch.

DERIVATIVES OF NEURAL CREST CELLS

Neural crest cells are ectodermal cells placed on the summit of the neural folds.

With the formation of neural tube these cells get buried to form a sheet / lamina between the skin and the neural tube.

The lamina breaks into fragments termed ganglia.

These ganglia cells migrate and differentiate into:

- Dorsal root ganglia of spinal nerves.
- Ganglia functionally attached to the cranial nerves. These are :

1. **Gasserian ganglion**: Vth cranial nerve
2. **Geniculate ganglion**: VIIth cranial nerve
3. **Superior ganglion**: IXth cranial nerve
4. **Middle ganglion**: Xth cranial nerve
5. **Inferior ganglion**: XIth cranial nerve

- Leptomeninges (Arachnoid and pia mater)
- Cartilages of branchial arches
  1. Meckel's cartilage
  2. Reichart's cartilage
  3. Laryngeal cartilages
- Melanocytes
- Sympathetic ganglia
- Adrenal medulla
- Schwann cells
- Odontoblasts

MORPHOGENESIS OF RHOMBENCEPHALON

Cranial part of rhombencephalon is termed metencephalon. It gives rise to:

- **Pons** – from the ventral part.
- **Cerebellum** – from the dorsal part.

The caudal part is termed myelencephalon. It gives rise to medulla.

Features of myelencephalon show:

- Extent: From pontine flexure to first spinal nerve.
- Central canal:
  - Gets splayed
  - Encloses IVth ventricle
  - Causes spreading of basal and alar laminae
  - The two laminae show subdivisions. Craniocaudal extent of these subdivisions referred to as columns
  - In horizontal disposition, collection of neuron is termed nucleus /group.

Fate of basal lamina: It is divided into three groups. From medial to lateral they are:

- Somatic efferent
- Special visceral efferent
- General visceral efferent

Features of each group are as under:

Somatic efferent (SE):

- Close to midline
- Innervates somatic musculature.
- At this level forms hypoglossal nerve nucleus (corresponding to hypoglossal triangle in floor of IVth ventricle.
- To supply muscles of tongue (derived from occipital myotomes)

Special visceral efferent / Branchial efferent : (SVE / BE)

- Lateral to somatic efferent.
- Innervates skeletal muscles (derived from branchial arches).
- At this level it forms nucleus ambiguous, which is functionally connected with 9th, 10th, and 11th cranial nerves.
- To supply the muscles of the larynx and pharynx.

General visceral efferent (GVE)

- Lateral most column of the basal lamina.
- Innervates glands (including salivary glands) and smooth muscles of respiratory gastrointestinal and cardiovascular systems.
- At this level it forms the dorsal nucleus of vagus.

Fate of alar lamina: It is divided into three groups that are mirror image of basal lamina. The fourth group is the lateral most. From medial to lateral, these are:

- General visceral afferent.
- Special visceral afferent.
- Somatic afferent.

- Special somatic afferent.

Features of each group are as under:

General visceral afferent (GVA)

- It is immediately lateral to sulcus limitans.
- It receives enteroceptive impulses.
- At this level with GVE group it forms dorsal nucleus of vagus (corresponding to vagal triangle in the floor of IVth ventricle). This nucleus is a fusion of afferent and efferent groups. Thus it has smaller sensory neurons and bigger motor neurons.

Special visceral afferent (SVA)

- It receives taste sensation from tongue and palate through 7th, 9th and 10th cranial nerves.
- At this level it forms nucleus of tractus solitarius. It lies ventrolateral to dorsal nucleus of vagus.

Somatic afferent (SA)

- It receives exteroceptive (Pain and temperature) impulses from head and face region. These impulses are carried in trigeminal (5th cranial) nerve.
- At this level it forms spinal nucleus of trigeminal nerve, which is placed ventrolateral to nucleus of tractus solitarius.

Special somatic afferent (SSA)

- It is associated with hearing and balance (**statoacoustic**). The impulses are carried in 8th cranial nerve.
- At this level it forms cochlear nuclei and vestibular nuclei and (corresponding to vestibular area in the floor of the IVth ventricle).

NEUROBIOTAXIS

The position of various nuclei indicates that their relative positions are not fixed. This active process of migration of cells / nucleus towards the source of a stimulus is termed Neurobiotaxis.

E.g., The shift of the motor nucleus of trigeminal nerve towards its sensory nucleus

MORPHOGENESIS OF VENTRAL PART OF METENCEPHALON

The features of metencephalon are ventral and dorsal parts, which give rise to pons and cerebellum respectively.

Fate of basal lamina:

Somatic efferent (SE)

- Medial most group close to midline.
- At this level forms abducent nerve nucleus, this is seen as facial colliculus in the floor of IVth ventricle. (The elevation is caused by the fibers of facial nerve surrounding the nucleus of abducent nerve.)

Special visceral efferent / Branchial efferent (SVE/BE)

- Innervates skeletal muscles derived from 1st and 2nd branchial arch.
- At this level forms motor nucleus of facial nerve and motor nucleus of trigeminal nerve.
- These are placed ventrolateral to the somatic efferent group.

General visceral efferent (GVE)

- It lies dorsolateral to branchial efferent group.
- It supplies nasal, lacrimal, pharyngeal and palatine glands through pterygopalatine ganglion.
- At this level forms lacrimatory nucleus (in upper part of pons), superior salivatory nucleus (in upper part of pons) and inferior salivatory nucleus (in lower part of pons).
- These nuclei are one below another.

Fate of alar lamina: The features of each group from medial lateral are as follows:

General visceral afferent (GVA)

- Absent as a separate entity.
- Merges with the dorsal nucleus of vagus

Special visceral afferent (SVA)

- Constitutes the cranial part of nucleus of tractus solitarius.

Somatic afferent (SA)

- At this level it forms main sensory nucleus of trigeminal nerve.
- It receives impulses for discrimination of touch from head and face.

Special somatic afferent (SSA)

- At this level it forms the vestibular nuclei (superior and medial), which appear in the lateral part of floor of IVth ventricle.

MORPHOGENESIS OF CEREBELLUM

Rhombic lip

From the dorsal part of metencephalon or roof plate rhombic lips arise from both the sides. They advance medialwords.

Cerebellar plate

It is formed by the fusion of the two rhombic lips. It grows and the transverse fissure divides it into:
- Flocculonodular lobe
- Corpus cerebelli
  - Vermis –median part
  - Cerebellar hemispheres- lateral part

Morphogenesis

The different layers of cerebellum start appearing in a sequential manner from the basic three layers of the neural tube.
- Molecular layer: It is formed from migration of cells of mantle layer into the marginal layer.

- Purkinje cell layer: Cells from mantle layer migrate and form this layer.
- Granular layer: These cells are also derived from migration of cells from mantle layer.
- Cerebellar nuclei: The various nuclei are formed from the differentiation of cells of mantle layer.

Laminae - They accommodate increasing cellular population. Thus, the outer layer gets folded. These folds appear like small leaves.

Medullary velum: A thinned out portion of the roof plate devoid of grey matter is termed the medullary velum.

MORPHOGENESIS OF MESENCEPHALON

The three layers of the mesencephalon show changes as under:

- **Ependymal layer** lines the cerebral aqueduct.
- **Mantle & marginal layers** together constitute:
  - Tegmentum in the ventral part
  - Tectum in the dorsal part

Alar lamina appears as raised eminences divided by a transverse sulcus into:

- Superior colliculi
- Inferior colliculi

The fate of basal lamina and alar lamina differs at the two levels as under:

AT SUPERIOR COLLICULUS:

Fate of basal lamina:

Somatic efferent

- It forms the medial-most group.
- At this level it forms motor nucleus of oculomotor nerve.

Special visceral efferent

- There is no representation of this group at this level.

General visceral efferent

- At this level it forms Edinger Westphal nucleus of oculomotor nerve.
- It issues preganglionic parasympathetic impulses for ciliary ganglion to innervate constrictor pupillae muscle.

Fate of alar lamina:

General visceral afferent & special visceral afferent:

- Have no representation at this level.

Somatic afferent

- It is placed along the lateral wall of cerebral aqueduct.
- At this level it forms mesencephalic nucleus of trigeminal nerve.
- It receives proprioceptive impulses from gums, teeth and muscles of mastication, face and eye.

Special somatic afferent

- At this level this group shows migration of cells which settle to form the following:
  - Nucleus of superior colliculus
  - Red nucleus.
  - Substantia nigra.

Marginal layer at the superior colliculus level forms the crus cerebri.

AT INFERIOR COLLICULUS LEVEL:

Fate of basal lamina:

Somatic efferent

- It forms the medial-most group.
- At this level it forms trochlear nerve nucleus.

Special visceral efferent & general visceral efferent

- These groups have no representation at this level.

Fate of alar lamina:

General visceral afferent, special visceral afferent & somatic afferent have no representation at this level.

Special somatic afferent

- Cells from this group migrate to form:
  - Nucleus of inferior colliculus
  - Substantia nigra.

Marginal layer at the level of inferior colliculus level forms:

- Crus cerebri
- Decussation of superior cerebellar peduncle
- Rubrospinal tract.

MORPHOGENESIS OF PROSENCEPHALON

The two components of prosencephalon give rise to the following:

- **Diencephalon** – forms thalamus and hypothalamus.
- **Telencephalon** – forms cerebral hemispheres and corpus striatum.

MORPHOGENESIS & FEATURES OF DIENCEPHALON

The diencephalon encloses the cavity of third ventricle.

Its lateral wall presents hypothalamic sulcus that divides the diencephalon into thalamus and hypothalamus.

Interthalamic adhesion (grey matter + bundle of fibers) is seen along the lateral wall.

Basal lamina is absent.

In relation to the diencephalon, the boundaries of third ventricle present:

- Roof plate
- Lateral walls (alar lamina of diencephalon)
- Floor

The features of these components of diencephalon (which explain the gross anatomical features) are as under:

- Roof plate
  - Choroid fissure with choroids plexus.
- **Anterior boundary** from above downwards.
  - Interventricular foramen of Monro.
  - Anterior column of fornix.
  - Anterior commissure
  - Lamina terminalis
  - Optic chiasma.
- **Floor** presents the following landmarks from anterior to posterior:
  - Infundibulum.
  - Tuber cinerium
  - Mamillary bodies
  - Crus cerebri
- **Posterior wall** presents from anterior to posterior:
  - Cerebral aqueduct
  - Pineal body
  - Posterior commissure

MORPHOGENESIS & FEATURES OF TELENCEPHALON

Lateral outpouching of the prosencephalon encloses the cavity of lateral ventricle while its wall forms cerebral cortex. (Telencephalon = cerebral cortex +corpus striatum.)

The wall of telencephalon is lined by the three layers, i.e.,

- Ependyma
- Mantle
- Marginal

This arrangement constitutes the paleocortex

Ependymal layer

- Part of medial wall of telencephalon, which is close to the roof plate of diencephalon, gets thinned out.
- Thinned out part of the wall encloses a tuft of capillaries within the pia mater. These form the choroid plexus.
- The choroid plexus invaginates into the cavity of lateral ventricle along the choroid fissure (seen above the thalamus and below the fornix).

Mantle layer

- The fate of mantle layer is different on medial and lateral aspect (base of the lateral ventricle).
- At the level of interventricular foramen the mantle layer proliferates to form layers of cells giving it a striated appearance termed corpus striatum.
- The cells of mantle layer along the remaining walls of lateral ventricle (Medial, superior, lateral) migrate in succession towards the marginal layer Thus, neopallium is formed.

Marginal layer

- The axons of cells of the mantle layer from frontal and parietal lobes pass as ascending and descending fibers.
- These fibers pass through the developing corpus striatum to divide it into caudate nucleus and lentiform nucleus.
- The collection of ascending and descending fibers between the thalamus, caudate nucleus and lentiform nucleus constitute the internal capsule.
- To understand the formation of posterior limb of internal capsule, a coronal section is to be taken passing through the third ventricle and middle of lateral ventricle. It illustrates the mantle and marginal layers of the diencephalon and the mantle and marginal layers along the medial surface of telencephalon coming closer.
- There is collection of marginal layers of the telencephalon and the diencephalon sandwiched between mantle layers of diencephalon (thalamus and hypothalamus) medially and of telencephalon (corpus striatum) laterally.

FORMATION OF INSULA & POSTERIOR RAMUS OF LATERAL SULCUS

- The cerebral hemispheres are expanding posteriorly and cover the diencephalon, mesencephalon and part of metencephalon.
- The continuous growth leads to formation of various lobes i.e. frontal, temporal and occipital.
- Part of the cerebral hemisphere lateral to corpus striatum is termed insula.
- Since the growth is slow in insular cortex than the neighbouring part, it gets buried between the overgrowing temporal and frontal lobes.
- This process forms posterior ramus of lateral sulcus wherein temporal and the frontal cortices form the lid (operculum) in the depth of which is the insular cortex.

FORMATION OF SULCI AND GYRI

- The growth of cerebral hemisphere is rapid. Hence in the limited available space it gets accommodated by getting folded.
- The depressions are termed as sulci and the raised areas between the sulci are termed gyri.
- The complete sulci are the deep sulci that cause indentation on the wall of lateral ventricle.

- Axial sulci are formed along the axis of the growth of cerebral hemisphere.

FORMATION OF CEREBRAL CORTEX

Allover, the cerebral cortex initially has three layers, i.e.

- Ependyma
- Mantle
- Marginal.

It is termed pallium

These three layers are retained immediately lateral to the corpus striatum termed as paleopallium. Here, from the mantle layer cells migrate to the marginal layer yet retaining the composition of the three layers. Thus hippocampal gyrus / limbic cortex is formed.

Rest of the cerebral hemisphere is called neopallium.

From mantle layer, cells migrate in successive waves and settle down at particular levels. These constitute six layered cortex.

The differentiation of cells occurs after the migration. Thus Betz cells, granular cells, pyramidal cells are formed.

FORMATION OF PHARYNGEAL CLEFTS, POUCHES & ARCHES

Cranial-most part of foregut is termed pharyngeal gut.

Buccopharyngeal membrane separates the pharyngeal gut from the stomodeum (future opening of oral cavity).

Buccopharyngeal membrane (BPM) ruptures and it corresponds to the future gum-line. Behind this line is endoderm while in front of it including the gums is lined by ectoderm.

Pharyngeal pouches are endodermal outpouchings from the lateral wall of pharyngeal gut.

Pharyngeal clefts are ectodermal invaginations towards the pharyngeal pouches from the external surface of the lateral wall of pharyngeal gut.

Pharyngeal arches are the mesodermal collections between ectoderm and endoderm of pharyngeal gut.

FATE OF PHARYNGEAL POUCHES

There are four pharyngeal pouches (fifth pouch is a part of fourth pouch). These are placed along the lateral wall of the foregut.

Each pouch has a ventral and dorsal part.

Ventral part of first and second pouch gets obliterated by the developing tongue.

Fate of first pharyngeal pouch:

- The pouch extends to reach the first cleft separated by a sheet of mesoderm.
- Ventral part gets obliterated by the developing tongue.
- Dorsal part elongates.
  - Its proximal narrow portion gives rise to the auditory tube / Eustachian tube.
  - Its distal dilated portion forms the middle ear.

Fate of second pharyngeal pouch:

- Ventral part gets obliterated by the developing tongue.
- Dorsal part thickens and is infiltrated with lymphoid tissue. Its endoderm and the lymphoid tissue give rise to palatine tonsil.

Fate of third pharyngeal pouch:

- Ventral part proliferates to form the primordium of thymus.
- Dorsal part differentiates to form the parathyroid.
- The communication of the thymic and the parathyroid primordia with the pharyngeal wall gets obliterated as these primordia enlarge.

DEVELOPMENT OF THYMUS

- Ventral parts of third pharyngeal pouches proliferate to form the primordia of thymus.
- The thymic primordia migrate downwards and anteriorly towards the thorax.

- The right and left thymic primordia fuse with each other in front of the foregut to form the thymus.
- The tail of the migrating thymic primordium may get caught during its descent. Thus accessory / aberrant thymic tissue may be seen in the lateral wall of the neck.

DEVELOPMENT OF PARATHYROID

Developmentally parathyroids are formed in two sets.

- Superior parathyroids derived from fourth pharyngeal pouch.
- Inferior parathyroids derived from third pharyngeal pouch.

They are differentiated from dorsal part of respective pouches.

The parathyroid primordia migrate caudally along with the thymic primordia.

The parathyroid primordia settle on the posterior aspect of the thyroid gland. Thus:

- Superior parathyroid: from fourth pouch.
- Inferior parathyroid: from third pouch.

The parathyroid primordia lose connection with the pharyngeal gut.

FATE OF FOURTH PHARYNGEAL POUCH

- Ventral part may give rise to thymus.
- Dorsal part proliferates, migrates down to settle on upper part of posterior surface of the lateral lobe of thyroid (superior parathyroid).

FATE OF FIFTH PHARYNGEAL POUCH

- The fifth pouch is not a separate entity.
- It is a part of the fourth pouch.
- It is termed Ultimo-branchial body.
- Its cells proliferate and infiltrate the thyroid tissue.

- It forms the parafollicular cells / clear cells of the thyroid gland.

FATE OF PHARYNGEAL CLEFTS

Out of the four pharyngeal clefts only first persists.

Second, third and fourth clefts get submerged by the overgrowing mesoderm of the second arch.

Fate of first pharyngeal cleft:

- The first cleft advances towards the first pouch.
- Its proximal narrow part forms external acoustic meatus.
- Its distal dilated part meets the first pouch with a thin layer of mesoderm in between.
- This forms the tympanic membrane (which is lined by endoderm and ectoderm on internal and external surfaces).

CONGENITAL ANOMALIES OF PHARYNGEAL CLEFTS / POUCHES

Lateral cervical sinus

Persistence of second, third and fourth pharyngeal clefts may remain submerged in the neck or may communicate with the exterior – **External cervical fistula**. The opening of external cervical fistula is always in front of sternocleidomastoid.

Internal cervical fistula – Second, third and fourth pharyngeal clefts may persist and communicate with the floor of second pouch.

DEVELOPMENT OF TONGUE

The mesoderm of first arch enlarges to form:

- Two lateral lingual swellings.
- A median swelling – Tuberculum impar

The second median swelling behind the tuberculum impar appears – termed as hypobranchial eminence or cupula of His. This is formed by mesoderm of second, third and ventral part of fourth arch.

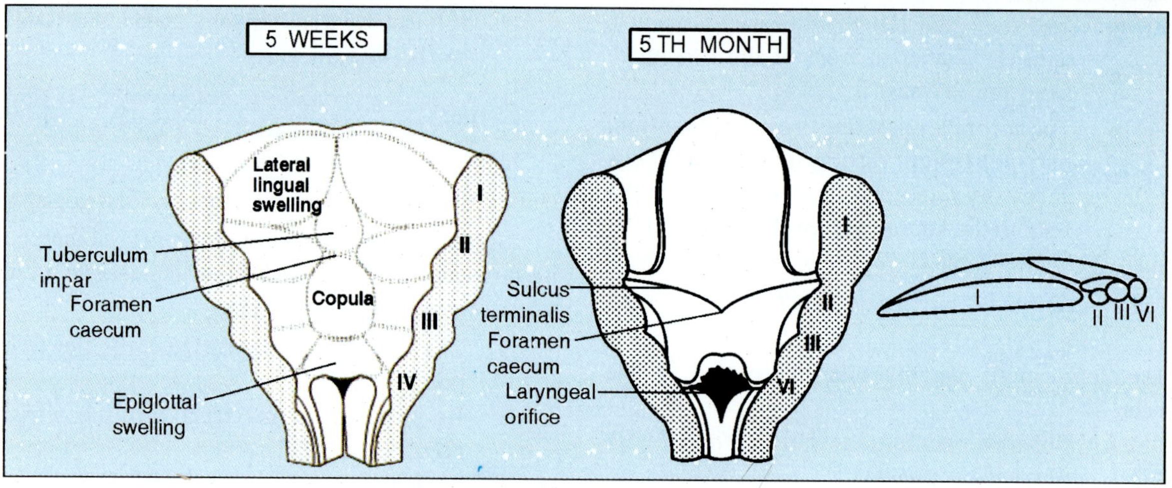

Fig. 79.1: Development of Tongue

The third median swelling appears behind the cupula – termed epiglottic swelling. It is formed by dorsal part of fourth arch.

Behind the epiglottic swelling appears the tracheobronchial groove, which is bounded by arytenoid swellings on the side.

Anterior two third of the tongue develops in a sequence:

- Lateral lingual swellings enlarge and fuse with each other.
- As these swellings grow, the tuberculum impar gets buried.
- Lateral to the lateral lingual swellings, linguo-gingival sulcus / groove appears.
- This sulcus deepens to separate the tongue from the floor of mouth.

Posterior one third of tongue: Develops as under:

- In the hypobranchial eminence, the mesoderm of third arch overgrows the mesoderm of second arch. Thereby second arch gets submerged.
- Thus the posterior one third of tongue develops from third arch.

Posterior-most part of the tongue develops from the ventral part of the fourth pharyngeal arch.

The epiglottis develops from dorsal part of the fourth arch.

Demarches of the tongue

Sulcus terminalis

- It is an inverted V shaped sulcus with apex directed posteriorly.
- It demarcates the anterior two third from the posterior one third of the tongue.

Foramen caecum

- It is a blind foramen seen at apex of the sulcus terminalis. Its endodermal lining forms the thyroid primordium.

Transverse sulcus

- It is placed behind the cupula and separates epiglottis from the posterior one third of the tongue.

Developmental components or parts of the tongue

The tongue is marked by:

- Epithelium
- Connective tissue
- Muscles

Epithelium

The mucosa of tongue is endodermal and differs in its origin in the anterior two third, posterior one third and the posterior-most part of the tongue.

Anterior two third of tongue

- The lining epithelium is derived from the endoderm overlying the first pharyngeal arch.
- It is supplied by:
  - Lingual nerve (general sensation)
  - Chorda tympani (taste sensation)

Posterior one third of tongue

- The lining epithelium is derived from the third pharyngeal arch.
- Mucosa of posterior one third of tongue including the circumvallate papillae is supplied by glossopharyngeal nerve (General and taste sensation)

Posterior-most part of tongue

- The epithelium is derived from endoderm overlying the fourth arch.
- It is supplied by internal laryngeal branch of vagus.

Connective tissue

- It is derived from the mesoderm of all the arches perhaps maximum from the second submerged pharyngeal arch.

Muscles

- The extrinsic and intrinsic muscles of the tongue are derived from occipital myotomes, which have migrated ventrally to reach and settle in the floor of mouth.
- This view explains the motor innervation of the tongue (Hypoglossal nerve)
- The other view is that all the muscles develop in situ to form the tongue.

DEVELOPMENT OF THYROID GLAND

- Thyroid primordium appears at the floor of foramen caecum as proliferation of endoderm.

- It invades the mesenchyme of the developing tongue.
- It descends in front of the hyoid bone and laryngeal cartilages to reach upper part of trachea.
- Its distal end enlarges to form the isthmus and the lateral lobes.
- The thyroid primordium is connected to the foramen caecum by thyroglossal duct.
- This duct regresses and is termed as levator glandulae thyroidae.

Anomalies of thyroid gland

Aberrant / ectopic thyroid

- Thyroid tissue found in tongue is termed lingual thyroid.
- It may also be found near hyoid bone and in superior mediastinum.

Thyroglossal cyst

A cyst may be found anywhere along the course of the thyroglossal duct. Hence thyroglossal cyst may be seen in relation to:

- Tongue
- Hyoid bone: Above, in front or behind the body
- In front of larynx

FATE OF PHARYNGEAL ARCHES

Each pharyngeal arch has following components:

- Cartilage
- Muscle
- Nerve
- Artery

Fate of cartilages:

- May get converted into bone or persist as ligament / cartilage.

Fate of muscles:

- All muscles derived from arches are skeletal muscles.

- These muscles migrate and settle in definite regions.
- During the course of migration these muscles drag their nerve supply.

Fate of nerves:
- Each arch has two nerves.
- These nerves arise from the brainstem.
- These nerves are related to the pharyngeal clefts, hence termed as pretrematic and post-trematic (trema = cleft) nerves.

Features of post-trematic nerve:
- It is a motor nerve.
- It runs along the upper border of an arch.

Features of pretrematic nerve:
- It is sensory nerve.
- It is placed along the lower border of arch.

DERIVATIVES OF 1st PHARYNGEAL ARCH

This can be traced under the following heads:
- Cartilage
- Muscles
- Nerve

Fate of cartilage of first arch:
- The first arch cartilage comprises dorsal part (Palato-pterygoquadrate bar) and ventral part (Meckel's cartilage).

Derivatives of dorsal part or PP bar:
- Maxilla
- Incus
- Greater wing of sphenoid

Derivatives of ventral part or Meckel's cartilage:
- Malleus
- Anterior ligament of Malleus
- Stylomandibular ligament
- Lingula of mandible
- Genial tubercles

Muscles derived from the first arch:
- Muscles of mastication.
  - Medial and lateral pterygoid muscles
  - Temporalis
  - Masseter
- Anterior belly of digastric
- Tensor tympani
- Tensor palati

The nerves of the first arch:
- Post-trematic (Motor) nerve is mandibular nerve. It supplies all the muscles derived from the first arch.
- Pretrematic (sensory) nerve is chorda tympani branch of facial nerve. It carries taste sensation from anterior two third of the tongue. The fibers run with the lingual nerve.

DERIVATIVES OF 2nd PHARYNGEAL ARCH

It is termed as Hyoid arch:

It also presents dorsal and ventral parts.

Dorsal part gives rise to:
- Stapes
- Styloid process
- Styloid ligament

Ventral part gives rise to:
- Lesser cornu of hyoid bone
- Upper half of body of hyoid bone

Muscles derived from the second arch are:
- Muscles of facial expression (Mimetic group of muscles including occipito-frontalis)
- Buccinator
- Platysma
- Posterior belly of digastric
- Stylohyoid
- Stapedius

Nerves of the second arch are:

- Post-trematic (motor) nerve is facial nerve. It supplies all the muscles derived from the second arch.
- Pretrematic (sensory) nerve is **Jacobson's nerve** - branch of glossopharyngeal nerve. It carries preganglionic parasympathetic fibers for the parotid gland.

DERIVATIVES OF 3rd PHARYNGEAL ARCH

Cartilage gives rise to:

- Greater cornu of hyoid bone.
- Lower half of body of hyoid bone.

Muscles derived are:

- Stylopharyngeus is the only muscle.

The nerves of the third arch are:

- Post-trematic (motor) nerve is glosso-pharyngeal nerve. It supplies only one muscle i.e. stylopharyngeus.
- Pretrematic (sensory) nerve is the Arnold's nerve - branch of vagus nerve. It is for sensory innervation of external acoustic meatus including tympanic membrane.

DERIVATIVES OF 4th PHARYNGEAL ARCH

Cartilage gives rise to:

- Thyroid cartilage.
- Arytenoid cartilages.
- Corniculate cartilages.
- Cuneiform cartilages.

Muscles derived are:

- Cricothyroid.
- Constrictors of pharynx.
- Levator palati.

Nerves of the fourth arch are:

- Post-trematic (motor) nerve is external laryngeal branch of vagus. It supplies all

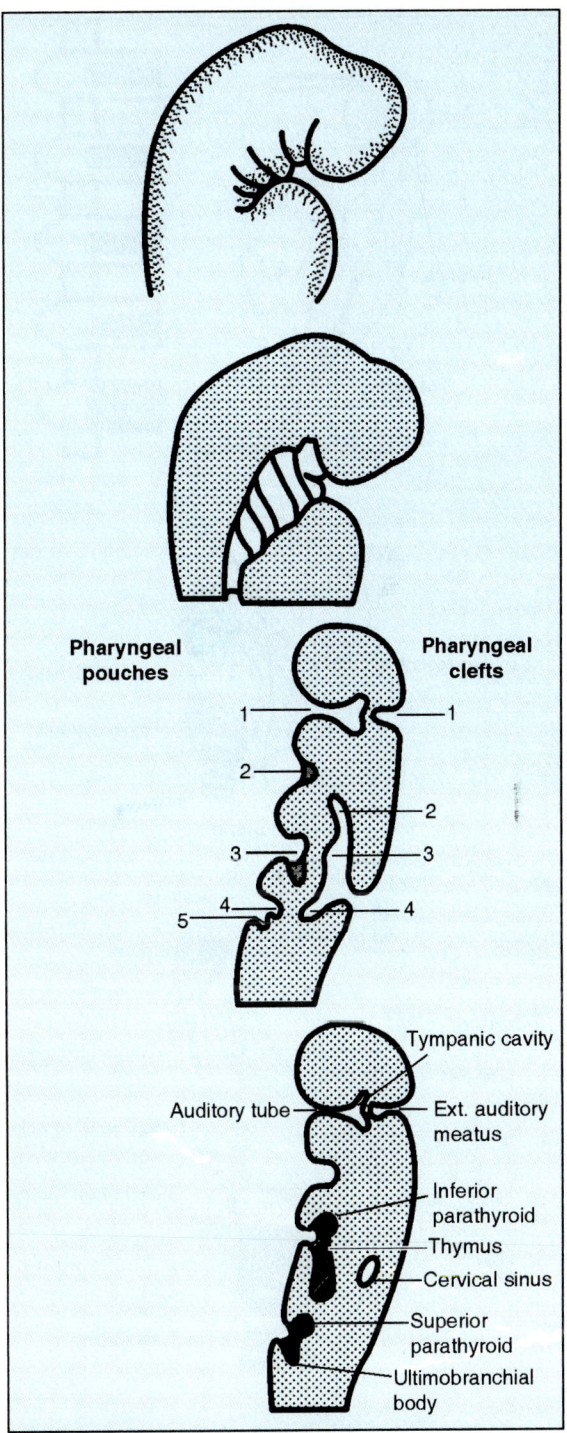

Fig. 79.2: Pharyngeal arches

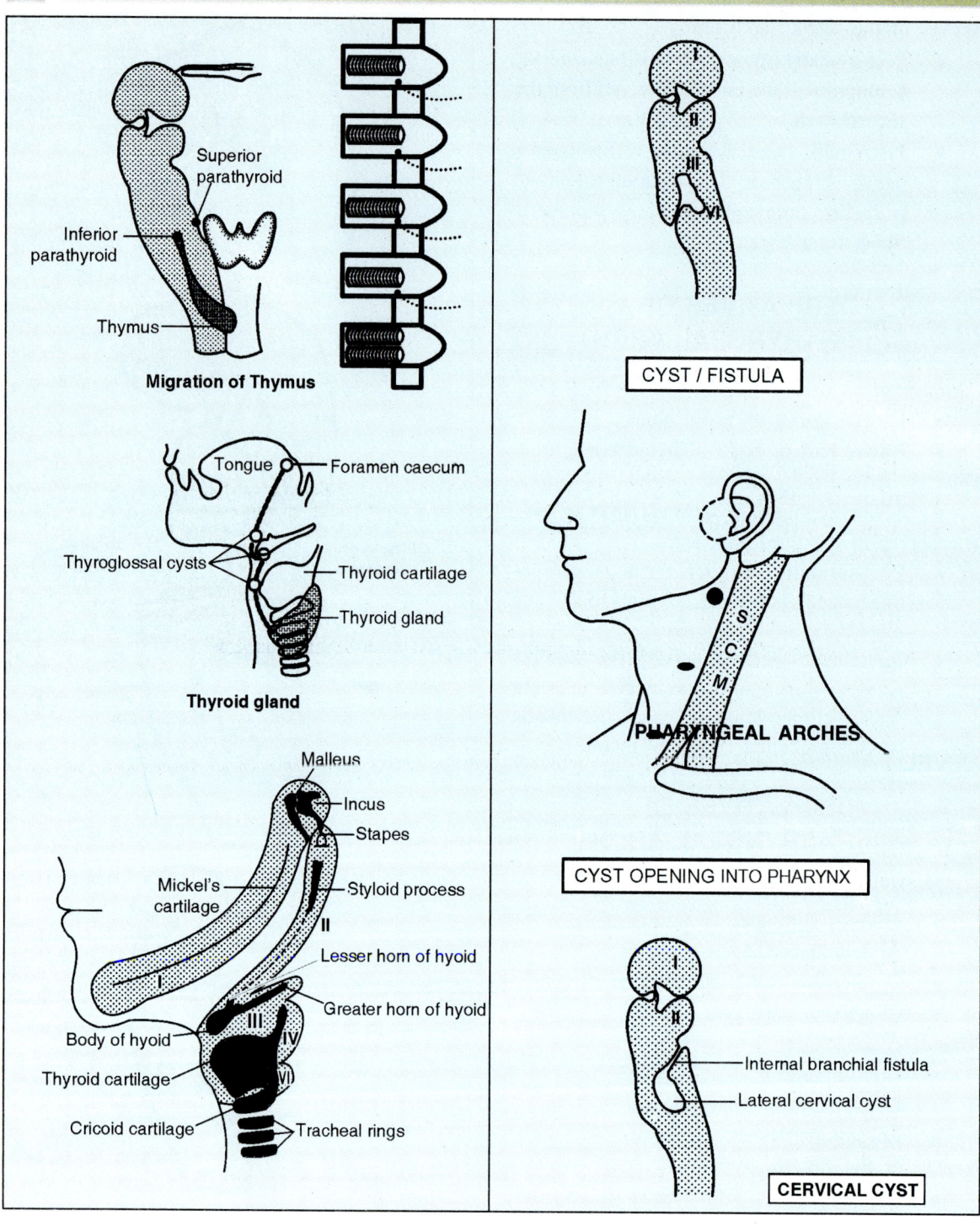

Fig. 79.3: Pharyngeal arches

Fig. 79.4: Derivatives of Pharyngeal arches

the muscles derived from the fourth arch.

- Pretrematic (sensory) nerve is internal laryngeal branch of vagus, which supplies the mucosa of the laryngopharynx uptill the vocal cords.

DERIVATIVES OF 6th PHARYNGEAL ARCH

The sixth arch gives rise to:
- Cricoid cartilage.

Muscles derived from the sixth arch are all the intrinsic muscles of the larynx (Except cricothyroid) that move the vocal cords namely:
- Adductors: Lateral cricoarytenoids
  Transverse and oblique interarytenoid
- Abductors: Posterior cricoarytenoid
- Tensors: Thyroarytenoid

Nerves of sixth arch are:
- Post-trematic (motor) nerve is recurrent laryngeal nerve. It supplies all the intrinsic muscles of larynx (Except cricothyroid).
- There is no pretrematic (sensory) nerve derived from this arch.

DEVELOPMENT OF FACE

The stomodeum is surrounded by different swellings of the first arch.

These swellings are in relation to the stomodeum.
- Caudally: Right and left mandibular swellings.
- Laterally: Right and left maxillary swellings.
- Cranially: Frontal prominence.

In the frontal prominence following features appear:
- Ectodermal thickenings – termed nasal placodes.
- Nasal placodes deepen to form nasal pits.
- Each nasal pit is surrounded by:
  – Lateral and medial nasal swellings

Each maxillary swelling advances medially resulting in:

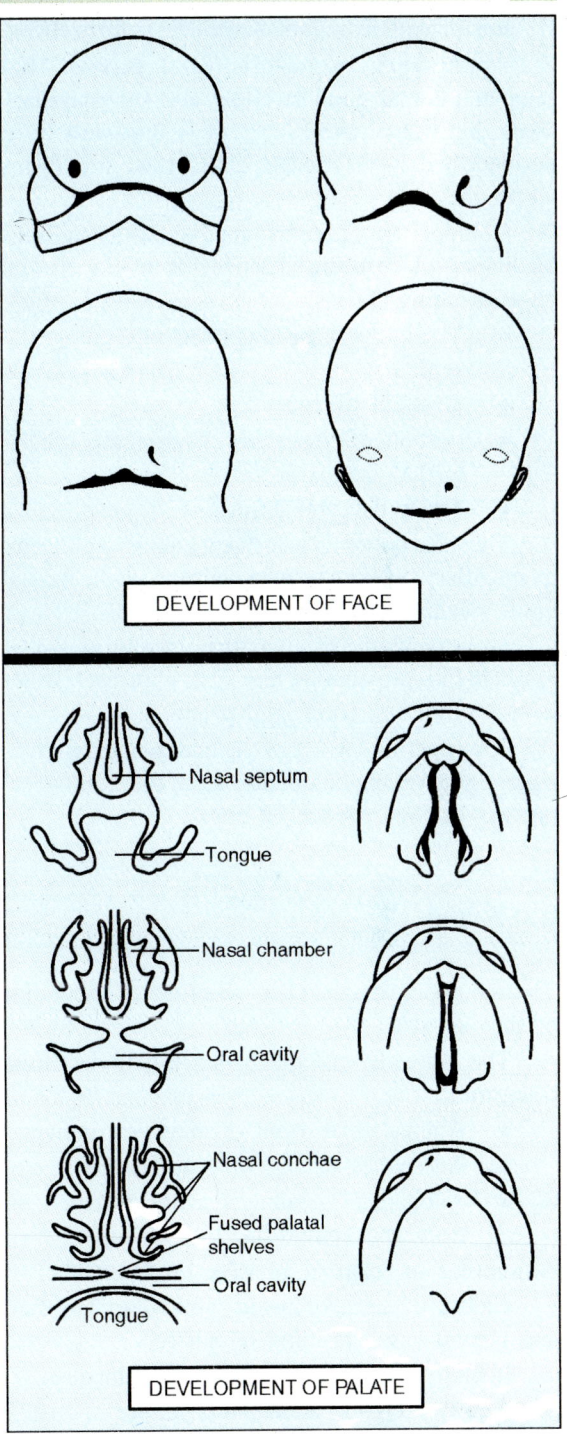

DEVELOPMENT OF FACE

Nasal septum
Tongue
Nasal chamber
Oral cavity
Nasal conchae
Fused palatal shelves
Oral cavity
Tongue

DEVELOPMENT OF PALATE

Fig. 79.5

Fusion with mandibular swelling to form cheek.

Appearance of nasolacrimal groove that separates lateral nasal swelling and the maxillary swelling. This groove gets converted into nasolacrimal duct. (The lateral nasal swelling forms ala of the nose.)

Compression of the two medial nasal swellings leading to their fusion. This fusion of the medial nasal swellings forms:

- Medial part of the nose excluding the septum.
- Philtrum of upper lip.
- Portion of upper jaw having the incisor teeth.
- Triangular premaxilla.

Thus, the upper lip is formed, lateral to philtrum by maxillary swelling and the philtrum by the medial nasal swelling.

In the depth the two maxillary swellings appear as shelf-like projections that fuse with each other in the midline to form hard palate.

The superior surface of the hard palate receives a globular swelling descending from the frontonasal process to form septum of nose.

CONGENITAL ANOMALIES OF FACE & PALATE

The anomalies of palate may manifest as anomalies of face as well.

The anomalies of the palate fall under three categories:

- Anomalies in front of incisive foramen.
- Anomalies behind incisive foramen.
- Anomalies including incisive foramen, in front and behind it.

Anomalies in front of incisive foramen are:

Cleft lip: Failure of fusion of maxillary swelling and medial nasal swelling on surface

It may be unilateral or bilateral (**Harelip**).

Anterior cleft jaw: There is failure of fusion of premaxilla (medial nasal swellings) and the palatine process of maxillary swelling(s).

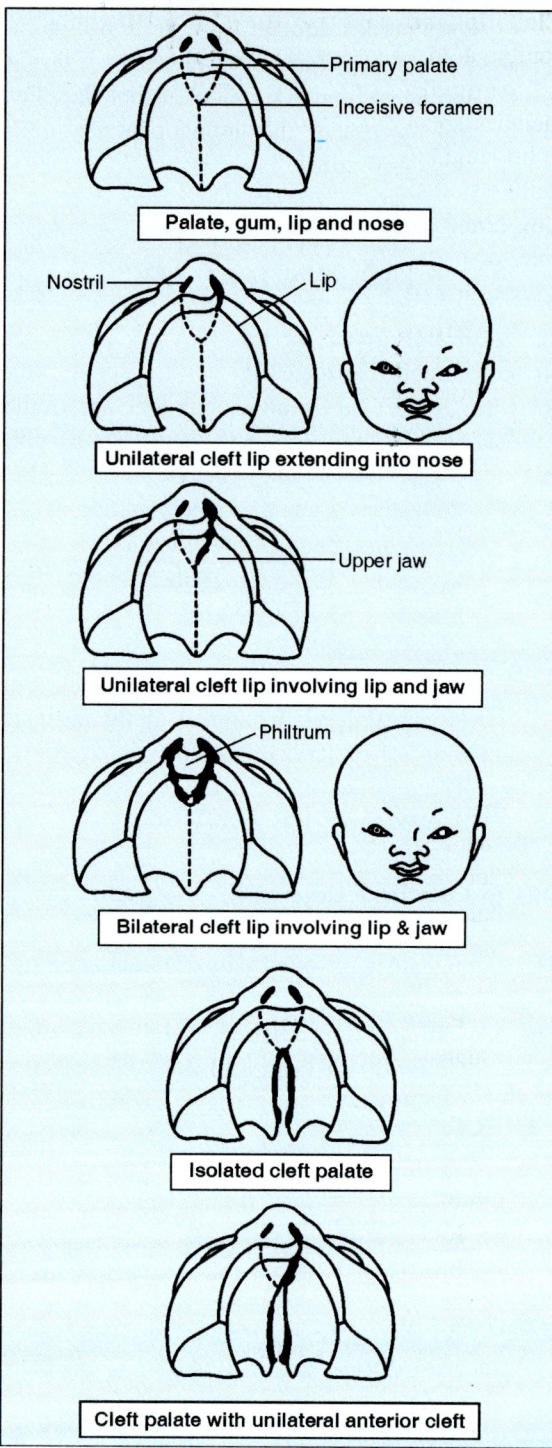

Primary palate
Inceisive foramen

Palate, gum, lip and nose

Nostril — Lip

Unilateral cleft lip extending into nose

Upper jaw

Unilateral cleft lip involving lip and jaw

Philtrum

Bilateral cleft lip involving lip & jaw

Isolated cleft palate

Cleft palate with unilateral anterior cleft

Fig. 79.6

Cleft lip and anterior cleft jaw: Here there is combination of cleft lip and anterior cleft jaw.

Anomalies behind incisive foramen: This includes isolated cleft palate. There is failure of fusion of horizontal (Palatine) plate of maxillary swelling. Failure of fusion could be of varying degrees.

Combined anomalies: Cleft palate with unilateral anterior cleft jaw and cleft lip.

Anomalies of face include:
- **Microstoma:** There is excessive fusion between maxillary and mandibular swellings.
- **Macrostoma:** Partial fusion between maxillary swelling and mandibular swelling.
- **Median cleft lip**: Failure of complete fusion of medial nasal swellings with each other.

FEATURES OF ANOMALIES OF FACE AND PALATE

These anomalies are compatible with life.

There is proved genetic bearing for some of these anomalies.

Cleft lips are more common (1 in 1000 births).

Males are more commonly affected.

The incidence of cleft lip increases with:
- Maternal age
- Parity

Cleft palate is common in females (**1 in 2500 births**)

DEVELOPMENT OF PITUITARY

The pituitary develops from two components:
- Rathke's pouch
- Infundibulum

Rathke's pouch

Cranial-ward ectodermal outpouching is seen
- From the roof of the stomodeum
- In front of the buccopharyngeal membrane
- Termed Rathke's pouch.

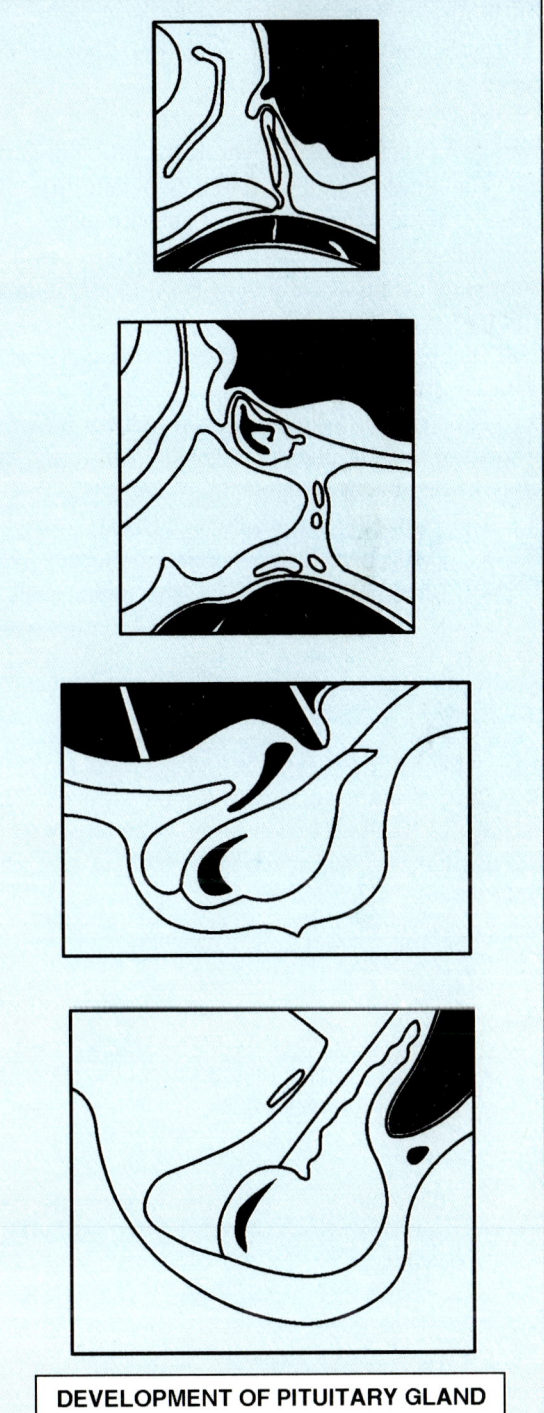

DEVELOPMENT OF PITUITARY GLAND

Fig. 79.7

Infundibulum

A downward growth seen from the floor of the diencephalon

The process of differentiation begins as the Rathke's pouch ascends towards the infundibulum.

The anterior wall of Rathke's pouch differentiates to form – pars anterior or anterior lobe.

The upward extension of Rathke's pouch surrounds the proximal part of the infundibulum to form pars tuberalis.

The posterior wall of Rathke's pouch forms pars intermedia.

The lumen of Rathke's pouch reduces with the growth of the adjoining components and forms the cleft in the anterior pituitary.

The infundibulum differentiates as:

- Distal part forms – Posterior lobe.
- Proximal part forms – The neural stalk.
- Neuroglial cells differentiate into pituicytes.

Anomalies associated with development of pituitary.

Craniopharyngeal tumour

It is seen in association with Rathke's pouch. The passage of Rathke's pouch forms craniopharyngeal canal which is at times seen in the body of sphenoid bone.

DEVELOPMENT OF EYE

Optic grooves

- Appear as two lateral outpouchings from the forebrain vesicle.

Optic vesicle

- With the closure of the neural tube the optic grooves are converted into optic vesicles.

Lens placode

- The surface ectoderm in contact with the optic vesicle gets thickened to form lens placode.
- It gives rise to lens.

Optic cup

- Further invagination by lens placode in optic vesicle leads to formation of optic cup.

Intraretinal space

- The lumen of optic cup is termed intraretinal space.

Choroid fissure

- The optic cup has an opening on lateral side which is continuous along ventral aspect with choroid fissure.

Pupil

- The lateral opening in the optic cup persists as pupil.

DEVELOPMENT OF LENS

Lens placode:

- It is thickened ectoderm in contact with optic vesicle
- It invaginates optic cup
- It acquires a lumen
- Subsequently it loses contact with surface ectoderm

The changes at the posterior wall of lens placode:

- The cells proliferate
- Give rise to - Primary lens fibers
- These form nucleus of lens.

The changes at equatorial part of the lens

- New fibers are laid down, termed – Secondary lens fibers.
- This continues till 20th year of age.
- Lumen of lens gets obliterated.

DEVELOPMENT OF IRIS, CILIARY BODY & RETINA

Invagination in the optic vesicle by the lens placode causes division of optic vesicle into:

- Outer layer
- Inner layer
- Intraretinal space.

Intraretinal space:

- It is the space between the two layers.
- The intraretinal space disappears with the fusion of outer and inner layers.

Outer layer of optic vesicle:

- Gives rise to the pigmented layer of retina.
- It is continued anteriorly into the iris and ciliary body.

Inner layer of optic vesicle:

- The fate of inner layer differs in the anterior 1/5th and posterior 4/5th parts.
- The junction between the two parts is demarcated by ora serrata.
- Anterior 1/5th : Presents following features:
  - Does not differentiate.
  - Remains one cell thick.
  - Forms iris and its posterior part gets folded to form ciliary body.
  - The mesodermal collection over the iris forms:
    - Constrictor pupillae.
    - Dilator pupillae.
- Posterior 4/5th : It differentiates into:
  - Ependymal layer.
  - Mantle layer.
  - Marginal layer.
  - Ependymal layer forms layer of rods and cones.
  - Mantle layer forms:
- Outer nuclear layer.
- Inner nuclear layer
- Ganglionic layer.
  - Marginal layer forms the optic nerve.

DEVELOPMENT OF CHOROID, SCLERA & CORNEA

The loose mesenchyme surrounding the developing eyeball posteriorly differentiates into two layers:

- Inner: Vascularised layer.
- Outer: Condensed layer.

Choroid is derived from vascular layer.

Sclera is derived from the outer layer which is continuous with dura mater over the optic nerve.

Cornea is also derived from the outer layer. Its different components are derived as under:

- Outer epithelial layer – From ectoderm.
- Inner epithelial layer – From mesenchyme.
- Intermediate stroma – From mesenchyme.

DEVELOPMENT OF MIDDLE EAR

The first pharyngeal pouch differentiates as:

- Proximal part: Forms auditory tube.
- Distal part: Forms primitive tympanic cavity.

Above the primitive tympanic cavity the dorsal tips of first and second branchial arches condense,

Into the condensed mass of mesoderm, the ossicles are embedded in the mesenchyme.

- Thereafter the mesenchyme dissolves.
- The endodermal lining of primitive tympanic cavity wraps around these ossicles.
- At places the double folds of the endodermal lining form ligaments of the ossicles.

DEVELOPMENTAL COMPONENTS OF TYMPANIC MEMBRANE

From outside in, the tympanic membrane has the following contributions:

- Ectoderm – Outer epithelium.
- Mesoderm – Middle fibrous layer.
- Endoderm – Inner epithelium.

DEVELOPMENT OF SUPRARENAL GLANDS

The suprarenal develops in two parts:

- Cortex
- Medulla

Cortex

- Mesothelium between the root of mesentery and the gonadal ridge proliferates.
- It invades the underlying mesoderm.
- These mesothelial cells form a large acidophilic mass termed primitive cortex or fetal cortex.
- The second wave of cells from mesenchyme differentiates and forms the three layers of cortex.
- After birth, the fetal cortex regresses.

Medulla

- The neural crest cells are ectodermal in origin.
- They form sympathetic ganglia.
- From these ganglia the cells migrate and invade the developing cortex of the suprarenal from medial aspect.
- These cells form cords and clusters.

DEVELOPMENT OF A VERTEBRA

The somite acquires a lumen.
The lumen divides it into two components:

- Dorsolateral part: Dermomyotome
- Ventromedial part: Sclerotome

Dermomyotome differentiates into two parts:

- Myotome: Forms muscles
- Dermatome: Forms dermis of skin

Sclerotome proliferates and the mesenchymal cells migrate to surround the neural tube and the notochord.

It presents following features:

- To start with, it is segmented.
- The two adjacent sclerotomes have an intersegmental portion in between them.
- Each sclerotome differentiates into cranial and caudal parts with a thin strip of mesenchyme in between.
- The caudal part and the cranial part of the adjacent sclerotomes fuse.
- Thus, the body of vertebra is formed with components from adjacent sclerotomes.

INTERVERTEBRAL DISC

- The notochord in the region of developing body of vertebra disappears.
- The notochord between the cranial and the caudal parts of sclerotome persists.
- It undergoes mucoid degeneration giving rise to nucleus pulposus.
- The loose mesenchyme around nucleus pulposus produces annulus fibrosus.

CONGENITAL ANOMALIES OF VERTEBRAL COLUMN

Scoliosis: When one half of a vertebra does not grow (Hemi-vertebra), it results in lateral bend in the vertebral column- termed scoliosis.

Kyphosis: When anterior part of the vertebra (body) does not grow, it leads to posterior bend in the vertebral column- termed kyphosis.

Spina bifida: The defect is in the vertebral arch.

- There is failure of fusion of laminae leading to deficient vertebral arch.
- The meninges and the spinal cord are placed under the skin.
- The condition may manifest as:
  - Spina bifida oculta
  - Meningocoele
  - Meningomyelocoele

DEVELOPMENT OF TOOTH

Dental lamina

- It is formed by thickening of epithelium over upper and lower jaw.

Dental buds

- These arise as outpouchings from the dental lamina into the underlying mesoderm.

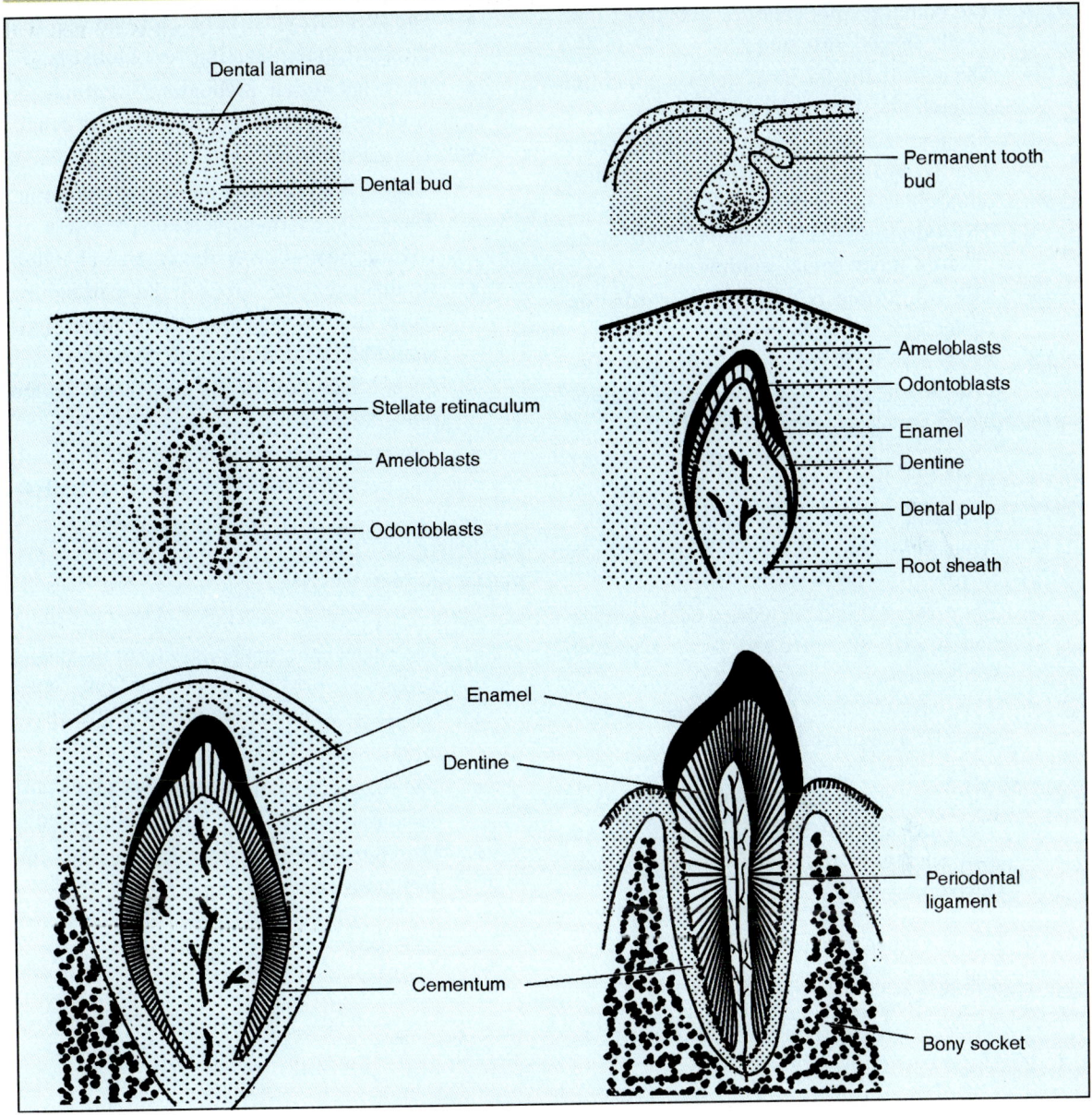

Fig. 79.8: Develpment of Tooth

- There are ten dental buds in each jaw.

Dental cap

- The dental bud gets indented by the mesenchyme to become bilayered giving it a shape of a cap.

Dental papilla

- The loose mesenchyme - stellate reticulum - in the depth of dental cap is termed dental papilla.

The subsequent development of tooth shows a series of differentiation grouped together as - **Bell Stage:**

- The dental papilla enlarges to convert into a bell shaped structure.
- The cells lining the inner dental epithelium differentiate into ameloblasts.
- The mesenchymal cells close to the inner dental epithelium differentiate into odontoblasts.
- The odontoblasts lay down predentine towards inner dental epithelium.
- The odontoblasts migrate towards the center of the dental papilla.
- Predentine gets calcified and the cytoplasmic processes of receding odontoblasts persist as dentinal channels.
- The ameloblasts deposit enamel first at the apex and then at the sides (towards the dentine layer).
- Ameloblasts migrate into stellate reticulum to reach the outer dental layer.
- They form a thin layer termed dental cuticle and it gets sloughed off when decidual teeth erupt.
- The odontoblasts (towards the centre) persist throughout life.

Root of tooth

- The inner and outer dental layers form the root sheath at the proximal end of the developing tooth.

- The mesenchymal cells close to the root sheath differentiate into odontoblasts.
- They lay down predentine/ dentine and migrate to line pulp canal/ dental canal.
- The mesenchyme on external aspect of root sheath differentiates into cementoblasts.
- These lay down cementum over dentine covering the root of the tooth.
- In mesenchyme around the cementum, there appears periodontal ligament. It is anchored to the wall of the alveolar socket on one side and to the cementum on the other side.
- The pulp cavity narrows and blood vessels and nerves appear in it.

PROCESS FOR APPEARANCE OF PERMANENT TEETH

- The permanent tooth arises from the dental bud.
- It appears on the inner aspect (towards the tongue) of the decidual bud.
- The sequence of formation is similar to the deciduous tooth.
- The permanent tooth-bud pushes the deciduous tooth to come out.

80

Glossary : Germ Layer Derivatives

ECTODERM

Surface ectoderm

- Epidermis
- Hair and nails
- Cutaneous and mammary glands
- Anterior pituitary gland
- Enamel of teeth
- Inner ear
- Lens of eye

NEUROECTODERM

Neural crest origin

- Cranial and sensory ganglia and nerves
- Medulla of adrenal gland
- Pigment cells

Neural tube origin

- Central nervous system
- Retina of eye
- Pineal body (gland)
- Posterior pituitary gland

MESODERM

Head mesoderm

- Skull
- Muscles and connective tissue of head
- Dentine of teeth

Paraxial mesoderm

- Muscles of trunk
- Skeleton, except for skull
- Dermis of skin
- Connective tissue

Intermediate mesoderm

- Urogenital system includes gonads, ducts and accessory glands

Lateral plate mesoderm

- Connective tissue and muscles (smooth and cardiac) of the viscera
- Serous membranes of pleura, pericardium and peritoneum
- Blood and lymph cells
- Cardiovascular and lymphatic systems

- Spleen
- Adrenal cortex
- Bone marrow

ENDODERM

Epithelium of

- Larynx and trachea
- Bronchi
- Lungs
- Pharynx
- Thyroid gland

- Tympanic cavity
- Pharyngotympanic tube
- Tonsils
- Parathyroid glands

Epithelium of

- Gastrointestinal tract and its glands
- Liver
- Pancreas
- Urinary bladder
- Urachus
- Vagina and vestibule
- Urethra and glands

81

Critical Periods of Human Development
(Sensitivity to Teratogens)

Major morphologic abnormalities occur during 3rd to 7th weeks.

Physiologic defects and minor morphologic abnormalities do occur from 8th week to term

1st and 2nd Weeks

This is the period of dividing zygote, implantation and bilaminar embryo.

The embryo is not normally susceptible to teratogens during this period.

A substance will damage either all or most of the cells at this time which results in prenatal death or the embryo will survive with few defects.

3rd Week

This is a highly sensitive period for the developing heart and CNS
- Highly sensitive for the heart from the middle of 3rd to 6th week
- Highly sensitive period for the CNS from the beginning of 3rd week 3 through early in 6th week

4th Week

During this period, the eyes, ears, arms, and legs begin to develop
- Sensitive period for the **eyes** - middle of 4th to middle of 8th week

- Sensitive period for the **ears** - middle of 4th to middle of 9th week
- Sensitive period for the **arms** - middle of 4th to the end of 7th week
- Sensitive period for the **legs** - middle of 4th to end of 7th week

6th Week

Teeth are most sensitive between the ends of 6th to 8th week

Palate is most sensitive between the end of 6th to early in 9th week

7th Week

External genitalia are most sensitive from the middle of 7th week until the end of 9th week

PERIODS OF LESSER SENSITIVITY TO TERATOGENS

- **CNS**: From early in 6th week to term
- **Heart**: From late in 6th week to the end of 8th week
- **Arms**: During 8th week
- **Eyes**: Middle of 8th week to term
- **Legs**: During 8th week
- **Teeth:** During 9th and 10th weeks
- **Palate**: During 9th week

- **External genitalia**: Late in 9th week to term
- **Ear**: Middle of 9th week to the end of 16th week

TERATOGENS KNOWN TO CAUSE HUMAN MALFORMATIONS

ANDROGENIC AGENTS

Ethisterone and Moresthisterone
Varying degrees of masculinization of female fetuses, e.g., most have labial fusion and clitoral hypertrophy

Diethylstilbestrol (DES)
May not be teratogenic (?) to the embryo or fetus, but is carcinogenic to female offspring in later life (16 to 22 years)

ANTI-TUMOR AGENTS

Aminopterin
Wide range of skeletal defects and malformations of the CNS, particularly anencephaly

Busulfan
Stunted growth, skeletal abnormalities, corneal opacities, cleft palate, and hypoplasia of various organs

Methotrexate
Multiple malformations, especially skeletal

SEDATIVE-HYPNOTICS

Thalidomide - Results in meromelia and other **limb** malformations, as well as malformations of the external ears, heart, and digestive tract

INFECTIOUS AGENTS

Cytomegalovirus
Microcephaly, hydrocephalus, microphthalmia, microgyria, and mental retardation

Rubella virus
Cataracts, chorioretinitis, deafness, microphthalmia, and congeni-tal heart defects

Toxoplasma gondii
Microcephaly, microphthalmia, hydrocephalus, and chorioretinitis

Herpes simplex virus
Microcephaly, microphthalmia, and retinal dysplasia

Varicella zoster virus
Congenital malformations similar to those from other viruses

Syphilis microorganism (Treponema pallidum)
- Wasting of fetal tissues, malformations of the teeth, fetal meningi-tis, mental retardation, hydrocephalus, deafness, and CNS dis-ease
- Pneumonia alba is a form of chronic pneumonia seen in stillborn and newborn infants dying of congenital syphilis

THERAPEUTIC RADIATION

- Microcephaly and skeletal malformations
- Mutations in fetal germ cells

ALKALOIDS

Caffeine
Implicated in congenital malformations of the human embryo

Nicotine

Effect on fetal growth, resulting in increased premature delivery, thus, lower weight infants

CHRONIC ALCOHOL

Prenatal and postnatal growth deficiency, mental retardation, microcephaly, short palpebral fissures, maxillary hypoplasia, ab-normal palmar creases, joint abnormalities, and congenital heart disease

ANTIBIOTICS

Tetracycline

In the second and third trimesters of pregnancy has been implicated with tooth enamel hypoplasia, yellow-brown discoloration of the deciduous teeth, distortion of bone growth, and possibly congenital cataract

Streptomycin

Deafness in infants

Penicillin

No teratogenic effects

ANTICOAGULANTS

Warfarin

- Foetal hemorrhage
- Hypoplasia of the nasal bones

ANTICONVULSANTS

Trimethadione (Tridone)
Paramethadione (Paradine)
Foetal dysmorphia, cardiac defects, cleft palate, intrauterine growth retardation, and digital hypoplasia
Dilantin, Phenytoin and Phenytoin with barbiturate

- Cleft palate
- Hypoplasia of the terminal phalanges

CORTICOSTEROIDS

Cleft palate and cardiac defects

INSULIN

Not teratogenic in the human embryo

THYROID DRUGS

Potassium iodide, 131 Iodine, and Propylthiouracil Congenital goiter

LSD AND MARIJUANA

Congenital defect formation has been conflicting and not fully proven. They may cause some limb malformations and some severe CNS abnormalities

ENVIRONMENTAL CHEMICALS (Industrial Pollutants and Food additives)

They have not been specifically shown to cause abnormal defects

MERCURY

Foetal Minamata disease (caused by eating fish contaminated with mercury) with neurologic and behavioral disturbances such as cerebral palsy, brain damage, mental retardation, and blindness

PHYSIOLOGIC DEVELOPMENT OF CNS

PRENATAL STAGES

Development of cellular function
Physiologic development of cells usually be-gins with and parallels their morphologic development.

The two processes continu-ally interact with one another

Typical enzyme systems appear in the spinal cord cells before they are seen in the brain. Examples of these are succinic dehydrogenase, ATPase, and cytochrome oxi-dase

Appearance of Nissl bodies (cytoplasmic RNA) marks the beginning of in-creased protein synthesis, resulting in the formation of axon and dendritic processes

Signs of functional activity, such as the onset of electrical activity and reactivity resulting in muscular contractions, as well as suppression of the related reflexes by cephalic structures, are superimposed on the morphologic and chemical changes with cerebral maturation

Cerebral maturation is slower and more gradual than that of the rest of the CNS and corresponds to the duration of cortical histogenesis. It may be physiologically evaluated by the spontaneous activity of the brain recorded from the skull by the electroencephalogram

- Electrical potentials recorded across the amniotic membrane suggest that this ac-tivity begins at about day 50 of intrauterine life
- Its maturation, which is a function of dendritic development of the neurons, as well as enzymatic development, is usually completed at about II years of age
- The fetus of seven months shows anarchic activity with interhemispheric asymmetry, indicating an immature cortex and commissures
- At birth, there is slow, more coordinated activity of about three to four cycles per second with the onset of some symmetry
- From two to three years of age, more rapid activity with alpha waves of about six to seven cycles per second are seen with symmetric activity of greater amplitude being well organized in the occipital

regions but less well in the frontal regions
- At 13 to 14 years of age, there is still more rapid activity of from eight to twelve cycles per second, and the alpha waves are well organized on the entire cerebral surface

During maturation of the brain, there are special needs and requirements for oxygen and glycogen

- The oxygen consumption in the adult is about 25% of that used by the entire body, whereas in the newborn and young child, it can be as high as 60%. Thus, neonatal anoxia is very serious and may result in intracranial hemorrhage, epilepsy, or even psychomotor retardation

Overall development

Physiologic development parallels histogenesis and begins in the spinal cord. It then follows in the derivatives of the rhombencephalon, the mesencephalon, and the prosencephalon to end with the development of the cerebral cortex. In a sense, it conforms to phylogenetic evolution

Foetal stages of development

- Muscular reactions to external stimuli are first seen at about 8th week
- Spontaneous movements, a sign of medullary maturation, are seen in 9th week
- Osteotendinous reflexes are seen in 6th month
- The respiratory centers of the medulla are functional at 5th month and, since maturation of pulmonary alveolar epithelium occurs at about 6th months of ges-tation, viability is theoretically possible at this age
- Archaic reflexes involving subcortical centers are possible

Sucking at 5th month of gestation

Grasping at 6th month of gestation

The inexcitability of the cerebral cortex until this time appears to indicate that these movements are independent of the cortex and may represent very rudimentary instinctive reactions, since they are also seen in anencephalics.

- Cerebral maturation begins between the 6th and 7th months of gestation, when the basic structures are all completed, although some disease processes may slow down this development, and newborns may then show a psychomotor retarda-tion of I to several months

POSTNATAL STAGES

The postnatal period is a continuation of the foetal state in terms of nervous system function. Behavior is predominantly reflex and purely subcortical. Movement is in-stinctual and rudimentary, consisting of flexion and extension or simple reflexes such as crying and coughing

- Neocortex becomes excitable about 10th day, but in a very weak and diffuse manner, and for a long time, movement is generalized and awkward
- Gradually, autonomic movements come under cortical control and are more elaborate, and behavior becomes progressively imitative and expressive
- Structural developments in the cortex foretell these activities: neural development coincides with myelinization which proceeds in a cephalocaudal direction

First fibers to be myelinated are those coming from the motor, visual, and auditory cortex areas

Last fibers to become myelinated at the end of gestation and just before birth are those coming from the association areas

Major clinical stages of development postnatally are

- Regression of the archaic reflexes is seen between the first and third months
- Ability to completely right one's head, with stability (head control), from a prone position is seen at about 3 months

- Sitting and development of prehension (use of thumb and index finger) usually occurs at about 8th or 9th months
- Standing usually occurs at about 9th or 10th months
- Walking takes place at about 12th to 15th months
- The first words are usually spoken between the 18th month and two years
- Cerebral maturation usually ends at about eleven years of age

GENERAL BRAIN DEVELOPMENT

Cerebral cortex has a surface of about 700 cm2 at birth, 950 cm2 at about 5 months, and about 1700 cm2 at about 2 years of age, after which time, the surface no longer increases

Brain weighs from 300gm to 350gm at birth or about one-tenth of its body weight, and its weight increases, as does its volume, mostly during the first two years of life. It weighs 800 gm at first year and 1350 gm at maturity.

- Growth of the brain takes place essentially in the hemispheres, particularly in the frontal lobes
- Increase of brain weight continues until about the age of fourteen years, but at a slower pace, and is due especially to the multiplication of the neuroglial cells and to the neuronal fiber growth. The central nervous system has most of its neurons at the time of birth
- In the adult, the brain represents only about 2.5% of its body weight as a result of general growth of the total body mass
- With growth, a complex pattern of sulci and gyri develops. These permit a considerable increase in the volume of the cerebral cortex without requiring an extensive increase in cranial volume or a reshaping of the cranial vault

Myelinization starts at the fourth foetal month
Cranial nerves are myelinized at birth, and the spinal nerves are completely myelinized by three years of age

CLINICAL CONSIDERATIONS

Normal Reflexes

Moro's reflex (embrace):

When the infant is startled by a jarring of the table or crib or by a loud noise, he draws his legs up and brings his arms around, as in an embrace

Tonic neck reflex:

In the resting state, the infant's posture is maintained by flexor tonicity of the arms and legs. Lateral rotation of the head to one side abolishes flexor tone on that side, causing extension of the arm and leg. This reflex is usually not developed fully until first month of age

Grasp reflexes

When the palm is stimulated by one's finger, the infant grasps and holds on; when the sole of the foot is stimulated from the heel forward, the toes turn downward

Deep tendon reflexes are present but tire easily

Abdominal reflexes are inconstant

Babinski's reflex is present, but there is no ankle clonus, and it disappears at about 10 to 16 months

Chvostek's sign is positive in 50% of newborn infants during the first week

Pupils react to light with contraction, but there may be secondary dilation

Swimming and walking reflexes are present during the first weeks

Rooting, sucking, and swallowing reflexes are important to feeding

Rooting reflex: when the infant smells milk, he turns his head to find the source, and when the cheek is touched by a smooth object, the mouth turns toward the object and the lips open as if to grasp a nipple

Development is related to myelinization and is not a steady process but a pat-tern of sequences of rapid and slow growth. Motor and sensory controls develop from above and proceed downward so that eye control develops before hand and leg control. Development is related to three functioning levels of the CNS: brainstem, archipallium, and neopallium

Newborn functions at brainstem levels

Archipallium - includes part of the temporal lobe, cingulate gyrus, and basal ganglia, supervenes on the brainstem and can be considered to be responsible for the basic emotions and some primitive motor and sensory control

Neopallium - includes most of the cerebral hemisphere, has intellectual rather than emotional function and is responsible for skill, discrimination, and fine movements

Clinical application of the above developmental patterns is important

Changes in physical signs in static brain lesions

- Upper limb paresis becomes apparent at five to six months
- Lower limb paresis becomes apparent at ten to twelve months
- Abnormalities of coordination, namely, athetoid and involuntary move-ments, become apparent between eighteen and twenty four months

Prematurity

Any newborn infant born alive who weighs 2500 gm or less is considered a premature infant.

This would include some infants of apparently full-term gestation

Signs of premature infancy (clinical and x-ray features)

- **Weight and length** are less than 2500 g and 47 cm at birth. The gestation period is usually 28 to 36 weeks

- **The cry** is feebler than that of a full-term infant, sucking is weaker, and there is general weakness with sluggish movements
- **Skin** is thin and wrinkled; there are abundance of lanugo and minimal amount of subcutaneous tissue, and the nails are soft
- **Head** appears large, but the circumference is less than 33 cm, with a characteristic wizened facies
- **Temperature** is low and unstable
- **Tendency** to cyanosis and irregular respirations
- **Jaundice** may be prominent and continue longer than in full-term infants
- **Feeding difficulties** are common with vomiting more frequent and a tendency to loose stools
- **Initially the weight loss** is often greater and weight recovery not rapid, in contrast to a full-term infant
- Distal femoral and proximal tibial ossification centers may be absent. in the full-term infant, these are present including those of the calcaneus, cuboid, talus, and proximal tibia

Complications of prematurity

A weak gag and cough reflex and an immature respiratory center that requires stronger afferent stimuli for response; incompletely developed alveoli; reduced vascu-larity of the pulmonary capillaries, sparse pulmonary elastic tissue; poor muscle tone and weak movements of the intercostal muscles and diaphragm plus softness and plia-bility of the bones of the thoracic cage which reduces intrathoracic pressure; and the presence of fetal hemoglobin which releases oxygen less readily to tissues

Cyanosis of the extremities and edema; paucity of vascular elastic tissue and low body reserves of vitamin C, resulting in capillary fragility and potential hemorrhage

Sucking reflex is very weak and hepatic immaturity predisposes to the development of increased bilirubinemia with jaundice. The slow rate of secretion of digestive en-zymes and gastric acid causes diminished tolerance, resulting in vomiting, diarrhea, and poor absorption of fats and minerals

Decreased renal function produces dehydration and acidosis

Faulty control of body temperature is associated with hypothermia and hy-perthermia due to inadequate function of the sweating mechanism, decreased body insulation (less fatty tissue), and low total heat production due to body inactivity and poor muscle development

Poor storage of minerals, vitamins, and immune materials makes the prema-ture infant subject to rickets, anemia, and a variety of infections

Prognosis

Survival rate is directly in proportion to the weight of the premature infant at birth, and the prognosis improves as the period of gestation is lengthened

Prematurity is one of the leading primary causes of neonatal deaths, and most of these occur in the first 24 hours, fewer in the second 24 hours, and even fewer after that.

Major contributing factors for death include

- Anoxia
- Intracranial hemor-rhage
- Hyaline membrane with resorption atelectasis
- Pneumonia and other infections
- Congenital malformations
- Blood dyscrasias

82

Correlated Human Development

Size (CR in mm): 1.5

- **Body form**: Embryonic disk flat. Primitive streak is prominent. Neural groove indicated
- **Mouth**: Not developed
- **Pharynx and derivatives**: Not developed
- **Digestive tube and glands**: Gut not as yet distinct from yolk sac
- **Respiratory system**: Not developed
- **Coelom and mesenteries**: Extraembryonic coelom present. Embryonic coelom al-most ready to make its appearance
- **Urogenital system**: Allantois present
- **Vascular system**: Blood islands appear on chorion and yolk sac. Cardiogenic plate reversing
- **Skeletal system**: Head process for notochordal plate is present
- **Muscular system**: Not developed
- **Integumentary system**: Ectoderm seen as a single layer
- **Nervous system**: Neural groove is indicated
- **Sense organs**: Not developed

Size (CR in mm): 2.5

- **Body form**: Neural groove deepens and closes except at ends. Somites 1-16 present. Cylindrical body constricting from yolk sac. First and second branchial arches are seen
- **Mouth**: Mandibular arch is prominent. Stomodeum a definitive pit. Oral membrane ruptures
- **Pharynx and derivatives**: Pharynx broad and flat. Pharyngeal pouches forming. Thyroid gland makes its appearance
- **Digestive tube and glands**: Foregut and hindgut present. Yolk sac broadly attached at midgut. Liver bud is present. Cloaca and cloacal membrane are seen
- **Respiratory system**: Respiratory primordium appears as a groove on pharyngeal floor
- **Coelom and mesenteries**: Embryonic coelom a U-shaped canal with a large pericar-dial cavity. Septum transversum seen. Mesenteries forming at this time. Mesocar-dium begins to atrophy
- **Urogenital system**: All pronephric tubules

are formed. Pronephric duct growing caudally as a blind tube. Cloaca and cloacal membrane are present

- **Vascular system**: Primitive blood cells and vessels are present. Embryonic blood vessels form a paired symmetric system. The heart tubes fuse, bend in an S-shape, and the heartbeat begins
- **Skeletal system**: Mesodermal segments are appearing (1-16). Older somites don't demonstrate sclerotomes. Notochord appears as a cellular rod
- **Muscular system**: Mesodermal segments appearing (I-16). Older somites begin to demonstrate myotome plates
- **Integumentary system**: No new developments
- **Nervous system**: Neural groove is prominent but rapidly closing. Neural crest is a continuous band
- **Sense organs:** optic vesicle and auditory placode are seen. Acoustic ganglia appearing]

AGE (WEEKS): 4.0

Size (CR in mm): 5.0

- **Body form**: Branchial arches completed. Flexed heart is prominent. Yolk stalk is slender. All 40 somites are present. Limb buds appear. Otocyst and eye are evident. Body is now C-shaped and flexed
- **Mouth**: Maxillary and mandibular processes are prominent. Tongue primordium is present. Rathke's pouch becomes evident
- **Pharynx and derivatives**: Five pharyngeal pouches are present. Pouches 1-4 have closing plates. The primary tympanic cavity is indicated. The thyroid gland is now a stalked sac

- **Digestive tube and glands**: Oesophagus is short. The stomach is spindle-shaped. Intestine is a simple tube. Liver cords, ducts, and gallbladder are forming. Both pancreatic buds appear. The cloaca is at its full development
- **Respiratory system**: Trachea and paired lung buds become prominent. Laryngeal opening is a simple slit
- **Coelom and mesenteries**: Coelom stills a continuous system of cavities. Dorsal mesentery is a complete median structure. Omental bursa is now indicated
- **Urogenital system**: Pronephros has degenerated. Pronephric (mesonephric) duct reaches the cloaca. Mesonephric tubules are differentiating rapidly. Metanephric bud is seen pushing into secretory primordium
- **Vascular system**: Hematopoiesis is seen on the yolk sac. The paired aortae fuse. The aortic arches and cardinal veins are completed. The dilated heart shows a sinus, atrium, ventricle, and bulbus
- **Skeletal system**: All 40 somites are present. Sclerotomes are massed as primitive vertebrae around the notochord
- **Muscular system**: All 40 so mites are present
- **Integumentary system**: Not remarkable
- **Nervous system**: Neural tube is closed. Three primary vesicles of brain are seen. Nerves and ganglia are forming. Ependymal, mantle, and marginal layers are seen
- **Sense organs**: Optic cup and lens pit are forming. Auditory pit becomes the closed detached otocyst. Olfactory placodes arise and differentiate nerve cells

AGE (WEEKS): 5.0

Size (CR in mm): 8.0

- **Body form**: Nasal pits are present. Tail is prominent. Heart, liver, and mesonephros are prominent. Umbilical cord organizes
- **Mouth**: Jaws are outlined. Rathke's pouch is now a stalked sac
- **Pharynx and derivatives**: Pharyngeal pouches develop dorsal and ventral diverticulae. Thyroid becomes bilobed. Thyroglossal duct atrophies
- **Digestive tube and glands**: Tail-gut atrophies. Yolk stalk detaches. Intestine elon-gates into a loop. Caecum is now evident
- **Respiratory system**: Bronchial buds presage future lung lobes. Arytenoid cartilage swellings and epiglottis are indicated
- **Coelom and mesenteries**: Pleuropericardial and pleuroperitoneal membranes are forming. Ventral mesogastrium pulls away from the septum
- **Urogenital system**: Mesonephros reaches its caudal limit. Ureteric and pelvic primordia become distinct. Genital ridge bulges
- **Vascular system**: Primitive vessels extend into head and limbs. Vitelline and umbilical veins are transforming. Myocardium is condensing. Cardiac septa appearing. Spleen becomes evident
- **Skeletal system**: Condensations of mesenchyme presage many future bones
- **Muscular system**: Pre-muscle masses are seen in head, trunk, and limbs
- **Integumentary system**: Epidermis acquiring a second layer (periderm)
- **Nervous system**: 5 brain vesicles are seen. Cerebral hemispheres bulging. Nerves and ganglia more clearly seen. Suprarenal cortex beginning to form
- **Sense organs**: Choroid fissure is prominent. Lens vesicle is free. Vitreous anlage is appearing. Otocyst elongates, and endolymphatic duct is budded off. Olfactory pit deepens

AGE (WEEKS): 6.0

Size (CR in mm): 12.0

- **Body form**: Upper jaw components are prominent but still separate. Lower jaw halves fuse. Head becomes dominant in size. Cervical flexure is marked. External ear appears. Limbs become more clearly recognizable
- **Mouth**: Lingual primordia fusing. Foramen caecum is established. Labio-dental laminae begin to appear. Parotid and submandibular gland buds appear
- **Pharynx and derivatives**: Thymic sacs, ultimobranchial sacs, and solid parathyroids are conspicuous and ready to detach. Thyroid gland becomes solid, converts into plates
- **Digestive tube and glands**: Stomach rotating, intestinal loop under torsion. Hepatic lobes are identifiable. Cloaca is subdividing
- **Respiratory system**: Definitive pulmonary lobes are indicated. Bronchi are sub branching. Laryngeal cavity temporarily obliterated
- **Coelom and mesenteries**: Pleuropericardial communications close. Mesentery ex-pands as the intestine forms a loop
- **Urogenital system**: Cloaca subdividing. Pelvic anlage sprouts pole tubules. Sexless gonads and genital tubercle are prominent. Mullerian duct appearing

- **Vascular system**: Hematopoiesis in the liver is seen. Aortic arches are transforming. Left umbilical vein and ductus venosus become important. Bulbus is absorbed into right ventricle. Heart acquires its general definitive shape
- **Skeletal system**: First appearance of chondrification centers. Desmocranium seen.
- **Muscular system**: Myotomes become fused into a continuous column and spread ventrally. Muscle segmentation generally lost
- **Integumentary system**: Milk line is now present
- **Nervous system**: Three primary flexures of brain are seen. Diencephalon is large. Nerve plexuses are present. Epiphysis recognizable. Sympathetic ganglia forming seg-mental masses. Meninges are beginning to appear
- **Sense organs**: Optic cup shows nervous and pigment layers. Lens vesicle thickens. Eyes are set at 1600. Nasolacrimal duct seen. Modeling of external, middle, and internal ear is beginning. Vomeronasal organ seen

AGE (WEEKS): 7.0

Size (CR in mm): 17.0

- **Body form**: Branchial arches are lost. Cervical sinus is obliterated. Face and neck are forming. Digits are evident. Back straightening. Heart and liver determine shape of body ventrally. Tail is now regressing
- **Mouth**: Lingual primordia merge into a single tongue. Separate labial and dental laminae are visible. Jaws are formed and begin to ossify. Palate folds are present and are separated by the tongue

- **Pharynx and derivatives**: Thymus becomes elongated and loses its lumen. Parathy-roids become trabeculate and associate with the thyroid. Ultimo branchial bodies fuse with the thyroid. Thyroid becomes crescentic
- **Digestive tube and glands**: Stomach attaining final shape and position. Duodenum is temporarily occluded. Intestinal loops herniate into cord. Rectum separates from bladder-urethra. Anal membrane ruptures. Dorsal and ventral pancreatic pri-mordia fuse
- **Respiratory system**: Larynx and epiglottis are well outlined with a T-shaped orifice. Laryngeal and tracheal cartilages are foreshadowed. Conchae begin to appear. Primary choanae are rupturing
- **Coelom and mesenteries**: Pericardium is extended by splitting from body wall. Mesentery is expanding rapidly as the intestine coils. Ligaments of the liver become very prominent
- **Urogenital system**: Mesonephros is at the height of its differentiation. Metanephric collecting tubules begin branching. Earliest metanephric secretory tubules differentiating. Bladder-urethra separates from the rectum. Urethral membrane is beginning to rupture
- **Vascular system**: Cardinal veins are transforming. Inferior vena cava is visible. Atrium, ventricle, and bulbus are partitioned. Cardiac valves are present. Stem of the pulmonary vein is absorbed into the left atrium. Anlage of the spleen is prominent
- **Skeletal system**: Chondrocranium is seen. Chondrification is now more general
- **Muscular system**: muscles are differentiating rapidly throughout body and are assuming their final shapes and relationships

- **Integumentary system**: Mammary thickening
- **Nervous system**: Cerebral hemispheres are becoming large. Corpus striatum and thalamus are prominent. Infundibulum and Rathke's pouch are in contact. Cho-roid plexuses are appearing. Suprarenal medulla begins to invade the cortex
- **Sense organs**: Choroid fissure closes, enclosing the central artery. Nerve fibers in-vade the optic stalk. Lens loses its cavity by elongating lens fibers. Eyelids are forming. Fibrous and vascular coats of the eye are beginning to form. Olfactory sacs open into the mouth

AGE (WEEKS): 8.0

Size (CR in mm): 23.0

- **Body form**: Nose is flat. Eyes are far apart. Digits are well formed. Growth of gut makes body evenly rotund. Head is elevating. Foetal state is now reached
- **Mouth**: Tongue muscles are well differentiated. Earliest taste buds are indi-cated. Rathke's pouch detaches from the mouth. Sublingual glands are now appearing
- **Pharynx and derivatives**: Auditory tube and tympanic cavity are evident. Sites of the tonsils and their fossae are evident. Thymic gland halves unite and become solid. Thyroid gland follicles are forming
- **Digestive tube and glands**: Small intestine is coiling within the cord. Intestinal villi are developing. Liver is very large in relative size
- **Respiratory system**: Lung is becoming gland like by branching of the bronchi-oles
- **Coelom and mesenteries**: Pleuroperitoneal communications close. Pericardium is a very large sac. Diaphragm is completed, including its musculature. Dia-phragm also completes its descent
- **Urogenital system**: Testis and ovary are now distinguishable as such. Mullerian ducts are nearing the urogenital sinus and are about ready to unite with the utero--vaginal primordium. Genital ligaments are indicated
- **Vascular system**: the main blood vessels are assuming their final plan. Primi-tive lymph sacs are present. Sinus venosus is absorbed into the right atrium. Atrioventricular bundle is present
- **Skeletal system**: First indications of ossification are evident
- **Muscular system**: Definitive muscles of the trunk, limbs, and head are well repre-sented. Foetus is now capable of some movement
- **Integumentary system**: Mammary primordia are seen as globular thickenings
- **Nervous system**: the cerebral cortex begins to acquire its typical cells. Olfactory lobes are visible. Dura and pia-arachnoid are distinct. Chromaffin bodies are seen
- **Sense organs**: Eyes are converging rapidly. External, middle, and internal ears are assuming their final form. Taste buds are appearing. External nares are plugged.

AGE (WEEKS): 10.0

Size (CR in mm): 40.0

- **Body form**: Head is erect. Limbs are well modeled. Nail folds are indicated. Umbilical hernia is reduced
- **Mouth**: Fungiform and vallate papillae are differentiating. Lips are separate from the jaws. Enamel organs and dental papillae are forming. Palate folds are fusing

- **Pharynx and derivatives**: Thymic epithelium is transforming into reticulum and thymic corpuscles. Ultimobranchial bodies disappear as such
- **Digestive tube and glands**: Intestines withdraw from the umbilical cord and assume their characteristic position. Anal canal is formed. Pancreatic alve-oli are present
- **Respiratory system**: Nasal passages are partitioned by fusion of the septum and palate. Nose is cartilaginous. Laryngeal cavity is reopened and the vocal folds appear
- **Coelom and mesenteries**: Processus (saccus) vaginales are forming. Intes-tine and its mesentery withdraw from the umbilical cord
- **Urogenital system**: Kidneys are able to secrete. Bladder expands as a sac. Genital ducts of the opposite sex are degenerating. Bulbourethral and vestibular glands are appearing. Vagina sacs are forming
- **Vascular system**: Thoracic duct and peripheral lymphatics are developed. Early lymph glands are appearing. Enucleated red blood cells predominate in the blood
- **Skeletal system**: Ossification centers are more common. Chondrocranium is at the height of its development
- **Muscular system**: Perineal muscles are developing slowly
- **Integumentary system**: Intermediate cells are added to the epidermis. Peri-derm cells are prominent. Nail fields are indicated. Earliest hair follicles begin developing on the face
- **Nervous system**: Spinal cord attains its definitive internal structure
- **Sense organs**: Iris and ciliary bodies are organizing. Eyelids are fused. Lacrimal glands are budding. Spiral organ of Corti begins to differentiate

AGE (WEEKS): 12.0

Size (CR in mm): 56.0

- **Body form**: Head is still a dominant feature. Nose acquires its bridge. Sex is readily determined by external inspection
- **Mouth**: Filiform and foliate papillae are elevating. Tooth primordia form prom-inent cups. Cheeks are seen. Fusion of the palate is complete
- **Pharynx and derivatives**: Tonsillar crypts begin to invaginate. Thymus forms its medulla and is becoming more lymphoid. Thyroid attains its typical form
- **Digestive tube and glands**: Muscle layers of the gut are present. Pancreatic islets are appearing. Bile is being secreted
- **Respiratory system**: Nasal conchae are prominent. Glands of the nasal cavity are forming. Lungs are acquiring their definitive form
- **Coelom and mesenteries**: Omentum has become an expansive apron which is partly fused to the dorsal body wall. Mesenteries are free and exhibit their usual relationships. Extension of the coelom into the umbilical cord is obliterated
- **Urogenital system**: Uterine horns are absorbed. External genitalia attain distinctive features. The mesonephric and rete tubules complete the male duct. The prostate and seminal vesicles begin to appear. Hollow viscera are beginning to form muscular walls
- **Vascular system**: Blood formation is beginning in the bone marrow. Blood vessels acquire accessory coats
- **Skeletal system**: Notochord is degenerating very rapidly. Ossification is

spread-ing rapidly. A number of bones are well defined

- **Muscular system**: Smooth muscle layers are becoming evident in the hollow viscera
- **Integumentary system**: Epidermis is now 3-layered. Corium and subcutane-ous tissue are now distinct
- **Nervous system**: Brain attains its general structural features. Spinal cord demonstrates cervical and lumbar enlargements. Cauda equina and filum ter-minale make their appearance. Neuroglial types are beginning to differentiate
- **Sense organs**: Characteristic organization of the eye is attained. Retina is now becoming layered. Nasal septum and plate fusions are completed

AGE (WEEKS): 16.0

Size (CR in mm): 112.0

- **Body form**: Face takes on a "human" appearance. Hair of the head is appearing. Muscles become spontaneously active. Body is beginning to outgrow head
- **Mouth**: hard and soft palates are differentiating. Hypophysis is acquiring its definitive structure
- **Pharynx and derivatives**: Lymphocytes are beginning to accumulate in the tonsils. Pharyngeal tonsil (adenoids) is beginning to develop
- **Digestive tube and glands**: Gastric and intestinal glands are developing. Duode-num and colon become affixed to the posterior abdominal wall. Meconium is collecting
- **Respiratory system**: Accessory nasal sinuses are developing. Tracheal glands appear. Mesoderm is still abundant between the pulmonary alveoli. Elastic fibers make their appearance in the lungs

- **Coelom and mesenteries**: Greater omentum is fusing with the transverse mesocolon and colon. Mesoduodenum, ascending mesocolon, and descending mesocolon are attaching to the posterior abdominal wall
- **Urogenital system**: Kidneys attain their characteristic shape. Testis is in position for its descent into the scrotum. Uterus and vagina are recognizable as entities. Mesonephros is involuted
- **Vascular system**: Blood formation is now active in the spleen. Heart muscla-ture is much condensed
- **Skeletal system**: Most bones are clearly indicated throughout the body. Joint cavi-ties appear
- **Muscular system**: Cardiac muscle which appeared in earlier weeks is now more condensed. Muscular movements in utero can be detected
- **Integumentary system**: Epidermis begins adding additional layers. Body hair begins to develop. Sweat glands appear. First sebaceous glands begin to differentiate
- **Nervous system**: Hemispheres now conceal much of the brain. Cerebral lobes are delimited. Corpora quadrigemina appear. Cerebellum attains some prominence
- **Sense organs**: Eye, ear, and nose are nearing their typical appearance. General sense organs are differentiating

AGE (WEEKS): 20.0- 40.0

Size (CR in mm): 160.0-350.0

- **Body form**: Lanugo hair appears in week 20. Vernix caseosa collects in week 20. Body becomes better proportioned but lean in week 24. Foetus is wrinkled, lean, and red, and eyelids reopen in week 28. Testes invade the scrotum in week 32. Body rounds out, fat collects, and wrinkling smoothes out in weeks 32 to 40

- **Mouth**: Enamel and dentine deposited in week 20. Lingual tonsil forming in week 20. Permanent teeth primordia indicated in weeks 24 to 32. Milk teeth are un-erupted at birth
- **Pharynx and derivatives**: Tonsils are structurally typical in week 20
- **Digestive tube and glands**: Lymph nodules and muscularis mucosae of the gut are present in week 20. Ascending colon becomes recognizable in week 24. Appendix lags behind the caecum in growth at week 24. Deep oesophageal glands are indicated in week 28. Plicae circulares are represented in week 32
- **Respiratory system**: Nose begins ossifying in week 20. Nostrils reopen in week 24. Cuboidal epithelium of the lung alveoli is disappearing in week 24. Pulmonary branching is only two-thirds completed by week 40. Frontal and sphenoidal sinuses are still quite incomplete by week 40
- **Coelom and mesenteries**: Mesenterial attachments are completed by week 20. Vaginal sacs are passing into the scrotal sacs between weeks 28 and 36
- **Urogenital system**: Female urogenital sinus is becoming a shallow vestibule by week 20. Vagina regains its lumen by week 20. Uterine glands appear in week 28. Scrotum is solid until sacs and testes descend in weeks 28 to 36. Tubules of the kidney cease forming at birth
- **Vascular system**: Blood formation is increasing in the bone marrow but is decreas-ing in the liver between weeks 20 and 40. Spleen acquires its typical structure

by week 28. A number of fetal blood vessels are discontinued by week 40

- **Skeletal system**: Carpal, tarsal, and sternal bones ossify late, some after birth. Most epiphyseal centers appear after birth, many during adolescence
- **Muscular system**: the perineal muscles finish their development by week 24
- **Integumentary system**: Vernix caseosa is seen in week 20. Epidermis cornifies by week 20. Nail plates begin in week 20. Hairs emerge by week 24. Mammary primordia bud in week 20 and the buds hollow out and branch by week 32. Nail reaches the fingertip by week 36. Lanugo hair is prominent in week 28 and is shed in week 40
- **Nervous system**: Commissures are completed by week 20. Myelinization of the cord begins in week 20. Cerebral cortex is typically layered by week 24. Cerebral fissures and convolutions appear rapidly in week 28. Myelinization of the brain begins in week 40
- **Sense organs**: Nose and ear ossify in week 20. Vascular tunic of the lens is at its greatest by week 28. Retinal layers are completed and light perception is possible by week 28. Taste sense is present in week 32. Eyelids reopen between 28 and 32. Mastoid cells are still unformed by week 40. At birth, the ear is still deaf to sounds.

DOWN'S SYNDROME

Trisomy 21

Chromosomal constitution 47, XY(X) + 21
Sex Ratio: Male: Female = 1: 1
Incidence: Overall incidence 1 in 700 live births. (Increases as maternal age advances)

Maternal age (years)	Incidence
20	1 in 1500
35	1 in 400
45	1 in 30

- High incidence is also found in very young mothers (age < 1 7 yrs)
- Increased incidence at extremes of age of fertility is probably due to low estrogen levels (oestrogen controls the rate of meiosis)
- Paternal age> 50 yrs: increased incidence

Cause

- Non-dysjunction of chromosome no. 21 in Meiosis I or Meiosis n in maternal or paternal gametes
- Translocation of long arm of chromosome number 21 to other chromosome

Clinical features

More than 300 external features are noted
Most common features are

Head

- Small round cranium with flat occiput-brachycephaly

Face

- Flat face with flat nasal bridge
- Small, low set dysplastic ears
- Upward and outward slanting palpebral fissures (mongoloid slant)
- Presence of epicanthic folds masking inner angles
- Breshfield spots on iris
- Protruding tongue

Neck

- Short nape of neck with excess of nuchal skin

Limbs

- Hypotonia of muscles
- Short fingers especially fifth digit and thumb
- Single transverse palmar (simian) crease
- Wide gap between 1st and 2nd toes

Heart

- Atrial septal defect (ASD)
- Ventricular septal defect (VSD)
- Patent ductus arteriosus (PDA)
- Common atrioventricular canal

Lungs

- Prone to respiratory infections

Mental status

- Mental retardation
- Delayed milestones - IQ 25 to 70
- Good sense of rhythm - music lovers

Life expectancy

- More than other trisomies and many patients reach adulthood.

Recurrence risk

- Related to maternal age (in 200 to 1 in 100 if a frank case of trisomy)
- 100% recurrence risk if 21 q/21 q translocation in either of the parent

KLINEFELTER'S SYNDROME

Chromosomal constitution: 47, XXY

Incidence

- 1 in 1000 live births
- Increases with advanced maternal age

Cause

- Nondysjunction of X chromosome during Meiosis I or Meiosis ll.

Clinical features

No significant dysmorphism is noted apart from symptoms pertaining to genital system.

Children

Non-specific associated malformations of genitalia may be present

- Ectopic testis
- Hypospadias
- Hypoplasia of testis and scrotum

The syndrome is usually diagnosed at puberty.

Adolescents

- Gynaecomastia
- Hypogonadism
- Testicular atrophy
- Azoospermia
- Sterility
- Weak facial hair growth
- Coarse voice

Hormonal status

- Low plasma testosterone and high gonadotrophins

Mental status

- Normal intelligence in majority of cases or mild mental retardation
- Abnormal sexual behaviour may be found in some cases

Cytogenetics

- Presence of Barr bodies in the cell nucleus of patients

Dermatoglyphics

Dermatoglyphic pattern shows

- Decreased total ridge count
- Increased frequency of arches
- Increased frequency of single transverse palmar crease

TURNER'S SYNDROME

It is the monosomy of X chromosome

Chromosomal constitution

- 45, XO
- Mosaics may be present i.e. 46XX/45XO

Incidence

- One in 2500 live births
- Frequency at conception is much higher (most of the zygotes with the 45, XO karyotype abort early in the first trimester)

Cause

- Non-dysjunction of X chromosome either paternal or maternal in Meiosis I or Meiosis II during gametogenesis

Clinical features

Many phenotypic variations are possible

Infant

- Small size
- Lymphoedema of hands and feet
- Excess skin at the nape of the neck

Adolescent

Face

- Triangular face
- Outward and downward slanted palpebral fissures
- High arched palate
- Hypoplasia of mandible
- Retrognathia
- Low set ears

Neck

- Short neck
- Webbing of the neck
- Low hairline on the nape

Thorax

- Widely spaced and hypoplastic nipples,
- Broad thorax,
- Biacromial diameter is excessively large

Limbs

- Short stature
- Cubitus valgus
- Shortening of 4th and 5th metacarpals

Genitalia

- Infantile external genitalia
- Scanty pubic and axillary hair
- Non development of secondary sex characters
- Streak gonads (gonadal atrophy) with infertility

Other anomalies

- **Cardiac**-coarctation of aorta
- **Renal** -horseshoe kidney
- **Ocular** –myopia and congenital cataracts
- **Auditory**-congenital deafness

Life expectancy

- In case of severe malformations- death in the neonatal period may occur
- Malformations are subdued and the survival rate is normal
- Disease is usually diagnosed at puberty

EDWARD'S SYNDROME

It is the trisomy of chromosome 18
Chromosomal constitution: 47, XY (X), + 18
Incidence: 1 in 8000 live births (increased with increase in maternal age)
Sex ratio: Male: Female 1: 4

Cause

- Non dysjunction of chromosome 18 in Meiosis I or Meiosis II during oogenesis

Clinical features

Head

- Dolichocephaly with prominent occiput

Face

- Low set ears
- Small mouth
- Receding chin
- Cleft lip-palate

Neck

- Webbed neck

Limbs

- Short thumb
- Index finger overlapping middle and ring finger
- Rocker bottom feet (protrusion of heel and convexity of sole)

Mental Status

- Severe mental retardation

Life Expectancy

- 2-3 months for males and 10 months for females

PATAU'S SYNDROME

It is the trisomy of chromosome 13.
Chromosomal constitution: 47, XX(Y), + 13

Incidence

- One per 10,000 live births

Sex ratio

- Females are slightly affected more than males

Cause

- Non-dysjunction of chromosome 13 during oogenesis in Meiosis I or Meiosis II

Clinical features

Head

- Small cranium
- Receding forehead
- Narrow temples
- Broad fontanelles and suture lines

Face

- Microphthalmia
- Harelip (bilateral cleft lip) accompanied by cleft palate
- Broad, flat nose
- Low set ears
- Haemangiomas on face, forehead and nape of the neck

Limbs

- Hexadactyly(uni-or bilateral) i.e. extra finger on the ulnar side of hand
- Rocker bottom feet (protrusion of heel and convexity of sole).

Other anomalies

- **Cardiac** (ASD & VSD)
- **Visceral** (Malrotation of gut)
- **Urinary** (Polycystic kidneys)

Mental status

- Mental retardation with seizures
- Hypotonia
- Failure to thrive

Life expectancy

- One to six months for both the sexes
- Survival beyond 3 years is exceptional

DIAPHRAGMATIC HERNIAS

Congenital diaphragmatic hernia is one of the more common malformations in the newborn. It is most frequently caused by failure of one or both of the pleuroperitoneal membranes to close the pericardioperitoneal canals. In such cases the peritoneal and pleural cavities are continuous with one another along the posterior body wall.

This hernia causes abdominal viscera to enter the pleural cavity. In 85 to 90 % cases, the hernia is seen on the left side. The loops of intestine, stomach, spleen, and part of the liver may enter the thoracic cavity.

The abdominal viscera in the chest push the heart anteriorly and compress the lungs, which are commonly hypoplastic. A large defect is associated with a high rate of mortality (**75%**) from pulmonary hypoplasia and dysfunction.

Occasionally a small part of the muscular fibers of the diaphragm fails to develop. This hernia may remain undiscovered until the child is several years old. Such defect which is frequently seen in the anterior part of the diaphragm is termed **parasternal hernia**. A small peritoneal sac containing intestinal loops may enter the chest between the sternal and costal portions of the diaphragm.

Oesophageal hernia - is due to congenital shortness of the oesophagus. The upper parts of the stomach are in the thorax and the stomach is constricted at the level of the diaphragm.

RDS SYNDROME

Surfactant is particularly important for survival of the premature infant. When surfactant is insufficient, the air-water (blood) surface membrane tension becomes high and alveoli collapse during expiration and respiratory distress syndrome (RDS) develops.

RDS is a common cause of death in the premature infant. In these cases the partially collapsed alveoli contain a fluid with high protein content, many hyaline membranes and lamellar bodies which are probably derived from the surfactant layer.

RDS (**Hyaline membrane disease**) accounts for approximately 20 % of deaths among newborns.

Recent development of artificial surfactant and treatment of premature babies with glucocorticoids to stimulate surfactant production have reduced the mortality associated with RDS. This has allowed survival of some babies as young as 5.5 months of gestation.

BIRTH DEFECTS AND PRENATAL DIAGNOSIS

STEM CELL TRANSPLANTATION AND GENE THERAPY

The foetus does not develop any immuno-competence before 18 weeks gestation. Therefore it may be possible to transplant tissues or cells before this time without rejection.

Research in this field is focusing on hematopoietic stem cells for the treatment of

- Immunodeficiency disorders
- Hematologic disorders

Gene therapy for inherited metabolic diseases, such as **Tay Sachs** and **cystic fibrosis** is also being investigated.

Summary

Many agents are known to produce congenital malformations in approximately 2 to 3 % of all live-births

These include

Viruses

- Rubella
- Cytomegalovirus

Radiation

Drugs

- Thalidomide
- Aminopterin
- Anticonvulsants
- Anti psychotics
- Antianxiety compounds

Social drugs

- Cigarettes and alcohol

Hormones

- diethylstilbestrol

Maternal diabetes

Effects of teratogens depend on

- Maternal and fetal genotype
- Stage of development when exposure occurs
- Dose and duration of exposure of the agent

Most major malformations are produced during the period of embryogenesis (teratogenic period – 3rd to 8th weeks).

But it should be noted that the foetus is also susceptible before and after the period of embryogenesis so that no period of gestation is completely free of risk.

Prevention of many birth defects is possible which depends on

- Preventative measures before conception
- Physicians' and women's awareness of the risks

Techniques available to assess the growth and developmental status of the foetus include

- **Ultrasound** - determines foetal age and growth parameters and detect many malformations
- **Maternal serum screening for alpha-fetoprotein** - indicate the presence of a neural tube defect or other abnormalities

- **Amniocentesis** – in this procedure a needle is placed into the amniotic cavity and a fluid sample is withdrawn. The fluid is analyzed and cells are used for culture and genetic analysis
- **Chorionic villus sampling** (CVS) – it involves aspirating a tissue sample directly from the placenta to obtain cells for genetic analysis

Many of these procedures involve a potential risk to the foetus and mother. Therefore they are generally only used for higher risk pregnancies (except ultrasound).

Risk factors include

- Advanced maternal age (35 years or older)
- History of neural tube defects in the family
- Previous gestation with a chromosome abnormality
- Chromosome abnormalities in either parent
- Mother who is a carrier for an X-linked disorder

With the advancement of modern medicine the foetus can receive treatment e.g.

- Transfusions
- Medications for disease
- Foetal surgery
- Gene therapy

Section-VII
Surface & Radiological Anatomy

CONTENTS

83. **Head and Neck**   491-502

84. **Conventional Radiology**   503-506

85. **Special Radiological Investigations**   507-512

Head and Neck

Pericraniocervical line extends from the symphysis menti anteriorly to the inion posteriorly - demarcates head from neck.

SKELETAL LANDMARKS OF HEAD

Posterior Aspect

- External occipital protuberance and inion

Lateral Aspect

- Mastoid process
- External acoustic meatus
- Zygomatic process of temporal bone, with temporal process of zygomatic bone - **zygomatic arch**
- Body of zygomatic bone
- **Pterion** - junction of frontal, sphenoid, parietal and temporal bones. It lies 4 cm above zygomatic arch and 3.5 cm behind fronto-zygomatic suture - marks anterior branch of middle meningeal artery and **Sylvian point** (stem of lateral sulcus) of the brain.
- **Suprameatal triangle** is posterosuperior to external acoustic meatus. Boundaries are:

Above - supramastoid crest

In front - posterosuperior margin of meatus

Behind - posterior vertical tangent to the margin of meatus.

The triangle forms the lateral wall of the mastoid antrum.

- Ramus of mandible
- Posterior border of the ramus, condylar process and head of the mandible
- During opening and closure of mouth the temporomandibular joint is felt.
- Angle of the mandible
- Mental tubercle

Anterior Aspect

- Superciliary arch above orbit
- Frontal tuberosity - above superciliary arch.
- Anterior fontanelle (**Bregma**) – at the junction of coronal and sagittal suture till 18 months of age.
- Between superciliary arches – **glabella**
- Nasal bones meet frontal bone (**nasion**) – at the root of nose.
- Canine eminence above canine socket. Incisor fossa lies anterior to it and posteriorly placed is canine fossa
- Frontal process of maxilla
- Zygomatic process of maxilla
- Alveolar process of maxilla
- Palatine process of the maxilla – palpable within the mouth

Orbital opening - Quadrangular in outline with following margins:

Supraorbital margin - frontal bone

Lateral margin - frontal process of zygomatic bone and zygomatic process of frontal bone

Inferior border - zygomatic bone laterally and maxilla medially

Medial margin - above by frontal bone and below by lacrimal crest of frontal process of maxilla

SOFT TISSUES

Posterior Aspect

- Epicranial aponeurosis

Lateral Aspect

- Auricle (pinna) surrounds external acoustic meatus
- With increasing age a fissure may be seen running obliquely downwards and backwards from the lobule of ear. This may be associated with cardiac insufficiency - **Frank's sign**
- Tympanic membrane is seen by auroscope
- Superficial temporal artery crosses in front of the tragus (pulsations felt)
- Muscles of mastication - palpable when the jaw is clenched
  Temporalis - lies in the temporal fossa covered by temporal fascia
  Masseter - palpable when the jaw is clenched, its anterior border becomes prominent
- Parotid duct emerges at the anterior border of masseter which can be palpated where it crosses the anterior border of masseter when the jaw is clenched

Anterior Aspect

- Opening of parotid duct is visible as a small papilla within the mouth at the level of the second upper molar tooth.
- Pulsation of facial artery - felt as it crosses lower margin of the body of mandible immediately in front of masseter.

- Palatine tonsil is marked by an oval area over the lower part of the masseter, just above and in front of the angle of the mandible.
- Inferior surface of tongue in the midline is connected to the floor of mouth by frenulum.
- Orifices of submandibular ducts may be seen each side of the base of frenulum.

NECK

Surface Landmarks

At the back of the neck the bones of the cervical vertebrae may be felt in the midline.

- C-1 vertebra (**atlas**) - not palpable
- Spine of C-2 vertebra can be felt on deep palpation.
- Spine of C-7 vertebra is prominent, can be palpated -**vertebra prominens**
- Below chin, hyoid is felt especially when the neck is extended. It is palpated between finger and thumb and can be moved from side to side.
- Thyroid cartilage and the midline fusion of its laminae - **laryngeal prominence (Adam's apple)**
- Curved upper border of thyroid cartilage and thyroid notch
- cricoid cartilage is felt, below inferior border of thyroid cartilage
- Posterior end of first rib is felt in the supraclavicular fossa in deep palpation.

Important vertebral levels

C-1 Dens, level of nasopharynx

C-2 Oropharynx and soft palate (with the mouth open)

C-3 Body of hyoid and its greater cornu

C-3 & 4 junction Upper border of thyroid cartilage & bifurcation of common carotid artery (CCA)

C-4 & 5 Thyroid cartilage

C-6 Cricoid cartilage

SOFT TISSUES

Neck is divided into two triangles by sternocleidomastoid (SCM)

These triangles are

- Anterior triangle
- Posterior triangle

Boundaries of anterior triangle

- Midline structures anteriorly
- Base of the mandible below
- Sternocleidomastoid (anterior border)

Anterior triangle is further subdivided into

1. Submental triangle
2. Muscular triangle
3. Carotid triangle
4. Digastric triangle

Boundaries of posterior triangle

- Sternocleidomastoid (posterior border)
- Middle one third of the clavicle below
- Anterior border of trapezius behind

Posterior triangle is further subdivided into

1. Occipital triangle (upper large)
2. Supraclavicular triangle (lower small)
   - Between two heads of SCM internal jugular vein (IJV) lies.
   - **Trachea** is palpated below the cricoid cartilage and its rings are felt. It lies in the midline.
   - Transverse process of the C-6 vertebra is prominent (**Chassaignac's tubercle**). The carotid artery may be compressed here and above this level it is superficial, where its pulsation can be easily felt.
   - **IJV** runs parallel and just lateral to the carotid artery.
   - **External jugular vein (EJV)** is demonstrated by forced expiration against a closed mouth and blocked nostrils-**Valsalva's manoeuvre**
   - Posterior end of 1st rib is felt in posterior aspect of supraclavicular fossa
   - Subclavian artery pulsations - as it crosses the 1st rib.
   - Above and behind subclavian artery - trunks of brachial plexus felt.

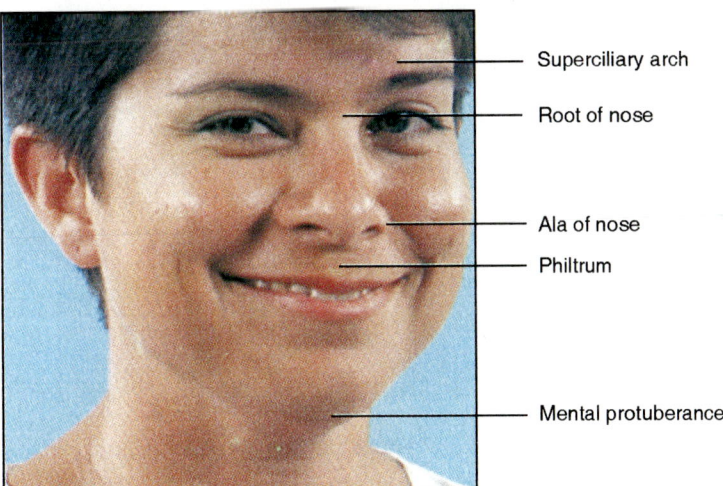

Fig. 83.1: Landmarks over face

Superciliary arch

Root of nose

Ala of nose

Philtrum

Mental protuberance

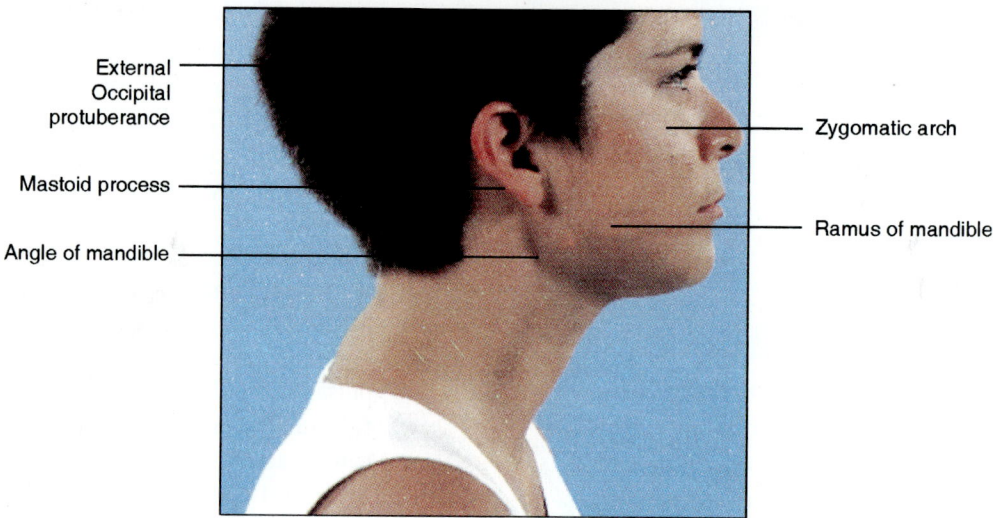

Fig. 83.2: Lateral Landmarks

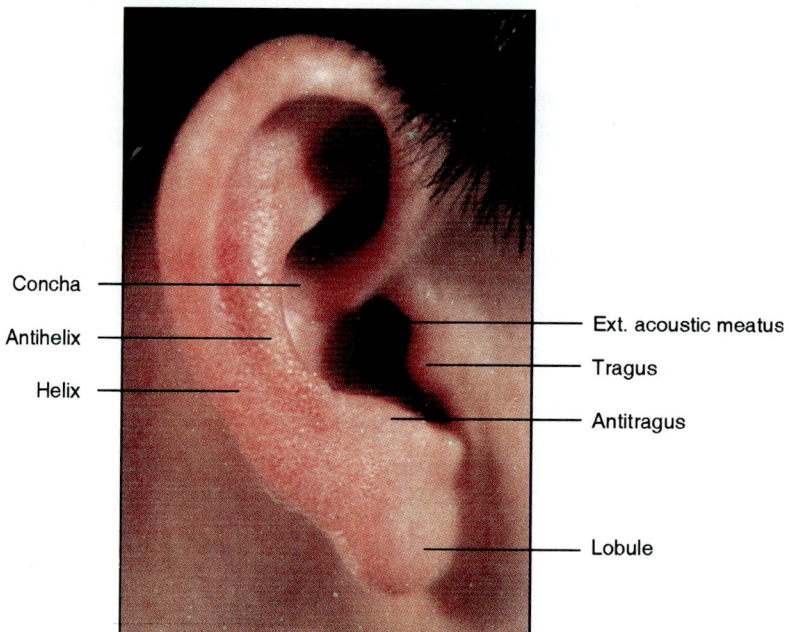

Fig. 83.3: Landmarks on Ear

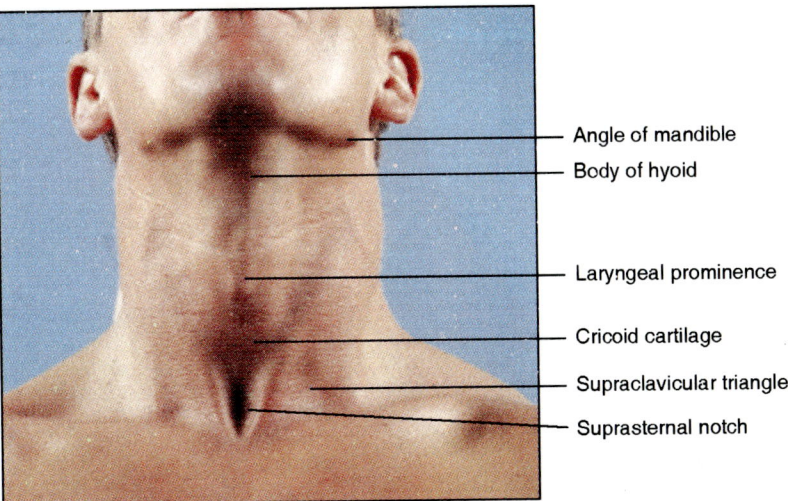

Angle of mandible
Body of hyoid

Laryngeal prominence

Cricoid cartilage

Supraclavicular triangle

Suprasternal notch

Fig. 83.4: Landmarks over anterior of neck

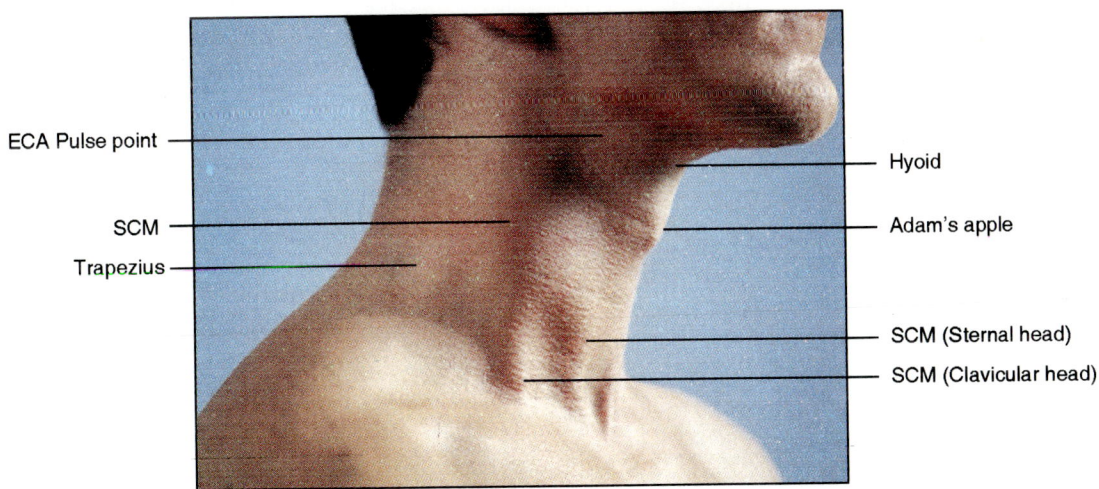

ECA Pulse point

SCM

Trapezius

Hyoid

Adam's apple

SCM (Sternal head)

SCM (Clavicular head)

Fig. 83.5: Landmarks on lateral side of neck

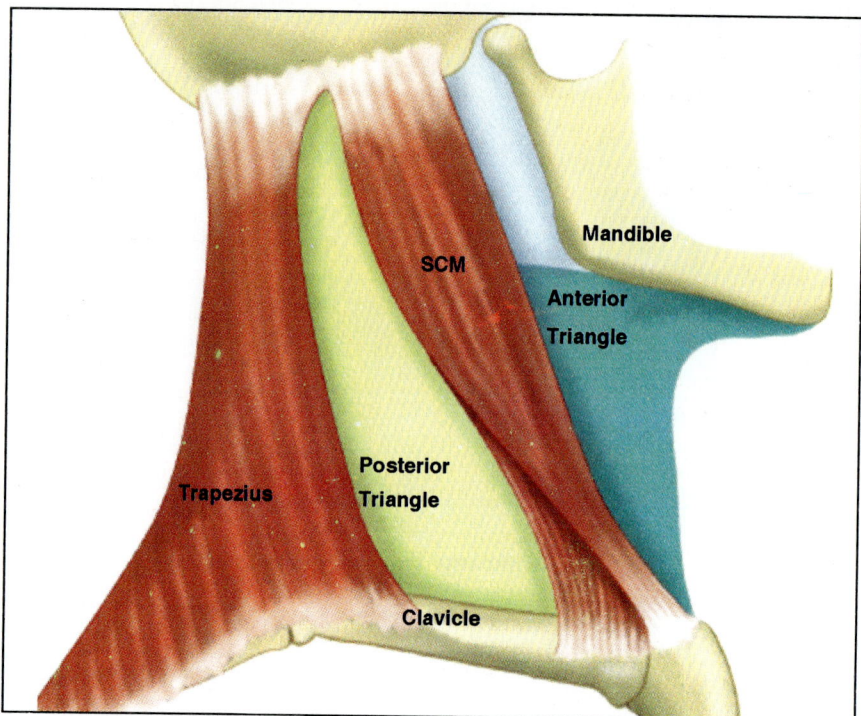

Fig. 83.6: Triangles of neck

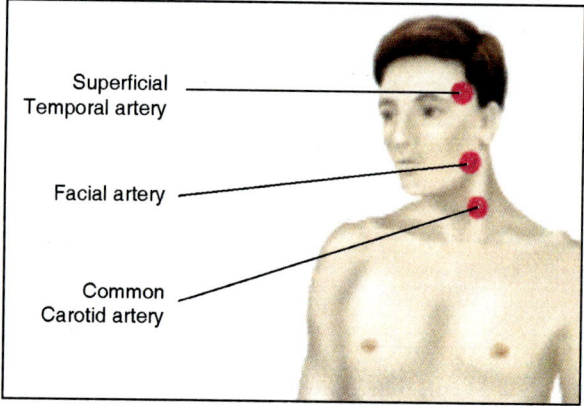

Fig. 83.7: Arterial palpation in head & neck

EXTERNAL JUGULAR VEIN

Take two points
- 1. Just below the angle of mandible
- 2. At the junction of medial one third and middle one third of the clavicle

Join these points by two parallel lines

INTERNAL JUGULAR VEIN

Take two points
- 1. On the ear lobule
- 2. At the medial end of the clavicle

Join these points by two parallel lines

COMMON CAROTID ARTERY

Take two points
- 1. At sternoclavicular joint
- 2. At the anterior border of SCM at the level of upper border of thyroid cartilage

Join these points by two parallel lines

INTERNAL CAROTID ARTERY

Take two points
- 1. At the anterior border of SCM at the level of upper border of thyroid cartilage
- 2. Just behind the condyle of the mandible

Join these points by two parallel lines

FACIAL ARTERY ON THE FACE

Take four points
- 1. Along the lower border of the mandible at the anteroinferior angle of the masseter muscle
- 2. One cm lateral to the angle of mouth
- 3. Just lateral to ala of nose
- 4. At the medial angle of mouth

Join these points by two parallel lines

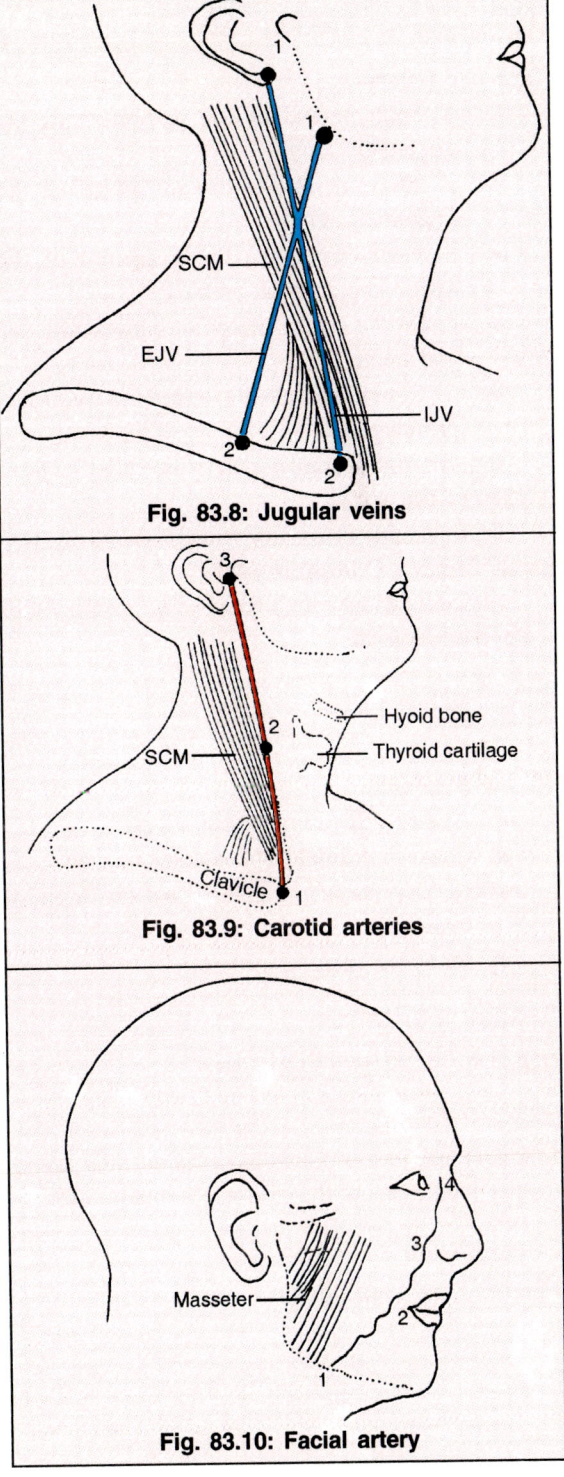

Fig. 83.8: Jugular veins

Fig. 83.9: Carotid arteries

Fig. 83.10: Facial artery

MIDDLE MENINGEAL ARTERY

Take five points

- 1. Just medial to the midpoint of the zygomatic arch
- 2. Two cm above the midpoint of the zygomatic arch
- 3. Four cm above the midpoint of the zygomatic arch (at pterion)
- 4. On the vertex midpoint between nasion and inion
- 5. Seven cm above external occipital protuberance

Join first and second points by two parallel lines – **Stem of the artery**

Join second, third and fourth points by two parallel lines – **Frontal branch**

Join second and fifth points by two parallel lines – **Parietal branch**

PAROTID GLAND

Take four points

- 1. Just in front of tragus of ear
- 2. At the middle of masseter muscle
- 3. Two cm below and behind the angle of mandible
- 4. At the mastoid process

Anterior border

Join first, second and third points

Superior border

Join first and fourth points by a curved line across the ear lobule below the external acoustic meatus

Posterior border

Join third and fourth points

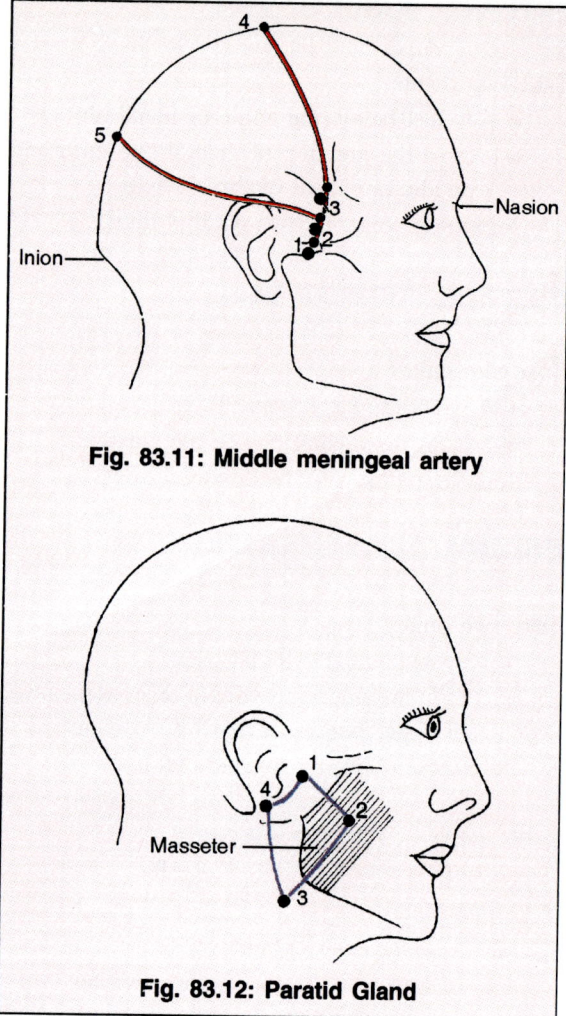

Fig. 83.11: Middle meningeal artery

Fig. 83.12: Paratid Gland

PAROTID DUCT

Take two points

- 1. At the lower border of tragus of ear
- 2. Midpoint between philtrum and red margin of upper lip

Join these two points by two parallel lines. Middle one third represents the parotid duct

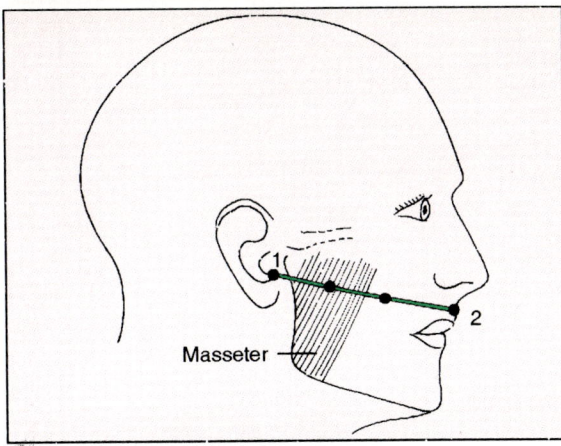

Fig. 83.13: Parotid duct

SUBMANDIBULAR GLAND

Take three points
- 1. At the angle of mandible
- 2. Midpoint between angle of mandible and the symphysis
- 3. Midway between the two points 1.5 cm above the lower border of mandible
- Mark greater cornu of hyoid

Join these points with an oval figure

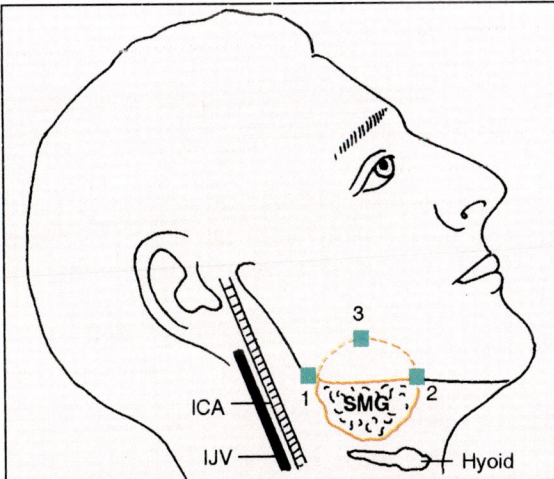

Fig. 83.14: Submandibular gland

THYROID GLAND

Isthmus

- **Upper border** is marked across the trachea, about 1 cm below the arch of cricoid cartilage by 1.5 cm long line
- **Lower border** is marked by another parallel line 2 cm below the first line

Lateral lobes

- Mark a point 1 cm below the lateral end of lower border
- Mark second point 2.5 cm below and lateral to the lateral end of lower border
- Mark third point just in front of anterior border of SCM muscle at the level of laryngeal prominence – level of upper pole of lateral lobe

Join third point and lateral end of upper border of isthmus to mark the upper border of lateral lobe

Join first, second third points by a curved line to mark the outline of lateral lobe

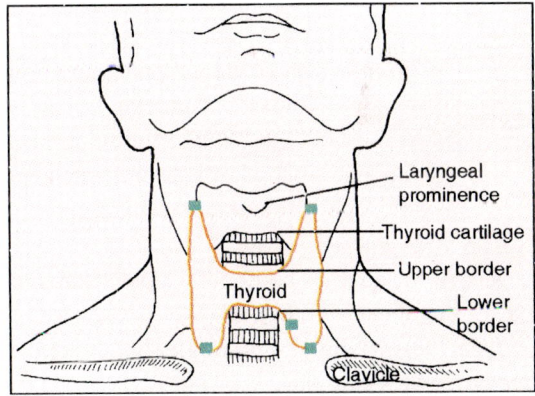

Fig. 83.15: Thyroid gland

GLOSSOPHARYNGEAL NERVE

Take two points
- At the anterior aspect of tragus of ear
- Just above the angle of mandible

Join the two points by a single line which is continued along the lower border of mandible for some distance

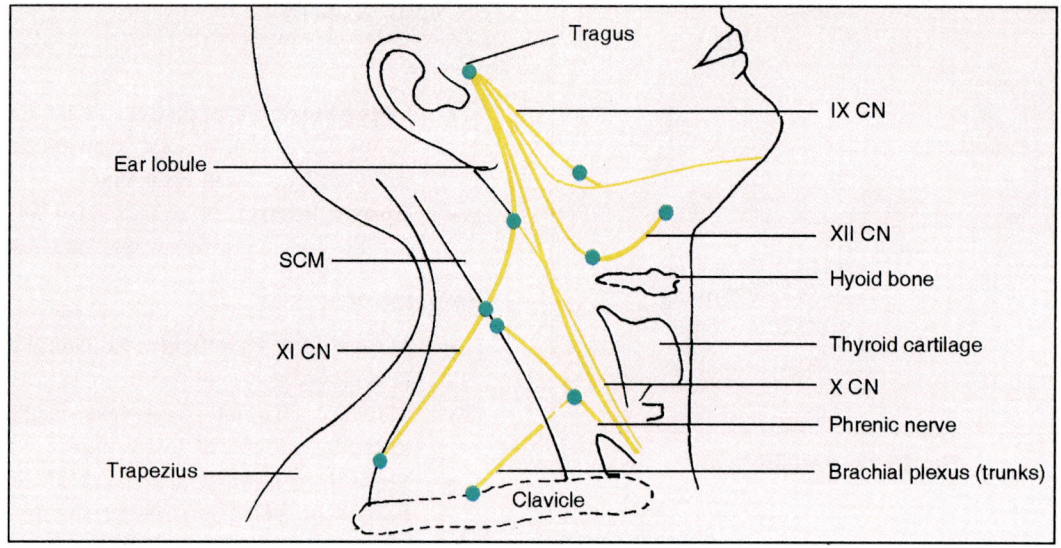

Fig. 83.16: Cranial nerves

SPINAL ACCESSORY NERVE

Take five points
- At the anterior aspect of tragus of ear
- At the tip of transverse process of atlas
- At the junction of upper one fourth and lower three fourth of anterior border of SCM muscle
- At the junction of upper one third and middle one third of posterior border of SCM muscle
- At the anterior border of Trapezius about 6 cm above of clavicle

Join these points by a single line which is directed downwards and backwards

HYPOGLOSSAL NERVE

Take three points
- At the anterior aspect of tragus of ear
- Just above and behind the greater cornu of hyoid bone
- Third point is midway between angle of mandible and symphysis menti

Join these points by a single line

VAGUS NERVE

Take two points
- At the anterior aspect of tragus of ear
- At the medial end of clavicle

Join these points by a single line

BRACHIAL PLEXUS (SUPRACLAVICULAR PART)

Take two points
- At midpoint between anterior and posterior borders of SCM at the level of cricoid cartilage
- At midpoint of clavicle

Join these points by a solid line to represent supraclavicular components of brachial plexus

PHRENIC NERVE

Take two points
- Point about 3.5 cm away from anterior median plane of neck at the level of upper border of thyroid cartilage

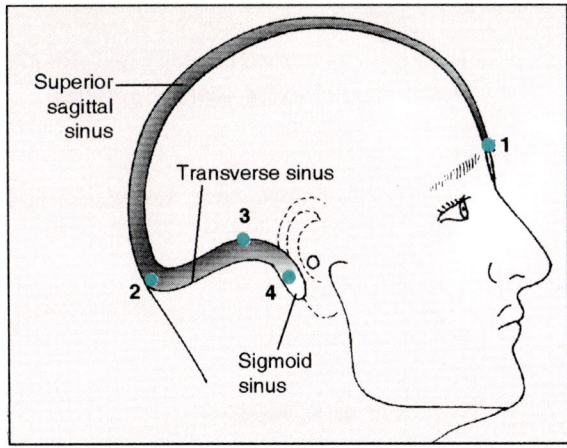

Fig. 83.17: Dural Venous Sinuses

- Second point between anterior and posterior borders of SCM at the level of cricoid cartilage
- Third point on at the medial end of clavicle

Join these points by a single line

SUPERIOR SAGITTAL SINUS

Take two points
- At the glabella
- At the inion

Join these points by two parallel lines

TRANSVERSE SINUS

Take two points
- At the inion
- At the base of mastoid process

Join these points by two parallel lines

SIGMOID SINUS

Take two points
- At the base of mastoid process
- Second point about 1.2 cm above the tip of mastoid process

Join these points by two parallel lines

NERVE BLOCKS

INTERSCALENE BLOCK

Landmarks

- SCM
- Interscalene groove
- Cricoid cartilage

Puncture site

- In the Interscalene groove at the level of cricoid cartilage

Direction of needle

- The needle is pushed medially and downwards (in an angle of 30 degree to the sagittal plane) and slightly backwards being directed to the transverse process of C-6 vertebra

Indications

1. Operations on clavicle, shoulder, upper arm and hand
2. Reduction of shoulder joint

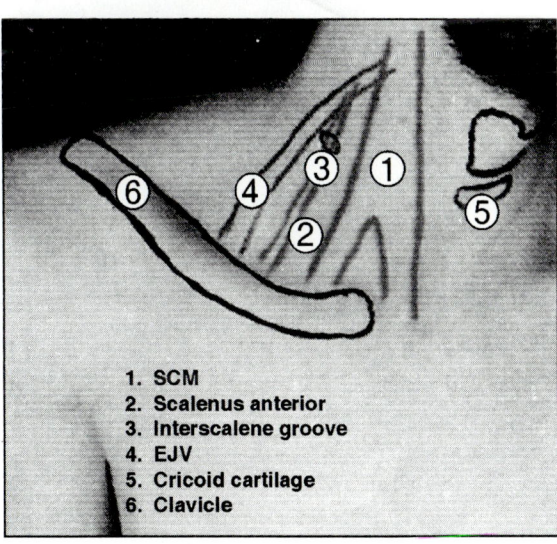

1. SCM
2. Scalenus anterior
3. Interscalene groove
4. EJV
5. Cricoid cartilage
6. Clavicle

Fig. 83.18: Interscalene block

Side effects

- Horner's syndrome
- Phrenic nerve block
- Recurrent nerve block

Complications

- Total spinal anaesthesia
- High epidural anaesthesia

Contraindications

- Contralateral phrenic nerve paralysis
- Contralateral recurrent laryngeal nerve paralysis

SUPRACLAVICULAR BLOCK

Landmarks

- Clavicle
- Subclavian artery

Puncture site

- Immediately dorsolateral from the palpated pulsation of the subclavian artery

Direction of needle

- The needle is pushed caudally and slightly lateral parallel to the scalene muscles

Indications

- Operations of upper arm, lower arm and hand

Side effects

- Horner's syndrome
- Phrenic nerve block
- Recurrent nerve block

Complications

- Pneumothorax
- Subclavian artery puncture

Contraindications

- Contralateral phrenic nerve paralysis
- Contralateral recurrent laryngeal nerve paralysis
- Contralateral pneumothorax
- Haemorragic disorders

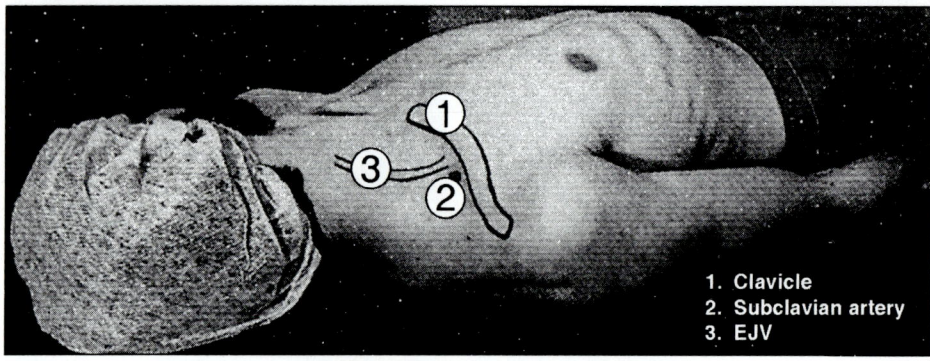

1. Clavicle
2. Subclavian artery
3. EJV

Fig. 83.19: Supraclavicular block

84

Conventional Radiology

INTRODUCTION

The Radiology and Imaging departments use a variety of different techniques to provide images of human internal organs and to demonstrate pathological lesions within them. These techniques can be classified into

Methods using ionizing radiation

- Simple X-ray
- Computed X-ray tomography (**C T scanning**)
- Radio isotope scanning (**Nuclear medicine**)

Other methods

- Ultrasound (**USG**)
- Magnetic Resonance Imaging (**MRI**)

X-Ray examination

- Roentgen (German physicist) discovered X-ray in 1895. This was the starting point for modern medical radiology and radiotherapy. These are part of electro-magnetic spectrum ranging from wireless waves to cosmic rays. They have short wave length so that they can penetrate materials not transmitting visible light.

- X-rays are produced by passing high voltage electric current across a vacuum tube. This induces a stream of electrons from an electrically heated metal element called cathode. This strikes a metal target called anode after passing across the vacuum. When the beam of electrons strikes the anode X-rays are produced.

Properties of X-rays:

1. **Penetrating power** depends on the density of the substance. Dense tissue like bones absorb X-rays more readily than the soft tissues. Thus the structure may be radiolucent (easily penetrated by X-rays) or radio-opaque (not penetrated by X-rays).
2. **Photogenic effect** causes photosensitive film to get photosensitized. Development of such film gives a radiographic image.
3. **Fluorescent effect** is used in fluoroscopy.
4. **Biological effect** is used in the treatment of various cancers to kill those cells.

SIMPLE RADIOGRAPHY

In this procedure the X-ray beam is passed through the patient on to a photographic plate.

MASS MINIATURE RADIOGRAPHY (MMR)

Miniature films are obtained by taking optical photographs of a fluorescent image. These films are cheap and used for large scale radiographic investigations such as tuberculosis.

XEORADIOGRAPHY

This procedure provides soft tissue contrast which is not obtained by conventional radiography. In this an aluminium plate is coated with a thin layer of selenium and electrically charged. An X-ray beam is passed through the patient to this plate. This results in alteration of the electrostatic charge corresponding with the image. The image is obtained by blowing a thin powder which adheres in proportion to the local charge on the plate. This is then transferred to a special paper.

TOMOGRAPHY

This has been in use for long and is a variant of the simple X- ray method in which tissue section radiographs are obtained.

Radiographic views

The view denotes the direction of the beam of X-ray. Thus, in AP view X-ray beam passes from anterior aspect and the radiography plate is placed posteriorly. In PA view it is other way round.

The part of the body closer to the plate is more clearly visualized.

HEAD AND NECK

AP VIEW OF THE SKULL

In this view, the petrous parts of the temporal bones are projected onto the orbits, almost completely obscuring the orbital features; however, maximal exposure of the cranial vault is obtained.

For this view

- Patient is placed in the upright position
- Chin is placed against the film tray
- Canthomeatal line forms a 37° angle with the film plane
- X-ray beam traverses the vertex posteriorly and the anterior nasal spine anteriorly.

The bony outlines of the orbits and frontal and maxillary sinuses are especially clear in this view.

Occipitofrontal view is

- Used mainly for sinus study
- For detecting blow-out fractures in orbital trauma

LATERAL VIEW OF THE SKULL

The X-ray beam passes through a point 1 inch above the midpoint of a line joining the lateral angle (canthus) of the eye with the tragus or the external acoustic meatus of the ear (canthomeatal line).This point lies just above the hypophyseal fossa.

- Two halves of the mandible are superimposed
- Cervical vertebrae are seen obliquely

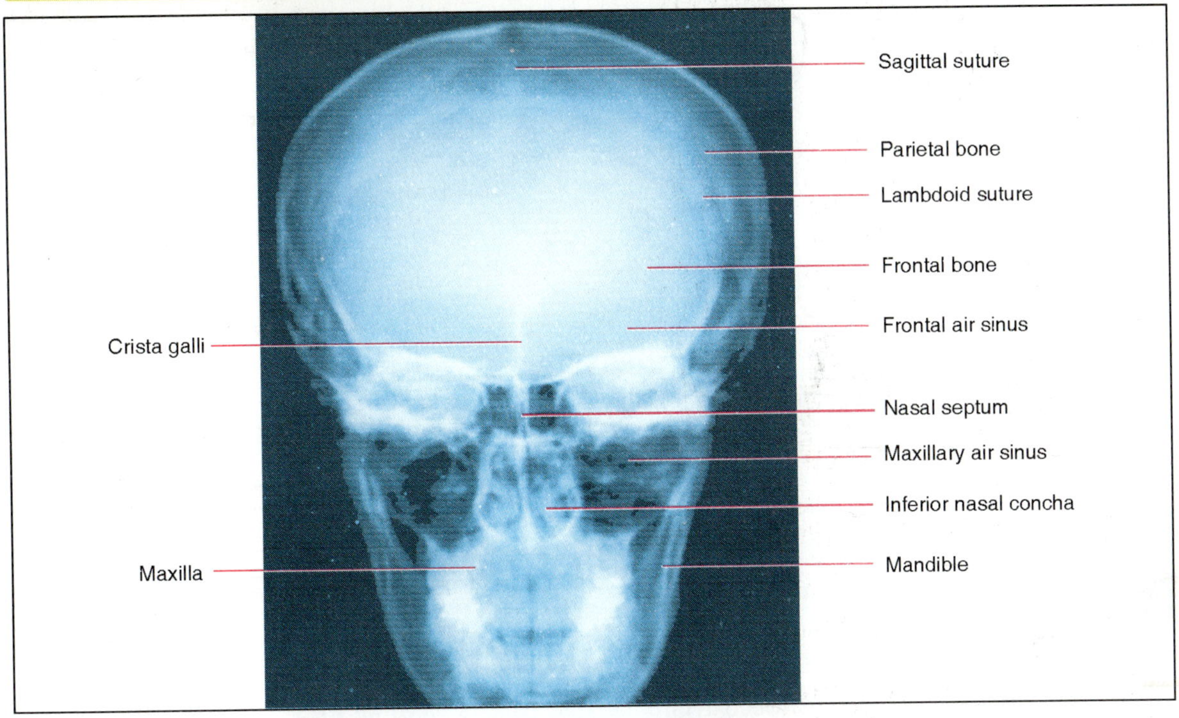

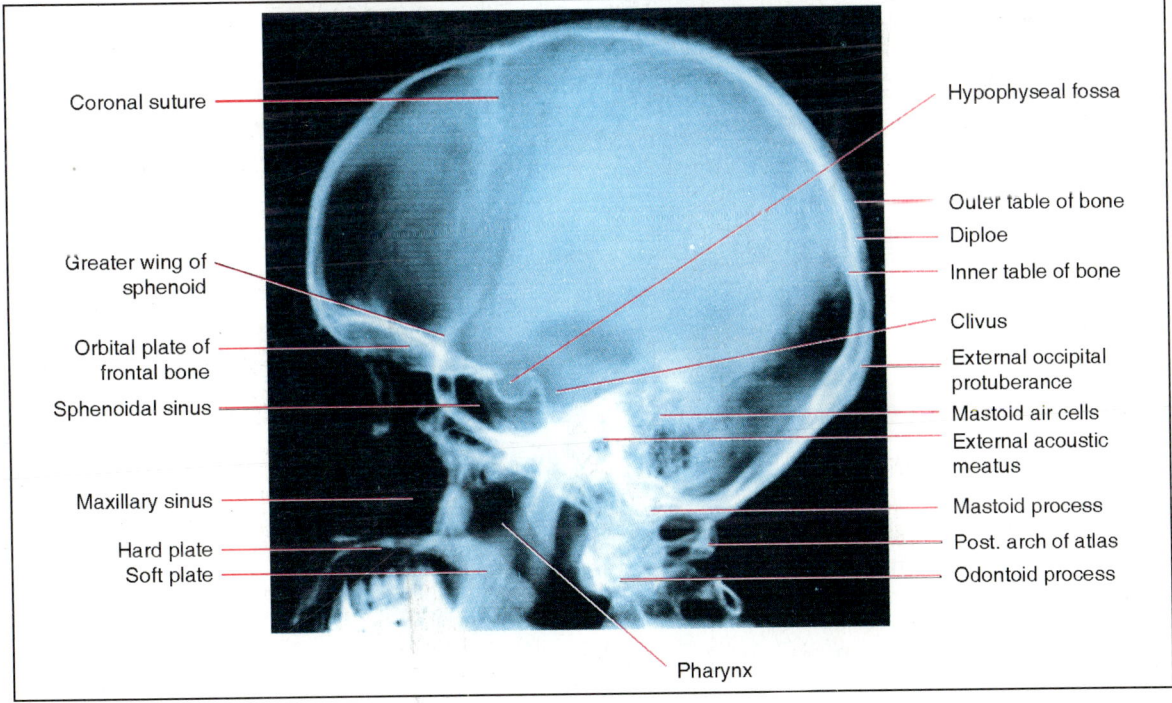

Fig. 84.1: Skull: AP view

Sagittal suture
Parietal bone
Lambdoid suture
Frontal bone
Frontal air sinus
Nasal septum
Maxillary air sinus
Inferior nasal concha
Mandible
Crista galli
Maxilla

Fig. 84.2: Skull: Left lateral view

Coronal suture
Hypophyseal fossa
Outer table of bone
Diploe
Inner table of bone
Greater wing of sphenoid
Orbital plate of frontal bone
Clivus
External occipital protuberance
Sphenoidal sinus
Mastoid air cells
External acoustic meatus
Maxillary sinus
Mastoid process
Hard plate
Post. arch of atlas
Soft plate
Odontoid process
Pharynx

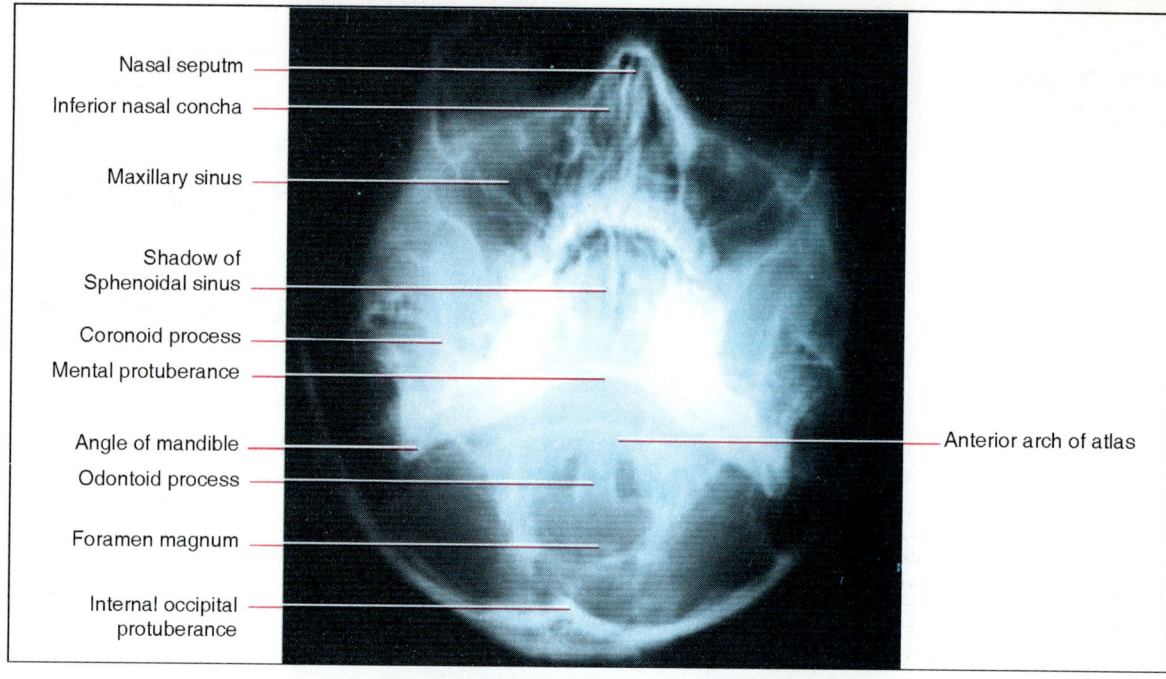

Nasal seputm
Inferior nasal concha
Maxillary sinus
Shadow of Sphenoidal sinus
Coronoid process
Mental protuberance
Angle of mandible
Odontoid process
Foramen magnum
Internal occipital protuberance
Anterior arch of atlas

Fig. 84.3: Occipityofrontal view (waters view) for PNS

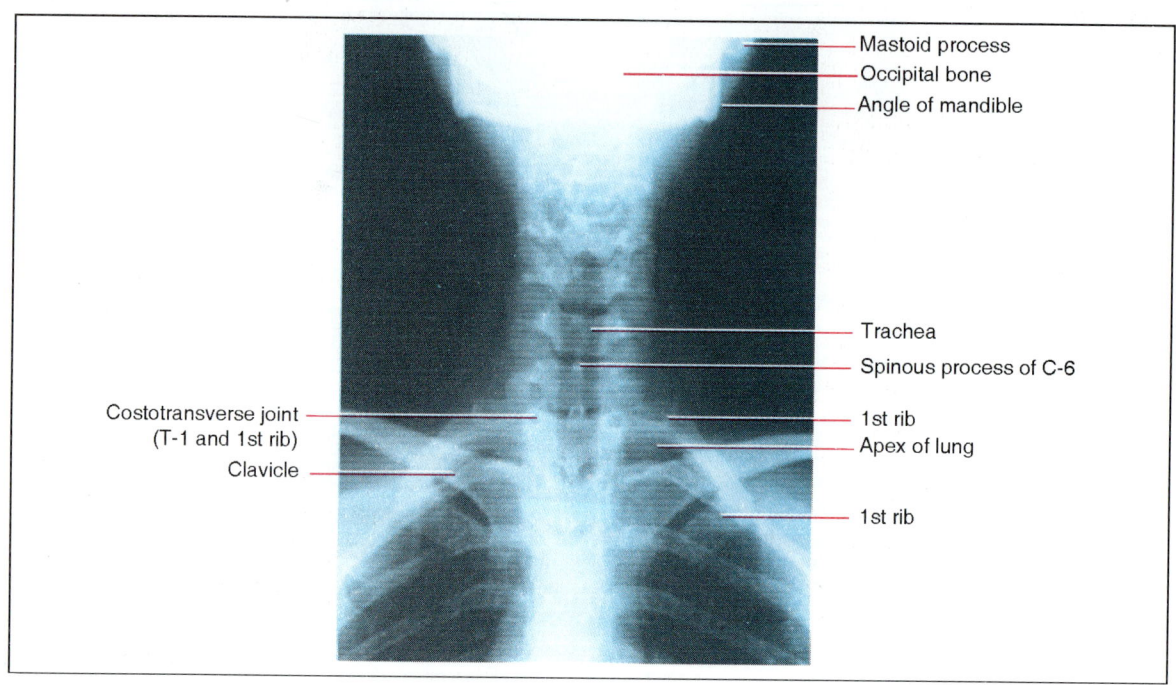

Mastoid process
Occipital bone
Angle of mandible
Trachea
Spinous process of C-6
Costotransverse joint (T-1 and 1st rib)
1st rib
Apex of lung
Clavicle
1st rib

Fig. 84.4: Cervical spine: AP view

85

Special Radiological Investigations

CONTRAST RADIOGRAPHY

Certain substances are used which have a different permeability to X-rays than that of the body. These contrast media can be introduced into body cavities, organs or blood vessels. Thus it is possible to get X-ray picture of the interior of the organ or blood vessel. Commonly used contrast media are:

Salts of heavy metals – Barium sulphate is most commonly used. Sodium iodide is used for cystography.

- Blood and lymph have same density as soft tissues on plain radiographs
- Vessels are seen only against:
  – Air back ground: lungs
  – Fat back ground: breast
- Vessels are also seen when their walls get calcified, as in atherosclerosis.

Thus we need to inject radio-opaque contrast medium into vessels to image them.

Femorocerebral angiography

This is used for evaluating the vessels of the head and upper limb. Under fluoroscopic control, a catheter is introduced into the femoral artery and guided through the iliac vessels up the descending aorta to the arch of aorta.

The catheter tip can be selectively placed into any of the three branches of the arch, and then into further divisions of the branch selected.

Once the tip is in position, radiopaque contrast medium is injected via the catheter. A series of radiographs are taken over eight to ten seconds time. This procedure demonstrates

- Structure and the functional state of the selected vessel and its branches
- Capillary beds they supply
- Veins draining them

COMPUTED TOMOGRAPHY (CT SCAN)

This was developed by a British physicist Godfrey Hounsfield in 1972. This is generally called as computed axial tomography (**CAT scan**). The conventional X-ray provides only a small proportion of data when X-ray beams are passed through human tissues. In CT scan by using multi-directional scanning of the patient multiple data are collected of all tissues in the path of X-ray beams. The X-rays are collected by detector which converts X-ray photons into scintillations. The scintillations are quantified and recorded digitally. The information is fed into a computer which produces different readings as the X-ray beam traverses round the

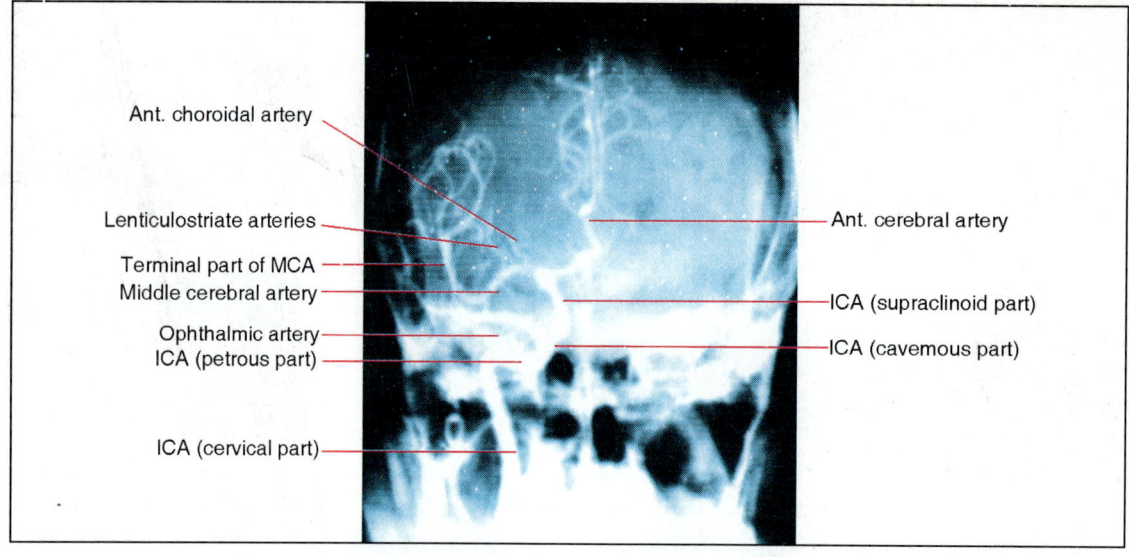

Fig. 85.1: Internal carotid artery: Angiogram

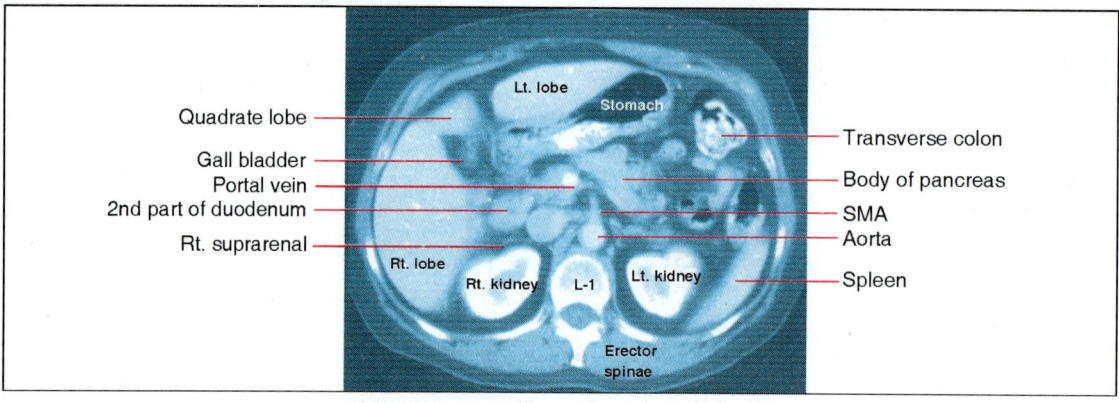

Fig. 85.2: CT scan (Axial section) ATL-1 Level

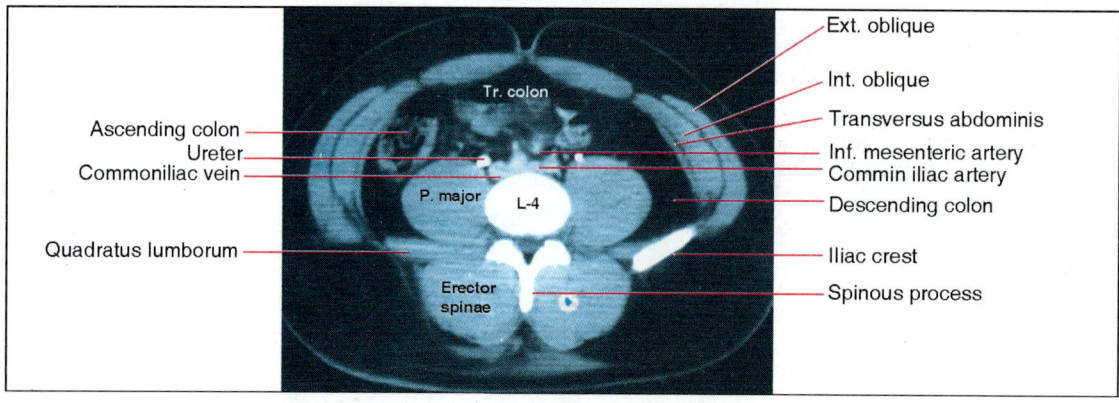

Fig. 85.3: CT scan (Axial section) ATL-4 Level

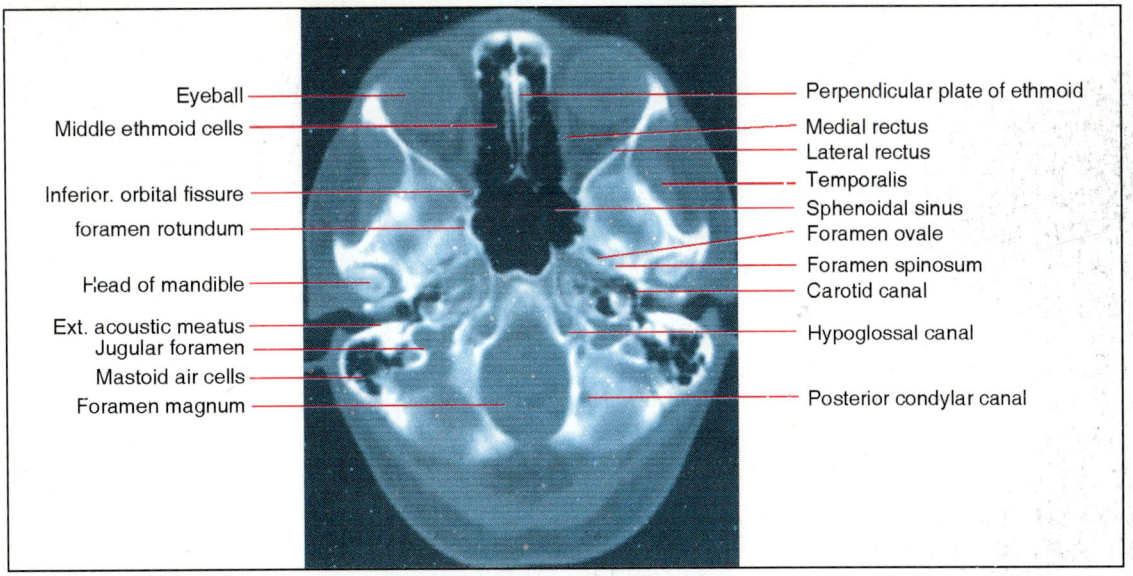

Fig. 85.4: Cranial base: CT scan (Oblique Axial Section)

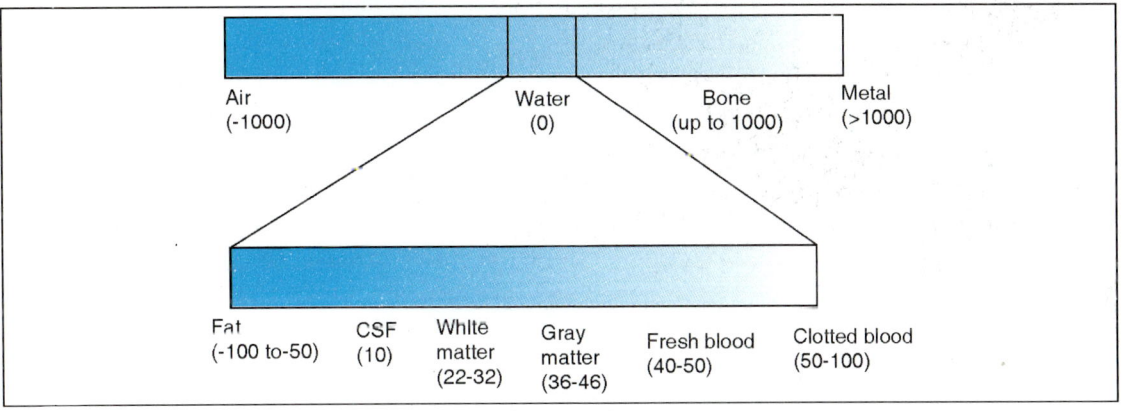

Fig. 85.5: X-ray attenuation of materials in the head

patient. The information can also be presented in analogue form as a two-dimensional display on a screen where each numerical value is represented by a single picture. The early machines were used for head scanning only. These days all parts of the body including the head can be examined.

Indications

1. Evaluation of intracranial lesions
2. Evaluation of intra-abdominal and pelvic masses
3. Evaluation of mediastinal pathologies
4. Soft tissue extension of bone tumours
5. Assessment of vascularity of organs

Contraindications

- Pregnancy
- Restless patient

SPIRAL CT

In this the patient moves longitudinally while the tube is moved in a continuous circular motion. This results in a spiral path for the X-ray beam through the organ being studied. The information obtained is manipulated by using computer system to get image which can be viewed from any angle. Computer manipulation can also remove unwanted tissues such as bone which are obstructing detail. The presentation can be improved by colour coding.

MAGNETIC RESONANCE IMAGING (MRI)

It is based on the fact that some nuclei behave like tiny magnets. The hydrogen nuclei (**protons**) are particularly suitable since they are present in vast numbers in the body tissues. When a strong external magnetic field is applied, this forces a proportion of these nuclei to align in a new magnetic axis from their previous random orientation.

The MRI uses a strong magnet and pulses of radio-waves. These are essential to excite and detect the magnetized protons. A pulse of radio-waves of the appropriate frequency displaces nuclei from their new alignment. They return to their position immediately after the pulse ceases. At the same time they release the energy absorbed as a radio signal of the same frequency which is detected. The signal returned is proportional to the concentration of the protons. This forms the basis for the digital record of the proton content of the tissues being examined. This is converted by the computer into an analogue image presented on a screen. MRI can produce axial images resembling those of CT. It has the great advantage that images can also be produced in any other plane. This is of special value in the study of the spinal cord and brain. This can also used for tissue characterization and blood flow imaging.

Advantages:

1. No ionizing radiation
2. Very high soft tissue resolution
3. Can image vessels without injection of intravascular contrast
4. Direct transverse, sagittal and normal imaging is possible
5. No bone or air artifact

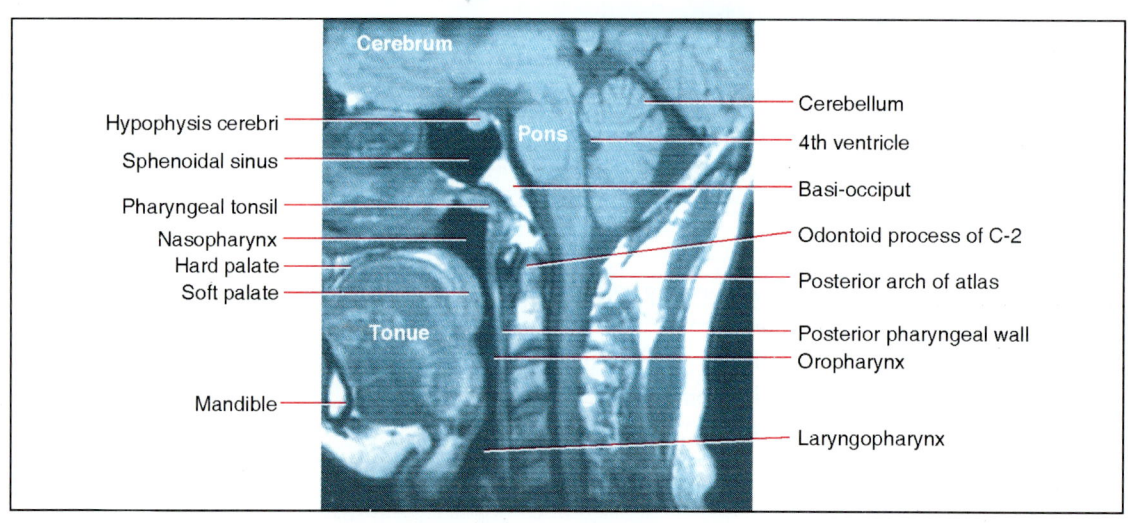

Fig. 85.6: MRI scan of head & neck: Midsagittal section

Disadvantages:

1. High cost
2. Inability to image bone
3. Unsuitable for patients with cardiac pacemakers which can be adversely affected by the magnetic fields.
4. Patient with pace-maker and critically ill patients can not be scanned

DIGITAL SUBTRACTION ANGIOGRAPHY (DSA)

This is also known as digital vascular imaging (**DVA**). It is a computerized image processing technique for improved visualization of vessels after the injection of contrast medium. The image contrast is improved by subtraction of images taken just before and during the injection of contrast medium, whereby image details common to both images are cancelled out. The contrast of this subtracted image is subsequently increased to display vascular ramifications with greater clarity.

Success depends on complete immobilization of the body part examined so that the two images are truly identical except for the injected contrast medium.

This technique is now frequently used for most cerebral angiography. It is also done to assess suspected cases of carotid artery stenosis or thrombosis. By using computer bones and soft tissues are subtracted. Thus the contrast enhanced blood vessels are better visualized.

Disadvantages

1. Expensive equipment
2. Requires OT environment
3. Ionizing radiation
4. Requires injection (minimally invasive)
5. Anaphylactic reaction to iodine can occur
6. Does not show surrounding soft tissue structures

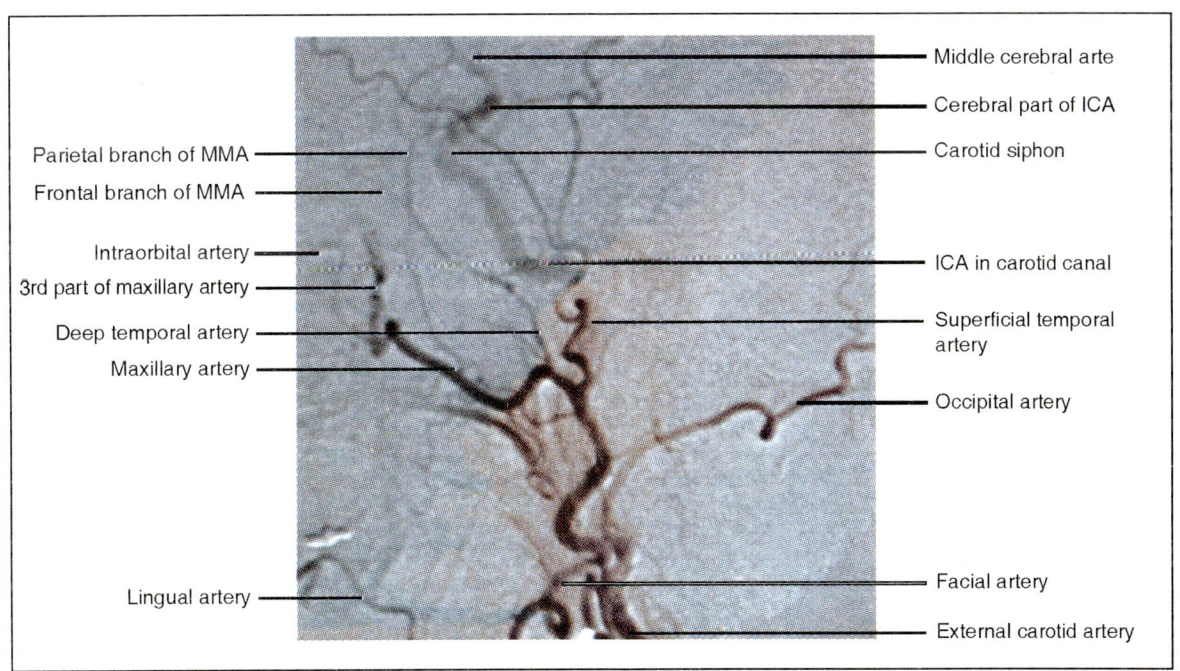

Fig. 85.7: DSA: External Carotid Artery

POSITRON EMISSION TOMOGRAPHY

PET scan combines computed tomography and nuclear scanning.

It is used to determine the biochemical activity of brain, heart or other organs by tracking the movements and concentration of a radioactive tracer which is injected into the blood.

A camera records the tracer's signals as it travels. A computer converts the signals into three dimensional images of the organ under examination. PET scan reveals the metabolic and functional changes at the cellular level in an organ. PET scan detects these changes very early while CT scan or MRI scan detects changes late when the disease process causes structural changes in the organ.

PICTURE ARCHIVING AND COMMUNICATIONS SYSTEM (PACS)

This is an attempt to replace conventional film based imaging, filing and reporting in radiology department by a film and paper-free system based on digital computing, recording, transporting and archiving of images.

Index

A

Abducent nerve, 58
Accessary nerve, 59
Achondroplasia, 37
Adenoidectomy, 250
Alveolar
   – arch of maxilla, 96
   – process, 107
Amyotrophic lateral sclerosis, 343
Angiography, 65
Anastomosis, 64
Anterior
   – condylar canal, 99
   – cord syndromes, 344
Apocrine sweat glands 18
Aponeorosis 28
Arthritis 47
Arnold chiary syndrome 100
Arcuate emimence 121
Articular disc 229
Ascending platine artery 207
Astrocytes 49
Auricular branch 209

B

Ball & socket joint, 46
Basal vein, 303
Biaxial, 44

Bilateral paralysis, 270
Blood
   – supply, 46
   – vessels, 371
Bone matrix, 29
Brachial plexus, 500
Bursitis, 47
Buccolabial muscles, 162

C

Cafe coronary phenomenon, 271
Caffeine, 468
Cancollous bone, 31
Canaliculus innominatus, 98
Carotene, 17
Cardiac muscle, 22, 24, 370
Cardiovascular system, 61
Carotid
   – canal, 98
   – seath, 155
   – sulcus, 90
Carcinoma
   – of thyroid, 201
   – of tongue, 264
Cavernous
   – sinus, 91, 282
   – sinus thrombosis, 282
   – sinus syndrome, 282

Central nervous system, 48
Cervical
– fascia, 154
– spondylosis, 145
– vertebral, 141
Cerebral hemispheres, 325
Cephalopelvic disproportion, 153
Cephalhaematoma, 152
Chondrodystrophy, 37
Circumorbital & palpebral muscles, 159
Ciliary ganglion, 275
Compact bone 31
Cachlear canaliculus & notch, 100
Common carotid artery, 497
Conjuctival reflex, 295
Conus medullaris syndrome, 344
Condylar joint, 45
Corneal
– grafting, 295
– reflex, 295
Cranial
– fossal, 88
– nerves, 57
Criocothyroid artery, 205
Cytomegalovirus, 468

D

Dentate suture, 39
Depressor septi, 161
Dermis, 16
Diethylstilbestrol, 468
Digastric
– fossa, 102
– muscle, 240
Digestive system, 437
Digital subtraction angiography, 511
Diognosis, 12
Diploic veins, 302
Dorsal root, 52
Dorsum sallae, 90
Dysphagia, 248
Dyspepsia, 248

E

Eccrine sweat glands, 18
Edward's syndrome, 484
Elastic cartilage, 35, 366
Ellipsoid joint, 45
Embrynic period, 430
Emissary veins, 308
Emissary sphenoidal foramen 92, 98
Endochondral growth, 139
Endotracheal intubation, 216
Endosteum, 30
Epidermis, 16
(e) Epindymal cells, 49
Epicranial muscles, 159
Epithelium, 353
Ethisterone & moresthisterone, 468
External occipital
– crest, 100
– protuberance, 100

F

Facial
– artery, 240
– nerve, 58
Fasciculi proprii, 343
Fibro cartilage, 35
Fibrous capsule, 42
Flat bones, 32
Foetal skull, 137
Foramen
– lacerum, 91, 98
– magnum, 93, 99
– ovale, 91, 98
– rotundum, 91
– spinosum, 91, 98
Fracture of spine of sphenoid, 100
Frankfort's plane, 73
Frontal process, 107

G

Gametogenesis, 408
General vicceral

– afferent, 445
– efferent, 445
Genial tubercles, 102
Geniohyoid, 188
Geniohyoid muscle, 240
Glandular branches, 207
Glossopharynged nerve, 58, 499
Gomphosis, 40
Gross anatomy, 3

H

Hassall's corpuscle, 385
Heimlich maneuver, 271
Hemoglobin, 17
Henle's layer, 389
Herpes simplex virus, 468
Hilton's law, 46
Horner's syndrome, 283
Hypertrophy, 28
Hypodermis, 16
Hyboglossal nerve, 59
Hyoid bone, 130
Hyper thyroidism, 201
Hypophyseal fossa, 90
Hypophyseal canal, 94
Hypoglossal nerve, 500
Hypophysis cerebri, 402
Huxley's layer, 389

I

Infratemporal surface & infratemporal crest, 98
Infrahyoid muscles, 188
Infrahyoid artery, 205
Inorganic portion, 29
Interior of larynx, 267
Internal
– acoustic meatus, 94
– jugular vein, 497

J
Jugular

– fossa, 100
– foramen, 94, 99
– process, 99
– tubercle, 94

L

Lamphatic system, 66
Laryngopharynx, 243
Laryngeal oedema, 270
Laryngoscopy, 271
Laryngectomy, 272
Lateral
– pterygoid, 233
– pterygoid plate, 98
Lesser cornua, 131
Ligaments, 44
Limbus suture, 39
Longus
– capitis, 190
– colli, 190
Lymphatic
– capillaries, 66
– drainage, 262
– organs, 68
– system, 436
– tissue, 67
– trunks, 67

M

Mammary glands, 18
Mandibular fossa, 99
Masseter, 232
Mastoid
– artery, 208
– process & notch, 100
Mastoidectomy, 290
Mastoiditis, 290
Maxillary
– artery, 225
– vein, 215
Maxilla, 105
McEvan's triangle, 121

Medial pterygoid, 234
Melanin, 17
Medial pterygoid plate, 97
Meningeal
 – branches, 208
 – veins, 303
Microglia, 49
Microgial cell, 375
Middle meningeal artery (MMA), 226
Mixed salivary gland, 380
Mobilization of gland, 200
Mucous salivary gland, 379
Muscles, 44
Muscular
 – branches, 208
 – spasm, 28
Mylohyoid, 188
Mylohyoid line, 102
Myopathy, 28
Myloyoid muscle, 240
Myringoplasty, 290

N

Nasal muscles, 161
Nasopharynx, 242
Nasotracheal intubation, 217
Nerve
 – plexuses, 52
 – supply, 46
Nervous
 – system, 48
 – tissue, 374
Neurol, 48
Neuropathic joint, 47
Neuroglial cells, 375
Neuroectoderm, 465
Neurobiotaxis, 445
Neurovascular hilum, 26

O

Occipital
 – branches, 208, 209

 – condyles, 99
 – vein, 215
Ocular myopathy, 284
Oculomotor nerve, 58
Olfactory nerve, 57
Oligodenrocytes, 50
Oligodendroglial cell, 375
Omohyoid, 189
Optic
 – canal, 90
 – cup, 460
 – externa, 289
 – grooves, 460
 – media, 289
 – vesicle, 460
Organic portion, 29
Orbicularis oculi, 159
Oropharynx, 243
Osteoblasts, 29
Osteocytes, 29
Osteoporosis, 34
Osteoclasts, 29
Osteomalacia, 34
Osteosarcoma, 34

P

Palatine
 – arch, 245
 – bone, 124
 – process, 107
 – tonsil, 245, 386
Papillary layer, 16
Papillae of tongue, 260
Paralysis, 27
Parasympathetic component, 53, 55
Paralysis of tongue, 264
Parasympathetic nervous system, 349
Parathyroid gland, 400
Parotid
 – duct, 498
 – gland, 498
Passavant's ridge, 245

Patau's syndrome, 484

Periosteum, 30

Peripheral nervous system, 48, 377

Pharyngeal arteries, 205

Pharygeal tonsil, 245

Pharyngitis, 248

Piriform fossa, 269

Plane suture, 39

Pneumatic bone, 32

Polyaxial, 44

Posterior
  – auricular vein, 215
  – clenoid process, 90
  – condylar fossa, 99

Preservation of parathyroid gland

Pretracheal fascia, 155

Prevertebral fascia, 155

Pterygoid
  – Hamulus, 98
  – process, 97
  – venous plexus, 215

R

Raphe, 28

Rectus capitis
  – anterior, 190
  – lateralis, 190

Reflex arc, 50

Regeneration, 28

Respiratory system, 436

Reticular layer, 16

Retrimandibular vein, 215

Rickets, 34

Rubella virus, 468

S

Salivary glands, 378

Satellite cells, 50

Schindylesis, 40

Schwann cells, 50

Scaphoid fossa, 97

Scaleness
  – anterior, 191
  – medius, 192
  – posterior, 192

Sella turcica, 90

Sesamoid bone, 32

Serrate suture, 39

Short bones, 32

Simon's law, 270

Skeletal muscle, 22, 369

Skin, 16

Smooth muscle, 22, 24, 370

Spasmodic torticollis 172, 186

Spine of sphenoid, 98

Spinal
  – accessary nerve, 500
  – cord, 51, 338
  – nerves, 52

Squamous suture, 39

Squamo-tympanic fissure, 98

Stapedectomy, 290

Sternocleidomastoid (SCM), 186

Sternohyoid, 188

Sternothyroid, 189

Sternocleidomastoid artery, 205

Stretch reflex, 52

Styloid process, 100

Stylomastoid foramen, 100

Stylohyoid, 187

Stylohyoid ligament, 187

Stylomandibular ligament, 229, 240

Stylohyoid muscle, 240

Sublingual fossa, 102

Submandibular fossa, 102

Suboccipital muscles, 178

Sublingual gland, 239, 499

Submandibular
  – ganglion, 239
  – gland 238
  – region 238

Sulcus chiasmaticus, 90
Sulcus tubal, 98
Sulci & guri, 327
Suprahyoid muscles, 187
Superior laryngeal artery, 205
Sutures, 39
Syndesmosis, 40
Synovial
   – fluid, 43
   – membrane, 42
Syringomyelia, 343

T

Tendonitis, 47
Tegmentympani, 121
Temporal fascia, 232
Temporalis, 232
Thyrohyoid, 189
Thyroid
   – capsules, 200
   – crisis, 201
   – gland, 195
   – swellings, 199
Thalamus & hypothalamus, 333
Tonsillar artery, 207
Tonsillitis, 250
Tonsillectomy, 250
Tomography, 504
Toxoplasma gondii, 468
Traumatic cephalhydrocele, 152
Trigeminal nerve, 58
Trigeminal impression, 121
Trochlear nerve, 58
Tubercle of root of zygoma 99
Tympanic
   – canaliculus, 100
   – membrane, 288
   – reflex, 289

U

Uniaxial, 44
Unilateral paralysis, 270
Urogenital system, 438
Uveitis, 295

V

Vagus nerve, 58, 500
Varicella zoster virus, 468
Venis of brain, 303
Venous system, 436
Ventral root, 52
Vertebral
   – arch, 142
   – foramen, 141
Vestibulo cochlear nerve, 58
Visceral reflexes, 55
Vitreous
   – degeneration, 295
   – humour, 294
Vocal
   – cords, 268, 269
   – palsy, 270

W

Wallarian degeneration, 342
White fibrocartilage, 366

X

Xeoradiography, 504

Z

Zygomatic
   – bone, 127
   – nerve, 222
   – process, 107
Zygomatico-orbital artery, 209